IRCVM-Medieval Cultures

15

IRCVM-Medieval Cultures

IRCVM-Medieval Cultures is the collection of interdisciplinary research monographs published by the Institut de Recerca en Cultures Medievals of the Universitat de Barcelona. Its purpose is to make known the leading research carried out by the members of the Institute and other international authors and research teams in its original language as well as in English, thus preserving Europe's own linguistic diversity.



IRCVM
Institut de Recerca en Cultures Medievals
Facultat de Geografia i Història
Universitat de Barcelona
carrer de Montalegre, 6 - 08001 Barcelona
www.ircvm.ub.edu

IRCVM Institut de Recerca en Cultures Medievals
UNIVERSITAT DE BARCELONA

Antoni Conejo da Pena, Pol Bridgewater Mateu

# Building the Historiography of the Medieval and Early Modern Hospital: New Perspectives on Its Physical and Symbolic Identity

The differentiating element of the Christian ideology on the duties towards others was its embodiment in concrete and lasting institutions, with their own legal identity and physical manifestations in buildings and spaces of care. The typologies and architectural forms varied through geography and time, with the underlaying and unifying principle of the fostering of the diverse universe of need. However, the physicality of hospital buildings and complexes went beyond the Vitruvian notion of *utilitas*: in addition to fostering, they also exhibited. In *De re aedificatoria* (1452), one of the first treatises that made references to hospital architecture, Leon Battista Alberti insisted on how great architectural structures acted as visual testimonies of the power and dignity of great men (and women, we might add today).

Hospitals acted as a vehicle for the visual expression of institutionalized charity, a space that reflected the identity and the ideological and moral traits of the founders, both public and private, as well as the prosperity and relevance of the towns or cities to which they belonged. Therefore, hospitals were not only spaces of care, but also of *venustas* and *decor*. Visible elements, such as sculpture, epigraphy, mural paintings, or the architectural form of hospital buildings and complexes, conveyed concise messages about their idealised functionality and, above all, virtue and political will. At the same time, hospitals functioned as the backbone of urban spaces, providing them with structure and charisma, and facilitating economic activity, human movement, and religious services.

With this volume, we intend to reflect on the physical dimension of hospitals, both as brick-and-mortar buildings and as spaces of symbolic expression, as well as their manifestations in urban and rural landscapes. But, beyond this thematic approach, this volume also serves as a vindication of the current vigour of hospital studies in (although not exclusively) the Iberian Peninsula and, more specifically, in the territories that were once part of the Crown of Aragon. Despite the weight of this specific regional reality, we have also included contributions on Northern and Central Italy and the Iberian Muslim world, both because of their enriching of the book's discourse and their comparative possibilities, but also to represent the links of scholarly collaboration that have been carefully built in the past decades.

Indeed, any approach to a transregional and long-lasting historical reality, such as the pre-modern hospital, is bound to assume more or less arbitrary limitations. In this sense, this weight of certain historical geographies is, above all, a modern development, created through shared academic spaces and relationships between researchers. This volume would have not been possible without the "Abrils de l'Hospital" symposium. The initiative began in 2012, and since then it has almost always been held during the month of April to commemorate the inauguration ceremony of the hospital of the Holy Cross in Barcelona on April 17, 1401. And, although the "Abrils" were born linked to the Institute for Resarch on Medieval Cultures (IRCVM) of the University of Barcelona and as a tribute to the great medieval hospital of the city, subsequent editions have taken place in other cities and towns that were part of the Crown of Aragon, such as Tarragona (2016), Saragossa (2017), Gandia (2020), Lleida (2021) or Cagliari (2022). And, what is more, the "Abrils" have also served as a meeting space for international scholars and a point of contact with the International Network for the History of Hospitals. Indeed, the 2019 edition of the "Abrils de l'Hospital" was celebrated together with the INHH and served as its 12th International Conference.

This character, both international but also rooted in the experience of the "Abrils", justifies the interdisciplinary and multilingual nature of the volume. This book includes chapters in Catalan, Spanish, Italian, and English. On the one hand, this linguistic diversity is testimony to the different origins of the scholars who, in recent years, have built networks of collaboration and knowledge transmission. On the other hand, the important presence of English, even among authors who are not native speakers, responds to the need to strengthen the presence of a historiographical tradition, that of the Iberian Peninsula and Southern Italy, that has remained mostly peripheral in the English-speaking world, at least in contrast with better known regions such as England, France, and Northern and Central Italy.

The volume is divided into four blocks. The first one functions as a preamble, as it proposes two iconographic and symbolic themes that are fully in line with the title and the spirit of the whole book. At the outset, Antoni Conejo reminds us of the historical changes in the perception of health. Nowadays, we associate health with the absence of disease and physical well-being. This is, of course, no novelty: within the Greek Olympus, the god Asclepius and his daughter Hygiea were already endowed with the virtue of healing the sick through rituals that were halfway between esotericism and shamanism. Conversely, in ancient Rome, the ideal of health took on a different hue. Without forgetting its physical aspect, it often became a metaphor for the supposed solidity of the state and its rulers and a form of rhetorical exaltation of public well-being. From these premises, Conejo delves into the search for the iconographic roots of the representations of health and how their meaning evolved from the ancient world into the dawn of the Middle Ages.

For their part, Fernando Serrano and Antonio González offer us an innovative approach to the popular devotion practises and the artistic representations associated with the Saints Cosmas and Damian in the Hispanic medieval world, from a longue durée perspective that stretches from the seventh century to the end of the fourteenth century. Both saints, martyred in the time of emperor Diocletian, have traditionally been linked to the practise of medicine, surgery, and pharmacy. For this reason, the authors focus on their attributes as miraculous healers and how their representations developed until forming an easily identifiable iconography. It's worth noting that this trend began to take shape spontaneously and involuntarily with the publication of works in which the two saints were represented, works that were then disseminated through informal social networks.

The second block is a miscellany consisting of seven articles, in which the reader will be able to find interesting contributions on hospital patrimonies, the impact of welfare institutions on the urban fabric, and reflections on the symbolic value of hospitals. Josep Barceló opens this section with a careful critical synthesis of the early stages of the processes of medicalization in the urban world of Western Europe at the end of the Middle Ages. Several circumstances gave rise to the implementation (and dissemination) of a new model of care based on the consolidation of what we know as the general hospital. This accelerated the pace of a process of health and disease management that became gradually dominated by the "medical gaze".

In turn, Jaume Marcé dwells on a topic that has been mostly forgotten by the historiography of the medieval hospital in Catalonia. His chapter studies the consequences, both economic and in urban planning, that came with the merger of six previously existing Barcelona hospitals and the subsequent creation of the hospital of the Holy Cross (1401). Marcé follows the evolution of one of such hospitals, the hospital of Pere Desvilar, and recreates the dismantling of its building after the merger of 1401. Indeed, the building and its premises were portioned into different plots and sold through emphyteutic establishments to generate income for the new hospital of the Holy Cross. Moreover, the chapter details how these sales triggered the transformation of a small area of the Barcelona neighbourhood of la Ribera, of which we were unaware until now.

Precisely, this urban perspective has a prominent role in the chapter signed by Fabio Gabbrielli. The hospital of Santa Maria della Scala in Siena was founded at the end of the 11th century as a religious institution dependent on the canons of the cathedral. Between the 13th and 15th centuries, it experienced a process of secularization that ended with its integration into the Sienese municipal government. In this context, between 1290 and 1338, the municipality of Siena promoted important initiatives that transformed the building and its immediate surroundings. The so-called *palazzo* del Rettore, the Gettatelli house, and the women's *pellegrinaio* were among such initiatives, as well as a pictorial cycle with Marian motifs. From a symbolic point of view, these works did not only beautify the hospital, but also consolidated its presence within the city and the process of municipalization of welfare.

In a similar vein, Salvatore Marino sets the main objective of his essay on the reconstruction of the origins of the urban welfare system in Naples, identifying the key moments of its evolution and underscoring the role played by hospitals in the development of new urban areas, especially outside the city walls.

The relationship between hospitals and cities is explored in its symbolic dimension by Pol Bridgewater. His study on the integration of the hospital of the Holy Cross into Barcelona's civic-religious ceremonies places the institution within the city's hierarchy of spaces, stressing how the city's municipal government made use of these ceremonies to display its commitment to the hospital. The understanding of the symbolic placement of the hospital shines some light on the apparent contradiction between the ideals of beauty, pride, and fear of uncleanliness that coexisted in relation to medieval hospitals.

Insisting on the indissociable pairing of city and hospital, Raúl Villagrasa shows how, at the end of the 15th century, the municipal authorities of Zaragoza used a procession honouring the hospital of Santa María de Gracia to reinforce the progressive separation between the false and true poor. It was not by chance that the council chose All Saints' Day to carry out the procession, since it was a date rooted in the transgressive winter holiday cycle, often related to childhood and dementia. Initiatives like this coincided with the institutional maturity of a hospital that was becoming the main welfare institution in the whole Kingdom of Aragon.

Pere Marquès closes this second block with a chapter that stands out, as it addresses the hospital within an Islamic medieval society. The author presents the *Māristān* of Granada, considered the most important Islamic hospital in the Iberian Peninsula and one of the best exponents of this type of architecture in the Islamic West. Heir to the Eastern *bīmāristānats*, the building founded between 1365-1367 was used for medical purposes until the Christian conquest of 1492. Subsequently, the property was significantly transformed until its demolition in the 19th century. At present, some recent restoration initiatives aim to recreate the original structure based on historical, artistic, and archaeological criteria. This chapter has its origins in his BA thesis in Art History, which was awarded the II IRCVM Award for the best TFG on medieval cultures (2022).

The third block is comprised of six chapters on the relation between hospitals and their surrounding territory. Ester Diana has made a relevant contribution on the hospital de la Misericordia e Dolce of Prato. The hospital cannot be understood without taking into account its location, in one of the main pilgrimage routes that connected Rome with French Burgundy, closely associated with the Via Francigena. The hospital's first registers of patients reveals that many of its inmates were travellers and pilgrims going from Rome to Vézelay and Santiago de Compostela.

Regarding the traffic of people and goods, Giuliana Albini illuminates the role of hospitals in the construction, maintenance, and management of bridges. Between the 12th and 13th centuries, new demands associated with trade and pilgrimages created the ideal climate for the construction of new bridges. Many of these bridges were built by lay powers, but they were often taken care of by religious communities, which, in turn, looked after and assisted the travellers who made use of them. Thus, the *domus pontis* were born spontaneously as works of charity supported by bequests, donations, and alms.

The contribution of Marina Gazzini shares a few similarities with the aforementioned chapter, since it also addresses the relationship between welfare institutions and their urban and rural contexts and, especially, the network of paths and ways built around them. Gazzini sets her focus on the analysis of how hospitals became important stops on different routes and answers a series of related questions: did certain people start a long journey to reach a specific hospital? Did they leave their towns to go to large urban hospitals in search of treatment, alms, or even paid employment? As the author herself states, in the Middle Ages many hospitals became the end point of processions, not to mention full-fledged pilgrimages.

Also stressing this territorial dimension, Frederic Aparisi proposes an interesting exercise of geolocation and mapping of the rural hospitals of the Kingdom of Valencia in the 13th-16th centuries. This is an issue that a usually urban-centric historiography has only dealt with in passing, but which is fundamental to understanding the territorial reality and the connections (also through the means of communication) of the non-urban hospitals.

The last two contributions in this block emphasise the study of documents. Anna Ester analyses the first years of the hospital of the Holy Cross in Vic from a series of unpublished inventories of goods (1388-1407) kept in the Episcopal Archives and Library of Vic. This type of source is essential for knowing the day-to-day life, economy, and management of these types of institutions. For their part, Mariangela Rapetti and Beatrice Artizzu co-sign a chapter on the old hospital of Sant'Antonio abate of Cagliari, consisting of two clearly differentiated parts. In the first, the authors delve into archival sources in order to redo the structure that the building must have had in the 16th century. To this end, a magnificent plan by Giuseppe Viana (1773), corresponding to a project that was never executed but that provides a lot of information to understand what the building must have looked like in the past, is of great interest. In the second part, Rapetti and Artizzu take a step forward by virtually recreating the environments of the complex through the study of its inventories and archival documents, a recreation in which students from the Liceo Artistico of Cagliari have also collaborated.

Finally, the fourth and last block is made up of four articles mostly focused, although not exclusively, on the medical aspect of hospitals and the impact that epidemic outbreaks had on them. Guillem Roca opens this block with an article focused on the evolution of the hospital network of Lleida between 1149, the year of the Christian conquest of the city, and 1454, the year of the foundation of the general hospital of Santa Maria. In his analysis, Roca emphasises the medical and health-related criteria that were taken into account when choosing the place where the city's welfare facilities were to be located. From the second half of the 14th century, the municipality understood the need to restructure the system, relocate some centres, and create new ones. These projects of reform were, to some extent, failures, forcing a renewed attempt at reform that resulted in the aforementioned hospital of Santa Maria. The hospital was built in a peripherical neighbourhood, following the sanitary and hygienic arguments prevailing at the time, but it soon became integrated in the city's urban fabric.

At the other end of the Iberian Peninsula, Joana Balsa shows us how, in the late 15th century, the construction of a hospital for plague patients in Lisbon was the result of specific urban needs. Since the city was the capital of the Kingdom and had an important commercial projection, the initiative fell to the monarchy, and counted on the support and approval of the municipal authorities. Different forms and locations were proposed for its erection; and even the famous master João Castilho contributed with a proposal in the mid-16th century. Balsa, based on the study of serialised documents, redoes the process of conception, projection, and construction of this Lisbon hospital, and sheds light on a little-studied phenomenon in the history of public health and Portuguese hospital architecture. At the same time, she contextualises the hospital within the development of emerging conceptions of health that defined plague and its contagious nature, thus developing a set of rules and laws aimed at preventing its contagion and spread.

Regarding the historiography of the hospitals of Valencia at the end of the Middle Ages and the beginning of the Renaissance, Carmel Ferragud and Marialuz López Terrada provide us with another example of their expertise in the subject. The apologetic and laudatory nature –to the taste of political, ecclesiastical, and, sometimes, academic authorities– has enjoyed a success that has often blurred the precise historical reality of what hospitals really were, as institutions with a prolonged continuity in time but which must always be understood in terms of their social and historical context. Starting from this premise, both authors delve into the analysis of the Valencian welfare landscape prior to the creation of the city's general hospital (1512), and give much needed nuance to some historiographical clichés such as the consideration of the Hospital dels Innocents (founded in 1409) as the first institution for the mentally ill in Europe. In this sense, they lament the lost opportunity that the commemoration of the five hundredth anniversary of the foundation could have meant for the study of the hospital's history. Consequently, they close the article with a statement of intentions and a roadmap of the current challenges that Valencian hospital historiography faces.

The final contribution and colophon of this book is an article by John Henderson. Most of his scientific career has been focused on the study of hospitals, illness, and the institutionalisation of care in Florence in the Middle and Early Modern Ages. This chapter is no exception, since in Henderson's opinion, during this period the "capital of the Renaissance" developed a hospital system with more than thirty-five institutions, ranging from the four large hospitals for the seriously ill and the famous hospital of Innocenti for foundlings, to numerous smaller hostels for the poor, pilgrims, and travellers. During the outbreak of epidemic episodes in the 15th century, hospitals were the main institutionalised answers to the disease, in a context in which isolation measures evolved slowly and gradually.

In conclusion, this volume serves as a representation of a tradition of hospital studies that combines the work of both consolidated scholars and emerging ones. But it is not only that. *The Medieval and Early Modern Hospital: A Physical and Symbolic Space* is a written testimony of the links (and, dare we say, also very pleasant companionship) that have been recently built among researchers of different universities and centres. It is almost a cliché to say that the history of hospitals is a discipline that cannot be ignored. Indeed, it has experienced an impressive degree of development. But this book contributes, without doubt, to consolidating this discipline as relevant.

# I
# *Iconography and Symbolism*

Antoni Conejo da Pena

# «Without You, no One is Happy». The Power of the Image of Health from Ancient Rome to Early Middle Ages*

Hygieia, most revered of the blessed gods,
May I dwell with you for the rest of my life.
And may you be the gracious inmate of my house,
For if there is any delight in wealth or in offspring,
Or in royal dominion which makes men equal to gods, or in those desires.
Which we seek to capture by Aphrodite's hidden nets
Or if any other joy or rest from toil has been revealed to men by the gods,
It is with your help, blessed Hygieia,
That they all flourish and shine in the Graces' discourse.
But without you, no man is happy.
Ariphron, *Hymn to Hygieia* (quoted in Athenaeus, *Deipnosophistae* 15.702)

The poet Ariphron of Sicyon composed this hymn in honour of the Greek goddess of health, Hygieia, whom he recognized as the «most revered of the blessed gods»; in his authoritative words, without her «no man is happy».[1] Almost 2400 years later, in 1948, the World Health Organization (WHO) defined health as «a state of complete physical, mental and social well-being and not merely the absence of disease or infirmity». Since then, this definition has headed the list of basic founding principles of the organization, but its wording has been criticized on more than one occasion. In the opinion of its detractors, it does not

* This present study is part of the project *Barcelona en el contexto del gótico meridional: arquitectura y ornamentación* at the Universitat de Barcelona (PGC2018-094265-B-I00). Some of its themes were already presented in a conference titled *Epidemics in Catalonia in the Middle Ages. Documentary Approach*, read at the *Simpósio Internacional: O testemunho da história para viver e superar a epidèmia no presente* (Lisbon, June 2020) and especially in my contribution to the round table *La representació de la salut (mon antic i medieval)* at the *XVII Congrés d'Història de Barcelona* (Barcelona, November 2021). I would like to thank Drs. Carles Buenacasa and Fernando Serrano Larráyoz for their review of the first draft and the subsequent comments that have allowed me to better this final version. Nevertheless, any possible mistakes are solely the author's responsibility.

1. Despite Ariphon was traditionally identified as a poet of the late classical period (c. 400 BCE), it has been proved that the hymn was actually composed in the 3rd century BCE (Lardinois et al. 2011: 220). This translation of the hymn is a modified version of C. D. Yonge's, who, in 1854, used the English term «Health», instead of the original Greek *Hygieia*. See: http://www.attalus.org/old/athenaeus15.html; link active September 2022.

refer only to physical health, but includes the achievement of complete social well-being, in such a way that any aspect of human life and its miseries, political or economic, including world peace, can be considered its responsibility (BICKENBACH 2015). Leaving this debate aside, it is clear that WHO aims to give health a global dimension, which goes beyond the individual to elevate it to something communal. A purpose that is not at all original and that finds its roots in the Greco-Roman world.

## 1. *Soteria, Hygieia and Salus: The Politicization of Public Health*

Rome occupies a distinguished placed in the publications on pre-modern public health, a merit fully justified if we consider the magnificent aqueducts, baths, latrines and sewers built in its time and whose ultimate goal was to guarantee hygiene and collective well-being (SCARBOROUGH 1981). Of these, the great Roman baths of the Eternal City stand out. They were multipurpose and salubrious spaces, so it is not surprising that the sick frequented them in large numbers, to the point that emperor Hadrian (2nd century) had to enact a law to prevent their entry after the eighth hour (in the afternoon, when there was a greater influx), certainly to prevent them from mixing with the healthy bathers (*Historia Augusta*, Hadrian, 22.7).[2] The most monumental baths are remembered for their architecture, but also for their excellent decoration. Among the deities that adorned them, the most common sculptures were those of Asclepius, the Greek god of medicine whom the Romans called Aesculapius, and his daughter Hygieia. For example, one of the apsidal environments that connected the *frigidarium* and the *natatio* of the famous *thermae* of Caracalla (beginning of the 3rd century) was presided over by a colossal figure of Aesculapius, the largest of the entire complex, about 4 meters high and of which only the head is still extant; probably another statue of Hygieia acted as its pendant, but it has been completely lost (MARVIN 2002: 363-364). This is no exceptional case, since in many other public and private baths in Italy, North Africa and Asia Minor, fragments of statues, inscriptions, mosaics and all kinds of representations have survived that feature this same divine pair, perhaps because they served as a reminder of the health benefits of frequenting baths (FAGAN 2002: 89). For all that, it is not surprising that the Greek Lucian of Samosata (2nd century; *Hippias seu balneum*, 5) only paid attention to the images of Asclepius and Hygieia and not to those of any other deity when describing certain *thermae*.[3]

2. In effect, ancient romans preferred to go to the baths from the eighth hour to sunrise (MARQUÉS 2018: part I).

3. The combined representation of Aesculapius-Salus was a constant throughout the empire. Not surprisingly, the Capitoline Museums of Rome (NCE 15) house a magnificent inscription that was discovered in the Testaccio in 1885 and which has been dated to the first half of the 2nd century CE. The text refers to the construction of a new seat for the *collegium Salutare,* which was dedicated to Aesculapio et saluti Aug(ustae).

The iconography of the Greek Asclepius and the Roman Aesculapius is identical. He is usually represented bearded, with his body covered by a himation tied to his shoulder and leaving part of his chest, abdomen and one of his arms bare, while holding a staff with a snake coiled around it.[4] His place of worship in Rome was on the Tiber Island, where a temple had been built c. 292 BCE in gratitude for the end of an epidemic that had ravaged the city (Renberg 2006). His daughter Hygieia, often identified with the Roman deity Salus, was a goddess linked to hygiene and health, and according to mythology she had the task of feeding and caring for her father's sacred snakes and to act as his assistant (fig. 1). Aesculapius-Asclepius' field of action was exclusively circumscribed to everything that had to do with health and physical healing (Compton 2002: 313).[5] On the other hand, Salus –one of the oldest deities in the Roman pantheon– had attributes that went beyond the physical body and referred to prosperity, wealth, safeguarding and the ability to restore the good order of things after a crisis or calamity (Saladino 1994: 556). In fact, his name's meaning is much closer to the Greek ideal of Σωτηρία (*Soteria*, cognate of the verb *sozien*, "to save", and of the adjective *soter*, "savior"), which alluded to salvation, security and community well-being (Jim 2022), principles analogous to what we understand today as public health and which remind us of the definition proposed by the WHO with which we headed these lines.

*Soteria* was an abstract concept that had neither a concrete personification nor its own attributes. We are aware of its existence thanks to inscriptions on altars and statue bases and literary mentions. Its first written evidence dates back to the 5th century BCE, in the midst of the Greco-Persian wars. From then on, it was invoked on multiple occasions to request divine intercession for the protection of any aspect of life. At an individual level, prayers were usually aimed at achieving good health, avoiding death, improving purchasing power, ensuring safety before embarking on a journey and giving birth without complications. *Soteria* was also collectively invoked in solemn supplications for military victories, freedom from the enemy and the end of an epidemic or a natural disaster. Under these circumstances the *hyper soterias* were understood as a cannel for receiving unearthly help in the here and now. For this reason, the epithet *soter* was added to the names of many Greek divinities, such as with Artemis, Athena, Hecate, Hera,[6] Hygieia, Isis, Persephone and Tyche (Jim 2015: 63; 2017: 256-257).[7] One of the most

4. On the multiple symbolism of the snake, see: Retief, Cilliers 2002.

5. Regarding the origins of the worship and identity of Hygieia, see Beumer 2016

6. Despite the risk of stablishing direct connections between the Greek Olympus and the Roman pantheon, the latter included Juno Sospita as an equivalent of the Greek Hera Soter. Her name came from the Latin *sospes* (liberator/protector, therefore having the same meaning as the Greek *soter*). In the capital she was worshiped at a temple in the Forum Holitorium and maybe at another one in the Palatine.

7. Some "male" gods were also deserving of this distinction, such as Zeus, Poseidon, Dionysus, Apollo, Hades, and of course Asclepius. Regarding the latter, I want to highlight the inscription in Greek characters on a votive vase from the 2nd quarter of the 2nd century, found in Tivoli but

common examples of this practice was Artemis, whose profile bust appears on the head of some coins minted in Syracuse (4th-3rd centuries BCE) together with the inscription ΣΩΤΗΡΙΑ. Many Hellenistic rulers also adopted the nickname "Soter" with a clear propagandistic intention and did not hesitate to disseminate it through inscriptions and coins, such as those minted by Ptolemy I (c. 367-283 BCE), Antiochus I (324-261 BCE) and Demetrius I (c. 185-150 BCE), among many others (fig. 3).

Salus was born as a syncretic deity, created ex novo from the fusion of a pre-existing Latin tradition, the influence of other Mediterranean cultures,[8] and the healing properties of Hygieia and the Greek ideal of *soteria*. Her cult has been attested in the Italian peninsula through epigraphy, at least since the 4th century BCE (Marwood 1988). In 302 BCE, at the end of the Second Samnite War, a temple was inaugurated in his honour on top of the Quirinal Hill in Rome.[9] According to Titus Livy (*Ab urbe condita*, 40.37), in 180 BCE, the decemvirs urged the consuls to commission golden statues of Apollo –another god related to medical practice–, Aesculapius and Salus to appease an epidemic. Later, Pliny the Elder (*Natural History*, 34.80) would postulate that after the reconstruction of the Temple of Concordia, promoted by emperor Tiberius, the interior of the temple's *cella* became a kind of museum with numerous Greek works, including images of Asclepius and Hygieia.

When looking for the iconographic origins of the anthropomorphic representation of Salus, we realize that the Romans literally replicated the sculptures and reliefs of Hygieia: a woman dressed in a tunic and a himation, who could be shown standing or seated, often holding a patera in her hand and almost always accompanied by a snake, a reptile that became her symbol par excellence (fig. 2). This archetype remained unchanged, beyond a few swaps of attributes with other deities, as was common in ancient statuary.[10] It is difficult to discern whether the ultimate intention of this representation was to evoke the old Greek Hygieia or the "newborn" Roman deity Salus. In contrast, numismatics offers a much more varied range of readings and visual stereotypes. Precisely, the oldest

originally made in North Africa. Under the god's name we can read, in large, capitalized letters, ΣΩΤΗΡΙ (Rome: Musei Vaticani, inv. 1249). I would like to thank Fernando Serrano Larráyoz for sharing some clues about this altar.

8. Occasionally, Salus has been associated with Sancus, a primitive god of Sabin origin, protector of marriage, hospitality and trade (Marqués 2018: part II). Likewise, it is known that the Romans also came into contact with the divine idea of health through the Phoenician deity Eshmun, whose attributes were health and healing. This is clear from a famous trilingual inscription of Sardinian origin (2nd century BCE) that identifies the aforementioned Eshmun with the Greek Asclepius and the Roman Aesculapius (Moriggi 2011). I would like to thank Carles Buenacasa for this last observation.

9. The choice of this site was not at random. One of the tops of the Quirinal Hill used to be known as the Collis Salutaris, a reference to the cult of the ancient god Sancus (Marqués 2018: part II). See note 8.

10. In due time, Salus came to be represented with other attributes, such as an egg, a rudder and even a cornucopia.

known example of the Latin personification of Salus is found on the obverse of a denarii issue of Junius Silanus (91 BCE), in which we see the profile bust of a woman, with her hair gathered in a bun and tied by a diadem, and wearing a pearl necklace and earrings. Her bust is accompanied by the inscription «SALVS», which dispels any doubt about her identity. The opposite side of the coin depicted a *biga* being guided by victory (RRC 337, 2; fig. 4). A few years later, around 49 BCE, we find other denarii minted in the midst of the civil war between Julius Caesar and Pompey the Great that stand out (RRC 442; fig. 5). On the obverse, the female portrait with a laurel wreath, bun, earrings and necklace is repeated, accompanied by the word «SALVTIS». As for the reverse, a full-body woman leaning on a small column holds with her right hand a sacred snake, to which she gazes directly, thus making her association with the Greek Hygieia very clear.[11] The composition is completed with the inscription «IIIVIR VALETV(do) M(a) N(ius) ACILIVS», in allusion to the *triumvir monetalis* Manius Acilius Glabrio, who was in charge of the minting of the coin at Caesar's request, in the context of a campaign destined at injecting cash into the public treasury and thus face the expenses generated by the civil war. However, its most relevant aspect is the use of the Latin word *valetudo* –very rare in Roman numismatics–, which can also be translated as a synonym for health. The reason why both words (*salus* and *valetudo*) were used is not entirely clear; perhaps, the former was meant to transmit a more political or symbolic message, while the latter emphasized the word's physical meaning (KOHLER 1965).[12] It has also been said that the aim of the coinage was to pay public tribute to the *gens* Acilia, a lineage of plebeian origin to whom tradition attributed the merit of having hosted the Greek physician Arcagathus in 219 BCE, who would have been the first man to practice medicine in ancient Rome. However, given the warlike context in which the coin was minted, the most logical interpretation would be to read the iconography and inscriptions as an explicit way of appealing to Caesar's victory and, by implication, to the good health of the republic in its broadest sense (CLARK 2007: 153-158). In fact, it was in the environment of the crisis of the late republican when the goddess Salus was definitively linked to the principles of salvation and community welfare which were inherent in the Greek ideal of *soteria*. Cicero even proposed raising it to the category of supreme law, as can be seen from these two maxims: «*salus populi suprema lex esto*»[13] (*De legibus* 3.3, 8) and «*salus civitatis in legibus sita est*»[14] (*Cluentius*, 53). Both precepts asserted that the obligatoriness of preserving

11. The presence of a snake is not exclusive of the imagery of Salus. For instance, different coin emissions of Lucius Roscius Fabatus (64-59 CE) show a standing lady feeding a snake (RRC 412). This is a representation of Juno Sospita, a goddess from the ancient city of Lanuvium, who, similarly to the Greek Hygieia, was associated with a sacred snake. See note 6.

12. We find an example of its usage in a few aurei of Augustus that appeal to «PRO VALETVDINE CAESARIS» (RIC I², aug. 369). Beyond the differences, if any, between the meanings of *salus* and *valetudo*, the latter was rarely seen in numismatic inscriptions.

13. «The health of the people should be the supreme law».

14. «Safety in the city comes from the law».

of the health of the people (*populus*)[15] and the republic, or, in other words, that the rights of the citizens had to be put before private interests, since acting in accordance with the common good contributed to strengthening the State (Farrés 2020: 10-11). The ceremony of the *augurium salutis* also evidences the duality of Salus-State. This ritual was celebrated every 5th of August during peace time, and its purpose was to pray for the health and prosperity of the people (Cassius Dio, *Roman History*, 37.24, 1). However, the continuous armed conflicts that ravaged both the republic and the empire that it could only be somehow regularly celebrated during the reign of Augustus, during which it served as propaganda for the *pax augusta* (Montero 2001).

Precisely, with the rise of Augustus (27 BCE-14 CE) and the centralization of all power in a single individual, the physical health of the *princeps* became a matter of State importance. However, this concern did not only apply to his person, but was extendable to the prosperity of the empire as a whole (González 2021: 347).[16] Not surprisingly, Augustus was understood as the "father" of a political system in which the emperor became the embodiment of the State, in such a way that his personal wellness and that of the empire were seen as the same. The inscription on the reverse of an issue of silver denarii c. 19-15 BCE called directly to Jupiter to make vows «PRO SAL(ute) CAES(aris)» (RIC I/2, Aug. 57),[17] a prayer that was also present in a good number of epigraphic inscriptions throughout the empire, and which seemed entirely reasonable given that Augustus was prone to illness. Suetonius gives testimony of this (*Augustus*, 57 and 81-82), together with similar public tributes paid to him, such as throwing coins into the famous Lacus Curtius, just in the middle of the Roman forum, for his health. During the first imperial stage, the assimilation of Salus with the emperor was consolidated (Saladino 1994: 556), which contributed to narrowing the fine line that separated the man from the god (Wardle 2012). Thus, in the numismatic traditions of the Julio-Claudian, Flavian and Antonine dynasties, it is common to find the female personification of health, sitting or standing and with various attributes and postures, sharing prominence with the portrait of the prince. This is the case of numerous aurei and denarii from the last years of Nero's reign, in which we find the enthroned woman, with her hair tied in a bun and holding a patera –but without a snake–[18] and accompanied by the word «SALVS» (65-66

15. Some Greek texts already understood health as a societal good (Stafford 2000: 149).

16. According to William York (2012: 16) Salus came to be understood as another of the emperor's virtues. It had a physical dimension, associated with the absence of illness and the convenience of following healthy habits, but also emotional and spiritual components.

17. Epigraphic inscriptions found across the Empire show that the messages related to the emperor's health were very common until the late 3rd century. The same thing happened in numismatics (Moralee 2004: 5-13 and 41).

18. In effect, Julio-Claudian and Flavian (until Titus) numismatics never displayed Salus with a snake. She was usually seated and holding the patera, a visual archetype that was identical to that of Concordia. The only difference lay on the inscription, but not in the image. Domitian, the last of the Flavians, reintroduced the image of the goddess feeding the reptile in an issue of denarii

CE; RIC I, 59-60). In this case, the representation of Salus was perhaps meant to restore some civic self-esteem after the cruel fire that had ravaged Rome in 64 CE (fig. 6). A few years later, in 68 CE, some denarii were minted in Gaul (RIC I, 72) which have been linked to the rebellion led by the *propraeator* of Lyon, Julius Vindex, who rose in arms against Nero (BRUNT 1959). Cassius Dio (*Roman History*, 63.22) highlights that at that time there were several provinces unhappy with the Roman government. Indeed, the obverse depicts a victory standing on an orb with the emphatic legend «SALVS GENERIS HVMANI» (fig. 7). The absence of the imperial portrait is completely exceptional and therefore it must be interpreted as a challenge to the current regime and, again, as a revolutionary manifesto aimed at pushing the rebels towards victory. Instead, the reverse is inspired by republican symbology: it includes the acronym «SPQR» (*Senatus Populusque Romanus*; the Senate and the People of Rome) surrounded by a *corona civica*, with the aim of pointing out that the beneficiaries of the insurrection would be citizenry of the empire. This reading coincides with the final harangue delivered by Vindex himself: «Arise at last against him; help yourselves and help the Romans; liberate the whole world» (Cassius Dio, *Roman History*, 63.22, 6). It was a call for the salvation of humanity, which is literally the motto that appears on the denarii that we have just mentioned. The strength of the image of victory protected by the aphorism «SALVS GENERIS HVMANI» was so powerful that Nero's successor, Galba, did not hesitate to replicate it on the reverse of some aurei as a way of symbolizing the end of tyranny. Of course, on the obverse, he hastened to restore the *statu quo ante* by showing his profile portrait that accredited him as a brand-new emperor, albeit only for a short period of time (RIC I, 147). The instability produced by the abrupt demise of Nero and the Julio-Claudian dynasty (68 CE) was put to an end with the rise of the Flavian dynasty. First with Vespasian (69-79 CE) and then with Titus (79-81 CE) coins reassumed their role as the best messengers for the allegorical marriage between Salus and the emperor. This is evidenced by some magnificent sesterces decorated with the anthropomorphic personification of the former –enthroned and veiled– and the forceful slogan «SALVS AVGVSTA» (divine health, already present on some coins from the time of Tiberius), all completed with the abbreviation «SC» (*Senatus Consulto*), which certified its senatorial support (RIC II, 1; fig. 8).[19] Other epithets were progressively added to the name of the goddess, which complimented their meaning depending on the context. The formulas we have just seen, such as

that announced his condition of *princeps iuventutis,* although in this case without the inscription «SALVS» (c. 79 CE; RIC 1084).

19. It was not the first usage of the formula «SALVS AVGVSTA», which was already present in a dupondius of Tiberius (c. 22-23 CE), together with the portrait of a woman in profile and with her hair tied in a bun, the typical hairstyle of the late republican and early imperial periods (RIC I, 47). According to some scholars, it functioned as a representation of the wife of Augustus, Livia Drusilla, known as Julia Augusta after the death of her husband. She got sick after 22 CE and, therefore, the coin could be understood as a rogation for her recovery. Others consider it is a conventional allusion to the empire's good health (BOATWRIGHT 2021: 128).

«GENERIS HVMANI» and «AVGVSTA» are an example among others. Nerva (96-98 CE), the old senator who took the reins of empire after the tumultuous assassination of the last of the Flavians, Domitian, issued a silver denarius with the classical figure of Salus enthroned and the motto «SALVS PVBLICA» (RIC II, 20), with the purpose of reminding the population that despite the difficulties they had experienced, he held the authority to preserve the order of all things, that is, the common good. Hadrian (117-138) and Antoninus Pius (138-161) also chose to repeat the same maxim as a means of continuing to instil public confidence in the well-being of society.

With the death of Antoninus and ascension of a diarchy composed by Marcus Aurelius and Lucius Verus (161-169), the corulers would be the focus of a renewed interest, as can be deduced from an issue of aurei that included the effigy of Salus, standing, holding a sceptre and making a sacrifice on an altar in the company of a snake. The textual inscription read «SALVTI AVGVSTOR(um) [...]» (RIC III, 493; fig. 9). In this case, it is an explicit call for the good health of the two dignitaries and, at the same time, a public exaltation of the bicephalic government model.[20] Coincidence or poetic irony, in this same period (165-170) the so-called "Antonine plague" broke out. It was one of the most famous pandemics of antiquity, which apparently was imported by the legionnaires from the Middle East. In the opinion of some authors, the plague was behind the obsessive representation of Salus in the numismatics of the time (Garzón 1989: 10). The premature death of Lucius Verus (169) and later that of Marcus Aurelius himself (180) have been associated with this pestilent scourge. The Greek physician Galen (*Medendi Methodus*, 12) specified the symptoms of the plague: high fever, inflammation of the hands and neck, diarrhoea, thirst and pustules; hence it is also known as the "plague of Galen". Other texts certify its virulence: «*tanta autem pestilentia fuit, ut vehiculis cadavera sint exportata serracisque*» (*Historia Augusta*, Marcus Aurelius, 13); not without reason, the most pessimistic interpretations have estimated that the mortality rate could have ranged between 5% and 15% of the global population (Lorente 2021: 226-228). Although the inscription of the aforementioned *aurei* appealed to the health of the Caesars, it surely has nothing to do with this epidemic outbreak but, as usual, with the solidity of the state apparatus. In contrast, a coin minted in Alexandria and dated c. 167-168 (RPC IV, 4) could indeed be related to the "Antonine plague" (fig. 10). On the obverse we see a profile portrait of Marcus Aurelius, while the reverse depicts a *lectisternium*, a ritual banquet that took place inside the temples. It was based around a set table, around which statues of deities –made of wood and with marble or bronze heads and covered with clothes– were placed,

20. The usage of this formula in favour of the emperor's health («SALVS AVGVSTI») was particularly intense in the issues of Hadrian's later reign (134-138), a fact that has been interpreted as a form of prayer for his recovery, due to the episodes of sickness that afflicted then and worsened over time (Garzón 1989: 11). However, the personification of Salus was another of the many allegories that were part of the reverses of coins and, therefore, her presence was not exclusively explainable in relation to the physical state of the emperor (González 2021: 358).

which were the symbolic recipients of a copious meal. This type of ceremony was usually conducted before a battle or in gratitude for a victory, but also to plead with the gods for the end of calamities and other situations of extreme gravity, such as an epidemic (CÊBE 1989).[21] Indeed, the biographer of Marcus Aurelius describes the celebration of a *lectisternium* that lasted seven days, together with the issue of severe regulations for the burial of the dead in order to stop the spread of the plague (GOZALBES, GARCÍA 2007: 13).[22]

## 2. *Times of Crisis, Times of Changes: New Images and Messages for Salus*

From the second quarter of the 3rd century onwards, the empire entered a spiral of crisis as a result of political, institutional, military and fiscal instability, border weakness and religious uncertainty. We know the names of up to seventy-four emperors –most of them soldiers with short-lived reigns– that ruled between 235 (the end of the Severan dynasty) and 284. In general, they unsuccessfully tried to find formulas that would keep them in power, with the main objective of regain the trust of their subjects. For this reason, they propagated the idea that they enjoyed divine protection. Galienus (260-268), for example, presented himself as the chosen one of Jupiter, while Aurelian (270-275) and his successors established the custom of associating their person with the Sun, a deity of Eastern origin whose cult of which would eventually prevail over that of the other members of the Roman pantheon (BUENACASA 2021a: 173-180). At the same time, some panegyrics from the 3rd-4th centuries exalted the emperors as the sole providers of salvation and security for the empire, a power that emanated from their ambiguous status as a figure that was half human, half divine. Thus, in a speech attributed to Maximian in 291, it is said that «the first days of your rule (...) mark the beginning of [the city of Rome's] salvation [*salus*]» and, further on, it is stated that he was to dedicate all his «nights and days in perpetual concern for the salvation of all [*pro omnium salute*]». A few years later, another speaker welcomed Constantine as a *salutifer*, i.e. a "bearer of salvation" (MORALEE 2004: 49), a clear Latin version of the Greek epithet *soter*, which had already been used by some Hellenistic princes.

Throughout this turbulent 3rd century, the female archetype of Salus as codified in the preceding centuries continued to occupy a place of honour in imperial monetary issues. Examples include a series of antoniniani from the reigns of Philip the Arab (244-249; RIC IV, 46b), Galienus (260-268; RIC

21. As we have already stated, the Greeks also made frequent use of the vows *hyper soterias* and *pro salute*, in their Latin translation, as a way of clamouring for divine intervention during periods of danger and uncertainty (MORALEE 2004: 2).

22. Almost a century later (249-270) another epidemy, even more severe, if possible, than the Antonine plague, struck the empire. It was documented by the North African bishop and martyr Cyprian of Carthage (LORENTE 2021).

581), Probus (276-282; RIC 499) and Maximian and Diocletian, as corulers (286-305; RIC V, 89, 422), among others, which show on the obverse the portrait of the emperor with a solar crown on his head, while on the reverse Salus, standing and feeding a serpent, invokes the «SALVS AVG(usti)» or «AVGG(ustorum)» (fig. 11). But with the turn of the century the situation changed. From the beginning of the 4th century onwards, the inscription «SALVS» would no longer be accompanied by the snake feeding woman, nor by the young lady with a diadem or veil and holding the patera, but by images hitherto unseen, which, of course, had to be similarly used to convey the sense that the emperors were the prime sources of welfare for the population. One of the reasons for this change was the proclamation of freedom of worship throughout the empire through the Edict of Milan (313), which meant the definitive rise of Christianity and the spread of its own symbols, which gradually cornered the pagan (Saladino 1994: 661). This is the case of the Chrismon, the anagram that Constantine had seen in a dream on the eve of the famous battle of the Milvian Bridge (312) and that apologists such as Lactantius and Eusebius of Caesarea interpreted as a salvific sign (Bisconti 2012: 63). Thus, the Chrismon is the only figure that appears on coins that called out for the health of Constantius II (353)[23] next to the inscription «SALVS AVG(usti) NOSTRI» (RIC VIII, 332; fig. 12). An eloquent alternative is offered by the reverses of an issue of solidi minted by Valentinian I (364-378; RIC IX, 1; RCW 214/12). The emperor appears standing, dressed as a general, as was customary since the last quarter of the third century. With this right hand he holds the labarum with the Chrismon, and with his left hand, a globe topped by a victory that offers hum a crown; in the middle, he tramples with his foot a kneeling captive, with his hands tied. The scene clearly portrays the subjugation of an enemy, but the inscription invokes the «SALVS REIP(ublicae)»,[24] so the idea of triumph must be understood here as a representation of the safety of the republic in the face of external threats, and the dependence on the army to maintain this same safety (fig. 13).[25] A similar reading emerges from a few issues of the empress Aelia Flaccilla, wife of Theodosius I (c. 383-384). In some of these coins she commissioned a personification of a seated victory drawing a Chrismon on a shield and protected by the text «SALVS REIPVBLICAE» (RIC IX, 61.1),

23. Constantius II, son of Constantine, is known for his opposition to traditional cults. In 354 he commanded the destruction of the pagan temples throughout the empire and the persecution of the worshipers of the old gods.

24. We find the precedent of this iconography in a series issued by Constantine, in which the reverse was prised by a labarum crowned by a Chrismon, which was crossed by a snake and accompanied by the inscription «SPES PVBLIC(a)» (RIC VII, 19). I would like to thank Carles Buenacasa for sharing this information.

25. To the contrary, other contemporary coins that shared an almost identical iconography went for what seems like a more adequate aphorism: «GLORIA ROMANORVM» (RIC IX, 5). It was repeated, in identical terms, in a few issues of his sons Gratian I (RIC IX, 14) and Valentinian III (RIC IX, 38).

in others her husband next to a cross (RIC IX, 82).[26] This iconography was used for a long time, and came to be replicated by most of the empresses of the Theodosian dynasty, both in the East and in the West, a fact that reflects the new role assumed by the imperial family as a "sacred family" chosen by a God, in which all its members, including women, were useful to the cause of the empire (BUENACASA 2021b).

Going back to the dawn of the century, we note that Emperor Constantine did not commission any coins depicting Salus. Conversely, his wife Fausta Augusta did. An issue of follis from the years 324-326 shows the message «SALVS REIPVBLICAE» (RIC VII, 39, 40), accompanied by a veiled matron with two children in her arms (fig. 14).[27] It was a new subject regarding these depictions, but it had precedents in other spheres of pagan iconography: the personification of Tellus (related to *abundantia* and *pax*) had also been solved with the figure of a woman protecting a couple of children, as we can see it in the Ara Pacis (c. 13-9 BCE) and in the cuirass of the Augustus of Prima Porta (c. 20 CE). However, the depiction shown in Fausta's coins is both clear and fully justified. The two babies are an allegory of the prolific offspring of the imperial marriage, showing that the mother had fulfilled her mission: to ensure the survival of the empire by giving birth to and protecting Constantine's potential successors. As a matter of fact, the presence or absence of empresses in later-imperial numismatics depended to a large extent on whether they were mothers or not, in the same way that when receiving the honorary title of Augusta, motherhood was a determining factor.[28] Over time, the visual archetype of the woman nursing her children would evolve to become one of the most common representations of the Christian theological virtue of charity.

## 3. *From the Obscurity of Salus to the Modern Revindication of the Motto «Salus Populi Romani»*

As we have seen, while evocations of health continued to be common in Roman numismatic and epigraphic messaging, the female personification of Salus, inspired by the Greek Hygieia, completely disappeared in the 4th century. In addition, in 380, Emperor Theodosius I made Christianity the official religion of the empire through the Edict of Thessalonica, and a few years later, in 391, he banned the celebration of all pagan cults and rites. This was the final coup de grace that

26. Concerning Aelia Flaccilla and the role of women in the Theodosian dynasty, see BUENACASA 2021b.

27. In other variants that include the same effigy of Fausta we read the text «SPES REIPVBLICAE» (RIC VII, 203). Furthermore, other issues minted to honour Fausta's stepsister, the empress Teodora, show her standing and breast feeding a baby, together with the inscription «PIETAS ROMANA» (RIC VIII, 43). I would like to thank Carles Buenacasa for sharing this information.

28. I would like to thank Carles Buencasa for this insight.

brought Salus and the rest of the deities of the Roman pantheon to an irrevocable ostracism. However, the process was not automatic, even more so at a time when cultural exchanges between pagans and Christians were commonplace.[29] For this reason, I want to dwell on three masterworks that perfectly reflect this moment of impasse.

The National Museums of Liverpool (c. 400-430) keep an ivory diptych decorated with carvings of Aesculapius and Salus, standing and escorted by snakes in accordance with their traditional Greek iconography (fig. 15). What does their presence in this piece mean? At the turn of the 4th-5th centuries and despite official prohibitions, some diptychs for private use still reproduced pagan myths and rites, so this could have been commissioned as a gift to celebrate, for example, a recovery from an illness or the birth of a child. Or, perhaps, it even belonged to a doctor. Other authors, such as Margaret Gibson (1994: 10-15), have proposed more complex readings that link the piece to Neoplatonic philosophical currents in vogue in Rome at the beginning of the 5th century.[30]

A different case, which was part of a private-professional environment, is an ivory box made to contain medical instruments that would later be recycled as a reliquary (late 5th century; Sion: Valais Historical Museum). The front is also decorated with the effigies of Aesculapius and Salus, accompanied by snakes. In this case, its reading does not seem to have anything to do with philosophical interpretations but is rather an explicit allusion to its owner's profession (fig. 16).

On the other hand, in the 1930s, excavations were carried out in the so-called baths of Apolausis, in ancient Antioch, which made it possible to unearth a splendid mosaic that adorned the pavement of its *frigidarium* (c. 400). In the very middle of a rich octagonal composition there is a female bust, dressed in a himation and stole, wearing a necklace, earrings and crown, and flaunting long hair. The inscription in Greek capital letters allows us to identify her with *Soteria*,

29. However, it should be pointed out that what disappeared was the traditional and feminine iconography of Salus, but not the abstract ideal of public welfare, which was very easy to Christianize. At the same time, it is necessary to value the message of the coins struck by the Theodosian empresses who, due to their status as mothers, guaranteed the continuity of the imperial lineage, at the same time that, with their good deeds, they also contributed to the spiritual health of the whole empire, in such a way that the concept of *salus* would end up merging with that of *pietas* (BUENACASA 2021b).

30. Gibson's thesis is based on a passage from the *Saturnalia* (I, 20, 1-4) of Macrobius, written c. 430, although set around 370 and, therefore, before the Edict of Thessalonica. For Macrobius, Aesculapius and Salus were directly related to the nature of the sun and the moon. He said of the former that he embodied the power of health, which came from his solar essence. Regarding the latter, he considered her responsible for the lunar influence with which animals were helped. For this reason, their statues were accompanied by snakes, because they showed human bodies as if they had shed the skin of disease to return to their old vigour. As Gibson (1994) reiterates, this diptych could be part of the intellectual currents that circulated in Rome in the first third of the 5th century, of which Macrobius was part, and which used to evoke the ancient pagan gods to express their Neoplatonic ideas.

a completely exceptional choice, since we do not know of other personifications of her figure neither in Greece nor in Rome (fig. 17). In the opinion of Jason Moralee (2004: 51-54) the model used was that of Salus Augusta, a proposal based on the crown on the head, made of gold leaves and decorated in the middle with a precious gem. Moralee argues that it was not a random ornament, but the *corona civica*, the prize which, in the words of Cicero and Cesar, was awarded to those who had saved the republic from internal and external threats. Later, from the times of August onwards, it became the symbol par excellence of the hierarchy of the *princeps* who, in the eyes of the people, had become the sole saviour of the state and its inhabitants. This crown continued to be used on bronze sculptures and in monetary portraiture until the mid-4th century, when it was progressively replaced by a diadem. Moralee therefore concludes that this successful rendering of Soteria's unique personification, with the *corona civica*, was inspired by the rich language of imperial representation. In fact, as we have seen, the earliest images of Salus on late Republican monuments consist of female portraits in profile, with a leafy crown, earrings and a pearl collar, the same attributes of the Soteria of Apollausis. As for the use of the Greek word *soteria*, instead of the Latin *salus*, it could easily be argued that it was rather natural, since the mosaic was located in an Eastern city, but in my opinion other motives cannot be ruled out. It is known that the first Christians gave Jesus the title of *soter* –saviour– in the same way that some Hellenistic princes had received it before (Kittel et al. 1985: 1140), as the Gospel of Luke (Lk, 2:11) and other sacred books show. Although its use was ephemeral,[31] the decision to write *soteria* in place of *salus* might have to do with its symbolic link with Christ, which, unlike the Latin concept, had implicit pagan connotations that were much more deeply rooted. As for its function, it has already been mentioned at the beginning of this article that the inside of the baths was usually decorated with images of Aesculapius/Asclepius and Hygieia/Salus. Therefore, the presence of this syncretic version of Soteria-Salus would be entirely logical.

Be that as it may, personifications such as those of Liverpool, Sion or Antioch are no more than twilight testimonies of a receding iconography. Nevertheless, the ideals and meanings that lay behind the pagan Salus continued to be relevant and Christian society could not ignore them. A good physical condition, to ward off death and illness, and to have a prosperous life continued to be the main aspirations of any person, regardless of their religious beliefs. In imperial times, these yearnings could be expressed through public or private prayers to the goddess Salus, but with the prohibition of pagan rites, a substitute or substitutes had to be found. In the first place, and beyond Christ himself, some of the martyr saints were associated with healing properties and, thus, became the object of the prayers of the faithful

31. Eventually, the usage of the formula of Jesus *soter* became less prevalent, due to the risk of associating it with the Jewish hope of liberation or an excessive identification with the pagan ideal of the political benefactor (Kittel et al. 1985: 1140).

(SALTER 2021).[32] However, it was Mary, mother of Jesus, who became the true queen of these kind of prayers. To a certain extent, she adopted the role of a new Christianised Salus Augusta, albeit freed of any kind of meaning that might link her to the solidity of the State or to the loyalty to its rulers.[33]

By way of conclusion, I find it appropriate to close this text by referring to a celebrated masterpiece. Since 1613, the so-called Pauline chapel of the Basilica of Saint Mary Major in Rome has housed a Byzantine icon with the Virgin and Child of the *acheiropoieta* type, in Latin *non manufactum*, that is, made by a non-human hand (fig 18). In this case, tradition has attributed its authorship to the evangelist Saint Luke, who, supposedly, would have recycled a piece of wood from the table of the Holy Supper to paint on it. In reality, its dating continues to be the subject of debate, despite the fact that certain consensus places it between the 5th and 6th centuries. It is also not known for certain when the image arrived in Rome from the east, but from the first moment it was surrounded by an aura of divinity. Thus, in 590, in order to free the city from a voracious epidemic, Pope Gregory the Great organized a penitential procession to place the icon to St. Peter's Basilica in the Vatican. When the procession reached Hadrian's ancient mausoleum –the current Castel Sant'Angelo– an angelic choir was heard singing «*Regina coeli laetare, alleluia*» and the pontiff saw how the holy archangel Michael, brandishing a sword, dispelled the plague (WOLF 1991). The miracle proved the protective effectiveness of the icon and in order to facilitate its devotion by all Romans, it was decided to move it from its first location, the *Sancta Sanctorum* of the Lateran Basilica, to the aforementioned basilica of Saint Mary Major. This was the best place to preserve the panel painting, because it was the first church dedicated to the Virgin, coinciding with her proclamation as *Theotokos* at the Council of Ephesus (431). The memory of the prodigy experienced in 590 was perpetuated throughout the centuries and the icon was commonly invoked during wars, pestilences and famines.[34] Until the 19th century, it was known by the popular name of *Regina coeli*, but from then on it began to be called *Salus Populi Romani*, a title that still remains today. It was not a simple exchange of names, since it rescued one of the most common slogans of pagan propaganda: the health of the people of Rome. A health that, as Ariphron said, is the main desire of any person and community, because without it «no one is happy».

32. We find an example of this in the figures of the saint-doctors Cosmas and Damian. On their iconography see the chapter, in this same volume, by Fernando Serrano Larráyoz and Antonio González Bueno.

33. There is no ancient or medieval word to name these strategies, although they are commonly grouped under the generic concept of the common good.

34. The icon of Saint Mary Major was the most important in Rome, but not the only one with miraculous healing properties. Among others, the *Madonna del Conforto* or *Imago Antiqua*, kept in the basilica of Santa Francesca Romana, is noteworthy, as it was considered to be the most ancient in the city (5th century). Another important icon was that of the *Madonna della Clemenza* (7th century), in the basilica of Saint Mary in Trastevere.

## *Bibliography*


Beumer, Mark, 2016. "Hygieia. Identity, Cult and Reception", *Kleio-Historia*, 3: 5-24.

Bisconti, Fabrizio, 2012. "Il vessillo, il critogramma: i segni della salvezza", Genna Sena (ed.), *Costantino 313 d.C.*, Milan, Electa: 60-64.

Boatwright, Mary T., 2021. *Imperial Women of Rome. Power, Gender, Context*, New York, Oxford University Press.

Brunt, P. A., 1959. "The Revolt of Vindex and the Fall of Nero", *Latomus*, 18/3: 531-559.

Buenacasa, Carles, 2021a. *Esplendor y ocaso de Roma. Apogeo, crisis y decadencia del Imperio*, [Barcelona], Schackleton.

Buenacasa, Carles, 2021b. "Poder y legitimación de las emperatrices teodosianas y su reflejo en la iconografía numismática", *Mujeres imperiales, mujeres reales. Representaciones públicas y representaciones del poder en la Antigüedad tardía y Bizancio*, Padeborn, Brill: 115-131.

Bickenbach, Jerome, 2015. "WHO's Definition of Health: Philosophical Analysis", ed. T. Schramme & S. Edwards. *Handbook of the Philosophy of Medicine*, Dordrecht, Springer. https://doi.org/10.1007/978-94-017-8706-2_48-1 [link visited in September 2022].

Cêbe, Jean-Pierre, 1989. "Les lectiscernes republicains", Anne-France Laurens (ed.), *Entre hommes et deux: le convive, le héros, le prophéte*, Paris, Les Belles Lettres: 27-40.

Clark, Anna J., 2007. *Divine Qualities. Cult and Community in Republican Rome*, Oxford, Oxford University Press.

Compton, Michael T., 2002. "The Association of Hygieia with Asklepios in Graeco-Roman Asklepieion Medicine", *Journal of the History of Medicine and Allied Sciences*, 57/3: 312-329.

Fagan, Garrett G., 2002. *Bathing in Public in the Roman World*, Ann Arbor (MI), University of Michigan Press.

Farrés, Oriol, 2020. "*Salus populi suprema lex*", *Revista de Bioética y Derecho*, 50: 5-17.

Garzón, José A., 1989. "Propaganda religiosa en acuñaciones de Adriano, Antonino Pío y sus familias (Tipos de *Pietas*, *Pudicitia*, *Salus*, *Virtus* y *Votus*)", *Analecta Malacitana*, 12: 5-22.

Gibson, Margaret T., 1994. *The Liverpool Ivories. Late Antique and Medieval Ivory and Bone Carving in Liverpool Museum and the Walker Art Gallery*, Liverpool, National Museums and Galleries on Merseyside.

Gozalbes, Enrique; García, Inmaculada, 2007. "La primera peste de los Antoninos (165-170). Una epidemia en la Roma imperial", *Asclepio. Revista de Historia de la Medicina y de la Ciencia*, 49: 7-22.

González, M. Pilar, 2021. "La fórmula *pro salute Hadriani* en la epigrafía: una perspectiva general a propósito del caso hispano", *Studia Historica. Historia Antigua*, 39: 355-376.

Jim, Theodora S. F., 2015. "Can Soteira be Named? The Problem of the Bare Trans-divine Epithet", *Zeitschrift für Papyrologie und Epigraphik*, 195: 63-74.

Jim, Theodora S. F., 2017. "«Salvation» (*Soteria*) and Ancient Mystery Cults", *Archiv für Religionsgeschichte*, 18-19: 255-281.

Jim, Theodora S. F., 2022. *Saviour Gods and Soteria in Ancient Greece*, New York, Oxford University Press.

Kittel, Gerhard; Friedrich, Gerhard; Bromiley, Geoffrey W., 1985. *Theological Dictionary of the New Testament*, Grands Rapids (MI), Eerdmans Publishing.

Köhler, W., 1965. "Salus", *Enciclopedia dell'Arte Antica*, Roma, Istituto Treccani (online): sv.

Lardinois, Andre; Blok, Josine H.; Van der Poel, Marc, 2011. *Sacred Words. Orality, Literacy and Religion*, Leiden-Boston, Brill (*Orality and Literacy in the Ancient World*, vol. 8).

Lorente, Mario, 2021. "La «Peste de Cipriano»: la primera gran pandemia de la Antigüedad Tardía (249-270)", *Espacio, Tiempo y Forma*, 34: 219-242.

Marqués, Néstor F., 2018. *Un año en la antigua Roma. La vida cotidiana de los romanos a través de su calendario*, Barcelona, Espasa (Kindle e-book).

Marvin, Miranda, 1983. "Freestanding Sculptures from the Baths of Caracalla", *American Journal of Archaeology*, 87/3: 347-384.

MARWOOD, Martin A., 1988. *Roman Cult of Salus*, Oxford, BAR.

MONTERO, Santiago, 2001. "El «augurium salutis» o la paz imposible", *Ilu. Revista de Ciencias de las Religiones. Anejos*, 6: 47-55.

MORALEE, Jason, 2004. *For Salvation's Sake. Provincial Loyalty, Personal Religion, and Epigraphic Production in the Roman and Late Antique Near East*, London, Routledge.

MORIGGI, Marco, 2011. "Phœnician and Punic Inscriptions in the Museo di Antichità di Torino (Turin, Italy)", *Egitto e Vicino Oriente*, 34: 81-94.

RENBERG, Gil H., 2006. "Public and Private Places of Worship in the Cult of Asclepius at Rome", *Memoirs of the American Academy in Rome*, 51/52: 87-172.

RETIEF, Francois P.; CILLIERS, Louise, 2002. "Snake and Staff Symbolism and Healing", *South African Medical Journal*, 92/7: 553-556.

SALADINO, Vincenzo, 1994. "Salus", P. Müller, P. Linant de Bellefonds (ed.), *Lexicon iconographicum mythologiae classicæ*, Zürich-München, Artemis: 656-661.

SALTER, Ruth J., 2021. *Saints, Cure-seekers and Miraculous Healing in Twelfth-century England*, York, York Medieval Press.

SCARBOROUGH, John, 1981. "Roman Medicine and Public Health", Teizo Ogawa (ed.), *Public Health*, Tokyo, Taniguchi Foundation: 33-74.

SEAR, David R., 1982. *Greek Imperial Coins and Their Values. The Local Coinages of the Roman Empire*, London, Seaby.

STAFFORD, Emma, 2000. *Worshipping Virtues. Personification and the Divine in Ancient Greece*, Swansea, Duckworth & The Classical Press of Wales.

WARDLE, David, 2012. "Suetonius on Augustus as God and Man", *The Classical Quarterly*, 62/1: 307-326.

WOLF, Gerhard, 1991. *«Salus Populi Romani». Die Geschicte römische Kultbilder im Mittelalter*, Weinheim, VCH Acta Humaniora.

YORK, William H., 2012. *Health and Wellness in Antiquity Through the Middle Ages*, Santa Barbara, Greenwood.

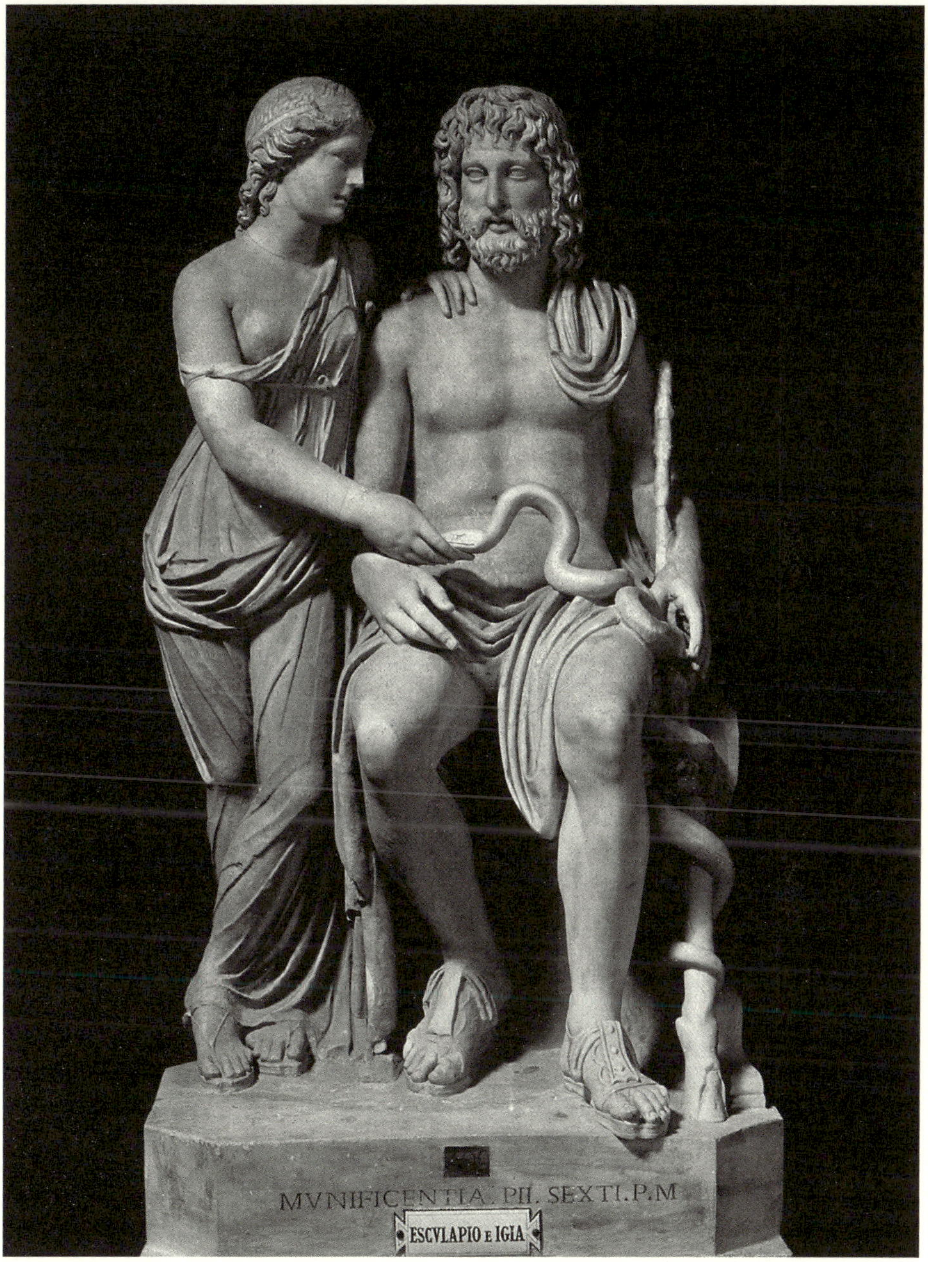


Fig. 1. Group with Asclepius and Hygieia. Roman marble copy from the time of emperor Hadrian, after a late Hellenistic original (Rome: Vatican Museums, Pius Clementine Museum, Gallery of statues, 33). Image: © Wellcome Collection, obtained from https://bit.ly/3rmz5BM.

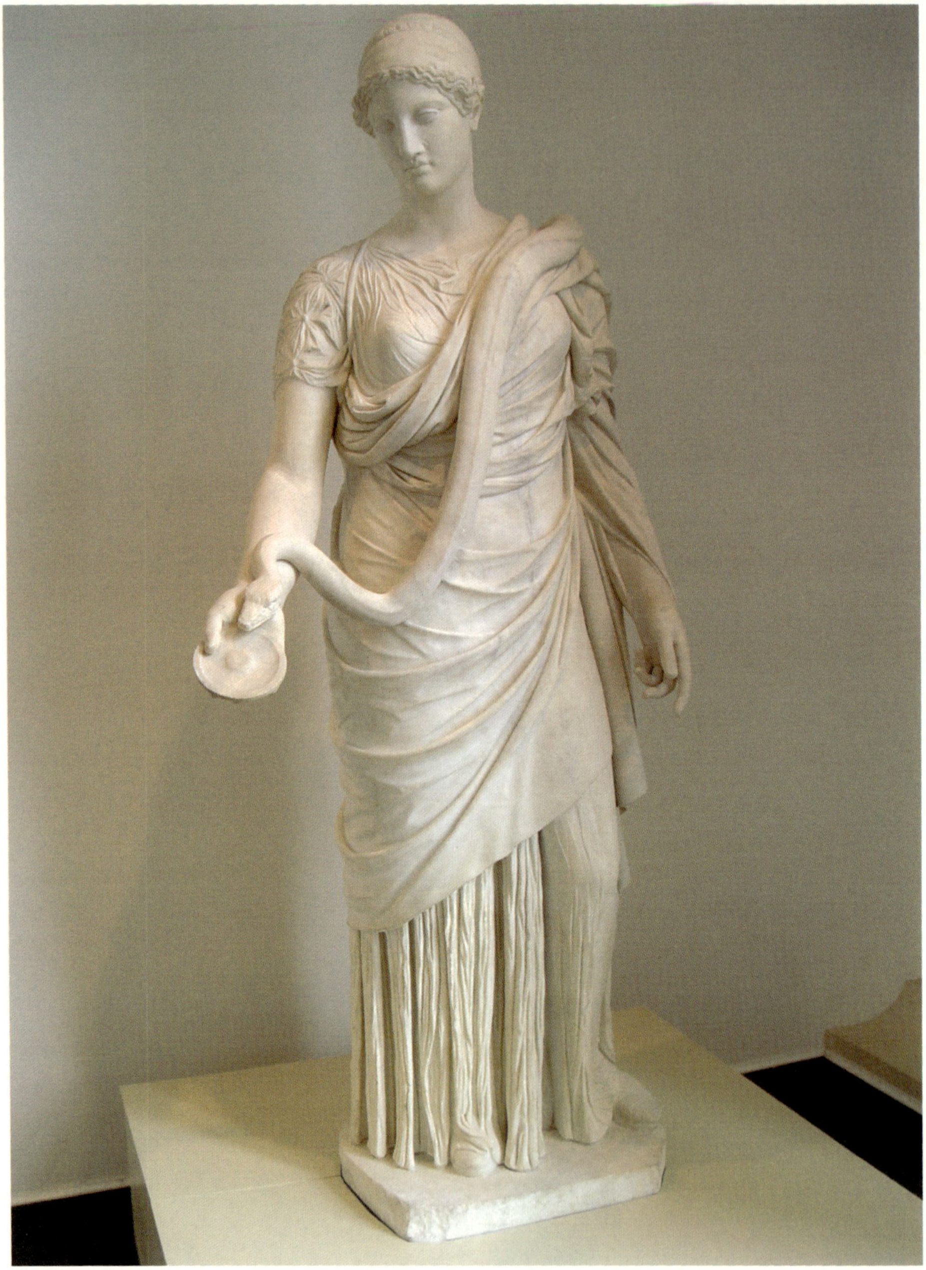

Fig. 2. "The Hygieia of Hope", Hygieia feeds a snake. Roman copy, c. 130-160, after a Greek original, c. 360 BCE. Excavated at Ostia, this is the only complete large example of the type (Los Angeles: County Museum of Art). Image obtained from https://bit.ly/3ys9iMv / Photograph by Howard Cheng / 

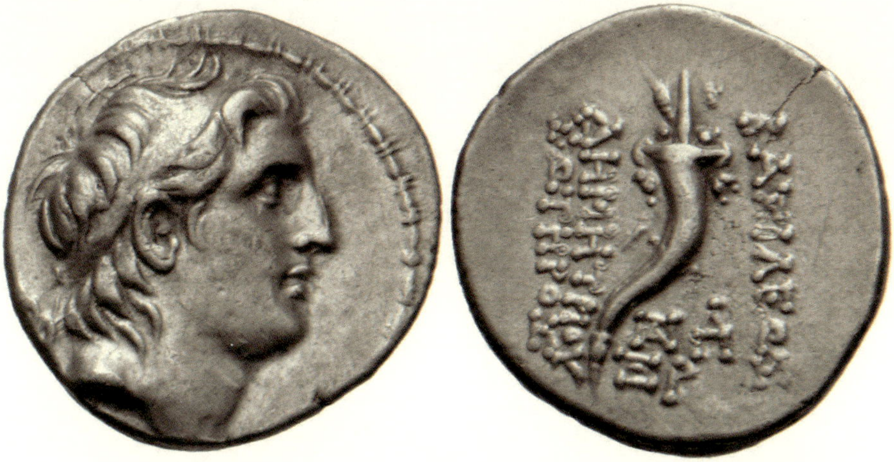

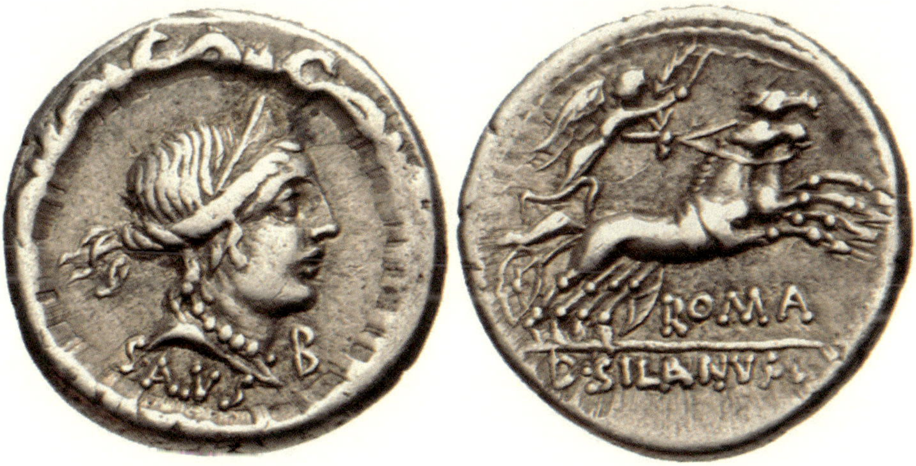


Fig. 3. Silver drachma of Demetrios I Soter, minted in Syria, c. 160 BCE (SC 1642.2). In the observe, diademed head of Demetrius I, right. In the reverse a cornucopia placed vertically with the inscription in Greek characters: ΒΑΣΙΛΕΩΣ ΔΗΜΗΤΡΙΟΥ ΣΩΤΗΡΟΣ; below, two monograms above ΞΡ. Image obtained from https://bit.ly/3y5OWbA.
Fig. 4. Silver denarius of D. Junius L.f. Silanus, minted in Rome, 91 BCE (RRC 337, 2c). Observe: diademed head of Salus within torque, right. Reverse: Victory driving biga, right, holding a palm-branch and reins in left hand and whip in right hand. Image obtained from https://bit.ly/3y51K21.

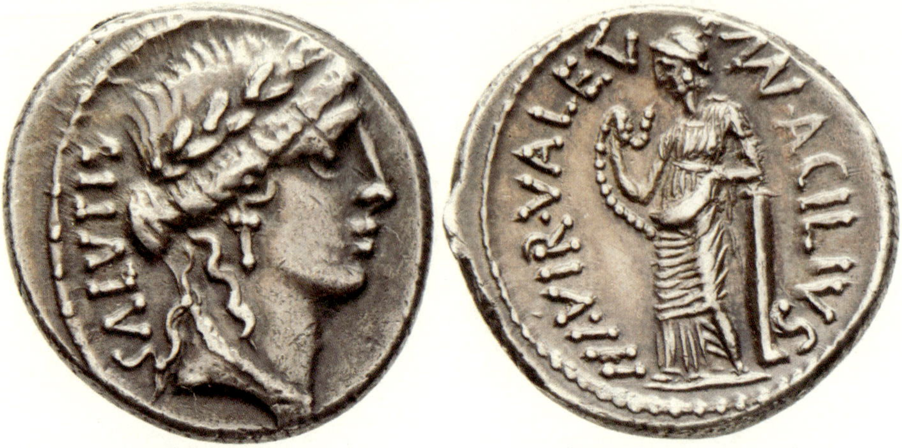


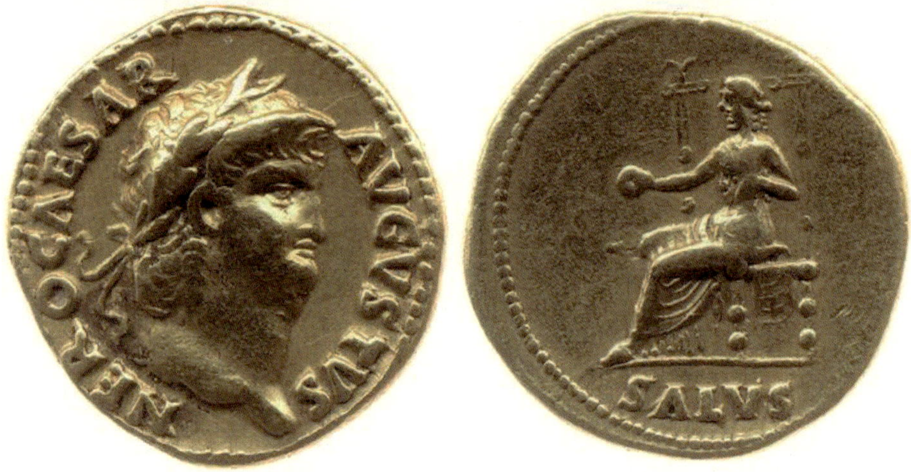


Fig. 5. Silver denarius of Manius Acilius Glabrio, minted in Rome, c. 49 BCE (RRC 442). Observe: diademed head of Salus, right. Reverse, Valetudo standing left, holding a snake and leaning on a column. Image obtained from https://bit.ly/3SDmi9K.

Fig. 6. Gold aureus of Nero, minted in Rome, c. 65-66 CE (RIC I, 59). Observe: head of Nero, laureate and with beard, right. Reverse: Salus, draped, seated left on an ornamental throne, holding a patera in her right hand and resting. Image obtained from https://bit.ly/3UMDN9r.

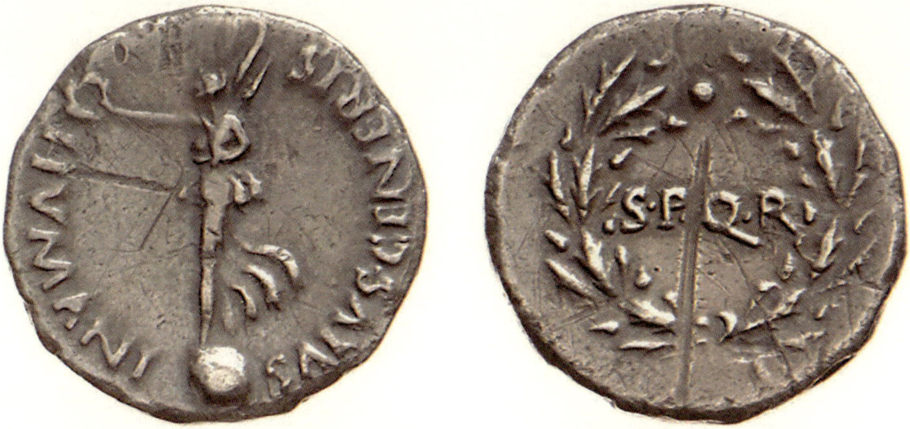


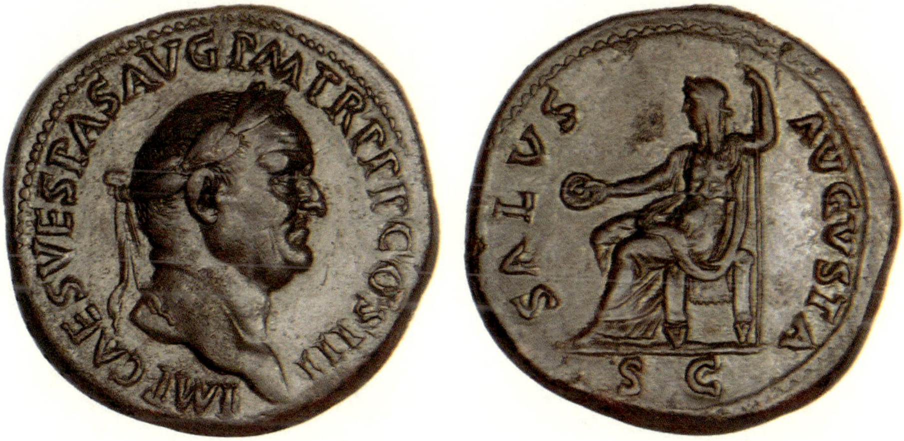


Fig. 7. Silver denarius minted in Gallia, c. 68-69 CE (RIC I, 72). Observe, Victory standing left on globe, holding a wreath in her right hand and a palm in her left and the legend «SALVS GENERIS HVMANI». Reverse, legend «SPQR» within oak-wreath. Image obtained from https://bit.ly/3UQZqFt.

Fig. 8. Bronze sestertius of Vespasian minted in Rome, 71 CE (RIC, II, 1). Observe: Head of Vespasian, laureate, right. Reverse: Salus, draped, seated left, holding a patera in her extended right hand and a vertical scepter in the left and the legend «SALVS AVGVSTA S(enatus) C(onsulto)». Image obtained from: https://bit.ly/3Tcxgng.

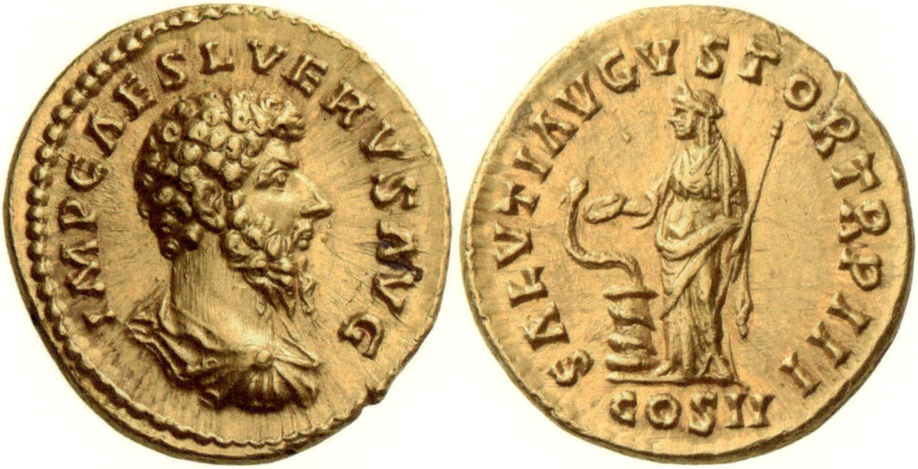

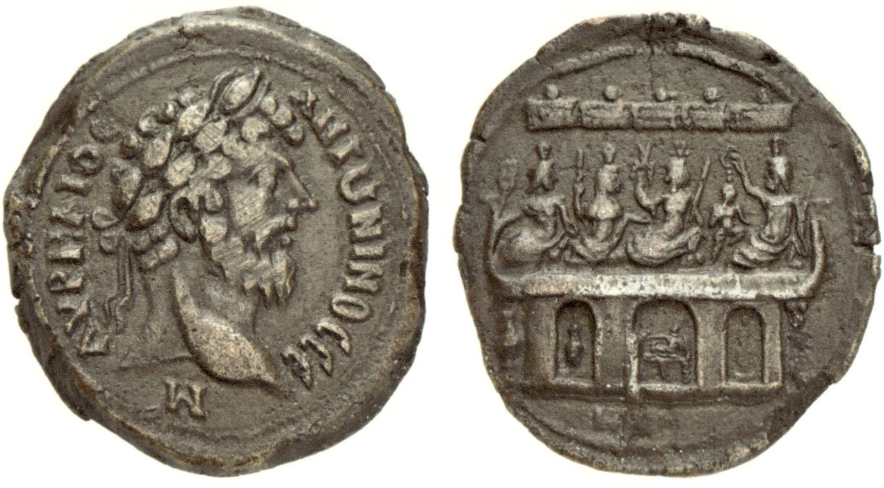

Fig. 9. Gold aureus of Lucius Verus, minted in Rome, 162-163 CE (RIC III, 493). Observe: bare-headed, draped and cuirassed bust of the emperor, right. Reverse: Salus, draped, seated left on an ornamental throne, holding a patera in her right hand and resting. Image obtained from https://bit.ly/3CHBn3s.
Fig. 10. Bronze coin of Marcus Aurelius, minted in Alexandria, 167-168 CE (RPC IV, 4). Observe: bare-headed bust of emperor, right. Reverse: representation of a meal of the gods (*lectisternium*): from right to left on a couch with three niches, Sarapis, Harpocrates, Isis, Demeter, Hermanubis. Above each deity a rectangular basket with a spherical top. In peripheral niches canopic jars, in the middle Tyche? Image obtained from https://bit.ly/3eB33iq.

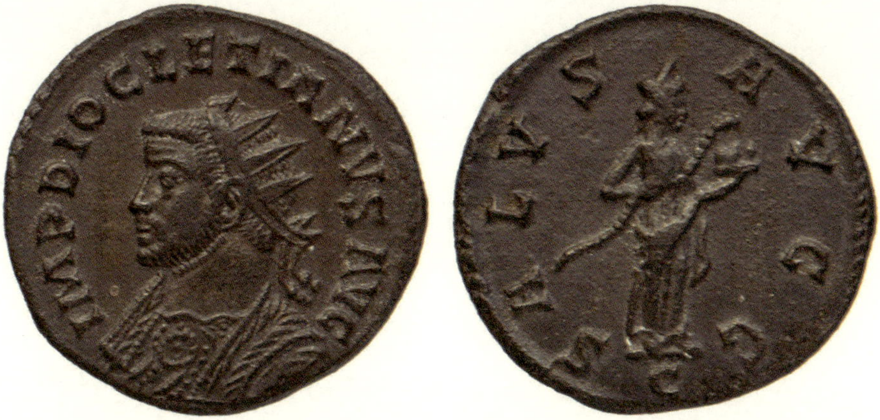


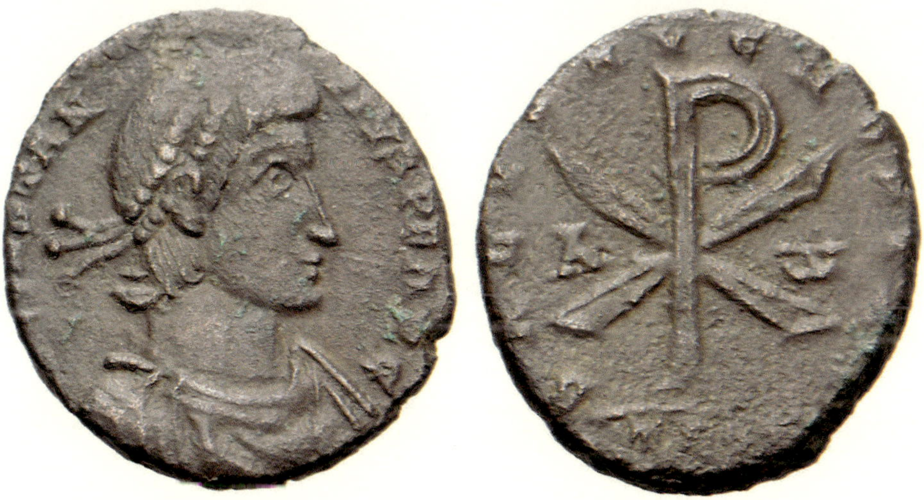

Fig. 11. Silver antonianus minted in Lyon, c. 291 CE (RIC, V, 89). Observe: bust of Diocletian, radiate, draped, cuirassed, right. Reverse: Salus, draped, standing right, feeding snake held in arms, and the legend «SALVS AVGG(ustorum)». Image obtained from https://bit.ly/3Vx6YgU.

Fig. 12. Bronze centenionalis of Constantius II, minted in Trier, 353 CE (RIC VIII, 332). Observe: diademed, draped and cuirassed bust of Constantius II, right. Reverse: Christogram between A and ω, and the legend «SALVS AVG(usti) NOSTRI». Image obtained from https://bit.ly/3g8haMB.

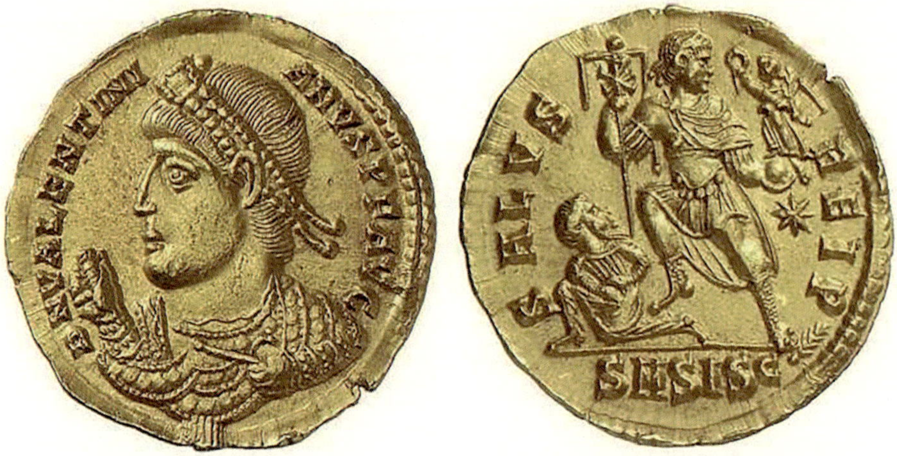

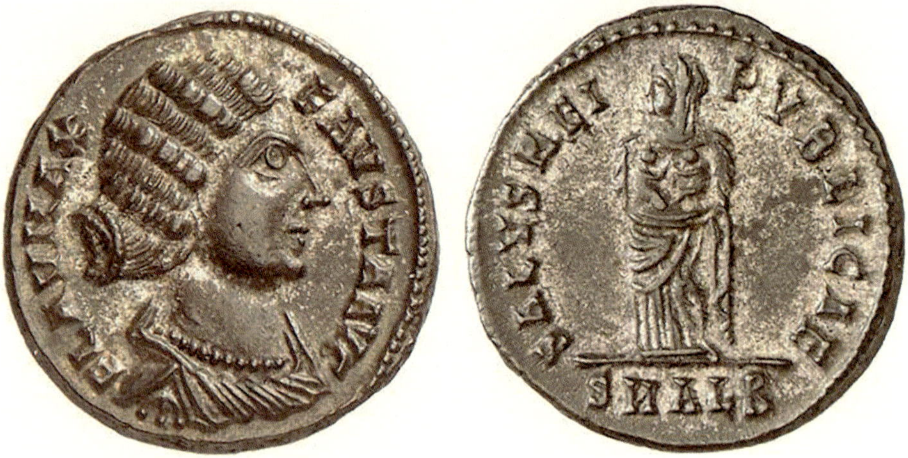

Fig. 13. Golden solidus of Valentinian I, minted in Siscia, c. 375 CE (RIC IX, 1). Observe: pearl-diademed bust of Valentinian I, left, wearing imperial mantle, holding mappa and sceptre. Reverse: emperor standing left, looking right, holding labarum and Victory on globe, right foot on a captive, half-kneeling, and legend «SALVS REIP(ublicae)». Image obtained from https://bit.ly/3SmOsVX.

Fig. 14. Bronze follis of Fausta Augusta, minted in Alexandria, 325-326 CE (RIC VII, 39). Observe: bare-headed bust of Fausta, hair waved hair, wearing necklace, right. Reverse: empress, veiled, standing left, holding two infants in her arms and the legend «SALVS REIPVBLICAE». Image obtained from https://bit.ly/3yXd4h5.

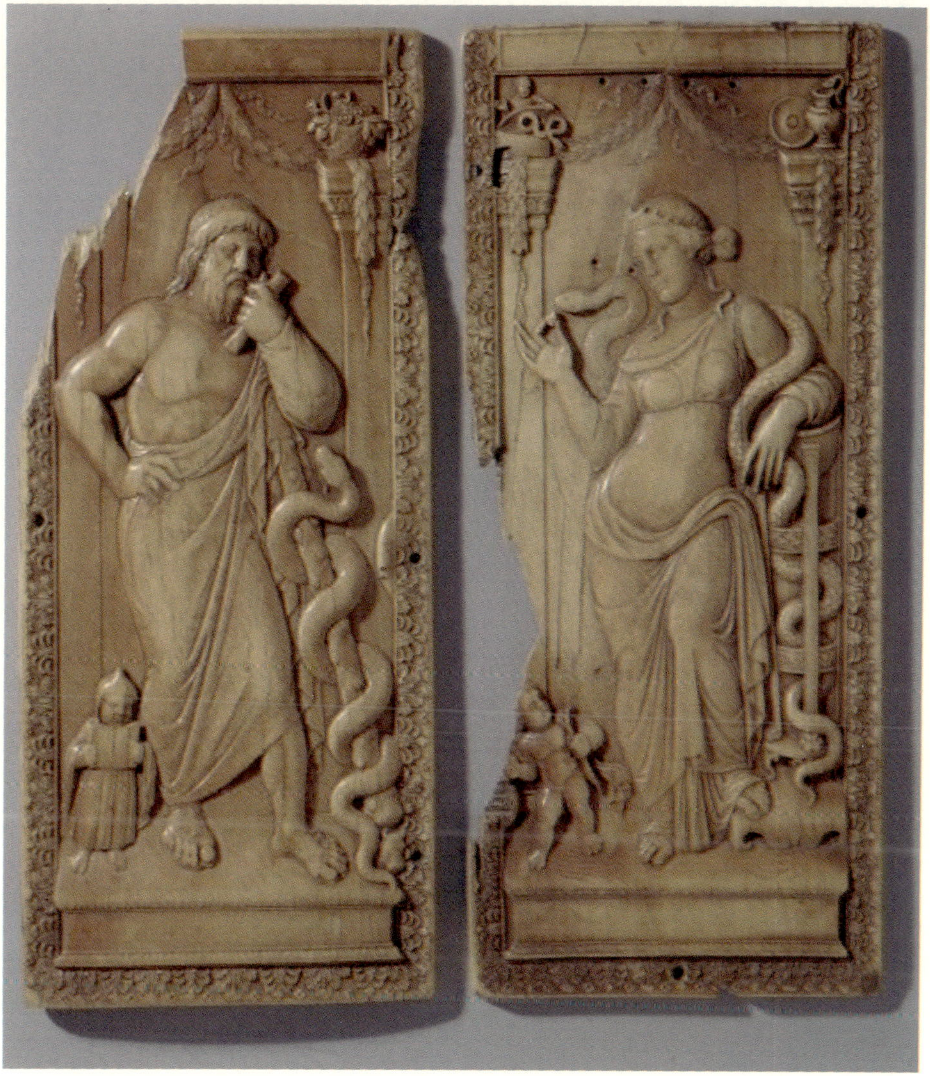

Fig. 15. Ivory "Asclepius-Hygieia Dyptich", 400-430 CE (Liverpool: National Museums). Image obtained from https://www.liverpoolmuseums.org.uk.

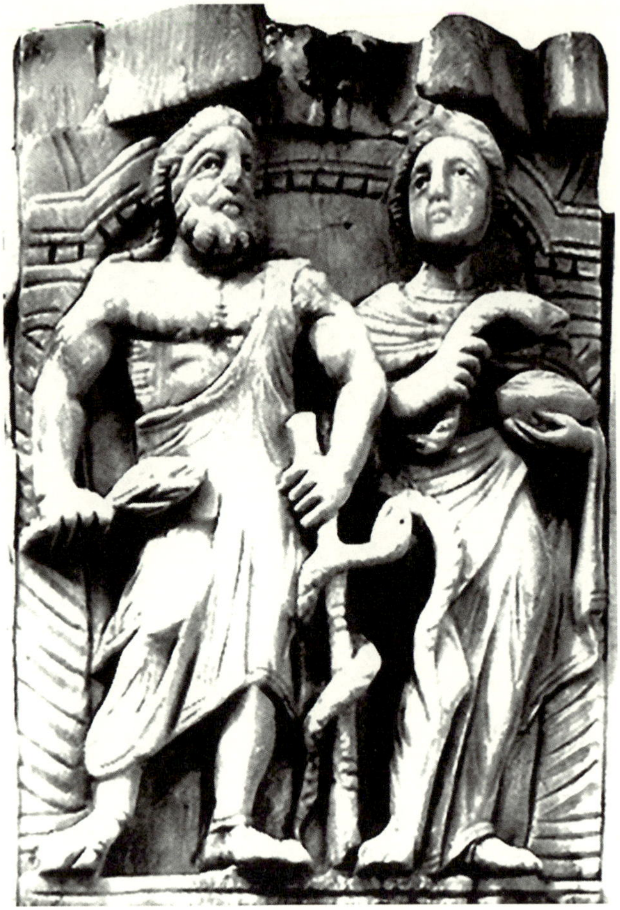

Fig. 16. Ivory medicine box with Asclepius and Hygeia, later converted to a reliquary, northern Italy; late 5th century (Sion: Valais Historical Museum). Drawing by the author.

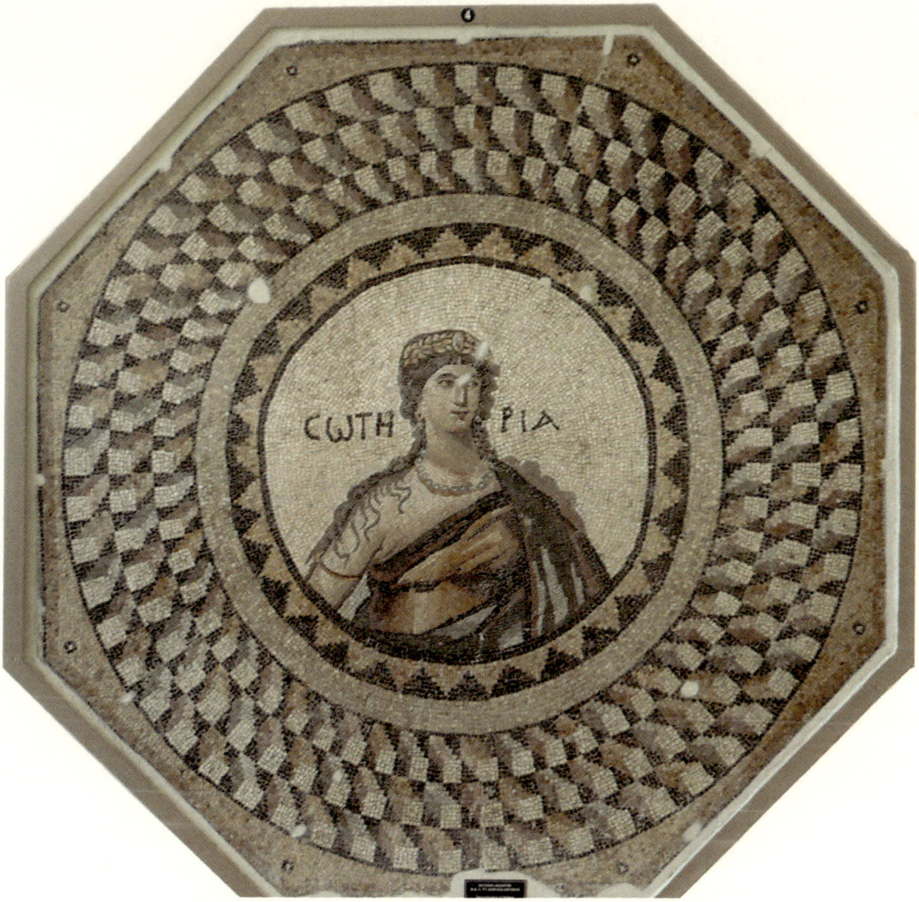


Fig. 17. Octagonal mosaic with a woman labeled with the Greek word *Soteria*, from the the bath of Apolausis, in Antioch (Syria), c. 400 CE (Antakya: Archaeological Museum). Image: © Wikimedia Commons, license CC BY-SA 3.0.

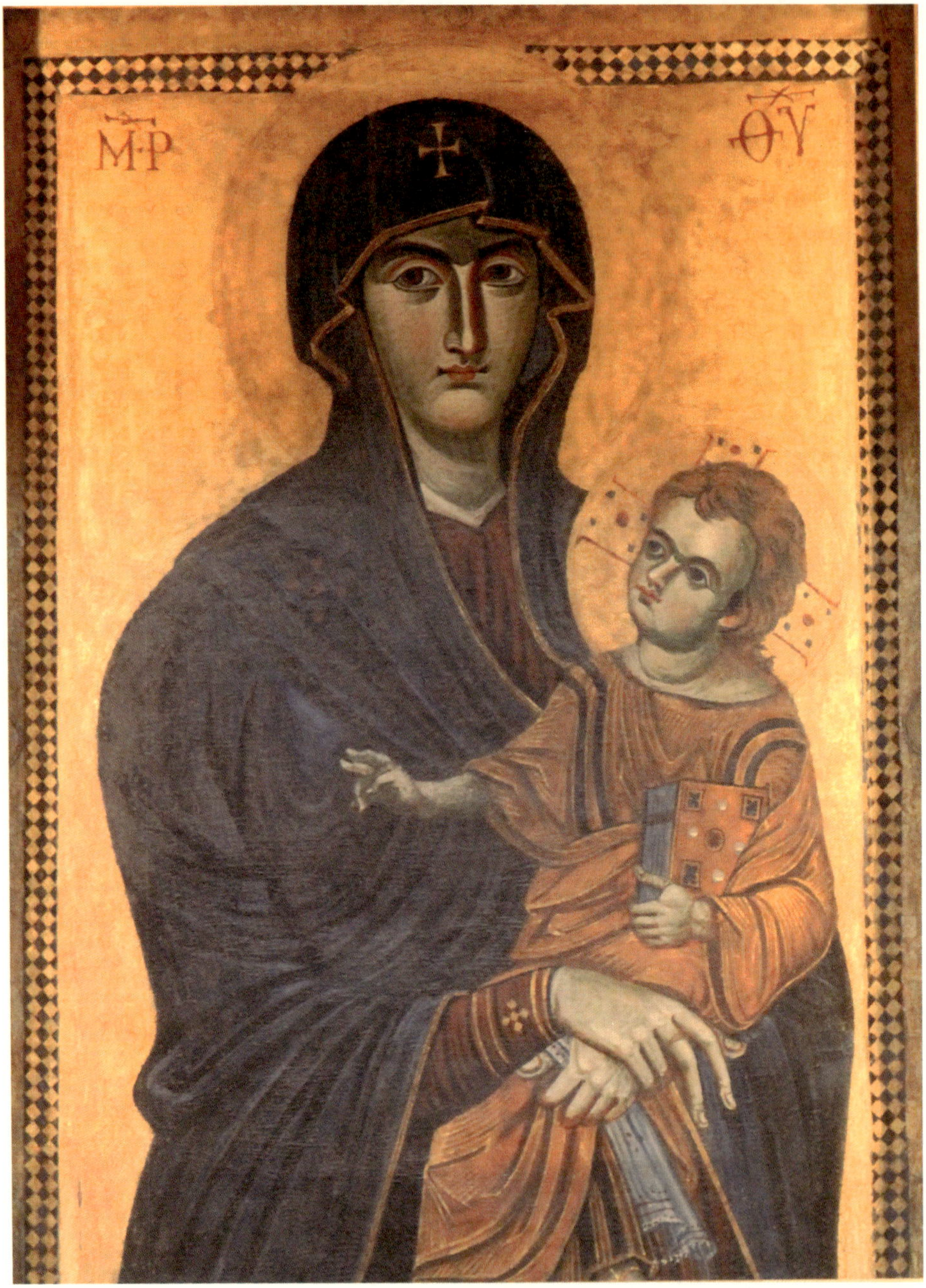


Fig. 18. Byzantine icon of "Salus Populi Romani", 5th-6th century (Rome: Santa Maria Maggiore, Pauline Chapel). Image: © Wikimedia Commons, license CC BY-SA 4.0.

Fernando Serrano Larráyoz, Antonio González Bueno

# The Tradition of the Worship and Iconography of Saints Cosmas and Damian in Hispanic Territory*

## 1. *Saints Cosmas and Damian: Their Lives and Miracles*

The hagiography of Saints Cosmas and Damian began spreading in the West in the 13th century (1264), chiefly through the *Golden Legend* of the Dominican Jacobus de Voragine (c. 1230-1298). Despite this, the oldest martyrologies, both the 5th century Greek version and the 6th century Latin version, allude to three pairs of saints with the same name, with different feast days: the 1st of November for those from Constantinople, the 1st of July for those from Rome, and the 17th of October those from Cyrrhestica (Festugière 1971: 93, n. 4; Bucci 2016: 17). The *Roman Martyrology* describes them as being of Arab origin and coming from a noble family. They were supposedly born in Aegeae (now Ayas), in Cilicia (although the text also ascribes them other origins), were educated as Christians and were also proficient in the arts and the sciences and especially medicine (Fracchia 2010: 132).

According to the text, they treated both people and animals. Their combined piety and technical knowledge guaranteed the success of their endeavours. This fact, together with their refusal to charge any fees for their services (which made them known as the *anargyroi*, or "unmercenaries") made them an example of Christian charity. In doing so, they were fulfilling the mandate of Christ (Mk 6: 7-14) when he sent his disciples out to preach in pairs, urging them not to take anything for the journey: «neither bread, nor knapsack, nor money» (Jong 2013: 37). According to tradition, they were executed on the orders of the prefect Lysias, during the persecution of Diocletian, in the year 287. After being tortured, beheaded and buried, their bodies were soon moved to the episcopal city of Cyrus, where a basilica was built for them (Nieto Ibáñez 2014: xi-xiii).

* This article is part of the research projects of the MICINN-AEI/ERDF *Vernacularidades en la ciencia medieval y renacentista: textos, creadores, profesionales* (PID2021-123419NB-I00, 2022-2025) and CECJA-ERDF *Recetarios, experimentación y ciencia. Los cuidados del cuerpo en la Edad Media y su aplicación en el siglo XXI* (1381195-R, 2022) (Fernando Serrano Larráyoz). For the help they have given us, we wish to thank Merche Osés Urricelqui, Juan Vicente García Marsilla, Raúl Villagrasa Elías, Manuel Ruiz de Luzuriaga Peña and Antoni Conejo da Pena.

Worship quickly spread from Aegeae to Syria and from Byzantium to Rome. In 423 they were mentioned by Theodoret of Cyrus, a member of the local aristocracy, who alluded to the pillaging and to an attempt to set fire to the basilica of Cyrus a few years after the Council of Ephesus. Other information comes from the Byzantine historian Procopius of Caesarea, who tells (*De Aedificis*, 1) of the miraculous healing of the Emperor Justinian and the redesigning of an old temple (or chapel) in Constantinople built by Theodosius II and dedicated to the saints: «completely changing the old building, which was anti-aesthetic and ignoble and was unworthy of being dedicated to such powerful saints» (López Campuzano, 1996: 257; Walker Vadillo 2011: 53). Later we know that, in Rome, in what is now the Via dei Fori Imperiali, Pope Felix IV (526-530) moved their relics and established a basilica in honour of the two saints, in the place where according to tradition Galen had lived (Matthews, 1968: 282; López Campuzano, 1996: 257).

We find numerous references to temples dedicated to the saints from the 4th century onwards (López Campuzano, 1996: 256-257; Bucci 2016: 71-152). We shall refer later to their dissemination and worship in Hispanic territory. It is more interesting now to study the important Greek collections of tales of miracles performed by Cosmas and Damian, 47 in total, to which we must add four more which appear in chapter 163 of Jacobus de Voragine's *Golden Legend*, along with the lives of the saints and their martyrdoms at the hands of the proconsul Lysias. The last of these four miracles was the most remembered and represented, due to the satisfactory conclusion of a surgical procedure that was unpracticable until very recently. This was the amputation of a black man's leg that was then grafted on to one of the people in charge of cleaning the aforementioned Roman basilica consecrated to the saints. This version does not appear in the Greek collections of miracles, but it is featured, with no indication of the race or position of neither the donor nor the patient, in one of the *Lives* of the saints (Nieto Ibáñez 2014: xv-xix):

> At the sixth hour of night, the angel Raphael appeared and told them: «Go to the church of the holy martyr cenobiarch, where there is a dead man. Take him to the tomb, as he has been dead for four days. Take his right foot and place it on the man who has a splinter, to thus help him» [...] He who had the splinter saw that some people had cut off his right foot and also that of the man there next to him [...] He also saw this in his dream. Damian says to Cosmas: «Brother Cosmas, I fear that the devil is deceiving us so that we might kill this man». Cosmas replies: «No, still your tongue, he was an angel of the Lord». Then, the angel of the Lord arrived and said to them: «Do as I have told you». The saints went and cut the dead man's right foot off. They also cut off, below the knee, the foot and the leg of the man who had the splinter and they placed on him the part they cut off the dead man in the name of the Father, the Son and the Holy Ghost [...] (Nieto Ibáñez 2014: 132-133).

The scene of the miracle of the leg, popularized by the *Golden Legend*, was already present in Hispanic territory in the 7th century, and its iconography was disseminated from the 14th century onwards. In the territories of the Crown of Aragon, but also in Castile to a lesser degree, the Greek version of the miracle, which makes no allusion to the donor's race, was the main source (Fracchia

2010: 131-132, 145-146; FRACCHIA 2013: 87-89).[1] It goes without saying that, in later versions, the donor's ethnicity would vary, between Moorish and Ethiopian, depending on the translations of Jacobus de Voragine's version (FRACCHIA 2010: 130). Nevertheless, in the Latin version the descriptors *Aethiops* and *Mauri* are used indistinctly, in a way that cannot be linked with a distinct Muslim identity that did not emerge until the early 7th century. Such words must be understood as a geographical designation, although at the end of the Middle Ages, and in Castile especially, their religious interpretation would gradually gain acceptance (GONZÁLEZ HERNANDO 2017). Some authors, for their part, trace the dissemination of the miracle back to the 9th century (JOVIC, THEOLOGOU 2015: 332).

## 2. *The Hispanic Genesis of a Tradition*

The oldest information regarding the Hispanic devotion to Saints Cosmas and Damian is associated with Saint Ildefonsus (607-667), a disciple of Saint Isidore and the abbot,[2] at a date close to 650, of the monastic community of Agali, located in the outskirts of Toledo, which was dedicated to Saints Cosmas and Damian. His signature as the abbot of this monastery, at the eighth and ninth Councils of Toledo, tells us of the existence of this monastic structure under this dedication, which, as far as we know, had no precedent in the ecclesiastical history of the Peninsula.[3] Ildefonso was apparently responsible for two masses composed in honour of these saints,[4] which regrettably have not

1. The image of the miracle of the black leg does not appear in the art of the Orthodox Church and, according to Jong (2013: 39), «it could hardly have appeared in the Catholic Church before *c.* 1270. The oldest known depiction of the miracle dates, in fact, from around 1300».

2. According to a tradition compiled by Nicolás Antonio: «[...] ad S. Isidorum Hispalim disciplinis omnibus instruendum remisit [...] & sub Helladio antistite monachale institutum in SS. Cosmee & Damiani monasterio, quod & Agaliense audit [...]» (1788 I: 388-410 – our citation on page 389 –).

3. This is how, in 1795, the informed pen of the Jesuit Rafael Casalbón (1785: 207) put it: «Spain too, already in this 7th century of the Church, was following the world in devotion to Saints Cosmas and Damian, and it already then had a famous monastery of this name. This is recorded in the eleventh Council of Toledo, in the year 675 [...]».

4. At least this is how it is related by their hagiographer, Cixilia, bishop of Toledo from 774 to 783, and the supposed author of *La Vita vel gesta S. Ildephonsi Sedis Toletanae Episcopi, atribuida a Cixila*, reproduced by Henrique Flórez in book V of his *España sagrada*, published with the title of *La provincia Cartaginense. Theatro geográphico-histórico de la Iglesia de España. Origen, divisiones, y límites de todas sus Provincias. Antigüedad, traslaciones, y estado antiguo, y presente de sus Sillas, en todos los Dominios de España, y Portugal. Con varias dissertaciones críticas, para ilustrar la Historia Eclesiástica de España*. «De la vida de S. Ildefonso, escrita por Cixilia, sacada del Código Emilianense, cotejada con otro de Toledo, y diversas ediciones» composes appendix VIII of its fifth book (1750 V: 501-520), in which it reads: «[...] in Ecclesia Sanctorum Cosme & Damiani, quae sita est in Suburbio Toletano, Abba praesiceretur. Ubi statim in officio clarens, duas Missas in laudem ipsorum, Dominorum suorum, quas in festivitate sua psallerent, miro modulationis modo perfecit [...]» (1750 V: 504).

survived. There is an extant Mozarabic Hispanic liturgical hymn, from those same dates in the 7th century, *Plebs Deo dicata pollens,* a cantus that has been preserved through a copy in a codex at the National Library in Madrid from between the end of the 9th century and the beginning of the 10th.[5] In the hymn, the medical aspect of the saints is made evident, and consequently that of the nature of their divine intercession.[6]

In Hispanic liturgy, the ritual of the blessing of the oils for the sick, the *unguentum*, which was undertaken during the feast of the holy Arabian physicians Cosmas and Damian, is probably Visigothic in origin.[7] Therefore, during the 7th century, shortly after it had been introduced in Rome, the Hispanic tradition of Saints Cosmas and Damian was already taking shape.[8]

The available testimonies allow us to extend their mark to not only Toledo, then the Visigothic centre of the Peninsula, but also to other localities; not for nothing, the first *Passionario Hispanico* in which the hagiography of these saints is referred to is a manuscript from the monastery of San Pedro de Cardeña,[9] in Burgos, dated to the middle years of the 10th century; and we know of their devotion in a Visigothic manuscript known as *Oracional de Verona*, dated to the turn of the 8th century –evidently prior to 711– from the Church of Tarragona, in Hispanic Catalonia.[10]

5. The cantus is included in the *Breviarium mozarabum*, a codex of 172 h. [2 columns, with 29 lines], with Visigothic-Mozarabe minuscule lettering and with musical pneumas at the start of each psalm, all of it written by the same hand, that of "Mauro p^rsro scriptor" for the "Abundantius p^br librum", bound in parchment and dated to the second half of the ninth or the first half of the 10th century. The codex, from the cathedral of Toledo, is kept in the National Library in Madrid (Mss/10001). It has been studied by, among others, Enciso 1943a: 189-211 and 1943b: 485-492.

6. The text of this hymn was established in the monumental work published by Guido María Dreves, Clemens Blume & Henry Marriot Bannister 1866-1922 (*cf.* hymn 104 "In ss. Cosmae et Damiani" in book XXVII of Blume 1897: 148-149). For its establishment both the aforementioned codex in the National Library in Madrid and the one conserved in the British Museum in London were used (Add. 30845).

7. Fábrega Grau 1953-1954 wrote about this tradition (cf. vol. 1: 213).

8. Cf. Fábrega Grau 1953-1954. (cf. vol. 1: 212-215).

9. Now conserved in the British Museum (Add. 25600), edited by Fábrega Grau 1953-1954 [volume 2] (with regard to Saints Cosmas and Damian *cf.* pp. 349-353); there is no doubt about their medical activity: «In diebus illis, sub Diocletiano et Maximiano imperatoribus sedente Lysio [preside] pro tribunali in civitae Egea, adstiterunt quidam de officio, et dixerum ei: Sunt quidam hic christiani industrii artis medicine, qui circumeuntes civitates et vicos, varios infirmos et spiritu inmundo vexatos sanant in nomine eius, qui dicitur Christus [...]».

10. Cf. the critical edition prepared by Vives (1946: 378) about the manuscript [Codex LXXXIX] conserved in the Capitular Library in Verona. Saints Cosmas and Damian have their celebration «XI kalendas novembris; its prayer is very expressive of the professional conduct of these martyrs in their lifetimes: Deus, medicina languentium, sanitas infirmorum, curator corporum, sanator providus animarum, qui beatissimos viros Cosmam et Damianum gemina medendi arte fecisti esse industrios; quo et verbo et opere humanis languoribus subvenirent, qui curatores et animarum et corporum eodem genere medendi gemino extitissent; dum et signis utraque curant, et in utrumque artificio manuum mirabiles extant; dum et mundiali arte corporibus, et caelesti medentur medicamine animabus: te quesumus, te rogamus, ut, eisdem patrocinantibus, vulneribus

From the 9th to the 14th centuries, coinciding with the Castilian resettlement of the Peninsula, a few monasteries dedicated to Saints Cosmas and Damian were built (LINAJE 1970). These are as follows: Pontacre, in the north of the present-day province of Burgos, at the beginning of the 9th century; Valderrama, in the vicinity of Frías (Burgos), which was founded around 865; Covarrubias, also in Burgos, at the start of the 10th century, associated from the last quarter of the century with the Counts of Covarrubias;[11] Cozuelos, in Palencia, in the middle of the 10th century; Congosto, in Burgos, also in the middle of the 10th century; Burbia, in the northwest of El Bierzo, near Los Ancares, recorded between 998 and 1218;[12] Abellar, in the vicinity of the city of León, founded in about 905 and active until the spring of 1120;[13] Viguera, in La Rioja on the border with Navarre, founded with certainty at the beginning of the 11th century and perhaps earlier.

Worship of the martyred physicians reached Pamplona at an early date, although it was widely spread between the 9th and 13th centuries. This period saw the dedication of the churches in Iriberri (Araguren), Cordovilla, possibly founded by Mozarabs, Astraín, dating back to the 13th century, and Ansoaín, founded in the 12th century, overlooking a small settlement. The relics of these saints were kept, along with those of many others, around the image of the Virgin in the presbytery of Pamplona Cathedral, according to a list written in 1511 (JIMENO ARANGUREN 2003: 233, 130, 142, 164, 51). We find the same dedication attached to the churches of Aspurz (1063) and Pioaona (1110), both dependent on the monastery of Leire (SERRANO LARRÁYOZ 1998: CD-Rom).

Beyond the list of specific monasteries dedicated to Saints Cosmas and Damian, we can find a rich record of toponyms that are also indicative of this same devotion, especially in Galicia and Asturias (LÓPEZ SANTOS 1952). This clearly shows the existence of strong centres that disseminated the fervour for these saints in those territories.

nostris providam medendi curam inpertias, internas externasque passiones removeas, quo, sanatis cordibus atque corporibus, dum in hac peregrinatione beneplacitam tibi persolvamus servitutem, consummatae salutis mereamur in futuro pervenire ad requiem».

11. For it, centuries later Pedro de Berruguete (1450-1504) painted the miracle of the leg transplant, in homage to its titular saints. The panel [102 x 94 cm], dated to about 1490, is now in the old collegiate church of Covarrubias; it was part of the high altarpiece of this church; we shall discuss it in greater detail below.

12. Dedicated to it are the studies by QUINTANA PRIETO 1957, UBIETO ARTETA 1959, QUINTANA PRIETO 1983 and COSMEN ALONSO 1986. Interesting facts about the history of this monastery are offered in *Códice 1195*B in the National Historical Archive (Madrid) and *Manuscrito 4357* in the National Library (Madrid).

13. Founded by the Mozarabe monk Cixila Recafredi, from Córdoba, whence he fled due to the Agarene persecution. It has been studied by: DÍAZ-JIMÉNEZ 1892; RODRÍGUEZ FERNÁNDEZ 1967; CARBAJO SERRANO 1988; CANAL SÁNCHEZ-PAGIN 1999.

### 3. *The Consolidation of the Tradition*

Devotion to Saints Cosmas and Damian spread rapidly among the population of Hispania; the arrival of some of their supposed relics from Rome helped it to grow even more. The presence, in the church of Encinacorva (Aragon), of a piece of the shoulder of Saint Cosmas, placed in a reliquary by the Grand Master of the Order of the Knights Hospitallers, fray Juan de Homedes, dates from 1545 (1477-1553).[14]

A good example of the relics of Cosmas and Damian moving around took place after Alfonso de Borja's accession to the papacy, with the name Callixtus III. In 1458 he sent a large number of relics from Rome to Valencia Cathedral, among which were those of the said saints (Martín Lloris 2010: 195). These relics are also recorded in the church of the General Hospital of Zaragoza (Carceller 1962: 22).

In 1560 Pope Pius IV granted a licence for the removal of the relics of Saints Cosmas and Damian from the Cistercian monastery of the Virgin of *Scala Dei*, outside the walls of Rome. This was done at the behest of Gaspar de Mendoza, and the relics were given to Antonio de Velasco y Zúñiga, Count of Nieva, who deposited them in the church of San Cosme y San Damián in Arnedo, in La Rioja, where they are still kept.[15]

In 1563 the Calced Mercedarian fray Gonzalo de Molina, the procurator general of his order, obtained new relics of Saints Cosmas and Damian from the Roman abbey delle Tre Fontane, with the express consent of Pope Pius IV. The relics had been requested from the Mercedarian by a brotherhood in Valladolid, created and dedicated to Saints Cosmas and Damian, that maintained a hospital and a hermitage outside the city walls.[16] In April 1602 the extramural hermitage

14. The information comes from Casalbón (1785: 186-187), who offers a small reconstruction of the route taken by the relics of these saints as they spread: «Generally it can be said that many of the relics that there are of St. Cosmas and St. Damian in Italy have been taken from Rome and Venice, and from there those that are loved in Spain have also come, such as those in the Sanctuary of S. Cosme in Guara, in the monastery of the Basilian Fathers in Madrid, and in other parts. From Bremen and Bamberg, and now from Munich, come the many that are scattered around Germany. And Luzarca has given to the particular churches of France the relics of these Saints, which worship them [...]».

15. The testimony of the Bull conserved along with the relics in the parish church of Arnedo was made in Alcalá de Henares, on 07/03/1566, is signed by the notary Martín de Frías; the relics passed, on 06/03/1566, into the hands of Sancho de Velasco –the count of Nieva's brother– so that he could take them to the town of Arnedo, of which he was the Lord (Abad León, 2005).

16. Of the presence in Valladolid and Madrid of the relics of Saint Cosmas and Saint Damian we have a detailed account by Pedro Paulin, abbot of the monastery of San Basilio in Madrid, who was responsible for looking after them (Paulin 1692: 259-315). The matter is the object of «Capítulo V. Declarase como la Religión de San Basilio Magno, en esta Provincia de Castilla, logró la fortuna de obtener las Reliquias de los gloriosos Mártyres, San Cosme, y San Damián; como fueron los monges Basilios los primeros que plantaron la devoción de estos Astros del Divino Sol en esta Coronada Villa de Madrid, y quan antigua sea esta devoción en la Religión de San Basilio"; sigue a este el "Capítulo VI. Apendix en que se refieren algunos de los muchos Milagros, que Dios ha

was ceded by royal order to the Basilian monks, who established a monastery in it dedicated to the holy healers, and the relics were moved there (BENITO 1979). A few years later the Basilian monks of the monastery of San Cosme y San Damián in Valladolid created an identically named one in Madrid, founded on 9 November 1608, where they placed some of the Saint's relics.[17] At the beginning of the 17th century, a brotherhood of surgeons and barbers was attached to the monastery in Madrid.[18] It was not unusual in Hispanic territory – and it is still common to some extent – for associations of physicians, surgeons, apothecaries and other similar professions to be set up and dedicated to these *anargyros* ("unmercenary") saints.

We have proof of the devotion to these saints in the *Ordinacions* (statutes) of the Barcelona Brotherhood of barbers, surgeons and apothecaries, already in existence in 1408 and attached to the church of Our Lady of Mount Carmel (ROMEU 1981: 107-108, 559);[19] that of barbers and surgeons in Zaragoza, created in 1455;[20] that of Saints Luke, Cosmas and Damian, of physicians, barbers and spice merchants in Huesca;[21] the Majorcan one of surgeons, named in honour of the *anargyros* saints, founded in 1489 and located in the church of the Virgin of

obrado por estos Astros del Divino Sol Encarnado, assí en el monasterio de Valladolid, del Orden de nuestro Gran Padre San Basilio, como en este Santuario del de Madrid» (PAULIN 1692: 316-364).

17. The monastery was founded, in 1608, next to the Abroñigal stream, a quarter of a league from Madrid; in February 1611 it was moved to the centre of Madrid, in a house in calle del Desengaño. Newly built in 1647 it was disentailed in 1836 and, after being used for various purposes, it was demolished in 1850.

18. Although not for long. Due to disagreements with the Basilian monks they broke away from it in the first third of the 18th century (PAULIN 1692: 259-315).

19. There is news of its public acts from 1424, the date when the dedication is present in a Corpus Christi procession, with Alfonso "the Magnanimous" in attendance; on 26 April 1458 the surgeons of the city made a solemn procession to translate the relics of these saints, from Tortosa (RIAL 1965). The Medical-pharmaceutical Brotherhood of Saints Cosmas and Damian, in Barcelona, markedly religious in nature, dates from 30 September 1884; its statutes were approved a few months later: on 12 May 1885 by the ecclesiastic authorities and on 19 June 1885 by the civil authorities. A brief reference to some Catalan brotherhoods of medieval origins, like those of Vic and Tarragona, and its corresponding bibliography, in BARCELÓ PRATS 2014: 196 (note 576). The former was re-founded in 1591. Its members were the surgeons, apothecaries, wax chandlers and shopkeepers of the town (SENA 1965: 182). The latter seems to have already been in existence in the 15th century, although we have to wait until the 16th century to find concrete references. Its statutes of 1578 served as the model for drafting those of the Brotherhood of Reus (SÁNCHEZ REAL 1976: 43-44). According to the privilege of Philip II, on 30 June 1599 the Brotherhood of Saint Cosmas and Saint Damian in Tarragona became the College of doctors, apothecaries and surgeons of Tarragona (BARCELÓ PRATS 2017: 116). With respect to the Brotherhood of the Holy Physicians of Reus it has been claimed that it could have been founded in 1471, although we have to wait until 1538 to have evidence of its functioning (VILASECA ANGUERA 1961: 164-165).

20. In 1488 the Brotherhood obtained, from King Ferdinand 'the Catholic', a privilege to examine those who wished to work in the profession (RUMEU 1981: 111, 555). On this date it is referred to as of *metges y cirujanos*, and it was also authorized to teach anatomy using human corpses (FALCÓN PÉREZ 1998: 138).

21. Under this triple dedication we know of some «Statutes of the Brotherhood and College of physicians, apothecaries and surgeons of the city of Huesca», dated in 1723, associated with the

Mercy;[22] the one in Pamplona of physicians, apothecaries, surgeons and barbers, dated from 1496 (Sánchez Álvarez 2010: 39-46); that of surgeons and barbers in Valladolid, attached to the parish church of Santiago, built on 19 September 1578 (Larruga 1787-1800. 23: 83); in Madrid the one of physicians, surgeons, bloodletters, veterinarians and barbers, with ordinances approved on 18 March 1563;[23] that of physicians and surgeons in Huesca, with ordinances of 1603, for purposes of mutual aid (Arco 1911: 199);[24] that of physicians and surgeons in Teruel, with ordinances drafted in 1634 (Javierre Mur 1950: 7-26); of physicians, surgeons and apothecaries in Burgos, founded in 1682 (López Gómez 1999); the brotherhood of bachelor surgeons in the city of Huesca, founded in 1683;[25] and that of surgeons and apothecaries in Calatayud (Folch, Eurquía 1953),[26] among others. All these examples show the establishment of this devotion among healthcare workers in Spain; although not all of these confraternities were concerned with controlling the professional aspects of their activity. Such brotherhoods, commonly known as "devotional brotherhoods", were mainly venues for the expression of religious piety

This is the case of the brotherhood of San Cosme y San Damián of Zamora, founded at the start of the 16th century and endowed with statutes in 1550. It was comprised of 100 laymen and a dozen clergymen;[27] and from the early 16th century we can document the celebration of processions, fraternal meals and devotional masses in honour of these saints. We know of their activity until the first third of the 18th century.[28] Another devotional brotherhood is the one in Arnedo of

monastery of Santo Domingo in Huesca (Vicente, 1962). The founding statutes date from the late 15th century (Pérez Galán 2009: 199).

22. A list of Spanish brotherhoods in the 15th and 16th centuries in annex III of Rumeu 1981: 541-577.

23. From the 18th century this Brotherhood was restricted to surgeons; it was initially associated with the convent of San Felipe el Real, but, from 1653, it had its own chapel in that of El Carmen Calzado. The Brotherhood combined an evident guild component with its devotional nature (Rumeu 1981: 207).

24. This Brotherhood, which also included the apothecaries, dedicated to Saints Cosmas, Damian, and Luke, was founded in 1480 (Carceller 1962: 8).

25. Its founding statutes, conserved in the Diocesan Archive of Huesca, have been studied by Abaurre 1981. Its *Libros de Estatutos y listas de cofrades* (1683, 1780, 1796), *Libro de Resoluciones de los Capítulos* (1744-1856), *Libro de Apocas* (1740), *Libro de Censales* (1694) survive, as well as a couple of *Libros de cuentas* (1682-1751; 1752-1892). The Brotherhood was active until 1892 at least, although it had been languishing since the early 19th century.

26. Its statutes, approved by the Castilian Court in 1381, were ratified by the Court of Justice of Aragon on 21 March 1631. Subsequently transformed into a professional association, they enjoyed the approval of the University of Calatayud, in 1654, and of the city itself, in 1705. This is a paradigmatic example of the transformation of an early religious group into a strictly professional one, adapting its statutes and ways of life to the changing times, maintaining in all of them the features characteristic of professional activity.

27. The number of women who were admitted to brotherhoods, either *per se* or for being members' wives, was not limited.

28. Its *Ordenanzas* of 1550, conserved in the Provincial Historical Archive of Zamora, section Protocols, have been transcribed and studied by Lorenzo 1992.

Saints Cosmas and Damian, formed through a bull issued by Pope Clement VIII (1592-1595) (Abad 2005).[29]

There is yet a third group of brotherhoods, formed by people unconnected to the healthcare professions, but whose devotional activity took the form of hospital care. This is the case of the old brotherhood in Burgos of San Cosme y San Damián, recorded between 1482 and 1740, and associated with the parish of the same name. It administered a small hospital for the poor, next to the parish church (López Martínez 1985). We find a similar case in Valladolid, with a brotherhood, active by 1563, that paid for the expenses of one of the city's hospitals (Paulin 1692: 259-315).

These three types of brotherhoods coexisted, not without difficulty, in time and space. Those created prior to the 18th century were especially common, coinciding with a period when the worship of the saints was especially intense, at least in Castile. In later periods, other forms of devotion became more prevalent, such as those dedicated to Christ and his Passion or, during the 18th century, the different devotions of the Virgin Mary (Christian 1981). Professional brotherhoods, although present on Hispanic soil in the 13th century, were banned by the monarchs of Castile in the 14th and 15th centuries; this did not happen in the Crown of Aragon, where they reached a high point in the 15th century.

Brotherhoods, either professional or devotional, experienced their particular moment of splendour after the Council of Trent (1545-1563), but they underwent an important crisis in 18th century Enlightened Spain. In the reign of Charles III, guild-based brotherhoods were affected by an intense process of reform and rationalization and, from 1783, only sacramental brotherhoods with ecclesiastical authorization were legally allowed in Spain.[30]

During the 19th century we witness a gradual deterioration in the life of pious brotherhoods, especially in the periods in which relations between Church and State were especially fraught; professional brotherhoods adapted to the new social trends, functioning more as mutual aid societies than as bodies capable of coordinating labour.[31] During the Second Spanish Republic, in reaction to the "secular atmosphere" advocated by the government, the Federación Nacional de Hermandades de San Cosme y San Damián was officially established in Madrid on 9 December 1932 (Federación Nacional de las Hermandades Médico-Farmacéuticas... 1960).[32]

29. This brotherhood survives today united to that of La Vera Cruz.

30. The decree of extinction of the brotherhoods was published on 25 June 1783 (Rumeu 1981: 387-413).

31. This is the case of the Hermandad de San Cosme y Damián founded in Madrid in 1849, whose statutes, approved at the general meeting held on 17 December of that year, define its regime of «illness, last rites and death», although they restrict its membership to «professors of medicine, surgery and pharmacy» (Hermandad de San Cosme y San Damián [Madrid] 1850).

32. These brotherhoods were recognized, as Spanish ecclesiastical associations, in 1970 (Hermandades Sanitarias... 1972).

After the end of the Spanish Civil War in 1939, public expressions of religious feeling were accentuated and new "worshipful brotherhoods" were created, including some dedicated to Saints Cosmas and Damian, in which large sectors of the population were grouped. This is the case of the brotherhoods in Abarán (Murcia) (Carrasco, Molina 1992) and Cuenca and its province (Hermandad de San Cosme y San Damián [Cuenca] 1944).[33] Others were restricted to doctors and pharmacists, despite the brotherhood's inability to interfere in professional aspects, as these brotherhoods created in Francoist Spain only functioned as "devotional brotherhoods". This is how, for example, the brotherhood of Mieres was created (Cerra 1992).[34] In general all of them were created in association with a hermitage, chapel or sanctuary dedicated to the healing saints.

The public expressions of fervour associated to these brotherhoods, of one kind or another, throughout their more than 800 years of history are made clear in the donation, for the chapel or the sanctuary to which the brotherhood was ascribed, of artistic elements in which the holy martyrs were represented.[35] This history of popular devotion has survived to the present day, as well as in these artistic manifestations, in two ways: the publication of novenas and the printing of flysheets, called *aleluyas* or *gozos*. We have a few 18th century examples of both typologies, but their high point was reached in the 19th century.[36] While the former seemed to be more common in Castile, we know of more Catalan examples of the latter.

## 4. *Medicine, Religion, Worship and Iconography*

Healing and miracles have always been closely related, and miraculous healing includes the presupposition that an illness is incurable by any earthly means.

33. A brotherhood created for religious, scientific-deontological, professional-deontological purposes and compassion «for those who profess the Catholic, Apostolic, Roman religion, and, having the legal capacity to practise medicine, pharmacy or odontology, reside in Cuenca or its Province», had its headquarters in the parish of San Esteban (Cuenca).

34. These medical-pharmaceutical brotherhoods had their periodic meetings, of which some minutes were published (Hermandades Médico-Farmacéuticas… 1960; Ibid. 1965; Ibid. 1972).

35. The iconographical representations of Saints Cosmas and Damian in Hispanic territory have been studied by, among others, Peyri 1932; Leal 1943; Jordi 1974; López Gómez 1982; López Campuzano 1996; some of them already surpassed in their interpretations. Far more complete, but with the emphasis on France, is the monograph by David-Daniel 1958.

36. Some of the flysheets printed in the 18th century contain hardly any more notes than the granting of indulgences to those who pray to the venerated images (cf. the chalcographic prayer card by Navarro (fl. 1759-1762) on the effigies of the convent of the Mercedarians in Granada, signed in 1761 [Biblioteca Nacional de Madrid (BN), inv.70377) reproduced by Manuel Jurado in 1795 [BN, inv. 70378]; the prayer card engraved by Anastasio Lleopart [Llopart] (*fl.* 1753-1791) for the monastery of San Basilio in Madrid, in 1784 [BN, inv. 14303] or the anonymous Parisian one engraved, for worship in the same monastery, in 1721 [BN, inv. 37908]); the later *gozos* usually include a prayer to the saints, adapted to local worship, with the engraving, generally with a worse line, reduced to a mere allusion identifying the dedication.

Namely, in the established pattern of a miraculous account, earthly medicine fails, is not available or is useless (KUULIALA 2020: 703). The early irruption of their worship and the miracles attributed to Cosmas and Damian have led some authors to suggest that they occupied a space that used to belong to the mythological twins and sons of Zeus, Castor and Pollux (or *Polydeukes* in Greek mythology). They have also been associated with the cult of Romulus and Remus or Jupiter Stator in Rome (BELDEKOS *et al.* 2015: 2021); a temple that, according to tradition, would have been in the Via Sacra of the Forum, close to the basilica built by Pope Felix IV.

Beyond these arguable claims, the fact is that their worship, like that of other saints, was superimposed from the 4th century onto pagan cults, in this case those typical of a religious medicine in which healing was closely linked to miracles performed through dreams, as happened at the temples of Asclepius (LÓPEZ CAMPUZANO 1996: 256). The interpretation of dreams was not just typical of religious medicine; Hippocratic-Galenic rational medicine had great respect for their therapeutic function. In a large number of sanctuaries there is evidence of the continuity of the pagan rite of *incubatio,* and in others Christian worship occupied the place of Asclepius and other deities who healed using this procedure (WALKER VADILLO 2011: 55; NIETO IBÁÑEZ 2014: xxviii-xxix).[37] Thus, arguable or not, the comparison of the Christian saints with the mythological twins and the parallels between the healing practices carried out in Greco-Roman temples and the therapeutic work of the Christian saints are obvious (NIETO IBÁÑEZ 2014: xxx).

The development of the worship of the physician saints in Europe brought with it a varied figurative representation, not just of them as individuals, but also showing some of their miraculous cures, as well as telling the story of their lives and martyrdoms. Depictions that very often, as we have already seen, were to be used by religious and professional corporations (brotherhoods and guilds of physicians, surgeons, barbers and apothecaries). In these contexts, the saints often appeared with a series of attributes that identified the professional activities of the members, who adopted them as their patron saints (figs. 1, 2). Similarly, these same attributes could also appear in votive or devotional artistic depictions unconnected with these corporations, materialized in paintings and sculptures, and in the miniatures of religious literature (figs. 3, 6), historical works (fig. 4), and medical engravings (figs. 13, 15).

The urinal, or the clear glass vessel that was used to analyse the colour, density and sediments of the sick person's urine before offering a diagnosis, was one of the identifying objects of physicians (figs. 1, 4, 5, 6, 8, 9, 12, 16, 26), as was the depiction of a book on which a prescription was written (figs. 15, 20); some consider that the book was a symbol of faith (CARMONA MUELA 2003: 91). Other habitual depictions were the medicine chest or case, with compartments in which to place medicines, and the spatula for mixing and applying medicine, which could

37. On the cult of health in Ancient Rome, see the chapter in this book by Antoni Conejo da Pena.

be contained in a jar (ointments) (figs. 1, 3, 4, 5, 8, 9, 11, 13, 15, 17, 18, 20, 21, 22, 24).[38] The rest of the elements, such as mortars, jars and other ceramic pots, mainly identify the apothecaries (figs. 6, 14), while the bag at the waist (figs. 6, 10, 14, 18, 23), a very common accessory in the clothing of the period, was used to keep the most diverse things in it, such as money, but also the instruments typical of some surgical operations, such as lancets and punches (figs. 2, 14),[39] which were used to bleed patients and were identified with surgeons and barbers. Other attributes, such as scissors, the comb and the knife were part of the iconography of barbers, who furthermore had the job of shaving and cutting hair as a practice of personal hygiene (fig. 7).[40]

The two brothers are usually depicted as beardless youths or middle-aged; they are more rarely identified with beards, although it is not exceptional. Hispanic imagery usually shows both physicians dressed in the clothes typical of the healthcare professionals of the time, although there are some exceptions in which they dress more classically, recalling the typical attire in which saints are generally shown (García Nieto, de Arana Murrio 2019: 11). Clothing typical of the late Middle Ages and the early Renaissance ranged from a loose-fitting sleeveless smock, from which the arms were removed by lifting the lower edge of the garment, combined with a collar, both of them lined with leather, to another closed, leather-lined smock, with hanging sleeves that covered the arms, called wings, with two small decorative tongues below the neckline, depicted by Jaume Huguet on the altarpiece of Saints Abdon and Sennen (c. 1460) from the church of Sant Pere in Terrassa (now kept in the church of Santa Maria, also in Terrassa). Both saints are wearing a biretta (fig. 8).

While attributed to the same painter, the depiction of the two brothers kept in the Wellcome Collection is completely different. They are both wearing a knee-length smock, open at the front and fastened with a belt. It is accompanied by a short cloak, placed over the shoulders but not fastened, and decorated with trim-

38. A case in which we can confirm the three aspects mentioned is the Navarrese altarpiece of Saint Lucy, Saint Cosmas and Saint Damian, dated to the first third of the 16th century, by the Master of Ororbia. It is now in the Museo de Bellas Artes in Bilbao: https://bit.ly/3NGLVmS (Consulted: 2 July 2022).

39. We can see another example in the panel of Saints Cosmas and Damian (*c.* 1527) by Miguel Esteve (c. 1485-1527), whose provenance is believed to have been the parish church of La Asunción de Nuestra Señora in Torrent (Valencia). Now conserved in the Serra de Alzaga Collection (Samper Embid 2015: 141).

40. After submitting the text for publication, we found, in the museum of the collegiate church of Santa María in Alquézar (Huesca), the depiction of the brothers Cosmas and Damian, each holding a book and a knife (or razor). This image, not at all usual in Hispanic iconography, appears on the predella of a lost altarpiece, which at a given moment was incorporated in another later altarpiece, in this town's chapel of Nuestra Señora de las Nieves. Due to the recent restoration of this altarpiece by the School of Restoration of Huesca, the predella is now exhibited in the said museum: https://cutt.ly/BVPyGrO (Consulted: 26 September 2022). Both saints are wearing a garment (probably a tunic) with wide sleeves, and over it a full-length smock with openings in the sides (called *maneras*) for the arms. On their heads they wear caps. The style of the clothes enables us to date the work to the second half of the 15th century. In this case, both saints are depicted as surgeons.

ming all around the edge, to match the cloak.[41] They are also wearing very tight-fitting hose with trimming below the knee and shoes. As in the previous example their heads are covered by a biretta, in this case trimmed (fig. 9).

On a panel attributed to the Castilian-Leonese school, painted circa 1460-1480 (fig. 20), the saintly physicians are wearing a full-length smock, with a small opening on the chest and others at the sides, called *maneras*, through which their arms poke out; underneath they wear clothes with tight-fitting sleeves. We can glimpse a black strap that corresponds to the collar of the jerkin. They also use a biretta, as in the previous examples.

The reinterpretation of the two physician brothers' clothes on a Valencian *socarrat* from the second half of the 15th century is exaggerated. On this occasion we see a reinterpretation of an item belonging to French fashion, the *cote-hardie*, in which sleeves fall from the elbow allowing us to see the shirt they are wearing underneath. They have been filled out quite noticeably, making them far more eye-catching than they must have been in reality (fig. 5). In fact, exaggeration was very common on this type of painted clay tiles.

It is not our aim to go into detail about these questions that fall outside our speciality, but we can observe the evolution of the clothing typical of these physicians, characterized as university doctors, from the 14th century onwards.

Another kind of garment is shown in a few paintings from earlier centuries, like the fresco in the apse of the monastery church of San Juan de la Peña (Huesca), dated from the 12th century.[42] Here Damian is wearing a long cloak, down to his ankles, with sleeves that get wider towards the cuff. The long cloak is placed over another cloak or tunic with tight-fitting sleeves. This clothing has nothing to do with the typical university attire cited above, since universities were a later development. One also must point out two works in which the saints do not appear with their heads covered, both in prayer cards depicting the miracle of the black leg. The older one is attributed to the Master of Rubió (second half of the 14th century) (fig. 29) and the more recent one was made in 1592 by Pedro de Raxis (fig. 25).

It is not always easy to identify which of the two brothers we are looking at, although when it is, Cosmas is habitually depicted with the typical instruments for examining urine,[43] while Damian is seen with a box containing medicine and

41. Surgeons are usually identified wearing short tunics, and university-trained physicians wearing long academic tunics (JONG 2013: 43). The clothing in the example referred to differs from all the other works consulted. Could the physician brothers be interpreted dressed as surgeons and with the symbols (medicine box and spatula, vessel with urine) of the physicians? It seems unlikely.

42. The depiction of the martyrdom of the saints, by an unknown painter (influence Soria-Silos) can be seen at: https://bit.ly/3I6WTkC (Consulted: 2 July 2022).

43. There are some authors who say just the opposite, claiming that Saint Damian «was the uroscopy technician, he was the 'internist', whereas Cosmas represented the other side of medicine, surgery» (GARCÍA NIETO, ARANA AMURRIO 2019: 13). This interpretation is backed up by some representations (fig. 4). A few depictions back up this opinion. Few Hispanic iconographies corroborate this option, like the late tiled depiction of Saint Damian with the urine jar in the church of Santa María in Piedraescrita (Toledo), dated to between the late 16th and the early 17th century

the spatula[44] (figs. 11, 12). Their attributes do not always provide an obvious identification. Thus, it was considered necessary to establish other forms of distinction (figs. 13, 14). Julien (1985: 48) says the following with respect to this matter:

> According to the legend, which makes no distinction between them, artists first depicted Cosmas and Damian identically as physicians with the common attribute essentially the medicine holder, indispensable for looking after patients. Then, as this was a utensil typical of the manual activity of surgeons and as these were placed systematically under the patronage of the two brothers to make surgeons as dignified as physicians, a distinction is introduced towards the end of the Middle Ages: Cosmas became more specially the university doctor, reluctant to perform manual healing, and Damian the surgeon, working with his hands and close to craftsmen; the former received as an attribute the receptacle for observing urine, the universally well-known symbol of medicine, and the latter the jar, the box or the case, often accompanied by a spatula or pincers.

The twins rarely appear identified with the palm leaf of martyrdom (fig. 14). The depiction of both saints with the cross is also infrequent. In a 15th century work by the Master of Palanquinos, now identified as Pedro de Mayorga, one of the brothers holds a book, while the other a bunch of arrows (Carmona Muela 2004: 90). The panels are exhibited in León Cathedral Museum (Ballesté Escorihuela 2019: 247).

As has already been said, the most iconic depiction of the miracles of Saints Cosmas and Damian in Hispanic imagery was undoubtedly the transplanting of the black leg of an Ethiopian/Moor (black African) onto the keeper of the basilica dedicated to both saints in Rome. Jacobus de Voragine, however, never alludes to the transplant as such but to the replacement of the sacristan's putrid flesh with the healthy flesh of a recently deceased man (David-Daniel 1958: 44).

Allusion to other miracles in Hispanic iconography, apart from those relating specifically to their martyrdom, is virtually non-existent. On at least two occasions a miracle is depicted, in which the saints bring a peasant back to life after removing a snake from his mouth that had entered it while he was asleep.[45] This

(https://bit.ly/3OOf80c) (Consulted: 10 January 2021). Along these lines there are a fair number of identifications that are not backed up by the iconographical depictions. One example can be seen in the 15th century panels attributed to the workshop of Martín Bernart or the workshop of Miguel Jiménez, which possibly belonged to an altarpiece dedicated to Saint Mary Magdalene, destined for the chapel of the same dedication in the Dominican convent in Huesca, conserved in the Museum of Huesca. The saint identified as Cosmas appears depicted with a box of ointments and its spatula, while Damian is with the glass vessel for observing urine. URL: https://bit.ly/39ZAnxy; https://bit.ly/3NskME5) (Consulted: 29 December 2021). Another example that corroborates our view is the image of Saint Cosmas on the altarpiece of Saint Lucy and Saints Cosmas and Damian, in the church of Santa María, in Ejea de los Caballeros (Zaragoza) (Bernis Madrazo 1979: 79).

44. The same attribution can be found in the woodcut engraving that depicts Saints Cosmas and Damian, by Hans Weiditz [the Younger] (*c.* 1495-*c.*1536) and conserved in the Wellcome Collection (London). URL: https://bit.ly/3Ox0wCB (Consulted: 26 December 2021).

45. Of their miraculous actions, the healing of the widow and the protection of the wife of a traveller were also quite popular (de la Vorágine, 1999 II: 615-618).

miracle was included in the *Golden Legend*, but not in the Greek texts. In these cases, the miracles are complementary parts of the main narrative:

> A husbandman resting in a field after reaping his ripe corn fell asleep with his mouth open, and as he slept a serpent entered it. When he awoke, without realizing what had happened to him he went home. That night he began to feel terrible pains, to cry out and call upon Saints Cosmas and Damian, begging them to help him. Since instead of remitting, the discomfort he felt was getting worse, he went to the church of the holy martyrs; shortly after he got there, he suddenly fell asleep and the serpent that had entered his mouth that afternoon left it (DE VORAGINE 1999 II: 617).

One of these miracles appears depicted on the far right of the predella of the altarpiece dedicated to both saints in Barcelona Cathedral, painted by Bernat Martorell and finished by his follower Miquel Nadal, dated to between 1453 and 1455 (fig. 16). In the case of the painting by Fernando del Rincón, dated to about 1510, from the convent of San Francisco in Guadalajara, the miracle is more explicitly shown. In both cases the husbandman is shown asleep, but in the depiction by Rincón the snake is shown leaving the sick man's mouth, something that is not reflected in the Catalan altarpiece (fig. 17). Fracchia (2013: 88), for his part, considers that the representation of the sleeping figure in Nadal's work is due to the Italian trend that, since the 14th century, used sleep to signify that the miracle of the leg transplant had taken place at night.[46]

The depiction of the miracle of the transplant of the cankered leg on the Catalan altarpiece, and in the terracotta sculpture by Niculoso Francisco Pisano (the modelling of the figures is by the sculptor Pedro Millán) on the doorway of the convent church of Santa Paula in Seville, made in 1504 (fig. 18), recalls the Greek version of the miracle, which does not specify the donor's skin colour.[47] Thus, the influence of the Catalan version of the miracle is felt in the image of the bleeding leg after the dissection of the sick man, in the first of the examples, and in the case (now with the black leg) of the depiction of the miracle on the predella of the altarpiece of Saints Abdon and Sennen in the church of Santa Maria in Terrassa (Barcelona), by Jaume Huguet and dated to 1459-1460 (fig. 19). This version, the oldest Catalan legend about the miracle, was one of the seven most archaic versions that were circulating in Europe[48] (FRACCHIA 2013: 88). A notable detail of this latter work is the painter's confusion when placing

46. He alludes to the panel by Mariotto di Nardo, active between 1394 and 1424, conserved in the Yale University Art Gallery in New Haven (USA), and to the painting by Fra Angelico (*c.* 1387-1455), dated to about 1434 (another dating is 1445), conserved in the Kunsthaus in Zürich (Switzerland) (FRACCHIA 2010: 146). In the last work referred to, the person asleep (or thinking, as Fracchia claims) represents a woman, not a man as in all the other examples.

47. Fracchia (2013: 88) interprets another version of the transplant in the work by a follower of Lluís Borrassà, dated sometime in the first half of the 15th century and kept in the Museo del Prado (Madrid). The current title is: *San Hipólito repone la pierna al boyero Pedro.* Nothing to do with Saints Cosmas and Damian. URL: https://bit.ly/3OC47Q0 (Consulted: 15 February 2022).

48. The depiction of the bleeding leg, the presence of surgical implements, or the help of others, is not common in Europe (JONG 2013: 43).

the legs. In the background we see the amputation of the dead black man's right leg, while in the foreground the left leg is being replaced (Jong 2013: 45).

From a chronological point of view the anonymous panel attributed to the Castilian-Leonese school, now privately owned, and dated to about 1460-1480, is the first to reflect the corpse of the black donor and to show the man who benefited from the miracle awake and having his pulse taken by the saints (fig. 20). In this work the gangrened leg is not depicted, as is the case in the examples alluded to so far, just like in the sculpture by Niculoso Francisco Pisano. From about the same time, the second half of the 15th century (dated by some to 1496) (Fracchia 2013: 88), we have the work by Pedro Berruguete (fig. 21), in the collegiate church of Saints Cosmas and Damian in Covarrubias (Burgos). Along the lines of the Castilian depictions, in this scene there is no reference to the angels that we see in the Catalan altarpieces, but it introduces the figure of the assistant and two women who are not mentioned in the Latin legend of the miracle (nor are the angels, it should be said), but who offer the work a certain degree of realism.[49] Fracchia states (2013: 80) that this painting could have been influenced by Italian artists, especially Tuscan, since their depictions of the miracle of the black leg started to gain popularity at the end of the 14th century. One example of the work of these Italian masters is the depiction of the miracle, dated to between 1370 and 1375, by the master of the Rinucini chapel (identified as Matteo di Pacino), who also includes other figures, like two women and two surgeons, one of them portrayed with scissors, who actually perform the transplant at the behest of Saints Cosmas and Damian.[50]

The depiction of the angels reappears in the work by the Master of Los Balbases, identified as Andrés Sánchez de Oña, dated to about 1495 (fig. 22), with no allusion whatsoever to the "black African" donor's corpse. Nor is there any reference to the latter in the panel kept in the hermitage of Nuestra Señora de las Vacas (Ávila), dated to the early 16th century (fig. 23). The sacristan is shown awake, an element that is not new, but the presence of another figure who has been identified as Saint Agatha is worthy of mention. Her presence does not correspond to the miracles of the holy physicians, so it has been interpreted as forming part of the donor's wishes. The donor seems to make an appearance as the smaller depiction of a woman praying, dressed in religious clothing, identified as Sor Constanza, the niece of Juan Núñez Dávila and the abbess of the convent of San Millán (Caballero Escamilla 2007: 7). The twice repeated depiction of both saints in the same scene, in the 15th century fresco in the parish church of Basconcillos de Tozo (Burgos), is strange: they appear next to the sick man and then again next to the donor (Fracchia 2013: 81) (fig. 28).

49. The depiction of the angels being associated with some literary source as yet unknown cannot be ruled out (Yarza Luaces 1994: 35).

50. Fracchia considers that those who we identify as surgeons are witnesses to the miracle (2010: 134). The image of the depiction of the miracle, whose work is kept in the North Carolina Museum of Art (Raleigh), can be consulted at: https://bit.ly/3Ic44Yw (Consulted: 7 February 2021).

During the 16th century the pictorial representation of the miracle is exemplified in the painting from the altarpiece of Bocos, commissioned by Burgos Cathedral in 1533 and painted by León Picardo (d. 1541), in which the image of the donor of the leg, shown through the amputation carried out in the cemetery by the two saints, is in the background with respect to the main scene, just as Jaume Huguet does in the middle of the 15th century (figs. 19, 24). We see a similar composition at the hands of Pedro de Raxis the Elder, who adapts Rincón's iconography, also depicting a pomegranate and the body of the Moor/Ethiopian in the foreground, in an oil painting destined for the convent of the Discalced Carmelite Martyrs in Granada.

The main novelty offered by this last work is that the donor is asleep, not dead, with the deacon's leg also grafted on (fig. 25), hence he is not covered with a shroud, as he is in the work by Fernando del Rincón (FRACCHIA 2010: 137), and in the painting by the Italian Matteo di Pacino. A restoration of the donor's body that some have wished to interpret as depicting his resurrection (FRACCHIA 2010: 137), but that also constitutes a correct assessment of the human body from an anatomical point of view (GONZÁLEZ HERNANDO 2017).

The depiction of the living donor is at its most realistic in the sculpture attributed to Isidro Villoldo, from the convent of San Francisco in Valladolid and dated to about 1539 or 1547[51] (fig. 26). Here he appears neither dead nor asleep but alive and mutilated, as in the sculptural scene from the chapel of San Gregorio in Palencia Cathedral, dated to 1533, and whose maker seems to be Juan Ortiz the Elder.[52] The depiction of the patient as being awake is not new, in this case in contrast to the figure of the donor, who has passed out due to his pain. Nor is the presence of women and servants of the saints new in the scene, as has already been seen in other examples, nor the depiction of other saints unconnected with the miracle, as in the case of Saint John the Baptist, and the praying donor of the altarpiece (fig. 27).

There is an interpretation of the evolution of the depiction of the "black African" figure in the miracle of Saints Cosmas and Damian in Spanish painting and sculpture, specifically Castilian, of the late 15th and 16th centuries. Thus, the expression of pain that gradually takes shape in some works corresponds to the image of the donor, when he is shown alive (now identified by some authors as a slave), and which for some reflects the racism existing in Castilian society, just as «the eyes of the viewers-the faithful are directed towards the pain, agony and death of their own slaves» (FRACCHIA 2010: 148), seeking to make the viewer aware of his suffering (TIELES FERRER 2014: 310).

Fracchia (2010: 131) thinks that the absence in some works of the depiction of the donor's body is curious, although it is true that it appears in the

51. By him is the design of a relief with the same subject, somewhat coarser, that is part of the choir stalls in Ávila Cathedral, dated to between 1534 and 1544 (FRACCHIA 2013: 86 and 93).

52. It has also been attributed to the French-born sculptor Felipe Vigarny (FRACCHIA 2010: 140).

great majority of them. Nevertheless, the scene of the miracle is understandable without the latter, so its omission could simply have been due to technical reasons (physical space) or artistic ones (iconographical preferences) (figs. 16, 18, 21, 22, 23, 30); to this we must add the preferences of the promotors of the works. A quite unusual example is the work by Juan Correa de Vivar, dated to 1540-1560, from the parish church of Muñoyerro (Ávila) and currently in the Museum of Navarre. The descriptions of the painting describe Saint Damian holding the sick man's thigh and Saint Cosmas blessing the black leg; both are being helped by a servant (fig. 10).

There are some iconographical elements, like the artichoke (fig. 21) or the pomegranate (figs. 17, 25), that some authors identify as symbols of the Hebrew and Muslim minorities, in the case of the artichoke (Ramos de Castro 2004: 85), while the pomegranate represents the heraldic device of the city of Granada and its conquest, even though it appears at dates as late as in those in the work by Pedro de Raxis. It is interpreted as «a connection between the legend of the healer saints and the violent repossession and Christianization of Granada» (Fracchia 2010: 136). Nevertheless, the pomegranate, besides possessing an important symbolic charge linked to the immortality of the soul, had numerous medicinal properties (Olivares Martínez 2017) that are not out of place, despite not being habitual, in the depiction of Saints Cosmas and Damian. Nor is it necessary to complicate the issue, since it could simply be a decorative element. Indeed, a sort of pumpkin or melon is also included in the work by Fernando del Rincón without any symbolism having been attributed to it. The same could be said of the miracle as depicted by León Picardo in which, on the window ledge, from where we observe the amputation of the leg of the "black African" donor, there is a sort of apple on a small plate (fig. 24). Equally mysterious is the symbolism of the flower (or plant) next to the sacristan – lilies? – and the flower next to the donor's corpse in the work by Rincón (González Hernando 2017).

If it is not easy to identify Saints Cosmas and Damian by the attributes assigned to them in the works where they are depicted singly or together, the same happens when trying to recognize them in the scene of the miracle. Neither the Greek nor the golden legend singles them out doing specific tasks during the miracle. Only in the Castilian depiction from the hermitage of Nuestra Señora de las Vacas is Cosmas identified as the saint who is grafting the leg on to the sick man, while his brother Damian, who is not identified as such, holds the gangrened leg in his hands (fig. 23). If we take the identification of Cosmas to be the holy physician who is doing the graft, due to him being depicted placing the leg on the sick man, his brother Damian would be personified with a medicine box or jar and a spatula for spreading ointments. Nevertheless, in the sculpture attributed to Isidro Villoldo, Damian is usually identified observing a jar of urine and taking the sacristan's pulse (fig. 26). A depiction, the taking of the pulse, that also appears in another panel, but in this case associated with Saint Cosmas (portrayed with an open book), while Damian appears with the classic medicine box and a spatula (fig. 20). Another identification of Cosmas as the author of the graft and Damian with a jar – of urine? – appears on the altarpiece dedicated to both of them in the church of San Pedro in Teruel, by the Frenchman Gabriel Joly, dated before 11 October 1537 (Arce Oliva 1995: 385) (fig. 30).

On other occasions, as in the abovementioned panel by Jaume Huguet from Terrassa, both physicians are concentrating on attaching the sacristan's leg, while it is two angels on the left of each saint who hold elements typical of surgical practice and the repetitive pot or box of ointments (fig. 19). This difficulty with identification also arises in the work by Pedro de Raxis, in which the saints handle the sick man's leg with no elements to characterize them (fig. 25). We have to say that in the individual depiction of the saints there is no defined iconographical pattern. In fact, López Campuzano (1996: 265) interprets that, in the work attributed to Fernando del Rincón, Saint Cosmas is standing, holding a box and a spatula, while Saint Damian is holding the transplanted leg.

## 5. *Corollary*

In the late 18th century, the Jesuit Rafael Casalbón (1729-1787), then in charge of the Library in the Royal Palace in Madrid, wrote:

> There can hardly be a kingdom or province in all Christendom that has not at one time or another experienced, in plagues and all sorts of ailments, the powerful intercession of these Holy Physicians; nor can there be any that in thanks has not built churches to them, where they may go as to the health office, and as an asylum against all disease [...] (Casalbón 1785: 207).

These words appear in a work dedicated to clarifying the "authentic" biographies of Saints Cosmas and Damian. The reasons that motivated this learned Jesuit to work on these hagiographies are strictly personal, as he was a faithful devotee of the monastery of Guara, in the mountains in Huesca of the same name, dedicated to venerating these saints.[53] During the 18th century 14 nearby villages went on processions to this sanctuary, returning also in procession, af-

53. «Los muchos beneficios recibidos de Dios por la intercesión de los gloriosos mártires de Christo San Cosme y Damián, venerados en la Sierra de Guara, que afuer de agradecido me han obligado a no excusarme como hubiera querido de esta obra, me fuerzan también a consagrársela toda como es justo, y á poner enteramente baxo su amparo este mi pequeño trabajo» (Casalbón 1785: [I-II]). The people of Huesca founded a brotherhood under the patronage of these saints in this Sanctuary, on 27/09/1396, with the permission of don Martín, king of Aragon; centuries later, Pope Clement X granted, through a Breve given in Rome, on 18/12/1672, the Apostolic graces. The monastery is now abandoned and in ruins. The primitive carvings of the patron saints, done, in the opinion of Rafael Casalbón, in cherry wood by craftsmen in the 11th century, and various paintings on copper, disappeared after the war of 1936-1939.

ter hearing the corresponding masses and sermons. The monastery was famous as a place of miraculous cures.[54]

And it was not the only one. Scattered all over Spain there are places in which the feast day of Saints Cosmas and Damian is celebrated with pilgrimages and processions, popular in nature and very old.

In Alberite (La Rioja) there is a communal meal in the village square in homage to the saints, who are taken out in procession; at it the people eat *bacochas*, pinto beans that are typical of the area. In the past, on the eve of the saints' feast day, the young people "stole" the *bacochas* from the fields in order to eat them afterwards in the *peñas* (clubs). The tradition of the theft has now been lost, but not the meal, which is still held, and all the local people take part in preparing it.

In Parres (Asturias), devotion to these saints goes back a very long way; Octavio Bellmunt (1900: 476) pointed out, at the end of the 19th century, that «in the festival of the Patron Saint and on other days there are many *ofrecidos* with a headache. The patients go up the belltower, put their heads inside the bell and give themselves a single knock with the clapper». The primitive church of Saint Cosmas, next to the parish cemetery, was burned down during the Spanish Civil War (1936-1939); the bell, dated 1630, was salvaged, and is now in the new church built in 1952.

In the vicinity of Mieres (Asturias), in the sanctuary located in the Cuna valley, after the solemn mass held on the saints' feast day, there is the *puya del ramu*, an auction of spelt loaves, followed by a traditional meal accompanied by sweet cider, and ending with some folk songs like this one, in which the intervention of the saints is requested to resolve sentimental matters: «Martyrs of Valdecuna / if you are saints and physicians / say, for a broken heart / do you not know any recipes?» (Cerra 1992: 60).[55]

Those interested in returning to good health follow an age-old rite in front of the figures of Saints Cosmas and Damian in the Sanctuary of Valdecuna; tradition dictates that a handkerchief that has previously been in contact with the sick person, or the aching limb, must be passed over the saints; when the handkerchief, now impregnated by the saints, is returned to the sick person, they will be cured (Brenes 1988). In this rite the Christianization of the magical healing practices is obvious, produced by sympathy of contact, a practice that was very much alive in archaic cultures.

54. In the same vein our Jesuit points out: «[…] los prodigios muy freqüentes que Dios se ha servido obrar en él […] que apenas se entrará en lugar alguno [de Aragón], en que no se halle quien cuente algún mal que por su intercesión de estos Santos en dicha Casa fue libre, y no acuerde así la memoria y excite la devoción […]» (Casalbón 1785: [V-VI]).

55. Saints Cosmas and Damian are the titular saints of at least ten parishes in Asturias: Bobes (Siero), Estacas (Belmonte), Rañeces (Grado), Tolinas (Grado), Villacondide (Coaña), Corias (Pravia), Llerandi (Arriendas), Villarmental (Cangas del Narcea), Nargenes (Peñamellera) and Tornón (Villaviciosa); in the villages of Rales, Tiñana de Laviana, Narciandi de Cangas de Onís and Tineo the patron saint's festivities are dedicated to them (Cerra 1992: 46).

In Abarán (Murcia) (CARRASCO, MOLINA 1992), Alberite de San Juan (Zaragoza), Covarrubias (Burgos), Gordexola (Basque Country), Poza de la Sal (Burgos), Rasines (Cantabria), Portillo de Toledo (Toledo), Narganes (Asturias), Palanques (Castellón), Torredonjimeno (Jaén), Aras de Alpuente (Valencia) (MARQUET 1975),[56] Almargen (Malaga) and Varea (La Rioja), the festivals, deeply rooted in history, combine religious fervour with the ludic aspect of popular pilgrimages. The religious part of the festival usually begins nine days before the big day, with a novena, and ends with a public procession of the images on their feast day. The popular part of the festival is celebrated on the big day, 27 September (according to the old Roman calendar), with traditional dances and country food in the fields around the hermitages that are dedicated to the "unmercenary" saints.

The festivals in Arnedo (La Rioja), celebrated since the middle of the 16th century, are particularly interesting.[57] They include a ritualized fight between the people of La Rioja and their neighbours from Navarre, both eager to possess the images-relics of the saints taken out in a procession. In specially designated places there are three attempted thefts. A town crier from Navarre shouts at the Riojans; he rebukes them for treating the saints badly and asks them to peacefully let them go to Navarre. The people of Arnedo refuse, and the town crier turns to the Navarrese, saying: «Navarrese, take the saints, and, to Navarre with them!» They then begin a race in the direction of Navarre but, a few metres farther on, they are stopped by the people of Arnedo and forced to go back to the procession; there is one last attempt at the doorway of the saints' church, with the same result. The procession ends with a solemn mass in the church of San Cosme y San Damián.

Spanish popular religiosity, since the 18th century in particular, has some special characteristics: it is collective, massive and usually takes place in public places; religious worship comes out of the churches, makes the public space sacred and externalizes devotion; these expressions of religion are also aesthetic manifestations and moments of playful expansion.[58] As in so many other popular expressions, the important thing is the ritual, the strength of the collective imaginary, the shared myth. The survival, throughout time, of the age-old traditions that, for more than three centuries, have connected the land, villages and people of Spain to Saints Cosmas and Damian.

56. The author mentions the local tradition that acknowledges them as «saints of the stone», protectors against hail, in memory of their martyrdom.

57. By Resolution of 27 October 2003, of the Councillor for Tourism, Environment and Territorial Policy of La Rioja, the festivities in honour of Saint Cosmas and Saint Damian in the locality of Arnedo are declared to be a festivity of regional touristic interest (*Boletín Oficial de la Rioja* 01/11/2003).

58. An opinion shared by those who have studied, in detail, the phenomenon of brotherhoods in Spain; among others, LÓPEZ MUÑOZ 1992: 19, Ibid. 1994 and SABE 2000: 16.

## *Bibliography*


Abad León, Felipe, 2005. "Las reliquias de los Santos Cosme y Damián, de San Jorge y otros santos", *A la sombra de su viejo Castillo. 25 temas de Arnedo,* Logroño, Ochoa: 173-182.

Abaurre Valencia, Miren-Maite, 1981. "Los estatutos de la cofradía de mancebos cirujanos de la ciudad de Huesca, fundada en 1683 bajo la advocación de los Santos Cosme y Damián", *Argensola. Revista del Instituto de Estudios Altoaragoneses*, 23/91, 115-122.

Antonio, Nicolás, 1788. *Bibliotheca Hispana Vetus,* vol. 1, Matriti, Viduam et heredes D. Iachimi Ibarrae.

Arce Oliva, Ernesto, 1995. "Una obra desconocida del taller de Gabriel Joly: las imágenes de los Santos Cosme y Damián en la iglesia de San Pedro de Teruel", *Artigrama*, 11: 381-388.

Arco, Ricardo del, 1911. *Antiguos gremios de Huesca*, Zaragoza, Tip. de P. Larra (Colección de documentos para la Historia de Aragón, 6).

Ballesté Escorihuela, Marc, 2019. "Tablas de nuevos maestros castellanos anteriormente atribuidas al maestro de Palanquinos (h. 1480-1500)", *Archivo Español de Arte,* 92/367: 245-260.

Barceló Prats, Josep, 2014. *Poder local, govern i assistència pública: el cas de Tarragona,* PhD tesis, Tarragona, Universitat Rovira i Virgili.

Barceló Prats, Josep, 2017. *Poder local, govern i assistència pública: l'Hospital de Sant Pau i Santa Tecla de Tarragona,* Tarragona, Arola.

Beldekos, Dimitris; Karamanou, Marianna; Poulakou-Rebelakou, Effie; Ploumpidis, Dimitris; Androutsos, George, 2015. "The Medical Vestments and Surgical Instruments of Saint Cosmas and Damian on Sinai Icons from the Seventh to the Eighteenth Century", *Journal of Religion and Health,* 54/6: 2020-2032.

Bellmunt Traver, Octavio, 1900. "Parres". Octavio Bellmunt Traver, Fermín Canella Secades, *Asturias,* vol. 3, Gijón, O. Bellmunt: 475-478.

Benito y Durán, Ángel, 1979. "Monasterio de San Cosme y San Damián de monjes basilios (Valladolid)", *Hispania Sacra*, 31/32: 201-283.

Bernis Madrazo, Carmen, 1979. *Trajes y modas en la España de los Reyes Católicos: II. Los hombres,* Madrid, Instituto Diego Velázquez (CSIC).

Blume, Clemens, 1897. *Hymnodia Godica. Die Mozarabischen Minen des alt-spanischen Ritus,* Leipzig, O. R. Reisland.

Brenes González, Rubén, 1998. "Cultura y sanación: San Cosme y San Damián", *Magister. Revista de la Escuela Universitaria de Magisterio de Oviedo*, 16: 9-25.

Brugeat, Celine, 2014. "The St. Cosmas and St. Damian capital: A Pyrenean sculpture at the Walters Art Museum", *The Journal of the Walters Art Museum,* 72: 43-53.

Bucci, Agapito, 2016. *I santi medici Cosma e Damiano,* Rome, Armando.

Carbajo Serrano, María J., 1988. "El monasterio de los Santos Cosme y Damián de Abellar", *Archivos Leoneses*, 81/82: 7-300.

Carceller, Mariano V., 1962. *Las Hermandades de Médicos y Farmacéuticos de San Cosme y San Damián en Aragón,* Valencia, Laboratorios Clariana.

Carrasco Molina, José; Molina Templado, José David, 1992. *Los santos médicos en Abarán. Arraigo de una devoción*, Abarán, Gráf. Templado.

Casalbón, Rafael, 1785. *Actas de S. Cosme y S. Damián, médicos árabes; y pruebas de la inverisimilitud con que se ha pretendido introducir otros santos con este nombre,* Madrid, Imprenta Real.

Caballero Escamilla, Sonia, 2007. "Nuevos descubrimientos en la Ermita de Nuestra Señora de las Vacas en Ávila: una talla Románica y la tabla de los Saints Cosmas and Damian", *Akobe,* 8: 4-8.

Canal Sánchez-Pagin, José M., 1999. "El monasterio de San Cosme y San Damián de Abellar. Su situación y entorno", *Studium Legionense,* 40: 305-320.

Carmona Muela, Juan, 2003. *Iconografía de los santos,* Madrid, Istmo.

Cerra Suárez, Silverio, 1992. *San Cosme y San Damián, Mártires de Cuna.* Valdecuna, Iglesia Parroquial de Santa María de Valdecuna.

CHRISTIAN Jr., William A., 1981. *Local Religion in Sixteenth-Century Spain,* Princeton, Princeton University Press.

COSMEN ALONSO, María C., 1986. "Los restos arquitectónicos de San Cosme y San Damián del Burbia (León)", *Estudios Humanísticos. Geografía, Historia y Arte*, 8: 201-209.

DAVID-DANEL, Marie-Louise, 1958. *Iconographie des Saints médecins Côme et Damien,* Lille, Imp. Morel & Corduant.

DE LA VORÁGINE, Santiago, 1999. *La leyenda dorada,* vol. 2, Madrid, Alianza.

DÍAZ-JIMÉNEZ, Juan Eloy, 1892. "Inmigración mozárabe en el Reino de León. El monasterio de Abellar o de los santos mártires Cosme y Damián", *Boletín de la Real Academia de la Historia*, 20: 123-151.

DREVES, Guido M.; BLUME, Clemens; BANNISTER, Henry M., 1866-1922. *Analecta Hymnica Medii Aevi,* Leipzig, Altenburg Stephan Geibe & Co. Fries, 55 books in 16 vols.

ENCISO, Jesús, 1943a. "Breviario mozárabe de la Biblioteca Nacional", *Estudios Bíblicos,* 2: 189-211.

ENCISO, Jesús 1943b. "El autor del prólogo en verso de los Himnos Mozárabes", *Revista Española de Teología,* 3: 485-492.

FÁBREGA GRAU, Ángel, 1953-1954. *Pasionario hispánico (siglos VII-XI),* Madrid, [Instituto de Historia Eclesiástica "Padre Enrique Flórez"], 2 vols.

FALCÓN, Isabel, 1998. "Aprovisionamiento y sanidad en Zaragoza en el siglo XV", *Acta Historica et Archaeologica Mediaevalia*, 19: 127-144.

FEDERACIÓN NACIONAL DE LAS HERMANDADES MÉDICO-FARMACÉUTICAS DE SAN COSME Y SAN DAMIÁN, 1960. *Actas de las sesiones de la X Asamblea Nacional de Hermandades de San Cosme y San Damián celebrada en Jerez de la Frontera (Cádiz), octubre 1959,* Jerez de la Frontera, Tipo-litografía Jerez Gráfico.

FESTUGIÈRE, André-Jean (trad.), 1971. *Saint Thècle. Saints Côme et Damien. Saints Cyr et Jean (extraits). Saint Georges,* Paris, Picard.

FLÓREZ, Henrique, 1750. *España sagrada*, published as *La provincia Cartaginense. Theatro geográphico-histórico de la Iglesia de España. Origen, divisiones, y límites de todas sus Provincias. Antigüedad, traslaciones, y estado antiguo, y presente de sus Sillas, en todos los Dominios de España, y Portugal. Con varias dissertaciones críticas, para ilustrar la Historia Eclesiástica de España,* vol. 5, Madrid, Antonio Marín.

FOLCH JOU, Guillermo; EURQUÍA MALO, Leopoldo de, 1953. "El Colegio de San Cosme y San Damián de médicos, cirujanos y boticarios de Calatayud", *Archivos Iberoamericanos de Historia de la Medicina*, 5/1: 215-227.

FRACCHIA, Carmen, 2010. "El esclavo negroafricano en las imágenes españolas de los santos Cosme y Damián", Aurelia Martín Casares, Margarita García Barranco (ed.), *La esclavitud negroafricana en la historia de España. Siglos XVI y XVII,* Granada, Comares: 127-149.

FRACCHIA, Carmen, 2013. "Spanish depictions of the Miracle of the Black Leg", Kees Wouter Zimmerman (ed.), *One Leg in the Grave Revisited. The Miracle of the Transplantation of the Black Leg by the Saints Cosmas and Damian,* Groningen, Barkhuis: 79-91.

GARCÍA NIETO, Víctor; ARANA AMURRIO, José I. de, 2019. "La uroscopia en España. A propósito de una imagen custodiada en el monasterio de Santa María de la Vid de Burgos", *Cuadernos de Historia de la Pediatría Española,* 17: 5-15.

GONZÁLEZ HERNANDO, Irene, 2017. *Conferencia: El Milagro de los santos Cosme y Damián, de Fernando del Rincón* [Video]. YouTube: https://www.youtube.com/watch?v=4GcD3hL3wQA (Consulted: 17 February 2022).

HERMANDAD DE SAN COSME Y SAN DAMIÁN [Cuenca], 1944. *Estatutos de la Hermandad de S. Cosme y S. Damián y su provincial*, Cuenca, [Imp. Moderna].

HERMANDAD DE SAN COSME Y SAN DAMIÁN [Madrid], 1850. *Reglamento para el gobierno y régimen de la Hermandad de S. Cosme y S. Damián, aprobado en Junta general de 17 de Noviembre de 1849*, Madrid, Vázquez Martínez e hijos.

HERMANDADES SANITARIAS DE SAN COSME Y SAN DAMIÁN, 1960. *Actas de las sesiones de la X Asamblea Nacional de Hermandades de San Cosme y San Damián celebrada en Jerez de la Frontera (Cádiz), octubre 1959*, Jerez de la Frontera, Tipo-Litografía Jerez Gráfico.

HERMANDADES SANITARIAS DE SAN COSME Y SAN DAMIÁN, 1965. *Actas del XIII Congreso Nacional de las Hermandades Medico-Farmacéuticas de San Cosme y San Damián, Alicante, octubre 1965,* Alicante, [s.n.]

HERMANDADES SANITARIAS DE SAN COSME Y SAN DAMIÁN, 1972. *Actas XV Congreso Nacional de Hermandades Sanitarias de San Cosme y San Damián*, Bilbao, Imprenta Marín.

JAVIERRE MUR, Aurea L., 1959. "Ordenanzas de la Cofradía de San Cosme y San Damián de médicos y cirujanos de la ciudad de Teruel", *Teruel*, 3: 7-26.

JIMENO ARANGUREN, Roldán, 2003. *El culto a los santos en la Cuenca de Pamplona (siglos V-XVI). Estratigrafía hagionímica de los espacios sagrados urbanos y rurales,* Pamplona, Gobierno de Navarra.

JONG, Jan L. de, 2013. "Transplantation and Salvation", Kees Wouter Zimmerman (ed.), *One Leg in the Grave Revisited. The Miracle of the Transplantation of the Black Leg by the Saints Cosmas and Damian,* Groningen, Barkhuis: 37-49.

JORDI GONZÁLEZ, Ramón, 1974. *Iconografía de los santos Cosme y Damián,* Barcelona, Colegio Oficial de Farmacéuticos de la Provincia de Barcelona.

JOVIĆ, Nebojša J.; THEOLOGOU, Marios, 2015. "The Miracle of the Black Leg: Eastern Neglect of Western Addition to the Hagiography of Saints Cosmas and Damian", *Acta Medica Historica Adriatica,* 13/2: 329-344.

JULIEN, Pierre, 1985. "Côme et Damien hier et aujourd'hui. Quelques questions", Pierre Julien, François Ledermann (ed.), *Saint Côme et saint Damien. Culte et iconographie / Die Heiligen Kosmas und Damian. Kult und Ikonographie / I Santi Cosma e Damiano. Culto e iconografia. Colloque / Kolloquium / Colloquio, Mendrisio 29-30 IX 1985,* Bern, Societé Suisse d'Histoire de la Pharmacie: 43-62.

KUULIALA, Jenni, 2020. "The Saint as Medicator: Medicine and the Miraculous in Fifteenth- and Sixteenth-Century Italy", *Social History of Medicine,* 34/3: 703-722.

LARRUGA, Eugenio, 1787-1800. *Memorias políticas y económicas sobre los frutos, comercios, fábricas y minas de España,* Madrid, Imprenta de Benito Cano, 45 vols.

LEAL, F., 1943, "San Cosme y San Damián en la hagiografía y en el arte", *El Monitor de la Farmacia y de la Terapéutica*, 49/1320: 193-200.

LINAJE CONDE, Antonio, 1970. "Monasterios altomedievales españoles de los santos Cosme y Damián", *Cuadernos de Historia de la Medicina Española*, 9: 15-74.

LÓPEZ CAMPUZANO, Julia, 1996. "Iconografía de los santos sanadores (II): san Cosme y san Damián", *Anales de Historia del Arte,* 6: 255-266.

LÓPEZ GÓMEZ, José Manuel, 1999. *Religiosidad y profesiones sanitarias en el Burgos del XVIII. La cofradía de San Cosme y San Damián y los médicos, cirujanos y boticarios burgaleses del primer cuarto del siglo XVIII*, Burgos, Hermandad Médico-Farmacéutica de San Cosme y San Damián.

LÓPEZ GÓMEZ, José Manuel, 1982. "Catálogo iconográfico de San Cosme y San Damián en la provincia de Burgos", *Minutos Menarini*, 14/112: 3-12, 22-23.

LÓPEZ MARTÍNEZ, Nicolás, 1985. "Regla de la hermandad médico-farmacéutica de San Cosme y San Damián", *Burgense*, 26/1: 273-293.

LÓPEZ MUÑOZ, Miguel Luis, 1992. *Las cofradías de la parroquia de Santa María Magdalena en Granada en los siglos XVII y XVIII*, Granada, Universidad de Granada.

LÓPEZ MUÑOZ, Miguel Luis, 1994. *La labor benéfico-social de las cofradías en la Granada moderna*, Granada, Universidad de Granada.

LÓPEZ SANTOS, Luis, 1952. *Influjo de la vida cristiana en los nombres de los pueblos españoles,* León, Centro de Estudios e Investigaciones de San Isidoro.

LORENZO PINAR, Francisco Javier, 1992. "La cofradía zamorana de San Cosme y San Damián. Ordenanzas de 1550", *Anuario Instituto de Estudios Zamoranos "Florián de Ocampo"*, 9: 565-579.

MARQUET, Louis, 1975. "Iconographie et culte des saints Côme et Damien", *Revue d'Histoire de la Pharmacie*, 63/224: 366.

MARTÍN LLORIS, Catalina, 2010. *Las reliquias de la capilla real en la Corona de Aragón y el santo cáliz de la catedral de Valencia (1396-1458),* PhD Thesis, Valencia, Universitat de València.

MATTHEWS, Leslie G., 1968. "SS Cosmas and Damian-Patron Saints of Medicine and Pharmacy: Their Cult in England", *Medical History,* 12/3: 281-288.

NIETO IBÁÑEZ, Jesús María, 2014. *San Cosme y san Damián: vida y milagros,* Madrid, Biblioteca de Artistes Cristianos & Universidad de León.

OLIVARES MARTÍNEZ, Diana, 2017. "Granada", *Base de datos digital de Iconografía Medieval.* Universidad Complutense de Madrid, https://www.ucm.es/bdiconografiamedieval/granada [consulted: 26 March 2022].

PAULIN, Pedro, 1692. *Los astros del divino sol encarnado, S. Cosme y S. Damián. Esclarecidos médicos, ínclitos mártyres de Jesucristo, que con sus heroycas virtudes luzieron en el Cielo de la Iglesia, para comunicar incendios de amor Divino a los hombres en la tierra. Su vida, milagros, y elogios, ponderados con algunos pensamientos; glosados los renombres con que los engrandecieron sus Panegiristas,* Madrid, Melchor Álvarez.

PÉREZ GALÁN, Cristina, 2009. "La Cofradía de médicos, cirujanos y boticarios de Huesca: un ejemplo de compromiso social con la pobreza", *Aragón en la Edad Media,* 21: 197-220.

PEYRI, Jaume, 1932. *Iconografia d'uns Metges Anargirs: Sant Cosme i Sant Damià* [Discurs inaugural de l'any acadèmic 1931-1932 a la Societat Mèdico-Farmaceutica dels Sants Cosme i Damià], Barcelona, Tip. Occitania.

QUINTANA PRIETO, Augusto, 1957. "Tebaida Berciana. San Cosme y San Damián del Burbia", *Archivos Leoneses,* 22: 77-109.

QUINTANA PRIETO, Augusto, 1983. "San Cosme y San Damián del Burbia", *Temas Bercianos,* 2: 149-153.

RAMOS DE CASTRO, Guadalupe, 2004. "Notas documentales y aspectos judíos e islámicos en Pedro Berruguete y su hijo Alonso Berruguete", Mª P. Silva Maroto (ed.), *Actas del simposium internacional Pedro Berruguete y su entorno, Palencia, 24-26 abril de 2003,* Palencia, Diputación de Palencia: 79-88.

RIAL, Juan, 1965. *Historia de la hermandad médico-farmacéutica de San Cosme y San Damián de Barcelona,* [Barcelona, Tip. Ars].

RODRÍGUEZ FERNÁNDEZ, Justiano, 1967. "En torno al desaparecido monasterio de Abellar", *Studium Legionense,* 8: 297-304.

RUMEU DE ARMAS, Antonio, 1981. *Historia de la Previsión Social en España. Cofradías, Gremios, Hermandades, Montepíos,* Barcelona, El Albir.

SABE ANDREU, Ana María, 2000. *Las cofradías en Ávila en la Edad Moderna,* Ávila, Institución Gran Duque de Alba.

SAMPER EMBIZ, Vicente, 2015. *Miguel Esteve (Xàtiva, h. 1485-Valencia, 1527) y algunas consideraciones más sobre la pintura valenciana de su época,* PhD Thesis, Valencia, Universitat de València.

SÁNCHEZ, Andrea, 2020. "La Unió de l'Art i la Ciència a la Col·lecció Pérez-Rosales", *Museus de Sitges: el Blog,* https://bit.ly/3QUdD2p [consulted: 30 June 30 2022].

SÁNCHEZ ÁLVAREZ, Julio, 2010. *El Protomedicato navarro y las cofradías sanitarias de San Cosme y San Damián. El control social de las profesiones sanitarias en Navarra (1496-1829),* Pamplona, Gobierno de Navarra.

SÁNCHEZ REAL, José, 1976. *Los médicos de Tarragona: siglos XIV-XVII,* Tarragona, Diputació Provincial de Tarragona.

SENA, Federico, 1965. "La pequeña historia de la Cofradía de San Cosme y San Damián", *Ausa,* 5/51: 181-191.

SERRANO LARRÁYOZ, Fernando, 1998. "El culto a los santos en Navarra (siglos XI-XIII)", *III Congreso General de Historia de Navarra, Pamplona, 20 al 23 septiembre de 1994,* Pamplona, Gobierno de Navarra: edition on CD ROM.

TIELES FERRER, Cecilio, 2014. "La imatge dels sants Cosme i Damià, reflex de les relacions entre la población negroafricana i la societat hispana entre els segles XVI-XVII", *Podall,* 4: 301-317.

Ubieto Arteta, Antonio, 1959. “Dos observaciones al abadologio de San Cosme y San Damián de Burbia”, *Archivos Leoneses*, 13: 163-165.

Vicente Carceller, Mariano, 1962. *Medicina. Una faceta de su historia. Las hermandades de médicos y farmacéuticos de San Cosme y San Damián en Aragón,* [Valencia, Laboratorios Clariana].

Vilaseca Anguera, Salvador, 1961. *Metges, cirurgians i apotecaris reusencs dels segles XIII-XVI. La Confraria dels Sants Metges, de Reus,* Reus, Asociación de Estudios Reusenses.

Vives, José (ed.), 1946. *Oracional visigótico* [estudio paleográfico de Jerónimo Claveras], Barcelona [San Feliú de Guíxols, J.M. Viader].

Walker Vadillo, Mónica Ann, 2011. “Los santos médicos Cosme y Damián”, *Revista Digital de Iconografía Medieval,* 3/5: 51-60.

Yarza Luaces, Joaquín, 1994. “Jaume Huguet i el retaule dels sants Abdó i Senén”, *Terme,* 9: 25-38.

Zimmerman, Kees W. (ed.), 2013. *One Leg in the Grave Revisited. The Miracle of the Transplantation of the Black Leg by the Saints Cosmas and Damian,* Groningen, Barkhuis.

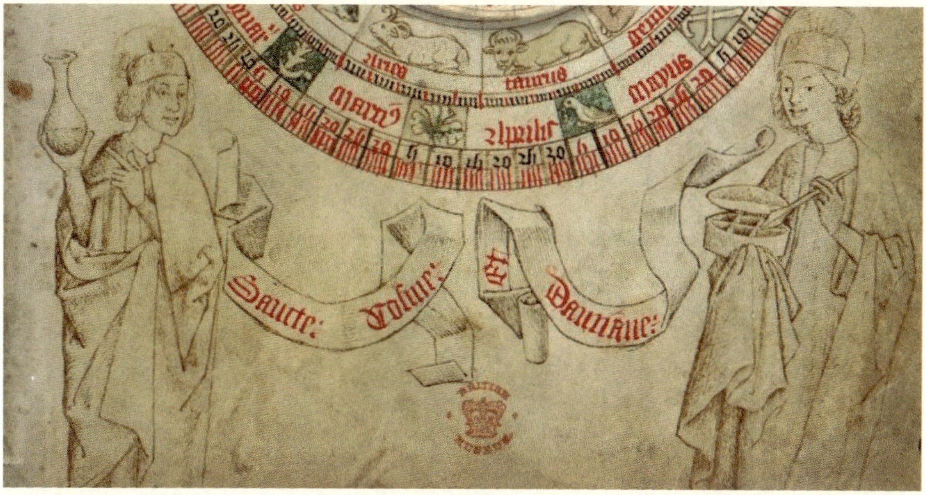

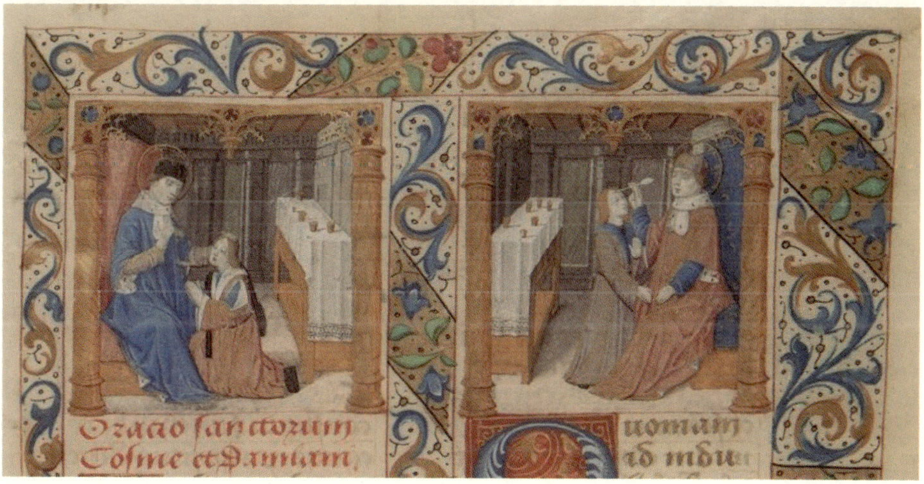

Fig. 1. "Saints Cosmas and Damian", detail. *Guild Book of the Barber Surgeons of York*, c.1486? (London. British Library, Egerton MS 2572, fol. 51r). Image obtained from https.//bit.ly/3HZIshY.
Fig. 2. "Saints Cosmas and Damian treating a patient (and trepanning)". *Statuts de la Confrèrie Saint-Côme-et-Saint-Damien* (of barber-surgeons) *de Paris* (page one of an illuminated manuscript, page from a 15th century missal), c. 1300-1400 (Paris. Musée Carnavalet - Histoire de Paris). Image obtained from https.//bit.ly/3Oz5izM / License CC0.

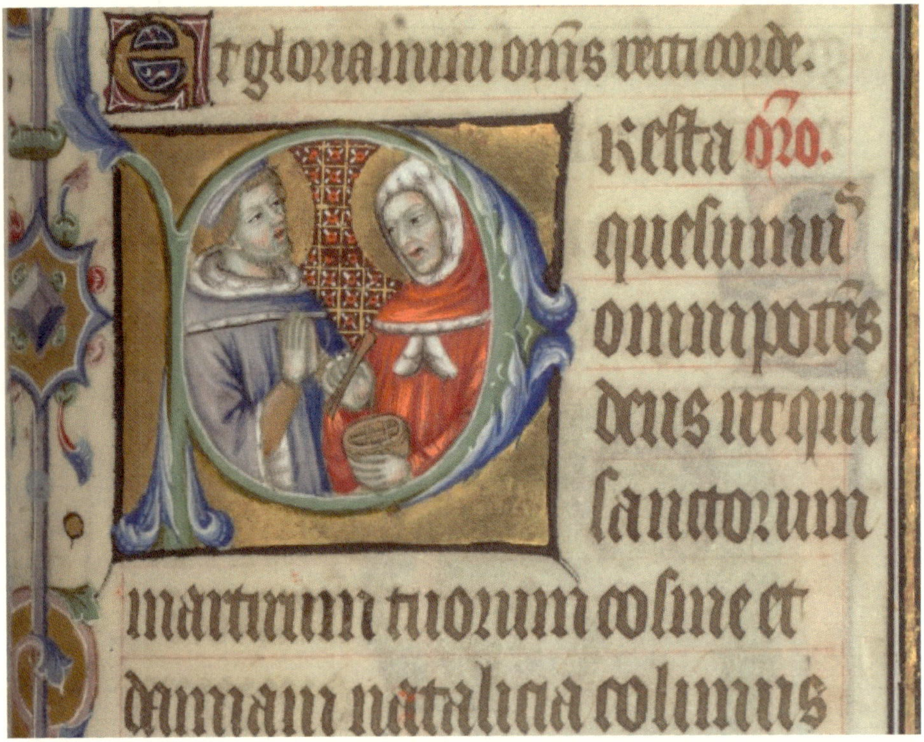

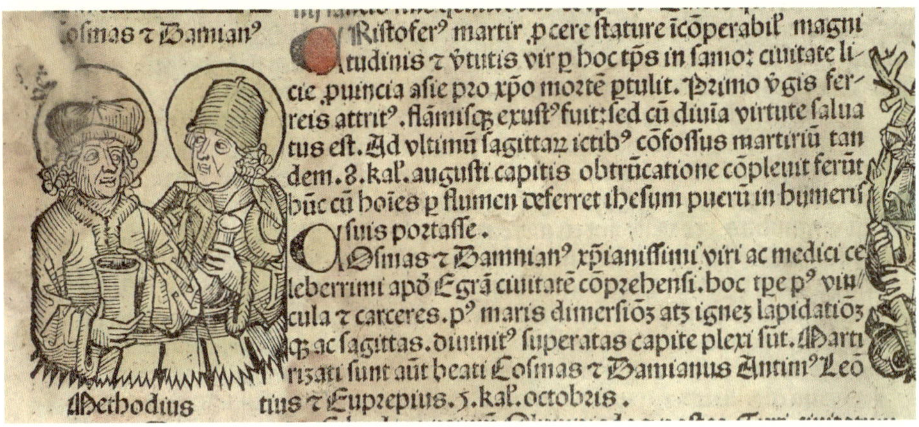

Fig. 3. Master of Brussels. "Saints Cosmas and Damian". *Book of Hours* of Charles III the Noble, King of Navarre (fol. 281r), c. 1405 (Cleveland, OH. The Cleveland Museum of Art). Image obtained from https.//bit.ly/3OMILiv / License CC0.
Fig. 4. Antonius Koberger (printer). "Saints Cosmas and Damian". *Liber chronicarum*, by Hartmann Schedel (fol. 124v), 1493 (Biblioteca Histórica Marqués de Valdecilla / Universidad Complutense de Madrid). Image obtained from https.//bit.ly/3ucpsap.

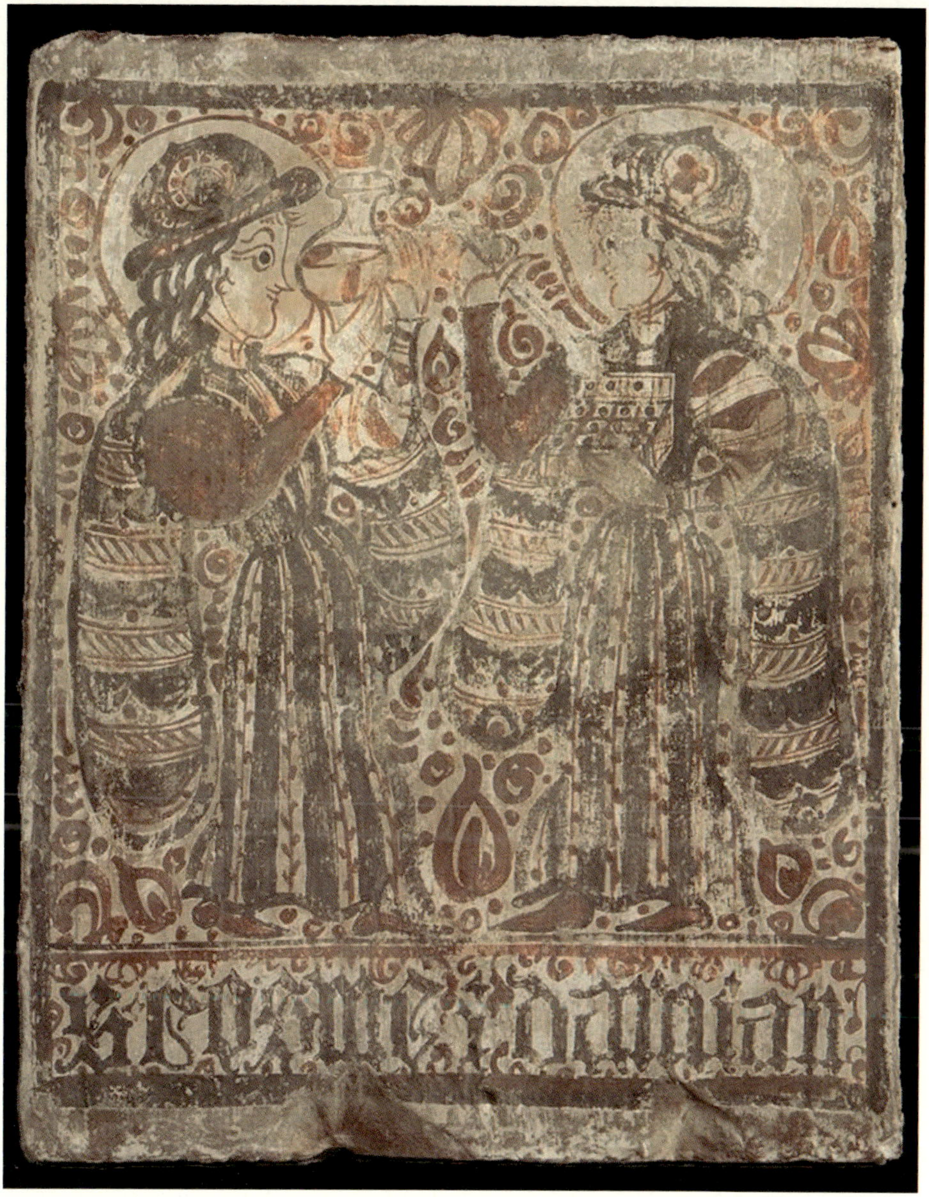

Fig. 5. "Saints Cosmas and Damian". *Socarrat* from Valencia (Paterna), c. 1450-1500 (London. Sam Fogg). Image obtained from https.//bit.ly/3A9pRy7.

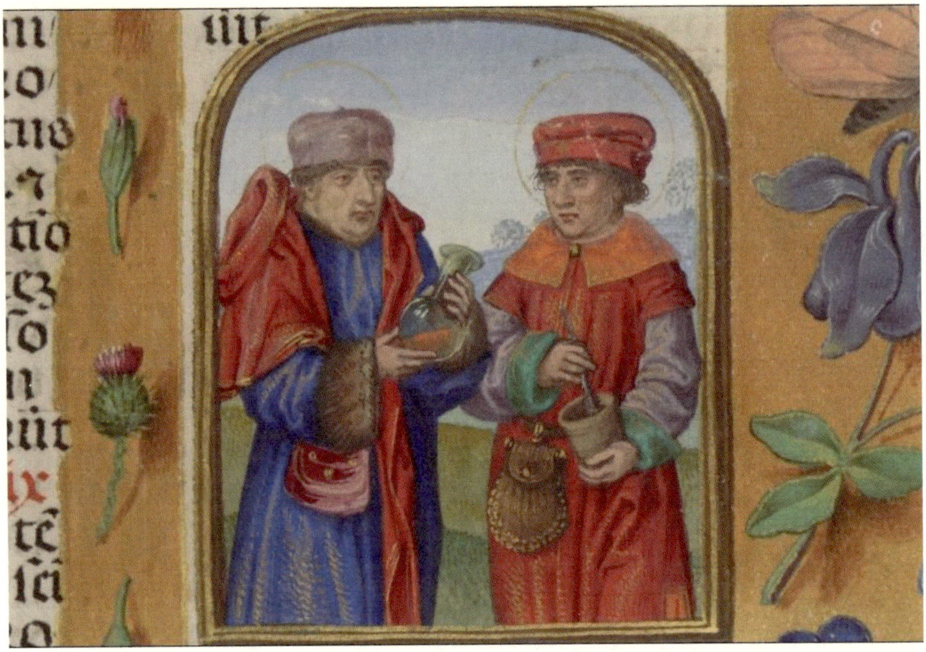

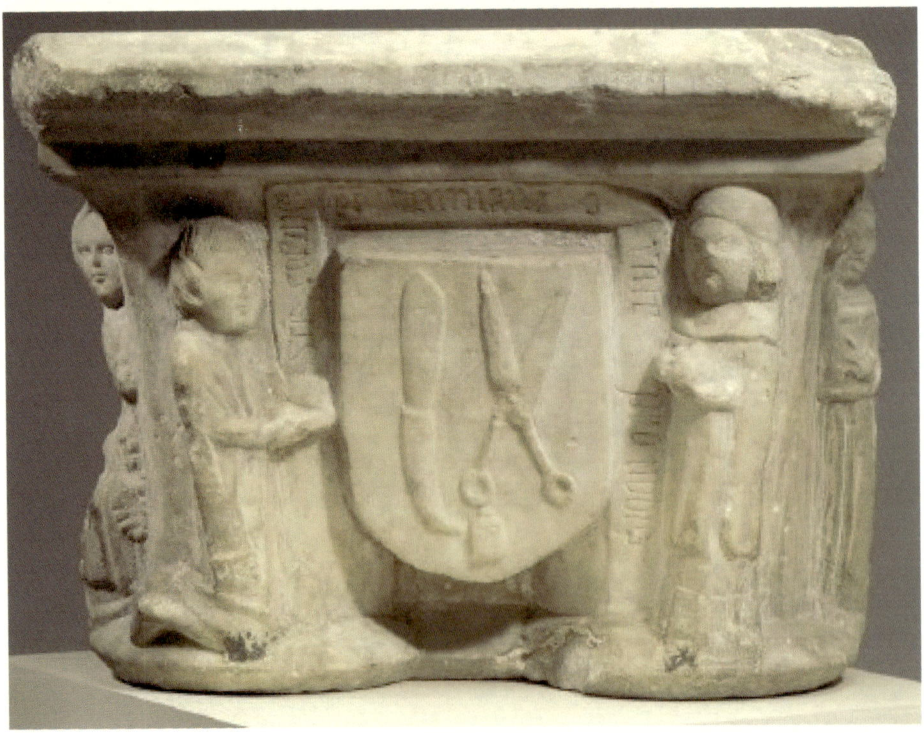

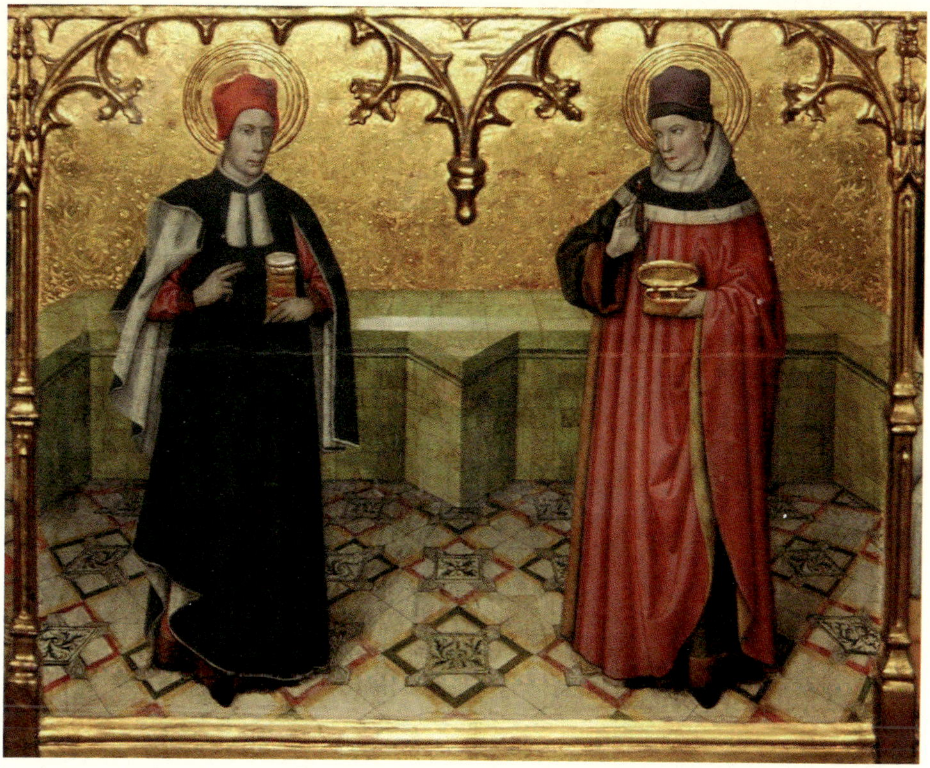

Fig. 6 (*on the other page, above*). Master of James IV of Scotland [identified as Gérard Horenbout]. "Saints Cosmas and Damian", detail. *Breviario de Isabel de Castilla,* c. 1447 (London. British Library Add, Ms 18851, fol. 462r) (detail). Image obtained from https.//bit.ly/3nrrUWY.
Fig. 7 (*on the other page, below*). Saints Cosmas and Damian flanked by a coat of arms in which are depicted a knife, some scissors and a box of ointments. Around the shield we see a pennant with a prayer to the two brothers martyred under Diocletian. *s[anc] te cosme et damiane orate pro nobis.* Double capital from the Carmelite monastery of Trie-sur-Baïse, near Tarbes, late 15th c. (Baltimore. Walters Art Museum). Image obtained from https.//bit.ly/3AdTsGU / License CC0.
Fig. 8. Jaume Huguet. "Saints Cosmas and Damian", central detail of the predella of the altarpiece dedicated to Saints Abdon and Sennen, 1460 (Terrassa. Church of Santa Maria in Terrassa. Image obtained from https.//bit.ly/3ucdxJE / Photograph by Amador Álvarez / License CC BY-SA 3.0.

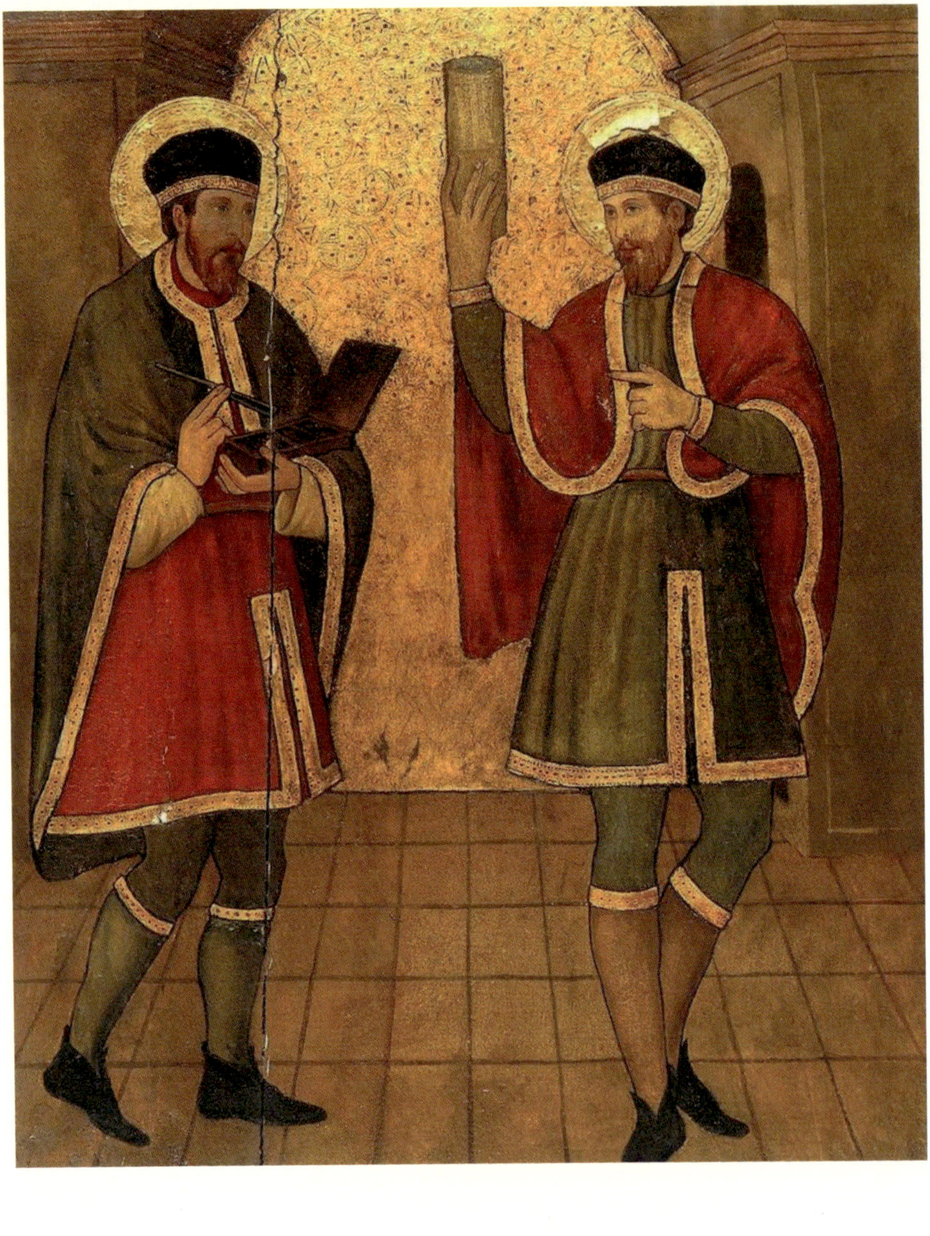

Fig. 9. Jaume Huguet (attr.). “Saints Cosmas and Damian”, detail altarpiece, 15th c. (London. Wellcome Collection). Image obtained from https.//bit.ly/3OtO9rd.

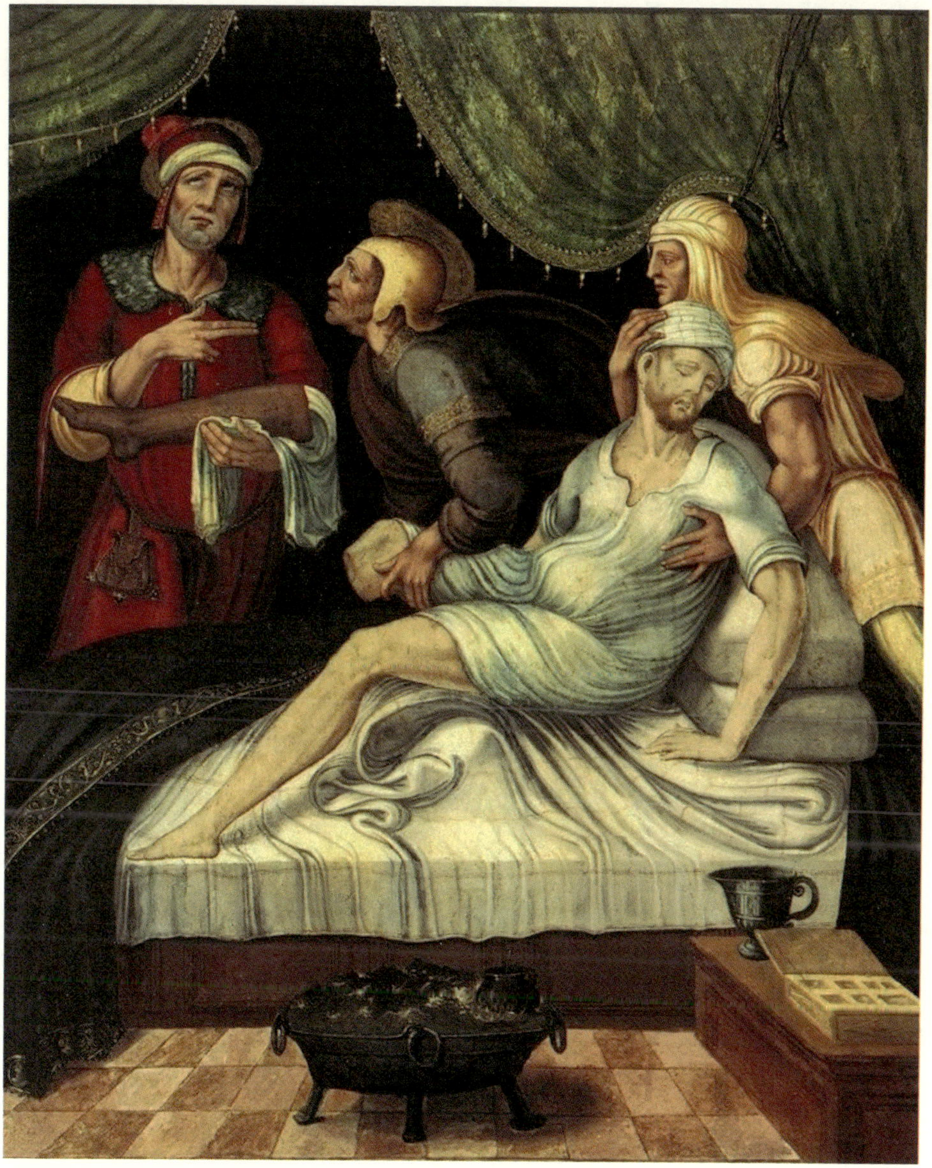

Fig. 10. Juan Correa de Vivar. "Miracle of Saints Cosmas and Damian (leg transplant)", c. 1540-1560 (Pamplona. Museo de Navarra). Image obtained from https.//bit.ly/3AaXkbF.

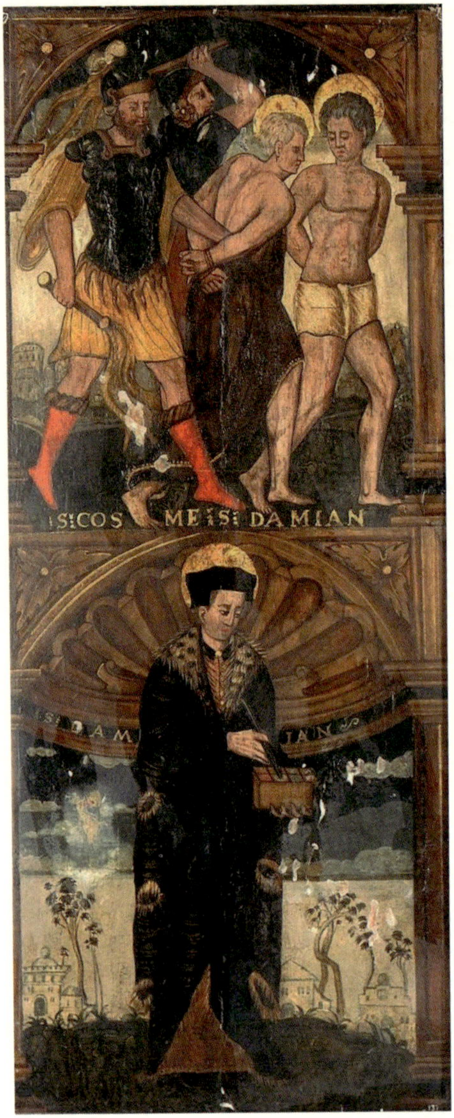

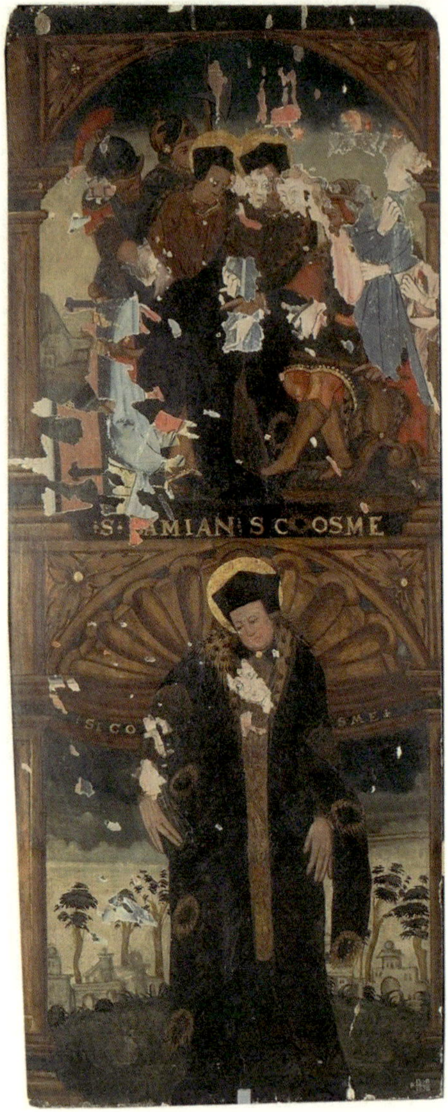

Fig. 11. “Saints Cosmas and Damian taken to their martyrdom (above) and Saint Damian (below)”, c. 1600 (London. Wellcome Collection). Image obtained from https.//bit.ly/3noUI22.
Fig. 12. “Saints Cosmas and Damian before the judge (?) (above) and Saint Cosmas (below)”, c. 1600 (London. Wellcome Collection). Image obtained from https.//bit.ly/3ysURb7.

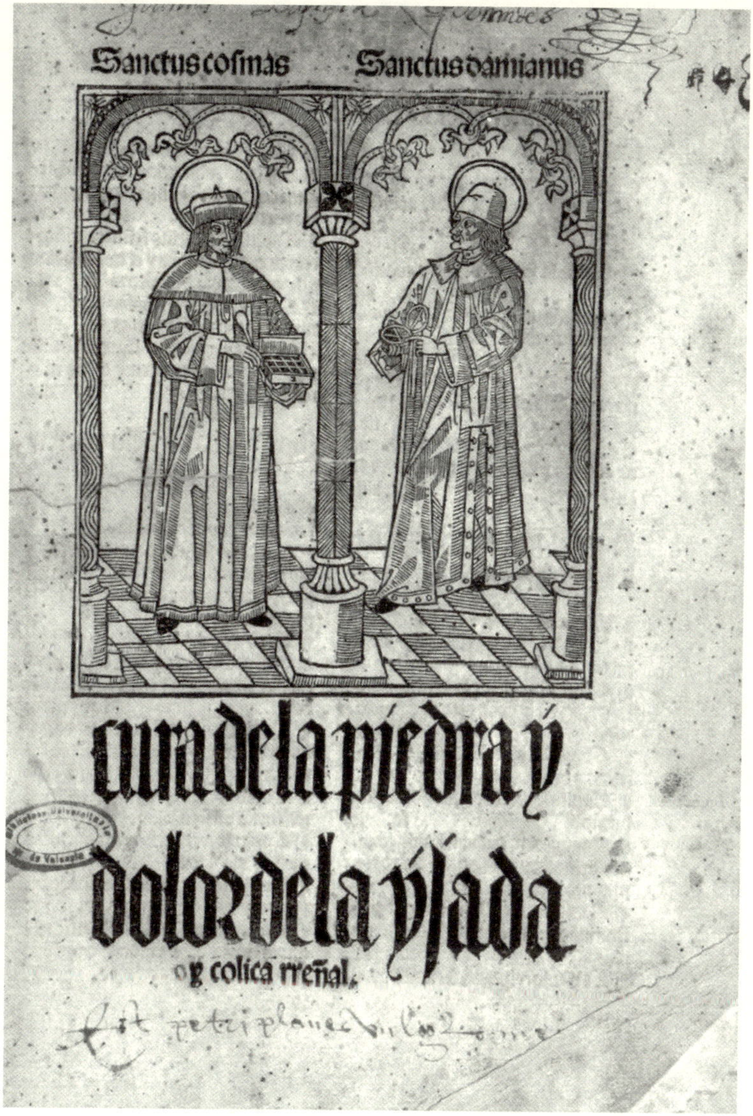


Fig. 13. Pedro Hagenbach (printer). "Saints Cosmas and Damian". Copy of the incunabulum *Cura de la piedra y dolor de la ijada* by Julián Gutiérrez, 1498 (València. Biblioteca Històrica, Universitat de València). Image obtained from https.//bit.ly/3bpVQjg / Roderic, Universitat de València / License CC BY-NC 3.0.

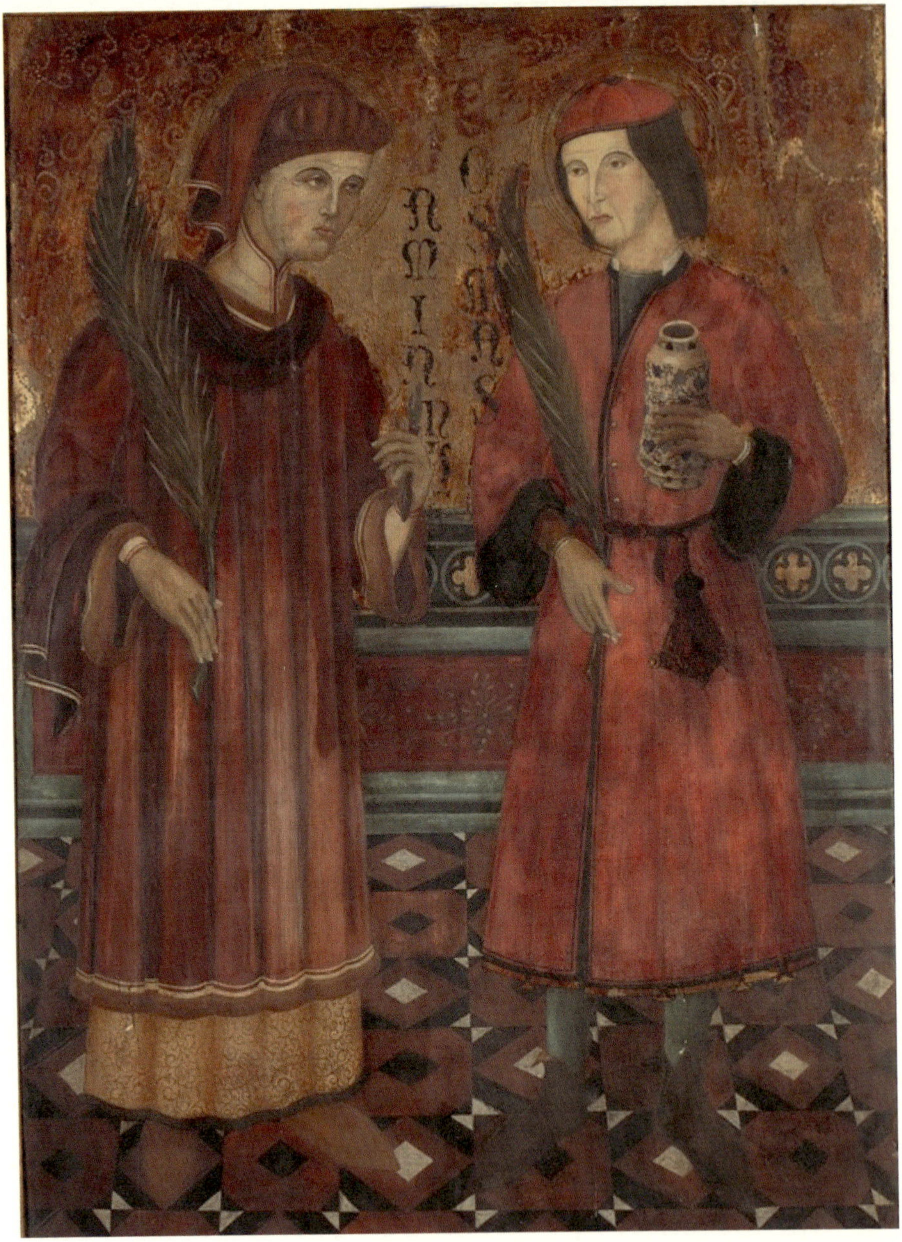

Fig. 14. "Saints Cosmas and Damian", 15th c. (Sitges. Museu de Maricel, col. Dr Jesús Pérez-Rosales). Image obtained from Sánchez 2020 / https.//bit.ly/3QUdD2p / Photograph. Arxiu Fotogràfic del Consorci del Patrimoni de Sitges.

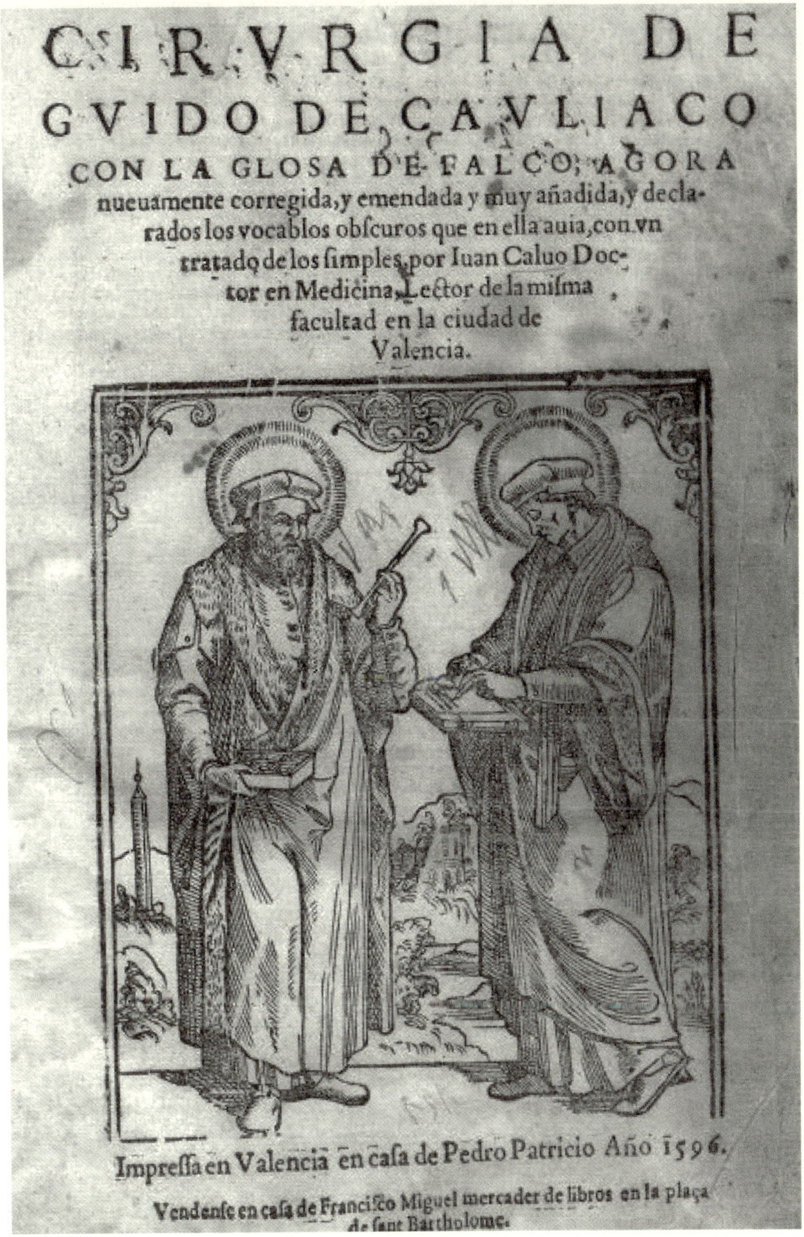

CIRVRGIA DE
GVIDO DE CAVLIACO
CON LA GLOSA DE FALCO, AGORA
nueuamente corregida, y emendada y muy añadida, y decla-
rados los vocablos obſcuros que en ella auia, con vn
tratado de los ſimples, por Iuan Caluo Doc-
tor en Medicina, Lector de la miſma
facultad en la ciudad de
Valencia.

Impreſſa en Valencia en caſa de Pedro Patricio Año 1596.
Vendenſe en caſa de Franciſco Miguel mercader de libros en la plaça
de ſant Bartholome.

Fig. 15. Pedro Patricio (printer). “Saints Cosmas and Damian”. Printed copy *Cirurgía de Guido de Cauliaco […] agora nuevamente corregida y enmendada y muy añadida, y declarados los vocablos obscuros que en ella avía, con un tratado de los simples de Juan Calvo* […], 1596. (Madrid. Biblioteca Nacional de España). Image from the collection of the National Library of Spain https.//bit.ly/3OvEQXE / License CCBY 4.0.

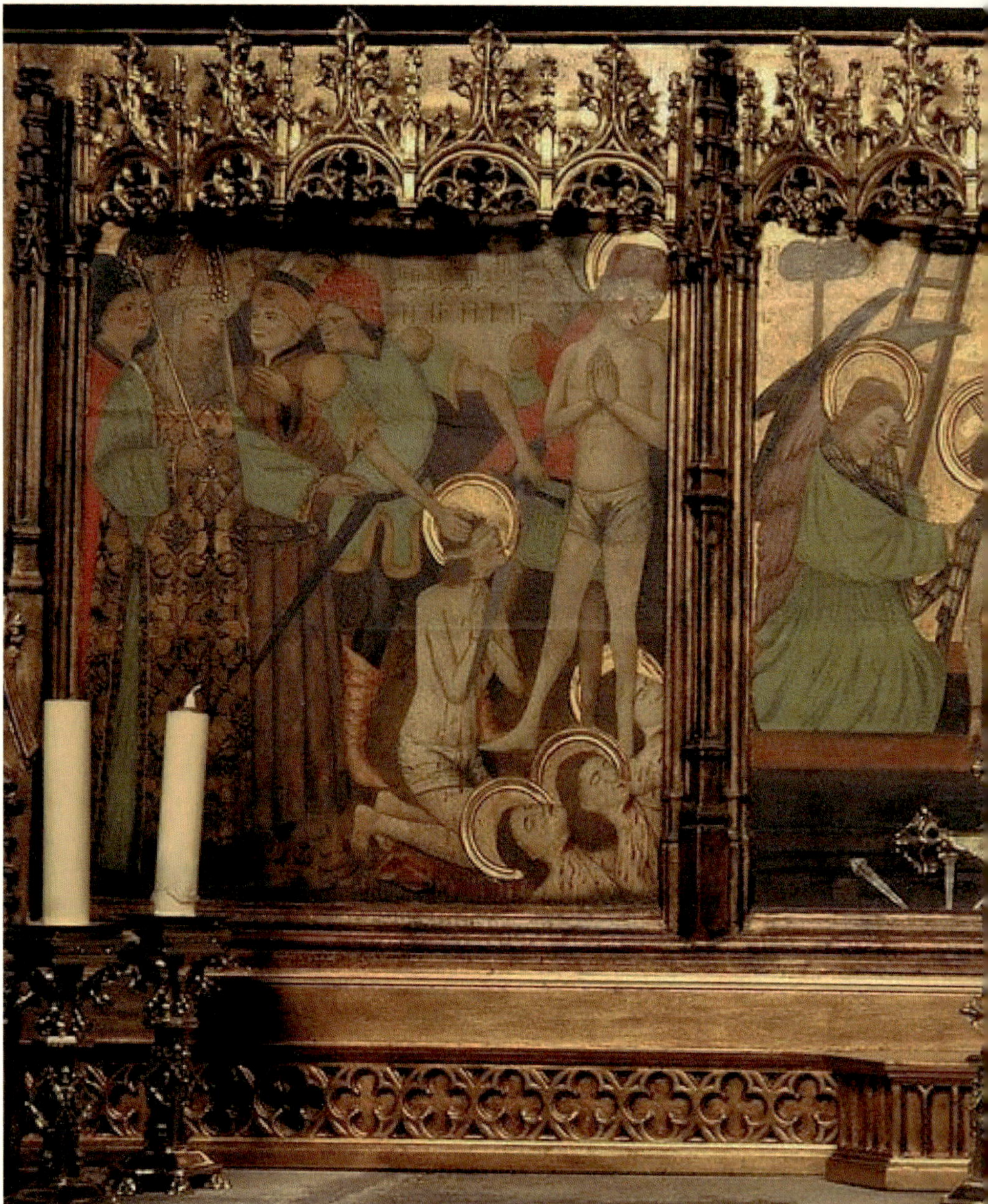

Fig. 16. Bernat Martorell and his follower Miquel Nadal. “Decapitation of the saints and their three brothers, *Ecce Homo*, and posthumous miracles of Saints Cosmas and Damian (leg transplant and miracle of the husbandman)”. Predella of the altarpiece dedicated to Saints Cosmas and Damian, 1453-1455 (Barcelona. Cathedral of Santa Cruz y Santa Eulalia). Image obtained from https.//bit.ly/3y2Lr4N / Photograph. Monestirs Puncat.

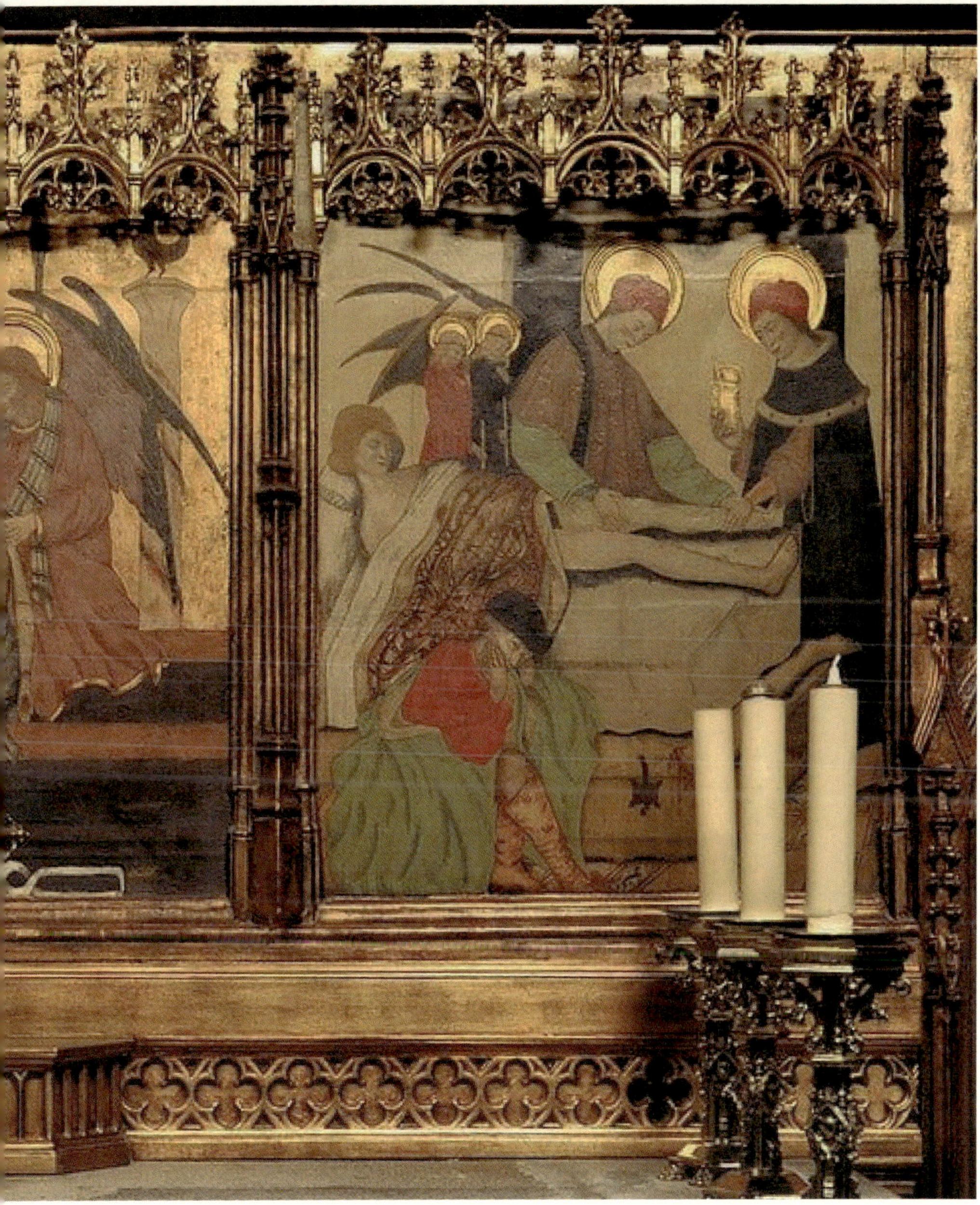

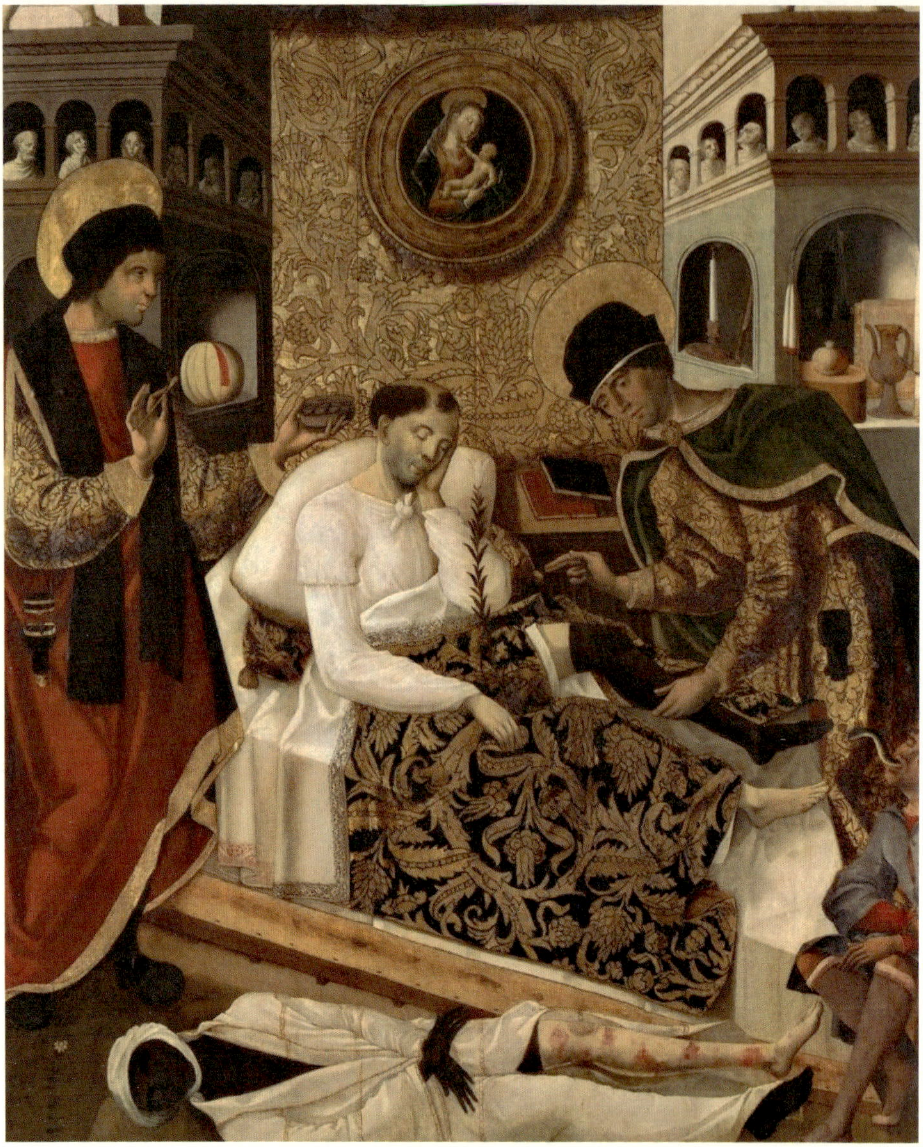

Fig. 17. Fernando del Rincón. "Miracles of Saints Cosmas and Damian (leg transplant and miracle of the husbandman)" from the monastery of San Francisco el Fuerte, Guadalajara, c. 1510 (Madrid. Museo Nacional del Prado). Image obtained from https.//bit.ly/3I2VR97.

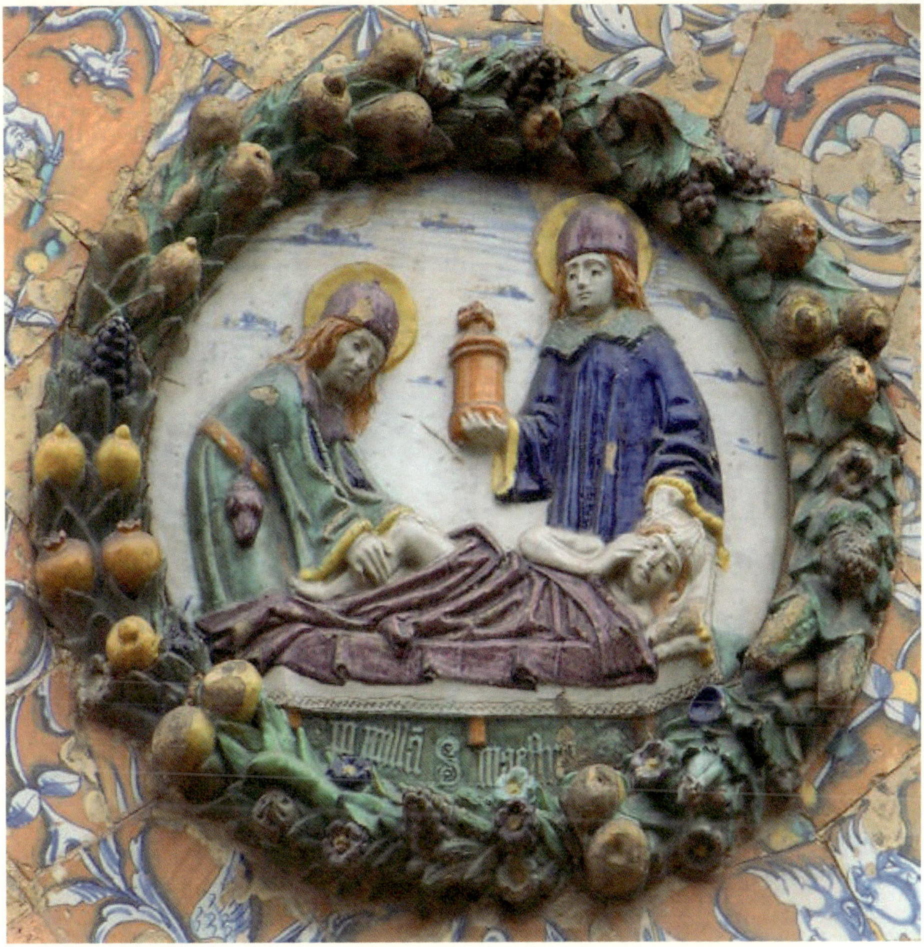

Fig. 18. Niculoso Francisco Pisano (the modelling of the figures is by the sculptor Pedro Millán). "Miracle of Saints Cosmas and Damian (leg transplant)". Doorway of the convent church of Santa Paula, 1504 (Seville. Plaza de Santa Paula). Image obtained from https.//bit.ly/3bBF4h8.

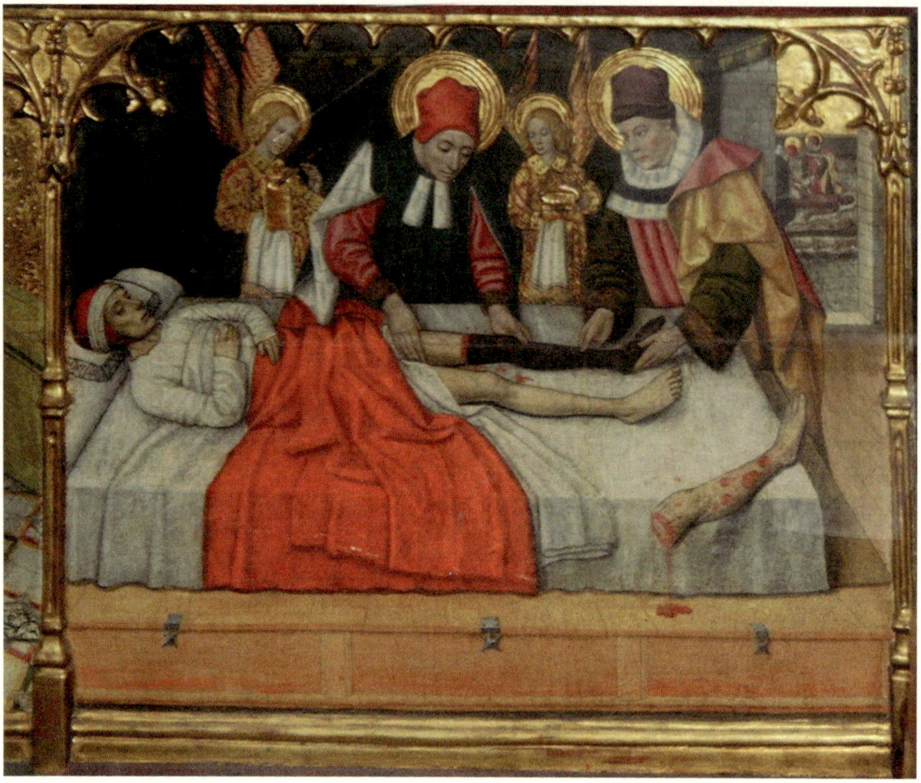

Fig. 19. Jaume Huguet. "Miracle of Saints Cosmas and Damian (leg transplant)". Detail on the right of the predella of the altarpiece dedicated to Saints Abdon and Sennen, 1460 (Terrassa. Church of Santa Maria). Image obtained from https.//bit.ly/3y3pylT / Photograph by Amador Álvarez / License CCBY-SA 3.0.

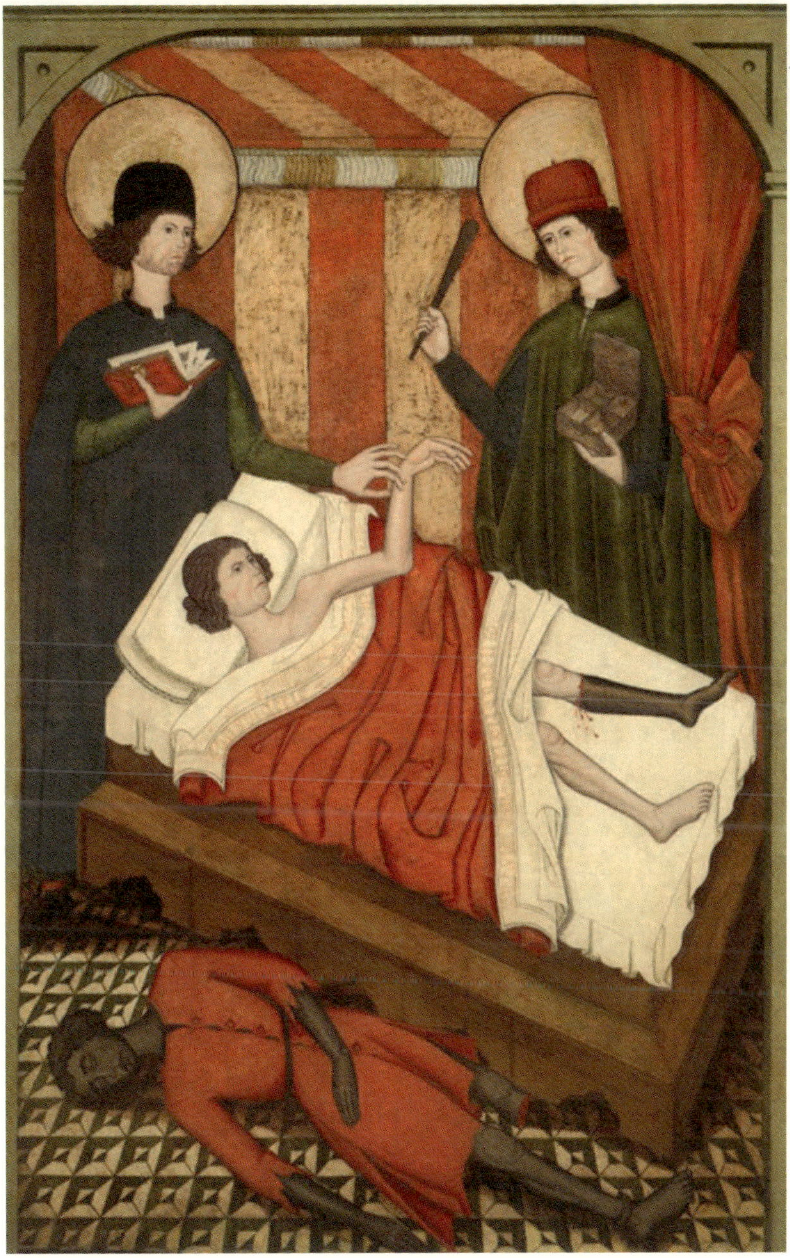

Fig. 20. School of Castile and León. "Miracle of Saints Cosmas and Damian (leg transplant)", c. 1460-1480 (Private collection). Image obtained from https.//bit.ly/3udybt8 / Photograph by Jesús Téllez Rubio.

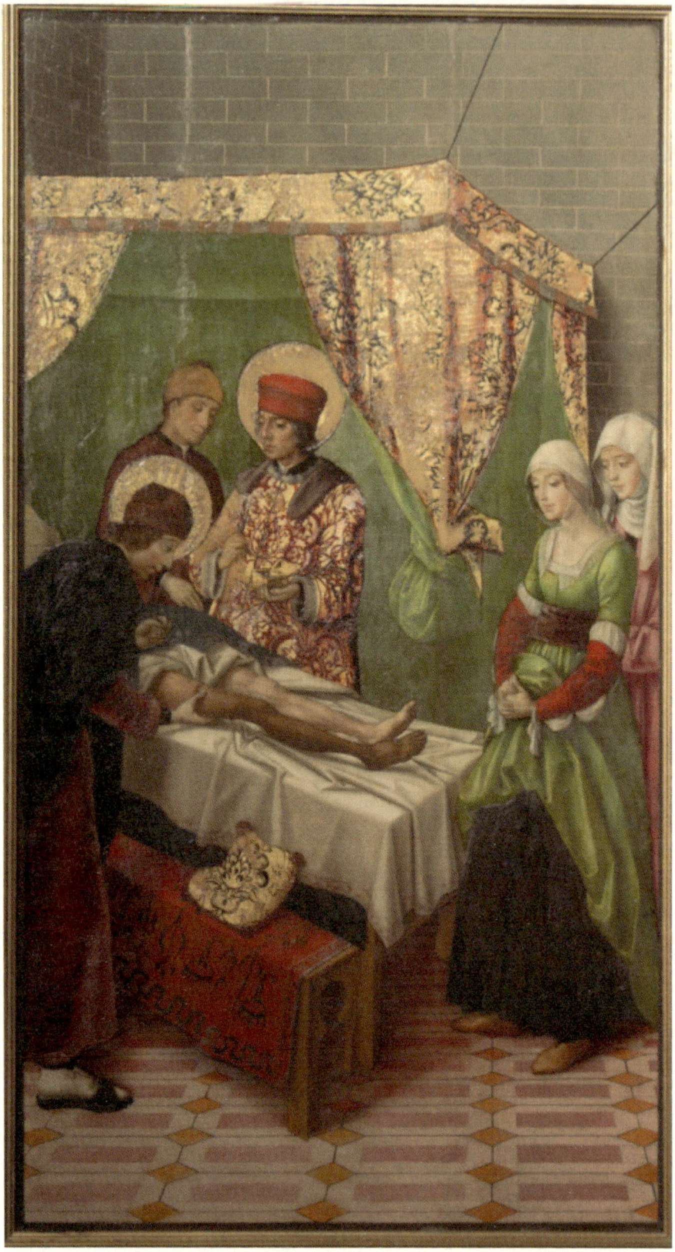

Fig. 21. Pedro Berruguete. "Miracle of Saints Cosmas and Damian (leg transplant)", second half of 15th c. (Real Colegiata de San Cosme y San Damián in Covarrubias, Burgos). Image obtained from https.//bit.ly/3HZhQxL.

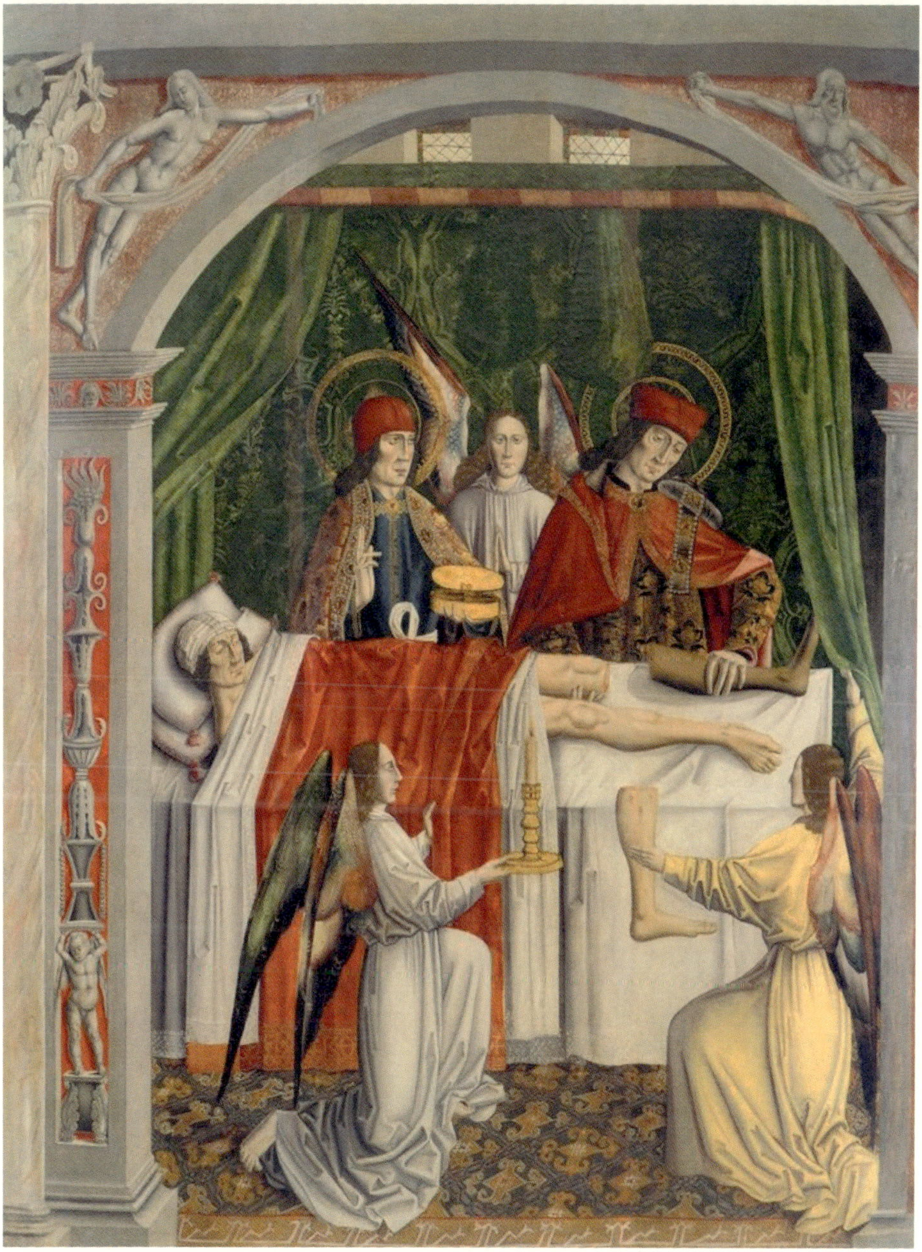

Fig. 22. Master of Los Balbases [Andrés Sánchez] (attr.). "Miracle of Saints Cosmas and Damian (leg transplant)", c. 1495 (London. Wellcome Collection). Image obtained from https.//bit.ly/3OShURY.

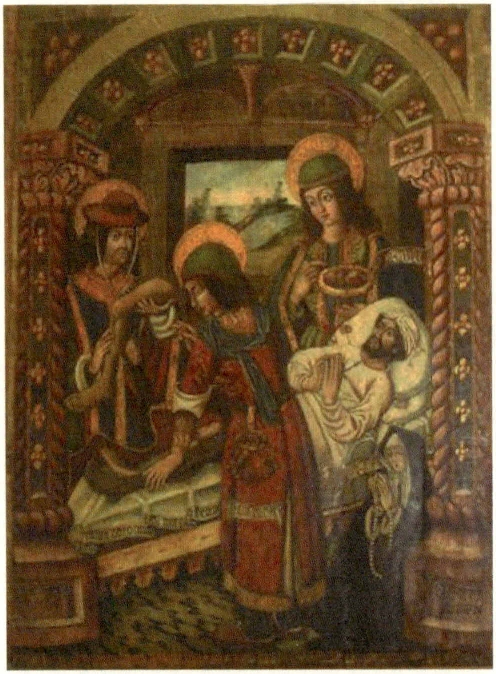

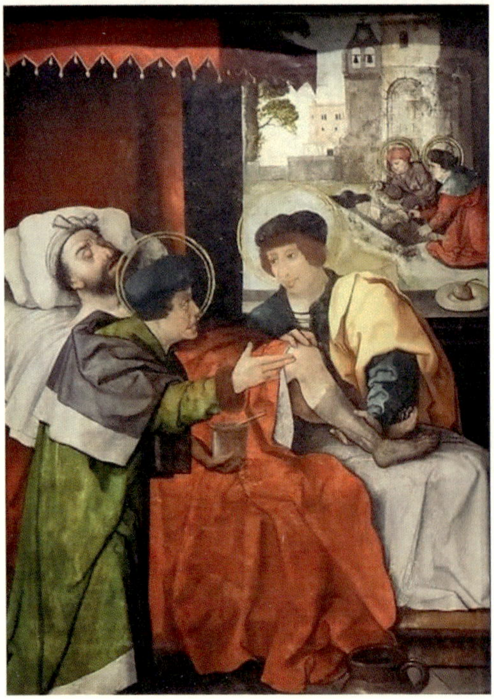

Fig. 23. "Miracle of Saints Cosmas and Damian (leg transplant)", early 16th c. (Chapel of Nuestra Señora de las Vacas, Ávila). Image obtained from https.//bit.ly/3Npe8Pa / Photograph. Patronato Virgen de las Vacas.
Fig. 24. León Picardo. "Miracle of Saints Cosmas and Damian (leg transplant)", first half of 16th c. (Burgos. Cathedral Museum). Image obtained from https.//bit.ly/3NwV9Sy / Photograph by Rafael Gómez.

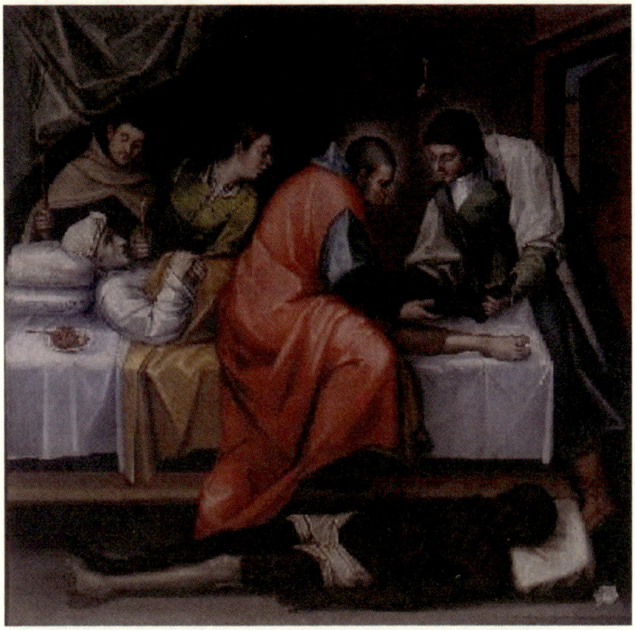

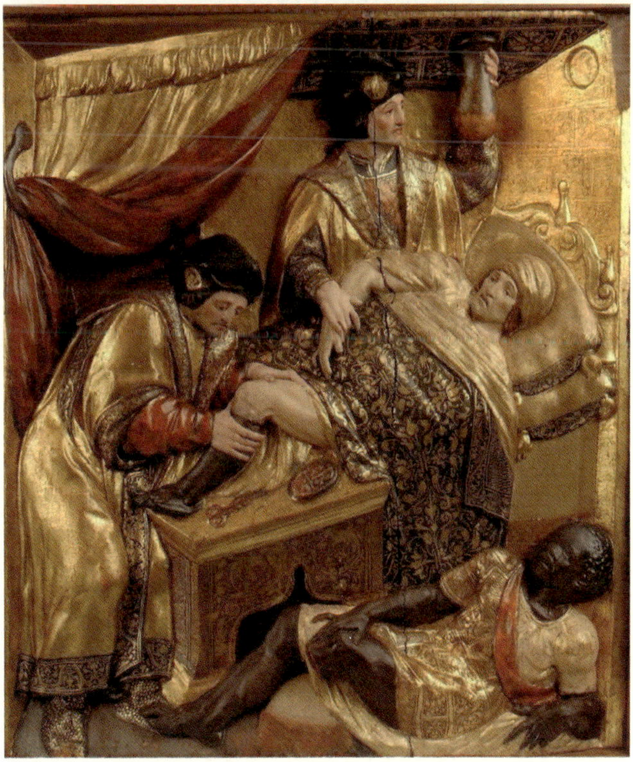

Fig. 25. Pedro de Raxis the Elder. "Miracle of Saints Cosmas and Damian (leg transplant)", 1592 (Granada. Museo de Bellas Artes). Image obtained from https.//bit.ly/3a3KktG.
Fig. 26. Isidro Villoldo (attr.). "Miracle of Saints Cosmas and Damian (leg transplant)", c. 1547 (Valladolid. Museo Nacional de Escultura). Image obtained from https.//bit.ly/3NoMP7D.

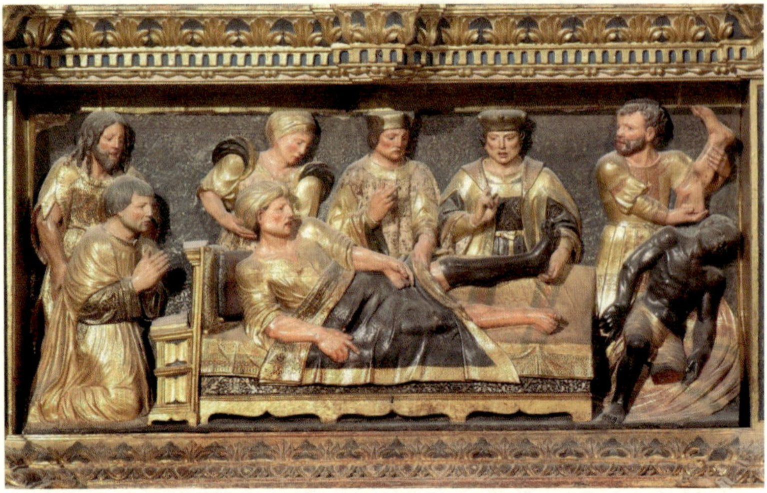

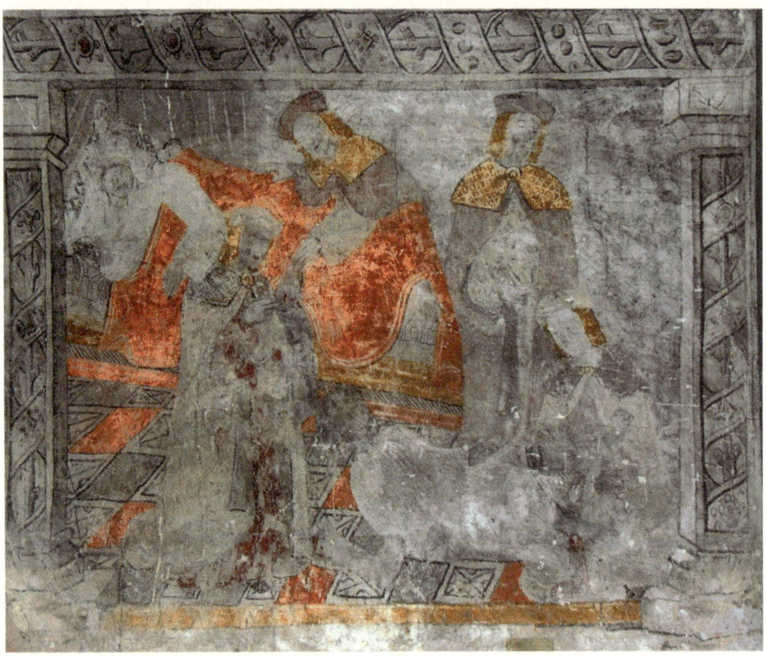

Fig. 27. Juan Ortiz the Elder I (attr.). "Miracle of Saints Cosmas and Damian (leg transplant)". Predella of the altarpiece dedicated to Saints Cosmas and Damian, 1533 (Palencia. Cathedral, Saint Gregory's chapel). Image obtained from https.//bit.ly/3Oz3YN2 / Photograph by Javier Ayarza.
Fig. 28. "Miracle of Saints Cosmas and Damian (leg transplant)", 15th c. (Basconcillos del Tozo [Burgos]. Church of San Cosme y San Damián). Image obtained from Zimmerman ed. 2013. 72.

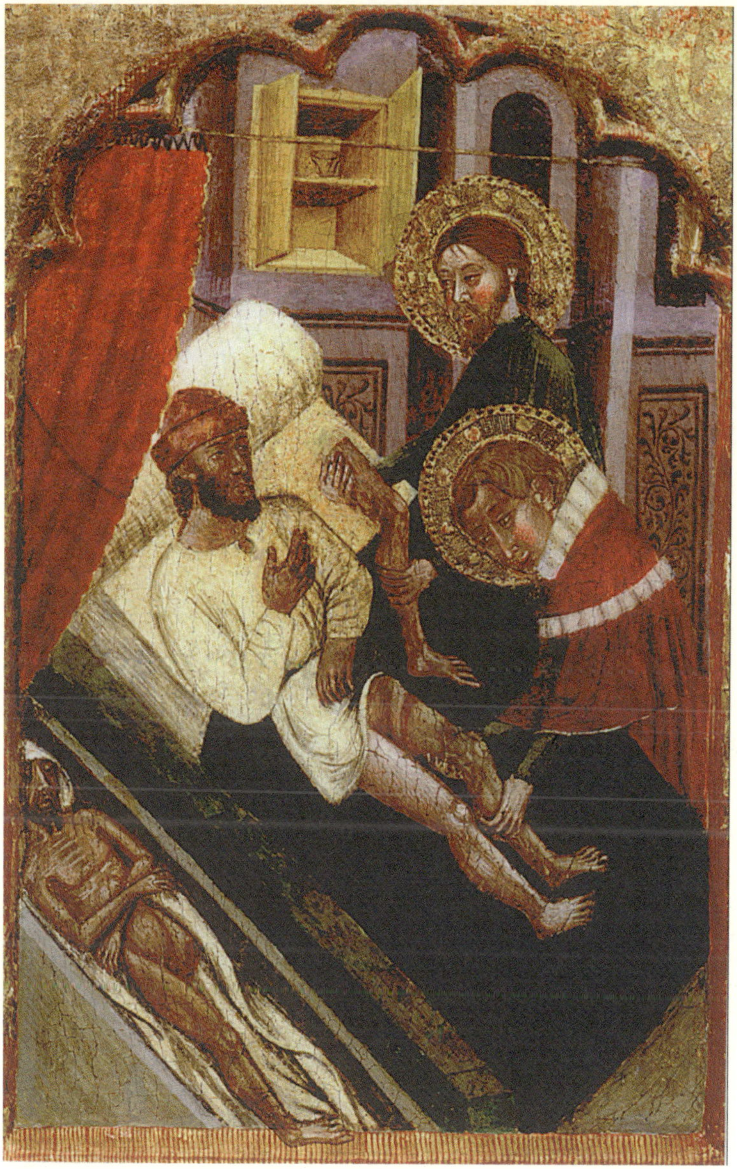

Fig. 29. Mestre de Rubió. "Miracle of Saints Cosmas and Damian (leg transplant)", c. 1351-1380 (Vic. Museu Episcopal). Image obtained from ZIMMERMAN ed. 2013. 52.

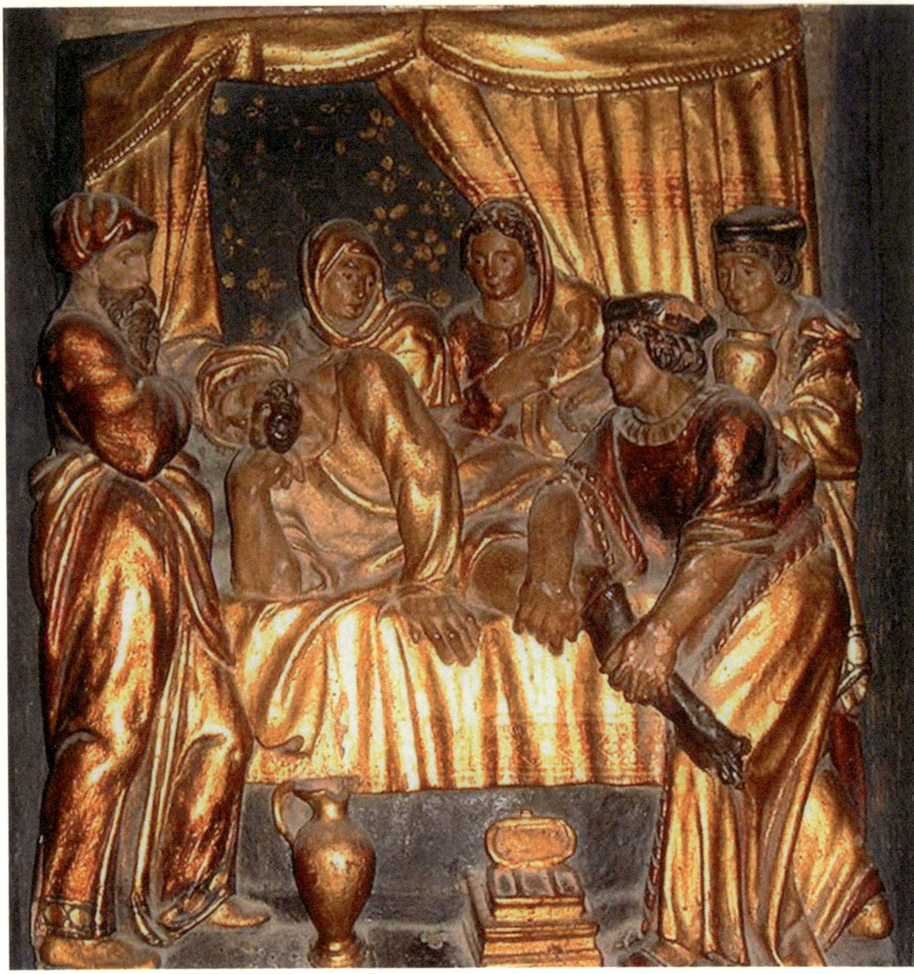

Fig. 30. Gabriel Joly. "Miracle of Saints Cosmas and Damian (leg transplant)". Detail on the right of the predella of the altarpiece dedicated to Saints Cosmas and Damian, c. 1537 (Teruel. Church of San Pedro). Image obtained from ZIMMERMAN ed. 2013. 108.

# II
# *Hospital Heritage and Symbolic Space*

Josep Barceló Prats

# The Birth of the General Hospital: Background and Development of a New Physical and Symbolic Space of Care in the Late Medieval City

## 1. *Introduction*

During the 1960s, various historiographical approaches began to affirm that the birth of modern hospital medicine was a sort of "Big Bang" which took place in Paris during the end of the 18th century. This interpretative model, inaugurated with the publication of the *Naissance de la Clinique* (Foucault 1963) and consolidated, although from a different approach, with the appearance of *Medicine at the Paris Hospital 1794-1848* (Ackerknecht 1967), idealized the technical progress of medicine, and questioned the medical significance of pre-modern hospitals. Thus, according to this historical "artefact", the pre-modern hospital could not be considered a medical institution, since during the *Ancien Régime* medicine was never a strictly hospital-related profession (Foucault 1977: 3-25).

Instead, it was argued that pre-modern hospitals should be studied as an important and even essential institution for urban life in the West during the Middle Ages, since they collected and assisted the poor materially and spiritually and, at the same time, protected the rest of society by being also a place of internment where vulnerable people could be isolated when they were carriers of diseases. In summary and according to these theories, during the late Middle Ages and the Renaissance the "general hospital" had to be understood as «a sort of mixed instrument of exclusion, care and spiritual transformation from which the medicine function is absent» (Foucault 1978: 23).

However, most recent historiographical reflections began to propose less restrictive interpretations of the hospital institution as a space of medicalization (Huguet 2004), affirming that the management of health and illness in pre-modern hospitals could not be explained solely through the analysis of «the archaeology of medical practice and institutional charity» (Comelles et al. 1991: 32). It was therefore necessary to highlight other meanings as legitimate (Horden 1988: 359-374), as those of a medical nature in post-revolutionary Paris, which situated the hospitals from the *Ancien Régime* in direct relation to the community that surrounded them and within the framework of a broad pluralism of care that monopolized the care of the hospitalized patient (Ferragud 2007).

It is for this reason that in recent decades, the study of hospitals in the *Ancien Régime* has allowed for a deeper understanding of different responses to phenomena such as poverty or, to cite another example, the relationships and motivation of the urban elites in the promotion of care (Huguet 2014: 13-26; Conejo 2013: 3-6). In this context, in which the therapeutic value of health regimens and religious consolation also played an important role (Henderson 2001: 188-216), the "general hospital", born at the dawn of the late Middle Ages, ceased to be interpreted simply as a type of "antechamber of death" or as an institution lacking a medical function simply because it did not include a doctor.

Consequently, analysis of the pre-modern "general hospital" have long since ceased to be based on the Foucauldian concept of "medicalization-artefact" –understood in presentist terms–. For more than three decades now, the medicalization of *Ancien Régime* hospitals has been conceived as a dynamic and dialectic process of production and diffusion of knowledge between different actors that has progressively affected care practices and different models of health policies and medical education (Martín, Comelles, Arnau 1993: 201-234). Similarly, the evolution of this process of medicalization cannot be considered without linking it to a much broader and more pluralistic curative and care context than that which characterized, at the end of the 18th century, the emergence of the modern hospital medicine, whose foundations were built on the so-called anatomic-clinical method: that is, the generalization of clinical experimentation, the performance of autopsies and medical statistics (Risse 1996: 75-96).

Emphasizing the notion of process also makes it possible to divide medicalization into phases that allow for better global comprehension of its evolution. Broadly speaking and from a *longue durée* perspective, one can document three main stages of medicalization (Barceló-Prats 2022: 30-32). The 1st stage, the development of which will be discussed in more detail in one of the sections of this chapter, began in the late Middle Ages and was characterized by the role that physicians, at the local level, played as experts not only in relation to disease but also in other social spheres.

The 2nd stage, which Foucault and other leading authors considered –on a "presentist" basis– as the origin of the process of medicalization, began at the end of the 18th century and was associated with a growing protagonism of states in the management of the health and illness of the population. It was in this second phase when the processes of naturalization and depoliticization of care began, leading to the hegemony of the so-called "medical model" (Menéndez 2005: 9-32), and resulting in the dominance of the biomedical approach, technology, and the rules of heredity (Perdiguero, Ruiz 2017: 248-249).

Finally, overlapping with this 2nd stage, we now find ourselves in the 3rd phase of medicalisation which, centred on the individual, is characterized by the generation of discourses around health that do not only come from the medical field but also from many other social spheres. Both the media and social networks, as well as the rest of information technologies, play a fundamental role in the dissemination of these messages to the population at large, the aim of which is to normalise certain supposedly healthy behaviours.

The complex articulation between the evolution of hospitals and the development of the process of medicalization, understood as an analytical tool for approaching the study of health and illness in past societies, justifies the objective of this text, firstly, to address the background that transformed the meanings of hospitality and hospitals during the Middle Ages. Secondly, it describes the first stage of medicalization in the western European urban space and its influence on the transformations in care. Finally, it analyses the "general hospital" model, highlighting the needs that led to the implementation of a new hospital policy in the late medieval city.

## 2. *Origin and Background of the "General Hospital"*

### 2.1. *Hospitality and Charity as the Basis for the Institutionalisation of Care in the Middle Ages*

The concepts of guardianship, asylum and, in general, hospitalization refer to social and cultural practices designed for caring for and attending to people who, affected by whichever type of misfortune or calamity, lacked social support or whose primary reference groups were unable or limited in their ability to cope with the management of misfortune (Gotman 2001). These notions have served as a basis for positing an eventual "medicalization process" in the ancient world and its relation to medical, but also political and legal practice (Corvisier 1985).

Within this interpretive scheme, in the ancient world, the origins of hospitality referred to the care of the barbarian, stranger or foreigner who lacked a primary reference group. It is not surprising, then, that its practice would be described in such different texts like Hesiod's *Works and Days* (Piñol 2013: 47-56), Homer's *Odyssey* (Hoces de la Guardia 1987: 43-56) –with the hospitality ritual by Alcinous, king of the Phaeacians on the island of Escheria (Corfu), and his daughter Nausicaa–,[1] or the New Testament (Ortega 2006: 83-94) with the parable of the good Samaritan.[2] All of them agree on the practices derived from the moral obligation to welcome and offer a warm place to stay to people in distress (Pitt-Rivers 1971) .

The development, both in the Judeo-Christian West and the Islamic context,[3] of these practices gave rise to an ethical, moral, and above all, cultural discourse

1. According to the *Odyssey*, Alcinous and Nausicaa took Odysseus into their palace after a shipwreck and, in return, he told them in front of an attentive audience who he was and where he came from (Marco 2006: 111-122).

2. The parable of the Good Samaritan, recounted in Luke's Gospel (10,29-37) illustrates how charity and mercy are virtues that guide men towards piety and holiness. The image of the Samaritan, who were considered a heretical people by the more orthodox sector of the Hebrew religion of that time, as the pious savior of a beaten Jew served to redefine the concept of neighbor at the time.

3. Hospitality in the Arabian world, in a similar way than in the Latin West with the emergence of Christianity, went from being a social virtue to having a character of a religious obligation. From pagan antiquity it was practiced as a form of welcome in such a hostile environment

on hospitality that would end up leading to the creation of hospital and asylum institutions (Miller 1985). This institutionalisation of hospitality should be understood as a civil response that had to guarantee the care and protection of those individuals who could no longer be cared for by their primary groups or who simply lacked these social networks.

Then, with the spread and expansion of Christianity during the first centuries after Christ, especially from the 4th century onwards,[4] the idea of hospitality was redefined on the base of traditional values present in pagan society. *Hospitalitas* [hospitality] went from being, in essence, a social virtue to having the character of a religious obligation. This was due to the impregnation of the concept of hospitality with a doctrinal foundation based, for example, on the Gospel injunctions to «love your neighbour as yourself» (Mt 22,39) or in the performance of the corporal works of mercy: «feed the hungry, give drink to the thirsty, welcome in the stranger, clothe the naked, visit the sick and imprisoned, and bury the dead» (Mt 25,35-46). That was how *hospitalitas*, along with *caritas* [charity], became the conceptual basis of the Christian hospital (Albini 2002).

However, we must not forget that all of this is a historical particularism whose genealogy can be described, without a break in continuity, from Late Antiquity, at the very least (Nutton 1981: 10-46), to the present day (Risse 1999). Nor should it be forgotten that the creation of all these institutions of care was simply not the product of individual action but of the meaning acquired, in certain cultural contexts, by this form of collective philanthropy, which was necessarily legally regulated. We must also consider that, even though hospitality and charity were fundamental for those who constructed the ideological framework of the Christian hospital, it would be biased to explain the medicalisation and institutionalisation process of care in Medieval Europe exclusively through these and other religious precepts.

It should be remembered that the necessity to institutionalise part of the processes of health/illness/care,[5] began, in a similar manner throughout Christian Europe, with slow economic growth and some urban development beginning to take shape from the mid-11th century onwards. This is the collective assumption of the management of what we nowadays call vulnerable social groups, which led to the foundation of a wide range of welfare institutions (Riu 1980). Thus, the first

as life in the desert. With the advent of Islam, much of the old Bedouin code of conduct was charged with new ethical values and with a humanistic and transcendent dimension (Abumalham 2006: 95-109).

4. One of the first specific reports of a Christian hospital is found in 360 AD, when Basil the Great founded a *nosokomeion* in Caesarea in Cappadocia. Everything suggests that the *nosokomeion*, or place of rest for the sick, has its roots in the *xenodokheion*, an ancient place of shelter for pilgrims, many of them located near the sanctuaries of Asclepius, whose purpose was to prepare them for the cathartic moment that was to heal through divine intervention (Miller 1985).

5. We define the health/illness/care process as the set of culturally structured representations and practices that any society is equipped with to respond to the crises derived from illness and death, where care processes are also incorporated (Menéndez 1978: 11-53).

medieval hospitals were small inns or hostels –with very unspecific functions in care– designed to provide shelter to a very diverse variety of groups with a common denominator: poverty, understood as a polysemic term (MOLLAT 1988; GEREMEK 1998). In this context, care of the poor –whether they were men or women in destitute situations, the sick of all kinds (VINYOLES 2013: 77-101), the disabled, orphans and abandoned children (ILLANES 2019), the elderly, vagrants and pilgrims, among others– became the hospital's mission. For example, in the Crown of Aragon, documents from the early 1300s often describe hospital residents collectively as *pauperes* et *infirmi*, and we would probably be right to think of them as "the helpless" rather than as just the sick, that is, as still having primarily a social rather than a specifically medical identity (McVAUGH 1993: 228).

Thus, the unspecificity of material and spiritual care offered in these early medieval hospitals made them, at the same time, hospices for travellers and pilgrims, asylums where all kinds of poor people could be taken in and maintained, and infirmaries where the sick could be cared for. Therefore, it was in the hospital «where the institutional response of medieval society to the problem of the poor was best reflected » (MARTÍNEZ-GARCÍA 2008: 80), together with everything related to the management of misfortune, hardship, and illness.

In short, during the first centuries of the Middle Ages, poverty and illness were a daily reality because of the growing development of cities which, within Feudalism, needed to put in place management instruments to help and assist their fellow citizens or outsiders in crisis situations (GOTMAN 2004). Thus, the hospital, more than being just an institution designed to protect and give refuge to individuals in vulnerable situations, also ended up becoming a tool for the social control of stigmatized groups, and, at the same time, an instrument of legitimization of local policies.

### 2.2. *The Medieval Hospital and its Relationship with the Common Good*

The concept of *bonum commune* [common good] was developed by philosophers and theologians, such as Thomas Aquinas, from the integration of Aristotelian ethics into the scholastic tradition, thus forming an ideological-political synthesis (FORMENT 1996: 51-85).

In medieval Latin Europe, this concept served as the basis for the construction, from the 13th century onwards, of a new ethic of responsibility that responded to the new challenges and problems arising from urban and economic growth in medieval society. Indeed, European cities became more and more attractive places of local exchange as different trades and urban economic and mercantile transactions developed. Consequently, these lucrative activities turned into an everyday occurrence, thus enriching the urban elites. However, the very act of enrichment could lead to a moral problem if it was considered as a potential source of societal poverty or simply a form of greed. The answer to this aforementioned problem came from the renewed Christian spirituality deployed throughout Europe by mendicant orders –especially Franciscans– (Todeschini 2008: 265-303), that emerged at the beginning of the 13th century (Arrizabalaga 2014: 27-48).

Influential authors such as Francesc Eiximenis and Ramon Llull articulated key words such as *caritas* [charity], *avaritia* [greed] and *infedilitas* [infidelity] with political concepts like *utilitas publica* [public utility] and *bonum commune* itself, which, in the end, ended up shaping the legal, economic, and moral limits of the *civitas* or community (Todeschini 2010: 225-236). In brief, what the mendicant orders, through their new ethic of responsibility, achieved towards communal problems was to «confront and finally demystify the taboo of commercial money transitions» (Rosenwein, Little 1974: 31), through the Christianising of the lucrative activities of medieval urban life. In other words, the enrichment of an individual could be tolerated if, to a certain point, part of these earnings ended up invested in the common good.

Obviously, the mendicant movement's proposals for spiritual renewal quicky became compatible with the interests of urban oligarchies, whose members began to make substantial donations, either during their lifetime or through bequests, in exchange for spiritual benefits (Albini 2013: 227-251). The beneficiaries of these practices were, logically, the mendicant orders and, in a similar manner, hospital institutions, transforming the way in which they assisted the most disadvantaged. This rationality led to the foundation of many hospitals through the 13th and 14th century, whose origin was «in the last will of a wealthy person who, driven by the desire for salvation beyond earth, earmarked part, or all, of his fortune in his will for the construction of a care centre dedicated for the poor» (Rubio Vela 1981: 17).

In conclusion, the notion of common good contributed to the configuration of a particular model of social organization which, between the 13th and 15th century, was decisive in defining, for example, the political and cultural identity of the Crown of Aragon (Comelles 2013: 183-208). Thus, this new ethic of collective responsibility for social problems spread by the mendicant orders, such as the Franciscans (Evangelisti 2006), ended up shaping a very particular way of administering a part of the *res publica* consisting of the foundation, government, and management of hospitals and other institutions of care.

## 3. *The First Stage of Medicalization and its Influence on the Transformation of Care*

### 3.1. *The Consolidation of Medicine as a Reference of Knowledge*

The book *Practical Medicine from Salerno to the Black Death* (García-Ballester et al. 1994), recounts how, from the 11th century until the outbreak of the Black Death in 1348, medicine was consolidated as a point of reference in the pursuit of knowledge. A new way of teaching medicine was able to develop thanks to the application of scholastic philosophy, which allowed the field of health and disease management to move towards a type of naturalistic thinking consistent with Aristotelian science, without contradicting the parallel evolution of theology (GARCÍA-BALLESTER 1992: 119-146). This increased the prestige of the care provided by university doctors, without detracting from the success of the rest of the healers that made up the broad pluralism of care which was characteristic of the period.[6]

Thus, in an economically expanding Europe, and especially in Mediterranean societies, this new medicine had a privileged place in the emerging universities (GARCÍA-BALLESTER 1994: 105-130), enabling their doctors to establish relations with the leading groups in European cities until, at the beginning of the 14th century, they became the true *artifices factivi sanitatis* (GARCÍA-BALLESTER 1995). Progressively, this new medicine, transmitted in universities, circulated among both popular and cultured channels. One of the most obvious proofs of this is to be found, for example, in the presence of medical language in poetic texts:

> One of the most explicit intersections between late medieval poetic and medical texts lies at the lexical level, as the language of healing becomes incorporated in verse, from descriptions of the sensory and cognitive faculties in Guido Cavalcanti's «*Dona me prega*» (late thirteenth century) to diagnoses of melancholy and playful allusions to uroscopy in the verse of Charles d'Orléans (mid-fifteenth century). The adoption of such language has been interpreted, in most of the critical literature, as evidence of the cultural capital of medical theory (SINGER 2011: 7).

From the end of the 13th century and the beginning of the 14th century onwards, the health discourses and practices of university medicine began to have a special impact in the construction of urban public policies, with particular emphasis on the defence of the city against epidemic crisis (ARRIZABALAGA 2001: 19-32). «The growing faith in medicine manifested by individuals» (McVAUGH 1993: 190) should be interpreted within what we know today as the process of medicalisation, since aspects of human behaviour that were previously perceived as normal or deviant –or good or bad– by the lay public, began to be controlled by the medical gaze and ended up being redefined as health or illness –relinquished of their moral overtones–.

The beginning of this first stage of medicalisation is already visible in the urban social order of the early 14th century. For example, the authorities of the Crown of Aragon were particularly keen to ensure the continued availability of medical advice for its inhabitants through the designation of municipal doctors and surgeons (FERRAGUD 2005).[7] This is one of the earliest signs of a swelling social conviction that medical learning carried authority and could be trusted, as from about 1300 on, local communities began to transfer jurisdiction over

6. For an overview of medical pluralism during the late Middle Ages, based on a case study centered on the Crown of Aragon, see: FERRAGUD 2007: 107-137.

7. These designations were the origin of medical assistance to the diseased by means of the *conductio* (GARCÍA-BALLESTER 1995).

various forms of social behaviour to the independent authority of physicians and surgeons (McVaugh 1993: 190).

Consequently, this type of medicalization was not only marked by the appropriation of medical language in clearly non-medical contexts, but also by the growing appointment of medical experts as supervisors of certain social aspects.

### 3.2. *The Biggest Medieval Epidemics and its Impact on the Development of the Medicalisation Process*

With the arrival of the Black Death in Europe, in the middle of the 14th century, health definitively converted into a common good as well as an individual one (Barceló-Prats, Bueno 2021: 107-135). This new collective significance began to be perceived, especially amongst the urban elites, as indispensable for the correct functioning of society and it had «repercusiones políticas y consecuencias prácticas en la vida cotidiana de las comunidades»[8] (Arrizabalaga 2014: 36).

One of these consequences was the definitive consolidation of the role of university doctors in the good governance of the *res publica* (Montford 2004). Indeed, one of the most eloquent examples of the growing notoriety acquired by these doctors in the preservation of *publicam valetudinem* can be found, in 1348, when Jaume d'Agramunt, a physician from the city of Lleida (Spain), wrote *Regiment de preservació a epidèmia e pestilència e mortaldats* (Agramunt [1348] 1998).[9] The significance of this treatise on protective measures against the Black Death, the first of its kind to be written in Europe, is that it was written for the instruction of the governing bodies and the residents of Lleida and not for other doctors (Roca-Cabau 2018: 22-37).

This is just one example of why, beyond the limited individual and social effectiveness of the technical care practised by university doctors, the Western urban population of the late Middle Ages came to identify this figure as a health provider (Legan 2015). The cyclical repetitions of the Black Death and the mortality that it caused put the medical university system and its credibility to the test. Despite this, is no less true to say that, in the end, it came out strongly consolidated (Cifuentes 2006: 105). In the same manner, although the ability of the great epidemic cycle that began in 1348 to transform the understanding of care for certain vulnerable groups is still a matter of dispute,[10] « the links between the various late medieval epidemics and the urban elites' concern for public health

8. English translation: «political repercussions and practical consequences in the daily life of the communities».

9. The part of the *Regiment* of Jaume d'Agramunt that is highlighted in this text is discussed in detail in (García-Ballester, Arrizabalaga 1998: 13-31).

10. *A priori*, it seems different to dissociate the impact of mortality on the structure of the labor market from the consequent laws to limit vagrancy and to reinforce public safety and health policies. However, based on the case study of Florence, it was argued that «there is little proof that in Florence the Black Death led to new distinctions between the worthy and unworthy poor» (Henderson 1994: 304).

and the perception of destitution as a source of disease and contagion are also evident» (BRIDGEWATER 2020: 201). Thus, during the 14th century, sordid, strident, and unpleasant groups began to be identified in the eyes of the leading members of a supposedly orderly urban society (MOLLAT 1988: 229; GEREMEK 1998: 56). Hence, the emergence of these new forms of poverty, intrinsically urban and associated with economic and demographic crises, exacerbated a distrust based on the fear of anonymity, idleness, disease, and turmoil. All this, put together, culminated in a series of transformations in both the ideology and practice of care in the late medieval world.

It was precisely the increase in this distrust of poverty that made hospitals indispensable tools for the proper functioning of the late medieval city (JETTER 1972).[11] However, the small hospitals that existed at the end of the 14th century, which were widely spread throughout the territory but lacking in coordination and medical supervision –as well as carrying out very unspecific care functions– were unable to adapt to the social and economic changes that emerged in the Late Middle Ages (ROCA-CABAU 2018: 40).

## 4. *The Necessity of a New Hospital Policy*

From the 15th century onwards, in the Crown of Aragon, this model of small hospitals with unspecific functions entered into a definitive crisis and was gradually substituted by a smaller number of larger institutions (GALLENT 2012: 41-60). Thus, the so-called general hospitals were a result of a political strategy intended to respond, through processes of hospital reduction, to the new social, welfare and economic challenges of the late medieval period. This forced a hospital reform through Latin Europe that had two notable characteristics (BIANCHI, SŁÓN 2006: 12-13). The first consisted of an incipient medicalization of hospital care, whereby medical care, whether provided by physicians of surgeons, was seen as of particular value to some hospital administrators and employers. This said "hospital medicalization", defined in these terms, had different rhythms in various medieval and modern European territories. While in some areas of Italy (PICCINNI 2016: 8-26) and the Crown of Aragon (FERRAGUD 2014: 305-324) the doctors became even more associated with hospitals after 1350, maybe as a reaction to the arrival of the Black Death, in England the first doctors attached to the London hospitals cannot be found until the beginning of the 16th century (MCVAUGH 1993: 229).

The development of this second characteristic led to the birth of a new institution of care –the general hospital–, which can be understood either as a product of the merger of small hospitals to create a unique institution or the creation of *ex-novo* large-scale care buildings. Thus, the strategy of the political authori-

11. LINDGREN (1977-1978: 32-53) provides an overview of the evolution of hospital care from antiquity to the 15th century.

ties, both civil (municipalities and the Crown) and ecclesiastical (bishops and religious orders), was to concentrate or merge the assets of the small hospitals of a city,[12] not only to be able to create and maintain a larger and more efficient hospital, but to also make it a symbol of pride for the citizens:

> The rise of large urban hospitals during the late Middle Ages can be explained by the ascription to a series of characteristics, not necessarily standardized, which we have brought together under the concept of referentiality. We use this concept to define the success of a number of large urban hospitals, capable of generating admiration and adherence. Large hospitals may be associated with certain desirable processes, such as administrative rationalization and economies of scale, but also with more diffuse epithets (which were certainly more important in the medieval imaginary) such as nobility, fame and beauty. Herein lies the potential to capture the attention of potential donors, both from the immediate environment and at the interregional level, in a historical context marked by medical pluralism and a non-hospital-centric healthcare culture. (Bridgewater 2020: 332).

A pioneering experience in the creation of the large general hospital took place in Barcelona, in 1401, with the inauguration of the Hospital of the Holy Cross (Lindgren 1980: 14-137). Founded from the merging of six of the city's pre-existing hospitals, its new building was praised as «*lum, noblesa, ornament, laor, gloria e amplitud*»[13] (Conejo 2014: 415). This hospital strategy quickly became a point of reference for the rest of the cities in the Crown of Aragon (Martínez-Vidal, 2002).

The consolidation of this hospital model in the Crown of Aragon took place throughout the 15th century and the first-half of the 16th century, not only in large cities, but also in smaller ones (López-Terrada 1999: 177-200). Thus, in 1425 Zaragoza inaugurated its general hospital; Lleida, in 1454; Mallorca, in 1456; Tarragona, in 1464; and Valencia did so in 1512. These processes of hospitals downsizing to make way for the creation of a large general hospital also occurred, to cite a couple of other examples, in the Crown of Castille (Arrizabalaga 1999) and in parts of northern Italy (Piccinni 2017: 319-152). However, even though some cases are also documented in the late 15th and early 16th centuries, in the latter two territories the extinction of small hospitals in order to create a "general hospital" did not become a common phenomenon until the mid-16th century, and it was sometimes delayed until the 17th century. This shows the chronological diversity of these processes.

In turn, the emergence of general hospitals opened the possibility of assisting more specific groups of poor people and providing more specialized care for their needs. In other words, the hospital for the poor gave way to the hospital for the sick poor (Arrizabalaga 2006: 204), in a context still marked by the pluralism of care and a medical culture that had still not thought of the hospital as a sanitary space.

12. An example, center in Barcelona, of how medieval hospitals managed their assets, can be found in (Lindgren 1987: 525-532).

13. English translation: «light, nobility, ornament, praiseworthiness, glory and breadth».

Nevertheless, there is yet another novelty to be noted in the European panorama of the 15th and 16th centuries. In addition to general hospitals, hospitals for the treatment of specific diseases such as the French disease –syphilis– also began to emerge (ARRIZABALAGA 2021: 277-293). In this respect, it is also important to remember the division that began to exist during the late medieval period, and which expanded in the early modern period, between general hospitals and the hospitals for the incurable such as those that catered to the insane (HUGUET, ARRIZABALAGA 2010). Different from general hospitals, these models of medicalization of care for certain groups of poor people suffering from a specific disease, whether infectious –like syphilis– or uncurable –madness– had important implications in the evolution of the concept of a hospital for the sick poor (ARRIZABALAGA 2006: 204). Beyond the result of this unstoppable trend towards an increasingly organized and systematic pattern of care, the fact remains that the poor continued to be, for the most part, the object of hospital care during the modern period (TOMASSETTI 2019: 91-127).

In conclusion, it can be stated that, independent of the various transformations that European hospitals experimented during the course of the late medieval and modern centuries, the model of the general hospital that emerged at the beginning of the 15th century remained essentially unchanged throughout the *Ancien Régime*. In this arena, it was the hospital administrators –as the legal representatives of the institution– who held and exercised power over the day-to-day running of the institution, while the doctors were only employed by them to practice in the hospital (CRANSHAW 1993, 1184-1186). As such, social rather than strictly medical criteria usually weighed more heavily in the admission process. Thus, as was already mentioned in the introduction, it was not until the end of the 18th century and throughout the 19th century that, in the context of the new bourgeois and liberal order, the hospital became a medical institution.

## 5. *Conclusions*

In the preceding pages, we have discussed the relationship between the development of the process of medicalisation and the changes in hospitals during the Middle Ages and the modern centuries from a historical perspective of longue durée. In this way, we have explored how the first phase of medicalisation consolidated medical expertise as an essential element in secularising the knowledge and meaning of illness, giving physicians the status of *artifex factivus sanitatis*, while at the same time a sanitary reorganisation of cities took place.

In the meantime, the traditional medieval hospitals –with very unspecific care functions for all kinds of poor people– showed their inability to respond to the socio-political changes that were taking place in the late Middle Ages. As a result, hospital institutions underwent two fundamental changes: concentration and an incipient medicalisation. On the one hand, the concentration of hospitals facilitated the emergence of a new architectural and care model of hospital

–the general hospital–. On the other hand, although hospital medicalisation did not take place in a decisive way until the end of the 18th century –with what Michel Foucault called the «birth of the clinic»– the hospital for the poor gradually evolved into the "hospital for the sick poor", acquiring increasingly specific care functions.

This text has also sought to highlight how medicalisation, if considered as a cultural process –without forgetting other facets–, can be a useful analytical tool, also from a historical perspective, to approach everything related to health and illness. That is, for example, the relations that occur between experts and non-experts, between the local and the global, between collectivities and individuals, and everything related to the roots that currently shape the logics of hegemony and subalternity inherent to any culture of health.

For this reason, this text has not only related hospitals to concepts such as hospitality, charity, epidemic management, and the shaping of medical knowledge, but also to notions indirectly related to health and illness, such as the common good and the governance of the *res publica*.

## *Bibliography*


Abumalham, Montserrat, 2006. "La hospitalidad en el Islam", *Scripta Fulgentina. Revista de Teología y Humanidades*, 16/31-32: 95-109.

Ackerknecht, Erwin H., 1967. *Medicine at the Paris hospital, 1794-1848,* Baltimore, The Johns Hopkins University Press.

Agramunt, Jaume, [1348] 1998. *Regiment de preservació de pestilencia (Lleida 1348)*, ed. Luis García-Ballester, Joan Veny, Jon Arrizabalaga, Barcelona, Enciclopèdia Catalana.

Albini, Giuliana, 2002. *Carità e governo delle povertà (seccoli XII-XV)*, Milan, Unicopli.

Albini, Giuliana, 2013. "L'Osservanza francescana e la practica della carità. Uno sguardo alle città dell'Italia centro-settentrionale", *I frati osservanti e la società in Italia nel sec. XV, Atti del XL convegno internazionale in occasionedel 550° anniversario della fondazione del Monte di Pietà di Perugia, Assisi-Perugia, 11-13 ottobre 2012*, Spoleto, Società Internazionale di Studi Francescani e Fondazione Centro Italiano Studi Sull'Alto Medioevo: 227-251.

Arrizabalaga, Jon, 1999. "Poor Relief in Counter-Reformation Castile: An Overview", Oleg Grell, Andrew Cunningham, Jon Arrizabalaga (ed.), *Health care and Poor Relief in Counter-Reformation Europe*, London-New York, Routledge: 151-76.

Arrizabalaga, Jon, 2001. "Discurso médico y prácticas sanitarias frente a la enfermedad epidémica en la Europa medieval", *Demografía y sociedad en la España bajomedieval,* Zaragoza, Universidad de Zaragoza: 19-32.

Arrizabalaga, Jon, 2006. "Hospitals, història i medicina: l'Hospital de la Santa Creu de Barcelona", *Actes de la VIII Trobada d'Història de la Ciència i de la Tècnica*, Barcelona, Institut d'Estudis Catalans: 203-209.

Arrizabalaga, Jon, 2014. "Asistencia, caridad y nueva ética de la responsabilidad colectiva ante la salud y la pobreza en el espacio urbano occidental del Antiguo Régimen", Teresa Huguet, Pere Verdés, Jon Arrizabalaga, Manuel Sánchez (ed.), *Ciudad y hospital en el Occidente Europeo (1300-1700)*, Lleida, Milenio: 27-48.

Arrizabalaga, Jon, 2021. "Hospital care of venereal disease patients in Mediterranean Europe, 1495-1700", Yann Ardagna, Benoît Pouget (ed.), *La syphilis. Itineraires croisés en Méditerranée et au-delà, XVI*e*-XXI*e *siècles*, Aix-en- Provence, Presses Universitaires de Provence: 277-293

Barceló-Prats, Josep; Bueno, Eduardo, 2021. "Epidemias, medicalización y evolución hospitalaria: bases para una historia de las culturas de la salud y de la enfermedad", *Anais de História de Além-Mar*, 22: 107-135

Barceló-Prats, Josep, 2022. "La influencia de las grandes epidemias en la configuración histórica del proceso de medicalización y en la evolución hospitalaria", Margarita Vilar, Jerònia Pons (ed.), *Los hospitales y las pandemias en España e Italia desde una perspectiva histórica*, Alicante, Universitat d'Alacant: 27-55.

Bianchi, Francesco; Slón, Marek, 2006, "Le riforme ospedaliere del quattrocento in Italia e nel-l'Europa centrale", *Ricerche di Storia Sociale e Religiosa*, 35/69: 7-45.

Bridgewater, Pol, 2020. *Car vosaltres havets a veure sobre hospitals: el Consell de Cent i la construcció de la primera política hospitalària a la Barcelona baixmedieval*. PhD thesis, Universitat de Barcelona.

Cifuentes, Lluis, 2006. *La ciència en català a l'Edat Mitjana i el Renaixement,* Barcelona, Universitat de Barcelona.

Comelles, Josep M., 2013. "Hospitals, political economy and the Catalan cultural identity", Christopher Bonfield, Jonathan Reinarz, Teresa Huguet (ed.), *Hospitals and Communities 1100-1960*, Oxford, Peter Lang: 183-208.

Comelles, Josep M.; Daura, Angelina; Arnau, Marina; Martín, Eduardo, 1991. *L'Hospital de Valls: assaig sobre l'estructura i transformacions de les institucions d'assistència*, Valls, Institut d'Estudis Vallencs.

Conejo, Antoni, 2013. "L'estudi dels hospitals a l'Edat Mitjana: una història sense punt i a banda", *Svmma. Revista de Cultures Medievals*, 2: 3-6.

Conejo, Antoni, 2014. "Lum, noblesa, ornament, laor, glòria e amplitud: los hospitales y la renovada imagen de la ciudad bajomedieval", Teresa Huguet, Pere Verdés, Jon Arrizabalaga, Manuel Sánchez (ed.), *Ciudad y hospital en el Occidente Europeo (1300-1700)*, Lleida, Milenio: 415-445.

Corvisier, Jean N., 1985. *Santé e société en Grèce ancienne*, Paris, Economica.

Cranshaw, Lindsay, 1993. "The Hospital", *Companion Encyclopedia of the History of Medicine*, vol. II, London, Routledge.

Evangelisti, Paolo, 2006. *I Francescani e la costruzione di uno Stato. Linguaggi politici, valori identitari progetti di governo in area catalano-aragonese*, Padua, Editrici Francescane.

Ferragud, Carmel, 2005. *Medicina i promoció social a la Baixa Edat Mitjana (Corona d'Aragó, 1350-1410)*, Madrid, CSIC.

Ferragud, Carmel. 2007. "Los oficios relacionados con la medicina durante la Baja Edad Media en la Corona de Aragón y su proyección social", *Anuario de Estudios Medievales*, 37: 107-37.

Ferragud, Carmel, 2014, "La introducción de los practicantes de la medicina en los hospitales del reino de Valencia durante la Baja Edad Media", Teresa Huguet, Pere Verdés, Jon Arrizabalaga, Manuel Sánchez (ed.), *Ciudad y hospital en el Occidente Europeo (1300-1700)*, Lleida, Milenio: 305-324.

Forment, Eudaldo, 1996. "La integración de la ética aristotélica en la síntesis escolástica", *Actas del II Congreso Nacional de Filosofía Medieval*, Zaragoza, Sociedad de Filosofía Medieval: 51-85.

Foucault, Michel, 1963. *Naissance de la clinique. Une archéologie du regard médical,* Paris, Presses Universitaires de France.

Foucault, Michel, 1977. "Historia de la medicalización", *Educación Médica y Salud*, 11/1: 3-25.

Foucault, Michel, 1978. "Incorporación del hospital a la tecnología moderna", *Educación Médica y Salud* 12/1: 20-35.

Gallent, Mercedes, 2012. "Los hospitales de la Santa Creu de Barcelona y Nuestra Señora de Gracia de Zaragoza, dos modelos asistenciales para el Hospital General de Valencia", *Aragón en la Edad Media*, 25: 41-60

García-Ballester, Luís, 1992. "Medicina y filosofía natural en la Europa latina de los siglos XII y XIII: un debate abierto", *Arbor. Ciencia, Pensamiento y Cultura*, 558-560: 119-146.

García-Ballester, Luís, 1994. "Universidad y nueva profesión médica en la Europa latina medieval: siglos XIII y XIV", Santiago Aguadé (ed.), *Universidad, cultura y sociedad en la Edad Media*, Alcalá de Henares, Universidad de Alcalá: 105-130.

García-Ballester, Luís, 1995. "Artifex factivus sanitatis: health and medical care in medieval Latin Galenism", Don Bates (ed.), *Knowledge and the Scholarly Medical Traditions*, Cambridge, Cambridge University Press: 127-150.

García-Ballester, Luís; French, Roger; Arrizabalaga, Jon; Cunningham, Andrew (ed.), 1994. *Practical Medicine from Salerno to the Black Death*, Cambridge, Cambridge University Press.

García-Ballester, Luís; Arrizabalaga, Jon, 1998. "El *Regiment* de Jacme d'Agramont y el *Estudi* de medicina de Lleida", Luis García-Ballester, Joan Veny, Jon Arrizabalaga (ed.), *Regiment de preservació de pestilencia (Lleida 1348)*, Barcelona, Enciclopedia Catalana: 13-31.

Geremek, Bronislaw, 1998. *La piedad y la horca. Historia de la miseria y la caridad en Europa*, Barcelona, Alianza.

Gotman, Anne, 2001. *Le sens de l'hospitalité. Essai sur les fondements sociaux de l'accueil de l'autre*, Paris, PUF.

Gotman, Anne (dir.), 2004. *Villes et hospitalité. Les municipalités et leurs «étrangers»*, Paris, Mansion des Sciences de l'Homme.

Henderson, John, 1994. *Piety and Charity in Late Medieval Florence*, Oxford, Clarendon Press.

Henderson, John, 2001. "Healing the Body and Saving the Soul: Hospitals in Renaissance Florence", *Renaissance Studies*, 15/2: 188-216.

Hoces de la Guardia, Ángel, 1987. "La hospitalidad en Homero", *Gerión*, 5: 43-56.

Horden, Peregrine, 1988. "A Discipline of Relevance: The Historiography of the Later Medieval Hospital", *Social History of Medicine*, 1/3: 359-374.

Huguet, Teresa, 2004. "Una reflexió historiogràfica sobre l'hospital com a espai de medicalització", *Gimbernat*, 42: 41-48.

Huguet, Teresa, 2014. "*Speculum hospitalis, speculum civitatis*. ¿Por qué estudiar la historia de los hospitales?", Teresa Huguet, Pere Verdés, Jon Arrizabalaga, Manuel Sánchez (ed.), *Ciudad y hospital en el Occidente Europeo (1300-1700)*, Lleida, Milenio: 13-26.

Huguet, Teresa; Arrizabalaga, Jon, 2010. "Hospital Care for the Insane in Barcelona, 1400-1700", *Bulletin of Spanish Studies*, 87/8: 81-104.

Illanes, Ximena, 2019. *En manos de los otros: infancia y abandono en la Barcelona del siglo XV*, Santiago de Chile, Pontificia Universidad Católica de Chile.

Jetter, Dieter, 1972. *Geschichte des Hospitals*, vol. III, Stuttgart, Franz Steiner.

Legan, Joseph A., 2015. *The Medical Response to the Black Death*, Virginia, James Madison University.

Lindgren, Uta, 1977-1978. "Frühformen abendländischer Hospitäler im Lichte einiger Bedingungen ihrer Entstehung", *Historia Hospitalum*, 12: 32-53.

Lindgren, Uta, 1980. *Bedürftigkeit, Armut, Not. Studien zur spätmittelalterlichen Sozialegeschichte Barcelonas*, Münster-Westfalen, Aschendorffsche Verlagsbuchhandlung.

Lindgren, Uta, 1987. "¿De qué vivían los hospitales? Los fundamentos económicos de los hospitales de Barcelona de 1375 a 1500", *Anuario de Estudios Medievales*, 17: 525-532.

López-Terrada, Marialuz, 1999. "Health Care and Poor relief in the Crown of Aragon", Oleg Grell, Andrew Cunningham, Jon Arrizabalaga (ed.), *Health Care and Poor Relief in Counter-Reformation Europe*, London-New York, Routledge: 177-200.

McVaugh, Michael, 1993. *Medicine Before the Plague: Practitioners and their Patients in the Crown of Aragon 1285-1345*, Cambridge, Cambridge University Press.

Marco, Antonio, 2006. "Homeric hospitality", *Scripta Fulgentina: Revista de Teología y Humanidades*, 16/31-32: 111-122.

Martín, Eduardo; Comelles, Josep M.; Arnau, Marina, 1993. "El proceso de medicalización de los hospitales catalanes: el caso del Pío Hospital de Valls", *Dynamis*, 13: 201-234.

Martínez-García, Luís, 2008. "Pobres, pobreza y asistencia en la Edad Media hispana. Balance y perspectivas", *Medievalismo*, 18: 67-107.

MARTÍNEZ-VIDAL, Àlvar, 2002. "L'Hospital General de la Santa Creu de Barcelona: una nova institución asistencial a la Corona d'Aragó", *Annals de Medicina*, 85/4: 236-239.

MENÉNDEZ, Eduardo, 1978. "El modelo médico y la salud de los trabajadores", ed. Franco Basaglia et al. *La salud de los trabajadores*, México, Nueva Imagen: 11-53.

MENÉNDEZ, Eduardo, 2005. "El modelo médico y la salud de los trabajadores", *Salud Colectiva*, 1/1: 9-32

MILLER, Timothy S., 1985. *The Birth of the Hospital in the Byzantine Empire*, Baltimore, Johns Hopkins University Press.

MOLLAT, Michel, 1988. *Pobres, humildes y miserables en la Edad Media*, México, Fondo de Cultura Económica.

MONTFORD, Angela, 2004. *Health, Sickness, Medicine and the Friars in the Thirteenth and Fourteenth Centuries*, Aldershot, Ashgate.

NUTTON, Vivian, 1981. "Continuity or rediscovery: the city physician in Classical Antiquity and in the Middle Ages", Andrew L. Russell (ed.), *The Town and State Physician in Europe, from the Middle Ages to Enlightenment*, Wolfenbüttel, Herzog August Bibliothek: 10-46.

PERDIGUERO, Enrique; RUIZ, Mª Dolores, 2017. "Medicalización ¿Un concepto útil? Reflexiones a propósito de la investigación histórica de la cultura de la salud", Alfons Zarzoso, Jon Arrizabalaga (ed.), *Al servicio de la salud humana. La historia de la medicina ante los retos del siglo XXI*, Sant Feliu de Guíxols, Sociedad Española de Historia de la Medicina: 247-252.

PICCINNI, Gabriella, 2016. "I modelli ospedalieri e la loro circolazione dall'Italia all'Europa alla fine del Medioevo", Gregoria Cavero (ed.), *Civitas Bendita. Encrucijada de las relaciones sociales y de poder en la ciudad medieval*, León, Universidad de León: 8-26.

PICCINNI, Gabriella, 2017. "I grandi ospedali urbani dell'Italia medievale: all'origine del 'welfare'", Flocel Sabaté (ed.), *L'assistència a l'Edat Mitjana*, Lleida, Pagès: 139-152.

PIÑOL, Adrià, 2013. "Hesíodo: de una hospitalidad heroica a una hospitalidad pragmática", *Faventia*, 2/extra: 47-56.

PITT-RIVERS, Julián, 1971. *Tres ensayos de antropología estructural. Contexto y modelo; La ley de la hospitalidad; Derecho de asilo y hospitalidad sexual en el Mediterráneo*, Barcelona, Anagrama.

ORTEGA, Alfonso, 2006. "La hospitalidad en el nuevo testamento", *Scripta Fulgentina. Revista de Teología y Humanidades*, 16/31-32: 83-94.

RISSE, Guenter B., 1996. "Before the Clinic was 'Born': Methodological Perspectives in Hospital History", Norbert Finzsch, Robert Jütte (ed.), *Institutions of Confinement. Hospitals, Asylums, and Prisons in Western Europe and North America, 1500-1950*, Cambridge, Cambridge University Press: 75-96.

RISSE, Guenter B., 1999. *Mending Bodies, Saving Souls. A History of Hospitals*, Oxford, Oxford University Press.

RIU, Manuel, 1980. *La pobreza y la asistencia a los pobres en la Cataluña medieval. Volumen misceláneo de estudios y documentos*, Barcelona, CSIC.

ROCA-CABAU, Guillem, 2018, "Medidas municipales contra la peste en la Lleida del siglo XIV e inicios del XV", *Dynamis*, 38/1: 15-39.

ROSENWEIN, Barbara H.; LITTLE, Lester K., 1974. "Social Meaning in the Monastic and Mendicant Spiritualities", *Past and Present*, 63: 4-32.

RUBIO VELA, Agustín, 1981. "Una fundación burguesa en la Valencia medieval: El Hospital de en Clapers (1311)", *Dynamis*, 1: 17-49.

SINGER, Julie, 2011. *Blindness and Therapy in Late Medieval French and Italian Poetry*, Cambridge, Boydell & Brewer.

TODESCHINI, Giacomo, 2008. "Le Bien commun de la civitas christiana dans la tradition textuelle franciscane (XIIIe-XV[e] siècle)", Henri Bresc, Georges Dagher & Christiane Veauvy (dir.), *Politique et religion en Méditerranée. Moyen Âge et époque contemporaine*, Paris, Bouchène: 265-303.

TODESCHINI, Giacomo, 2010. "Participer au bien commun: la notion franciscaine d'appartenance à la *civitas*", Élodie Lecuppre, Anne-Laure Van Bruaene (dir.), *De bono comuni. The Discourse* *and Practice of the Common Good in the European City ($13^{th}$-$16^{th}$ c.)*, Turnhout, Brepols: 225-236.

Tomassetti, Stefano, 2019. "Dentro e fuori l'ospedale di età moderna. Idee, pratiche, contesti", *Storica,* 25/74: 91-127.

Vinyoles, Teresa, 2013. "El rastre dels més desvalguts entre els papers de l'Hospital de Barcelona", *Svmma: Revista de Cultures Medievals*, 2: 77-101.

Pol Bridgewater Mateu

# The Integration of the Hospital of the Holy Cross in the Urban Ceremonial of Medieval Barcelona*

The medieval hospital is a strange object of study. On a superficial glance, medieval hospitals often evoke images of poverty, sickness, and filth, but seldomly of beauty. This is, of course, a somehow unperceptive appreciation, mostly rooted in popular perceptions of the Middle Ages as a whole. Despite this, it is not totally lacking in base. Indeed, fear of contagion, or at least a vague understanding of physical undesirableness, is perfectly documentable when it comes to the medieval common sense on hospitals. Francesc Eiximenis (1330-1409), one of the most widely read author of the Catalan late Middle Ages (Wittlin 1993:441-459; Hernando 2007; Juncosa 2011:156), wrote that hospitals had to be placed, together with brothels, leprosariums, places of gambling, and sewage systems, far from the city centre and contrary to the direction of the most common winds, so their stench, both material and spiritual, would not contaminate the city itself.[1]

This theoretic approach coincided with private initiatives and public policies alike that tended to place, or even relocate, hospitals to the periphery of more or less dense urban centres.[2] But, beyond this apparent trend, a more complex reality emerges: on the one hand, the relegation of hospitals into the urban outskirts was far from absolute in the Middle Ages. One of the best-known hospitals of Central Italy, that of Santa Maria della Scala in Siena, was nowhere else but right in front of the city's *duomo*, and therefore in the very centre of the city's symbolic and ceremonial heart.[3] On the other hand, in the cases in which this peripheric placement did occur, its reasons could go beyond the fear of contagion. Aspects such as the control of gates and entry and exit routes, achieving a more fluid contact with pilgrims, or the availability of land and resources such as water could be as important in the placement of a hospital, if not more.

*This present study is part of the research project *De Ipsos Kastellos: Hàbitat i fortaleses de muntanya a la Catalunya Medieval (S. IX-XIII).* ARQ001SOL-161-2022 (2022-2025).

1. Eiximenis, *Lo Crestià*. book. xii, chap. cx, ed. Hauf 1983: 190: «Hospitals, llocs de llebrosos, bordells e tafureries, e escorriments de clavegueres, deuen estar a la part contrària d'aquell vent qui més s'usa en la ciutat, per tal que lo vent aquell no tir les infections del dit lloc, ans les lluny e no les hi lleix acostar».

2. We can see some examples of this trend in this same book, with the contributions of Guillem Roca on the case of Lleida or Esther Diana on the case of Prato.

3. On the hospital of Santa Maria della Scala of Siena, see Fabio Gabbrielli's contribution in this volume.

The case of the hospital of the Holy Cross of Barcelona fits within this complexity. Created as the merger of six previously existing hospitals in 1401 (Bridgewater 2020: 178-228), its location was mediated by different factors, such as the necessity of space or the possibility of reusing some of the aforementioned hospital structures. Indeed, the new hospital, conceived as a large, impactful building, was built in the Raval of Barcelona, a peripheral and relatively sparsely populated part of the city, and on top of the hospital d'en Colom, one of the institutions that took part in the 1401 merger. However, this relatively peripheral location did not entail that the hospital was relegated to the margins of the urban self-imagination. As we have already said, the new hospital was created as an intendedly great institution, that had to provoke admiration among Barcelonians and foreigners alike. In fact, this capacity to create emulation and capture the attention of its contemporaries was one of the keys to its survival across the centuries. A large, beautified, well-governed hospital was the ideal vehicle for enterprises of collective salvation that materialised in alms and bequests (Conejo 2017; 2018; 2020; Sánchez 2014).[4] Therefore, a dignified placement of the hospital into the city's symbolic landscape was of great importance: it did not only facilitate the hospital's thriving, but it served to represent the political community as an intrinsically pious association (Evangelisti 2015: 136). This symbolic integration could happen in different ways, chief among them through urban civic-religious ceremonies.

We can identify two main types of ceremonies that interacted, on several levels, with the Hospital of the Holy Cross: on the one hand, ceremonies that had the hospital at their very centre. On the other hand, those that, despite having a different raison d'être, interacted with the hospital in some capacity. In both cases, the ceremonies themselves could be of very different nature: religious processions, the entry of a king or a member of the royal family, or a gift of rich cloths or relics. Similarly, both types of ceremonies put the hospital in contact with a variety of actors and institutions, such as the bishop and chapter of Barcelona, the municipal government, and, on a more abstract level, the embodiment of the city itself.

Taking this into account, in this chapter we will describe and analyse the most important urban ceremonies that interacted with the hospital of the Holy Cross of Barcelona during the 15th century and dwell on their importance for the inclusion of the hospital into the city's symbolic landscape.

## 1. *The Hospital as Protagonist: Hospital-centric Ceremonies in 15th Century Barcelona*

The first urban ceremony associated with the hospital was related to nothing else than its founding. The aforementioned process of hospital fusion was re-

4. The recent thesis of Jaume Marcé (2023: 283-318) has dwelled more deeply in the role of alms in the funding mechanisms of the hospital of the Holy Cross.

markably swift: its first references appear in February of 1401 and, a few months later, in 17 April 1401, Barcelona saw its ceremony of foundation: a procession left from the cathedral, the city's most noble church and ceremonial heart, exited the 13th century walls through the gate of the *Boqueria*, and reached its objective, where the hospital's first stones were solemnly laid (fig. 1). The event served as a physical manifestation of the public's commitment towards the hospital and, especially, the dedication of the institutions that had promoted and benefited the initiative. Indeed, the laying of the four stones weaved a tapestry of the powers that be of 15th century Barcelona. Significantly, three of the four stones were laid by members of the royal house of Aragon: King Martin I; his wife, Queen Maria; and Count James of Prades, on behalf of Martin of Sicily, the King's son and heir. The fourth stone was laid by the *consellers* of Barcelona,[5] and, according to some sources, the city's bishop.[6] The strong presence of the monarchy has surprised some scholars (HUGUET-TERMES 2010), since the hospital merger was promoted and directed by the city council and the bishop and chapter of Barcelona. In this sense, the representative nature of the ceremony helps us dissipate some doubts. On the one hand, it stressed the natural hierarchy of powers of medieval society and Barcelona and the Crown of Aragon more specifically: if present, the King and his royal family took preference in all civic ceremonies, independently of their reason or nature (RAUFAST 2006-2007: 94). On the other hand, Martin I and his family were among the earliest and most important benefactors of the hospital, granting it privileges, donations, and bequests (CONEJO 2002: 165, 295-297). In all, the ceremony represented the commitment of the city's secular and ecclesiastical power towards the hospital, and more importantly, gave a solemn opening to a welfare institution that was meant as different, and elevated from the rest.

Beyond the foundation ceremony, other rites, festivities, and processions directly linked the hospital with the city and its government. In the mid-15th century, the hospital of the Holy Cross was once again the privileged protagonist of an extraordinary procession, organized to bestow the hospital with a relic.[7] In 1450, Barcelona's ambassadors to Naples obtained a finger of Saint Candida, one of the city's patrons, from Archbishop Gaspar de Diano.[8] The gift was not necessarily

5. The five *consellers* (councillors) were five citizens who constituted the elected holders of the city's executive power. They were also the main representatives of the city and hold places of priority in urban ceremonies.

6. Arxiu de l'Hospital de la Santa Creu i Sant Pau (from now on AHSCP), *Privilegis reials, doc. papals, doc. particulars*. Vol. VIII. Inv. 8. Carpeta 6/1/4. Confirmació reial de la confraria de la Santa Creu. Edited at ROCA 1920: 110-121.

7. Urban processions can be divided into ordinary and extraordinary. The former were repeated regularly in commemoration of a significant date, usually religious. The later were ceremonies that happened on exceptional occasions and with specific forms that did not have an immediate precedent (FERNÁNDEZ-CUADRENCH 2005: 404-405).

8. See the document of reception, signed in Naples, in the AHSCP, *Privilegis reials, doc. papals, doc. particulars.* Vol. VIII. Inv. 8. Folder 6/3/10. A second document of reception, this time signed by the Barcelonian notary Francesc Terrassa, can be found in the Arxiu Històric de Protocols of Barcelona (AHPB), Francesc Terrassa, leg. 2, man 5. 1450-1451. See the edited document in

rare. Barcelona and Naples had enjoyed a privileged relationship since the accession of King Alfonso the Magnanimous to the Neapolitan throne in 1442, and the great Italian city counted with a strong presence of Barcelonians and Catalans more generally. These Catalans acted both as political and commercial agents, linking both cities that now shared the same monarch and strengthening political ties (Carrère 1977: 481-482; Riera 2003: 65-83). In this context, the exchange and circulation of relics was part of the normal practice of medieval diplomacy (Castillo 1994: 65-83).

The relevance of the gift laid in the fact that the *consellers* of Barcelona opted, nine years later, to donate it to the hospital. The reasons behind the government's decision are not entirely clear in the extant documentation: it is possible that the cult of Saint Candida had hospital reminiscences, since it was linked with the Saint's welcoming of the apostle Peter during his passage through Naples, who, at the same time, would have cured Candida of a serious illness (Lucherini 2010: 533, 543-544). Beyond the dubious specific symbolism of the relic,[9] it is more likely that the aldermen simply intended to signify their link with the hospital as a privileged depository of public piety, and to imbue the Holy Cross and its church with a new symbolic and spiritual weight through the giving of a sacred and precious object.

Indeed, on 17 November 1459, after almost a decade since the arrival of the relic in the city, the municipal government agreed that the finger of the Neapolitan saint should be kept in a «beautiful reliquary» (fig. 2), in order to be deposited in a chapel of the hospital's church.[10] The handover ceremony, which was also carefully planned, was held on November 23. The event shared some characteristics with the city's main processional routes, but it also had particularities that betrayed its reason for being, which was strictly linked to the hospital. The docu-

Madurell 1963: 356, doc. 320. On 5 January 1451 the councillors of Barcelona sent a letter to the bishop of Naples, in which they thanked him for sending the relic. Arxiu Històric de la Ciutat de Barcelona (AHCB), *Rúbriques de Bruniquer*, vol 3, chap. 43, f. 112v.

9. Both the document that describes the delivery of the relic in 1450 and the documentation generated around its final transfer to the hospital make repeated references to the great devotion that Barcelonians had towards the Neapolitan saint. Similarly, Madurell (1963: 55-56) attributes the solemnity of the ceremony to the «traditional devotion in Catalonia» towards the saint and mentions some avocations, including a chapel and hospital in Santa Eulàlia de Provençana. Despite this, it is difficult to demonstrate a prominent presence of the cult of Saint Candida in 15th century Barcelona, beyond these anecdotal reports.

10. References to the planning of the ceremony appear in AHCB, *Deliberacions* 12, f. 180v, 182r. 1459, November 16-17; *Registre d'ordinacions* 8, f. 106. 1459, November 21. As for the handing over ceremony, we have extensive accounts of the event in the *Manual de Novells i Ardits*, the *Dietari de la Generalitat de Catalunya*, and the *Llibre de Jornades*, the last two by notary Jaume Safont, who included a drawing of the reliquary. Both the *Manual of Novells i Ardits* and the Safont versions are fully compatible, although they have some differences: the *Manual* was written from a perspective that clearly placed the municipal government at the centre of the ceremony and included the presence of the hospital administrators, which was ignored by Safont. AHCB, *Manual de Novells i Ardits*, edited by Schwartz, Carreras-Candi 1893, vol. I: 322-323; Arxiu Nacional de Catalunya (ANC), *Dietari de la Generalitat de Catalunya*, vol I, f. 40r, dir. Sans-Travé 1994: 151-152; Biblioteca de Catalunya (BC), *Dietari o llibre de jornades*, f. 62v.

mentation contemporaneous with the events records a processional itinerary that began at the city's cathedral, with a solemn mass officiated by Arnau Roger de Pallars, bishop of d'Urgell and patriarch of Alexandria (BATLLE 1978: 215-236; 2006-2007: 569-625), in representation of the absent bishop of Barcelona. After leaving the cathedral, the procession passed through the gate of the *Boqueria,* entered the Raval and deposited the relic in the hospital, from where it returned to the old city centre through the *carrer del Carme* (fig. 3).

As with other solemn processions, the event brought together a large representation of Barcelona's citizenship, hierarchically ordered according to their station, but it was also accompanied by a more diffuse mass, a «great crowd of people», attracted by the spectacle of the event and the promises of indulgence and forgiveness, either granted directly by the bishop and patriarch or through the miraculous intercession of the saint. At the head of the procession, musicians played string and wind instruments that gave the act its necessary air of festivity and solemnity, and made way for the main authorities, civil and religious, of the city and the country, who occupied the most prominent positions: the five councillors of Barcelona and Galceran de Requesens, governor of Catalonia, held the six staffs on which rested the golden cloth that, like a pall, housed the relic, accompanied by the bishop. By his side, the administrators occupied a significant central place.[11]

It is difficult to ignore, however, that despite the inclusivity and wide scope of the procession, the documentation powerfully conveys a sense of municipal agency. Certainly, the bishop and the Cathedral's clergy were privileged participants. However, and always according to the documentation generated by the municipality, the arrival of the precious relic had been the result, above all, of the efforts of the secular government of the city. It must be said that the ambassadors had obtained the saint's finger from Naples with the support of the bishop of Barcelona. Indeed, the notarial document of reception specifies that the donation had happened «*cum consensu tamen reverendissimi domini Barchinone episcopi, si et in quantum facere potest quadraginta dies indulgencia*».[12] Despite this, the decision to transfer it to the hospital had been taken by the city's secular government. In the *Manual de Novells i Ardits*, the recognition of municipal agency takes perhaps its most explicit form:

> In the light of the presence of the honourable ser Joan de Marimon and ser Bernat ça Pila, citizens, in Naples with our lord the King, acting as messengers of this city, they obtained one finger of the Virgin Saint Candida, which was kept in the House of the City, where it was not being shown [to the public].[13]

11. AHCB, *Manual de Novells i Ardits*, edited by SCHWARTZ, CARRERAS-CANDI 1893, vol. I: 323. «E finit lo dit offici precedents XIIJ trompetes e IIJ tabalers e ab sobrevestes e panons de la Ciutat anant sonant ab llurs trompes e fluviols, e VJ sonadors de corde qui sonaven devant la custòdia de la relíquia isqueren de la dita Seu per lo portal maior».

12. AHPB, Francesc Terrassa, leg. 2, man 5. 1450-1451. Edited at MADURELL 1963: 356, doc. 320.

13. AHCB, *Manual de Novells i Ardits*, edited by SCHWARTZ, CARRERAS-CANDI 1893, vol. II: 323.

As the city's chronicler reminds us, the arrival of the relic in Barcelona was the result of an embassy from its secular, municipal government. The same government that had jealously guarded it in its headquarters until it thought it fit to transfer it to the hospital, where it could be adored by the citizens of Barcelona and the hospital's patients alike.

Beyond the opulence of these great ceremonies, the bond between the city and the hospital of the Holy Cross was also expressed in more modest ways. From the mid-15th century on, we can document the regular delivery of liturgical cloths to the hospital, on behalf of the municipal councillors:

> On the said day, by order of the honourable councillors, VIIII long cloth pieces and VI table and bench covers, two of the new ones depicting angels and four depicting savage men, were delivered to the honourable Bertran Desvalls, citizen, one of the administrators of the hospital of the Holy Cross, by me, Joan Oliver, notary and scribe of the office of the *racional,* so they could decorate the chapel of said hospital of the Holy Cross. They were subsequently restored.[14]

The delivery of cloths continued over time, with very similar forms, throughout the 15th century. In fact, it is very likely that the same pieces were routinely delivered, with the same embroidered motifs of angels and wild men.[15] In some cases, we can document additions or substitutions and even the reuse of other fabrics that were already in the hands of the government: in the delivery of May 24th, 1454 a municipal officer gave to the hospital, in addition to the usual cloths embroidered with angels and wild men, four bench covers «*dels brots*», probably with floral motifs, and other pieces of fabric.[16]

The giving of these ceremonial cloths, although simple, had several layers of symbolic meaning. It recalled the link between the municipal government and the hospital, this time centred around key dates in the festive calendar of both the city and the hospital itself. The transfer of the pieces of cloth and covers was a key part of the mass that commemorated the Invention of the True Cross, the sacred object that gave its name to the hospital, and therefore allowed for the participation of the municipal government, one of the institution's two co-patrons, in the celebration of such an important day. In the delivery of 5 May 1456, it was specified that the set of textiles had to be displayed «for the feast of said hospital, which will be on the first coming Sunday».[17] At the same time, more exception-

14. AHCB, *Manual de Novells i Ardits*, edited by Schwartz, Carreras-Candi 1893, vol. II: 32. In the original Catalan: «Lo dit die de manament dels honorables consellers fforen lliurats al honorable mossenyor Bertran dez Vall, ciutadà, I dels administradors del Hospital de Sancta Creu per mi Johan Oliver notari e scriva del offici de Racional VIIII draps de peus e VI bancals, los II nous dels Àngels, e los IIII dels homens salvatges, los quals dix havia mester per enpaliar la cappella del dit hospital de Sancta Creu. Après foren restituhits».

15. AHCB, *Manual de Novells i Ardits*, edited by Schwartz, Carreras-Candi 1893, vol. II: 67, 143, 164, 182, 230

16. *Ibidem*: 182.

17. «A ops de la feste del dit hospital, qui serà digmenge primer vinent» (AHCB, *Manual de Novells i Ardits*, edited by Schwartz, Carreras-Candi 1893, vol. II: 230).

ally, we can document deliveries on significant days of the liturgical calendar and on the occasion of other solemn acts, such as the aforementioned procession of the relic of Saint Candida.[18]

## 2. *The Hospital as a Guest: The Inclusion of the Hospital of the Holy Cross in Barcelona's Ceremonies*

In Barcelona, processions, as the urban ceremony par excellence, used to start at the Cathedral and, from there, they took specific paths that, despite a certain variability, generally responded to the appropriateness, both symbolic and physical, of the spaces and milestones of the route. Wide and beautified streets, as specified in public announcements, were obviously preferred to tortuous, narrow, and disreputable roads. Likewise, the sacred and civic landscape of the city, made up mainly of churches, monasteries, and convents, marked stopping and passing points. If we look at the itineraries of the main late medieval processions, a hierarchy of the urban space becomes evident. Referring to the procession of the Corpus Christi, Miguel Raufast (2006: 136-137) states that:

> [The ceremonial circuit] has as its gravitational centre the first temple of the city, the cathedral, with the monastic centres (Franciscans, Dominicans, Augustinians and Carmelites, especially) or the church of Santa Maria del Mar as its main satellites, and the city walls as its limits. This draws a primordial itinerary, a rut deeper than the rest, which seems to have a powerful attraction on any other festive occasion.[19]

The Raval was therefore relegated to a peripheral space, far from the Cathedral and the City's House and even more so from Santa Maria del Mar, the second most important temple in the city, and some of the largest, most prestigious streets, such as Ample, Moncada, de la Bòria, or Regomir (BANKS 2003: 23, 31).

This, however, did not mean the complete marginalization of the hospital of the Holy Cross from the urban ceremonial. The hospital was in the centre of this periphery, in the most urbanized area of the Raval, and close to the monasteries of el Carme and, from the late 15th century, els Àngels. Moreover, the hospital's location, next to one of the main access roads into the city, the *portal* (gate) of Sant Antoni, turned it into an important stop for visitors who ceremonially entered Barcelona.

It is true that the hospital was a poor candidate as a stop in some of the more established processional itineraries, such as the Corpus Christi. But other extraor-

18. AHCB, *Manual de Novells i Ardits*, edited by SCHWARTZ, CARRERAS-CANDI 1893, vol. II: 122, 182

19. In the original Catalan: «Té com a centre gravitacional el primer temple de la ciutat –la catedral–, amb els centres monàstics (franciscans, dominicans, augustinians i carmelitans, especialment) o l'església de Santa Maria del Mar com a principals satèl·lits, i les muralles urbanes com a límits, se'ns dibuixa immediatament una mena d'itinerari mare, un solc més profund que la resta i que sembla atraure poderosament qualsevol altra iniciativa festiva».

dinary processions, while highly influenced by the traditional itineraries, had a little more flexibility to include stops that went beyond the city's symbolic centre, marked by the limits of the 13th century walls (Fernández-Cuadrench 2005: 408-409). For example, in April 1458, a solemn procession handed over a set of relics of Saints Cosmas and Damian to the confraternity of surgeons in Barcelona (fig. 4).[20] It was a gift from the bishop and cathedral chapter of Tortosa, and, like most of the traffic that entered Barcelona from the south and west, the procession came through the *portal* of Sant Antoni, «making through the street of the hospital of the Holy Cross», until it reached its final destination at the Church of Santa Maria del Pi.[21] In this case, the role assumed by the hospital was not related to the association of the saints with medicine and surgery, but by the hospital's closeness to one of the city's main gates. Similarly, in October 1482, during a period of severe drought, a rain invoking procession also passed through the hospital.[22]

In the case of the ceremonial practises related to Royal Entries and the reception of guests of high status, the participation of the hospital was strongly mediated, as we have already indicated, by its location. There was a well-established ceremonial tradition that defined the forms, tempos, and spaces through which the act took place. Undoubtedly, the monarch's first entry into Barcelona was an event with heavy symbolic weight, «the staging, in its most solemn form, of the city-visitor relationship, and, on the other hand, the visualisation of the socio-political structure of the city» (Raufast 2008: 1047). Broadly speaking, the protocol required that the royal entourage staid outside of the city walls, usually in the monastery of Valldonzella, from where, accompanied by the urban authorities, it entered the city through the Drassanes portal until arriving in plaça de Framenors, where the pact between the monarch and the *res publica* of Barcelona was solemnly represented on a scaffold (Raufast 2016: 357, 367). This route made the interaction between the city's royal guests and the hospital unlikely. However, the specific circumstances of each entry allowed, or rather required, a certain degree of protocol flexibility. The long and repeated absences of Alfonso the Magnanimous and the convulsions typical of the Catalan Civil War (1462-1472) resulted in a 15th century filled with ceremonial exceptionalism (Raufast 2016: 32; 2008: 1038). In addition, after the significant moment of the first entrance, the subsequent receptions, both of the monarch and other members of the royal family, allowed for more diverse urban routes in which the hospital had a role to play.

20. On the saints Cosmas and Damian see Fernando Serrano and Antonio González's contribution in this volume.

21. «E més avant los dits honorables consellers preguen e encarreguen a tots los stants o habitants en los carrers davall nomenats que vullen scombrar, denejar, reguar e anremar com millor poran les vies e carreres per hon passarà la dita processó, ço és, començant del portal de Sanct Anthoni, tirant la via del hospital de Sancta Creu, e d'aquí irà al portal de la Bocaria, e passarà tirant dreta via devant lo portal maior de la església del Pi» (AHCB, *Registre d'ordinacions* 8, f. 62v, 1458, April 26).

22. AHCB, *Registre d'ordinacions* 11, f. 30v, 1482, October 26.

However, the hospital could participate in the Royal Entries even when the building itself was not included in the ceremonial circuit. In 1423, after his first Neapolitan victory, Alfonso the Magnanimous entered Barcelona through the Drassanes gate without setting foot on the Raval.[23] Among several acts of great solemnity, the councillors of Barcelona donated their *gramalles*, the ceremonial robes that were the ultimate symbol of their municipal power, to churches, monasteries, and other relevant individuals and institutions, including the city's general hospital. Joan Bussot, one of the councillors, handed over his *gramalla,* to the hospital of the Holy Cross, a gesture that reminds us of Martin of Tours and his partition of the cape (Raufast 2014; 2016: 449).[24] Similarly, in February 1462, on the occasion of the arrival of Queen Joana of Castile and her firstborn and future king, Ferdinand, the city government agreed to give a few luxurious red clothes to the hospital. These robes, as one of the city's scribes dutifully recalled, had been bought to decorate the scaffold on which the Queen and the *Infante* swore to respect the privileges of the city.[25] We document once again the coming and going of luxurious fabrics, this time associated with both the municipal and royal powers.

The role of the hospital in the ceremonies of reception of distinguished guests went, however, beyond this dignified periphery. During the second half of the 15th century, numerous Royal Entries were made through the portal of Sant Antoni, closer to the border with Aragon and Castile. A standardised route was thus outlined, in which kings, queens, and Infantes, always duly accompanied, entered the city through the gate of Sant Antoni and crossed the Raval towards the gate of la Boqueria, meeting the hospital along the way (Kovács 2003: 79). Throughout the 15th century, several royals passed through the hospital: in the years 1460 and 1461, the *Infante* Charles of Viana; in 1479 and 1481, King Ferdinand and, later on, Queen Isabel; in 1488, the *Infante* Henry of Aragon; and in 1492, the Catholic Kings and their son, the *Infante* John. In most cases, contemporary documentation says very little about their interaction with the hospital. Most likely, they took at least one look, and who knows if a stop, to the magnificent building that was the «light, nobility, ornament, glory and spaciousness» of the city (Conejo 2014: 415-445).

However, there are two clear exceptions in this panorama of vague references. The second entry of Charles of Viana, in 1461, and the first entry of Isabel of Castile, twenty years later, present some interesting parallels due to the interactive and theatrical nature of their passage through the hospital. As described by Francesc Massip, a Royal Entry can be understood as a "linear scene" that took

23. AHCB, *Llibre d'Algunes Coses Assenyalades*, chap. 1, f. 1-8.

24. AHCB, *Llibre d'Algunes Coses Assenyalades*, chap. 1, f. 7bis.

25. «Lo dit cadeffal fou fet an lo pla de Fframenors devant la casa de Muncada, loch acustumat, en lo qual cadeffal foren fets XIII sacalons, e en lo mig del dit cadeffal fou fet un replà o sitial ab un scaló, lo qual cadeffal, sitial e scalons fou cubert de VIII draps vermells de lana, pagats per la ciutat, los quals draps foren donats al hospital de Santa Creu» (AHCB, *Llibre de les solemnitats de Barcelona*, ed. Duran i Sanpere, Sanabre 1930, vol. I: 257).

place within a city that was turned into a large theatrical space, in which each stop or point of reference was to be defined by a series of dramatic arrangements, either fixed or mobile: the static scaffold fits into the first category, on which «a series of actions, mimicked or dialogued, that the spectator will contemplate moving from one place to another» took place (MASSIP 1991: 117-118; KOVÁCS 2003: 74). The hospital was thus integrated as another (fixed) stage within the large (and mobile) welcoming ceremony.

On his passage through the hospital (fig. 5), Charles of Viana was able to contemplate «all the madmen and the innocents, high on a scaffold, with their faces painted red and other colours, armed with spears and lances, and mitres of white paper on their heads, as if they were bishops».[26] Conversly, the queen was recieved by a more peaceful sceen, framed by a scaffold on which the hospital's wetnurses, foundlings, and the «innocent» rested, this time disarmed.[27]

Once again, these were strongly ritualised acts, with multiple layers of interpretation. The small entertainments, known in Catalan as entremesos, that accompanied the entourage of the honoured visitor took on symbolic or allegorical meanings that went beyond playful enjoyment and mere spectacularity. Some of these deeply layered ceremonies refered to universal themes within Medieval mentality: the performing children with white paper mitres powerfully remind us of the Catalan *bisbetó*, the English Boy-Bishop or the Castilian *Obispillo*, along with the *Festum Stultorum*: these were festive events that revolved around the exaltation of the humble and the parody of the powerful, and, in the case of the *orats*, the sacralization of madness as an approach to mystery (MASSIP 2012).[28] But they also had specific meanings that were keenly adapted to the political reality of their time: for the *Infante* Charles, so loved by the Barcelonians, the performing foundlings and madmen could potentially serve as a reminder of the emptiness of earthly glory, just as the wheel of fortune that had followed his ancestor, King Martin I, who had entered Barcelona half a century earlier (RAUFAST 2016: 22). At the same time, the display of paper swords and spears functioned as a counterpoint to the steel weapons that the people of Barcelona had defiantly raised to protect the *Infante* from his father in the prelude to the Catalan Civil War. The second entry of Charles of Viana into Barcelona had a double meaning: firstly, as a manifestation of joy at his liberation and the apparent reconciliation with his father. Secondly, as a display of the city's military muscle. The *Infante* passed through the streets of Barcelona accompanied by the city in arms, «while children with reeds, wooden swords, and paper flags interrupted the first-born's

26. ANC, *Dietari de la Generalitat de Catalunya*, vol I, f. 40r, dir. SANS-TRAVÉ 1994: 160. In the original Catalan: «tots los horats e ignoscents, alt, sobre un cadefal, ab les cares pintades de vermelló e d'altres colors, armats ab llançes e cervelleres e ab mitres de paper blanch sobre lur cap a forme de bisbes».

27. AHCB, *Llibre de les solemnitats de Barcelona*, ed. DURAN I SANPERE, SANABRE 1930, vol. I: 330.

28. On the different meaning of the innocent in the Iberian late Middle Ages see Raúl Villagrasa's contribution in this same volume.

passage by praising him and censuring the attitude of John II's wicked advisers» (Raufast 2008: 1055, 1067). A few years later, war, ceremony, and marginality would interact once again when, in the midst of the civil war, King Peter of Portugal was received into Barcelona by slaves with painted faces, banging on drums, and accompanying the usual entourage of armed men.

Beyond the specific political context, and both in times of war and peace, the presence of the hospital's infants, wetnurses, and *orats* represented, after all, some of the central elements in the human landscape of the hospital of the Holy Cross, refuge of «poor men and women, the insane and the infirm, the wounded, and other various human miseries, abandoned children and other miserable people of various nations and conditions».[29] Thus, the hospital, as a setting, took on a meaning of its own, as a simple allegory of its welfare mission and, at the end of the day, utility for the Barcelona public. However, it was also integrated into wider ceremonial contexts, which linked it with the city as a whole.

## 3. *Conclusion*

This deployment of urban ceremonies showed how the hospital, despite its peripheral location in the urban landscape of Barcelona, was able to carry its own symbolic weight and gain a dignified space in the city's symbolic landscape. This was no accident: it was, of course, the direct consequence of the efforts of the institution's patrons, namely the bishop and chapter of Barcelona, the monarchy, and especially the city council.

The position of the hospital within Barcelona's civic-religious ceremonies pales in comparison with more established institutions, mostly the main churches and convents of the city, placed in the very centre of its sacred space, enclosed by the 13th century walls. This is, thought, a rather unfair comparison. Conversely, if we compare the ceremonial displays attached to the hospital of the Holy Cross with other welfare institutions in the city, either previous or coetaneous, the marked difference of the large, monumental hospital built in 1401 becomes apparent. And, nowhere more than in its foundational ceremony. The dignity of this festive event indicated the qualitative difference that the new hospital acquired. Where were the monarchy, the bishop, the councillors in the ceremonial past of the hospitals that would merge into the Holy Cross? Did they relate with similar magnificence to the alms-houses and other small hospitals that populated the 15th century city? Once again, the concept of a large, magnificent hospital is key. In due time, the denomination of "general" hospital would refer to this notion of referentially, this ability to hoard resources and attention, also in the symbolic horizon. From 1401, the hospital of the Holy Cross was not one of the

29. AHSCP, *Llibre d'ordinacions de l'Hospital* , f. 1r, ed. Marcé 2017: 119. In the original Catalan: «homens e dones pobres, afollats, contrets, orats, nafrats e havents altres diverses misèries humanes, infants gitats e altres persones miserables de diverses nacions e condicions».

city's hospitals, but *the* hospital of the city. The merger had created a qualitatively different institutions, not only larger, but holier and more magnificent than its predecessors.

## *Bibliography*


BANKS, Philip, 2003. "El creixement físic de Barcelona, segles X-XIII", *Barcelona Quaderns d'Història*, 8: 11-33.

BATLLE, Carme, 1978. "El bisbe Arnau Roger de Pallars i la Seu d' Urgell (1473-1461)", *Estudios Históricos y Documentos de los Archivos de Protocolos*, 6: 215-236.

BRIDGEWATER, Pol, 2020. *"Car vosaltres havets a veure sobre hospitals": el Consell de Cent i la construcció de la primera política hospitalària a la Barcelona baixmedieval*, PhD thesis, Universitat de Barcelona.

CARRÈRE, Claude, 1977. *Barcelona 1380-1462. Un centre econòmic en època de crisi*, Barcelona, Curial.

CASTILLO, José, 1994, "Funciones sociales del consumo: un caso extremo", *Reis*, 67/94: 65-85.

CONEJO, Antoni, 2002, *Assistència i hospitalitat a l'edat mitjana. L'arquitectura dels hospitals catalans: del gòtic al primer renaixement,* PhD Thesis, Universitat de Barcelona.

CONEJO, Antoni, 2014, "«Lum, noblesa, ornament, laor, glòria e amplitud»: los hospitales y la renovada imagen de la ciudad bajomedieval", Teresa Huguet, Pere Verdés, Jon Arrizabalaga, Manuel Sánchez (ed.), *Ciudad y hospital en el Occidente europeo. 1300-1700*, Lleida, Milenio: 415-445.

CONEJO, Antoni, 2017, "«En la present ciutat hun devot e solempne spital». Un estudi a quatre bandes sobre l'esplendor artístic i arquitectònic dels hospitals baixmedievals", Flocel Sabaté (ed.), *L'assistència a l'edat mitjana*, Balaguer, Pagès Editors, 2017, 99-137.

CONEJO, Antoni. "«El orgullo y la vanidad han construido más hospitales que todas las virtudes juntas». Patronazgo artístico y patrimonio hospitalario en la Corona de Aragón (siglos XIV-XV)". *Revista de la CECEL*, 18, 2018 [Los hospitales y su entorno II]: 91-120.

CONEJO, Antoni, "«La present casa, molt Illustre y magnífica per la grandeza de son edifici». L'hospital de la Santa Creu de Barcelona: 1401-1417". *Lambard. Estudis d'Art Medieval*, 28. 2020: 9-56.

DURAN I SANPERE, Agustí; SANABRE, Josep (ed.), 1930. *Llibre de les solemnitats de Barcelona,* Institut d'Estudis Catalans.

EIXIMENIS, Francesc, 1983. *Lo Crestià*, Albert Hauf (ed.), Barcelona, Edicions 62.

EVANGELISTI, Paolo, 2015. "*Construir una identidad: Francesc Eiximenis y una idea europea de 'civilitas'*", Julián Acebrón, Isabel Grifoll, Flocel Sabaté (ed.), *La construcció d'identitats imaginades*, Lleida, Pagès Editors: 125-166.

FERNÁNDEZ-CUADRENCH, Jordi, 2005. "Les processons extraordinàries a la Barcelona baixmedieval (1339-1498). Assaig tipològic", *Acta Historica et Archaeologica Mediaevalia*, 26: 403-428.

HERNANDO, Josep, 2007. "Obres de Francesc Eiximenis en biblioteques privades de la Barcelona del segle XV", *Arxiu de Textos Catalans Antics*, 26: 385-568.

HUGUET-TERMES, Teresa, 2010. "Un petit univers de miralls. Barcelona, l'Hospital de la Santa Creu i el rei Martí", *Lambard. Estudis d'Art Medieval*, 21: 99-114.

JUNCOSA, Eduard, 2011. "Pensar el pacto en la corona de Aragón: Francesc Eiximenis y el Dotzè del cristià", François Foronda 8 dir.), *Avant le contrat social. Le contrat politique dans l'Occident médiéval XIIIe-XVe siècle,* Paris, Publications de la Sorbonne: 451-480.

KOVÁCS, Lenke, 2003. "La ciutat com a escenari: les entrades reials i la festa urbana", *Barcelona. Quaderns d'Història*, 9: 71-82.

LUCHERINI, Vinni, 2010. "Il Chronicon di Santa Maria del Principio (1313 circa) e la messa in scena della liturgia nel cuore della cattedrale di Napoli", Carlo Gasparri, Giovanna Greco, Raffaella

Pierobon (ed.), *Dall'immagine alla storia. Studi per ricordare Stefania Adamo Muscettola*, Pozzuoli, Naus: 521-549.

MADURELL, Josep Maria, 1963. *Mensajeros barceloneses en la corte de Nápoles de Alfonso V de Aragón (1435-1458)*, Barcelona, Escuela Estudios Medievales, CSIC.

MARCÉ, Jaume, 2017. *El llibre d'ordinacions de l'Hospital de la Santa Creu de Barcelona (1416-1505). Estudi i reedició*, Masters Thesis, Universitat de Barcelona.

MARCÉ, Jaume, 2023. *«Pro succurrendo necessitatibus dicti hospitalis» Els orígens del patrimoni i els mecanismes de finançament de l'hospital de la Santa Creu de Barcelona (s. XV)*, PhD Thesis, Universitat de Barcelona.

MASSIP, Francesc, 1991. *La festa d'Elx i els misteris medievals europeus,* Alacant, Ajuntament d'Alcant.

MASSIP, Francesc, 2012. "El personaje del loco en el espectáculo medieval y en las cortes principescas del renacimiento", *Babel*, 25: 71-96.

RAUFAST, Miguel, 2006. "Itineraris processionals a la Barcelona baixmedieval", *Revista d'Etnologia de Catalunya*, 29: 134-146.

RAUFAST, Miguel (2006-2007), "La entrada real de Martín el Joven, rey de Sicilia en Barcelona (1405): solemnidad, economía y conflicto", *Acta Historica et Archaeologica Mediaevalia*, 27- 28: 89-120.

RAUFAST, Miguel, 2008. "Ceremonia y conflicto: entradas reales en Barcelona en el contexto de la Guerra Civil catalana (1460-1473)", *Anuario de Estudios Medievales*, 38/2: 1037-1085.

RAUFAST, Miguel, 2014. "Las ceremonias de la caridad: Asistencia, marginación y pobreza en el escenario urbano bajomedieval", Teresa Huguet, Pere Verdés, Jon Arrizabalaga, Manuel Sánchez (ed.), *Ciudad y hospital en el Occidente europeo. 1300- 1700*, Lleida, Milenio: 401-414.

RAUFAST, Miguel, 2016. *Entradas reales y ceremonias de recepción en la Barcelona bajomedieval,* PhD Thesis, Universitat de Barcelona.

RIERA, Antoni, 2003. "Barcelona en els segles XIV-XV, un mercat internacional a escala mediterrània", *Barcelona. Quaderns d'Història*, 8: 65-83.

ROCA, Josep Maria (ed.), 1920. *Ordinacions del Hospital General de la Santa Creu de Barcelona (any MCCCCXVII)*, Barcelona, Fidel Giró.

SÁNCHEZ, Manuel, 2014. "Las cuentas de un hospital medieval: la Santa Creu de Barcelona (1430-1431)", Teresa Huguet, Pere Verdés, Jon Arrizabalaga, Manuel Sánchez (ed.), *Ciudad y hospital en el Occidente europeo. 1300-1700*, Lleida, Milenio 177-209.

SANS-TRAVÉ, Josep Maria (dir.), 1994. *Dietaris de la Generalitat de Catalunya. Volum I,* Barcelona, Generalitat de Catalunya.

SCHWARTZ, Frederic; CARRERAS-CANDI, Francesc, 1893. *Manual de Novells Ardits, vulgarment apellat Dietari del Antich Consell Barceloní*, Barcelona, Ajuntament de Barcelona.

WITTLIN, Curt, 1993. "L'edició del 1499 del Regiment de la cosa pública: les revisions i ampliacions al text, a l'endreça i al comiat escrits per Francesc Eiximenis el 1383", *Boletín de la Sociedad Castellonense de Cultura*, 69: 441-459.

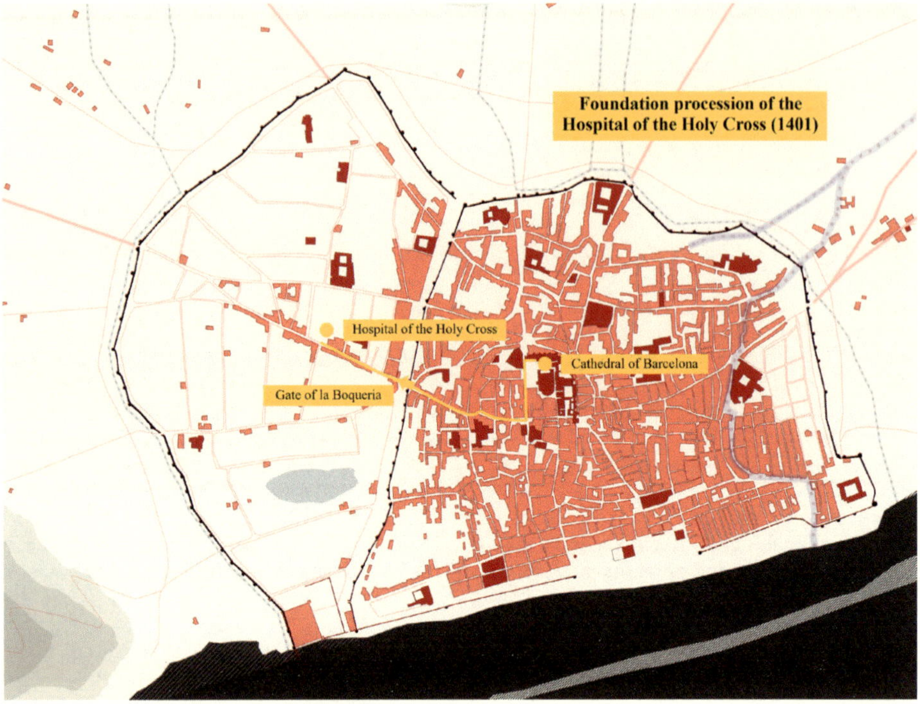


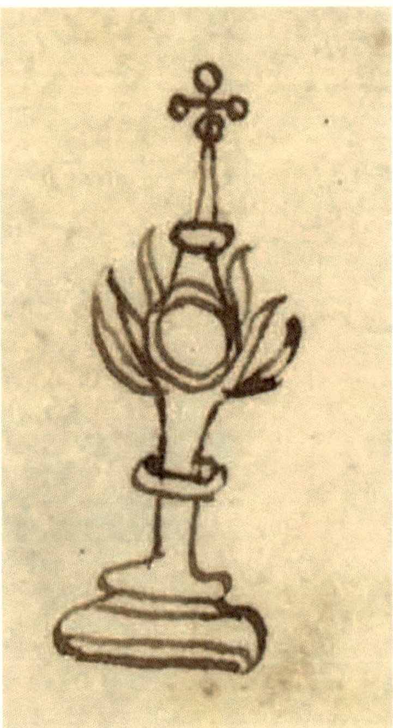

Fig. 1. The foundational procession of the Hospital of the Holy Cross. Map based on the *Carta Històrica de Barcelona* (Barcelona: Arxiu Històric de la Ciutat de Barcelona).

Fig. 2. Reliquary of Saint Candida as depicted by notary Jaume Safont in his dietary (Barcelona: Biblioteca de Catalunya, ms. 978, *Dietari de las turbacions de Catallunya,* f. 62v).

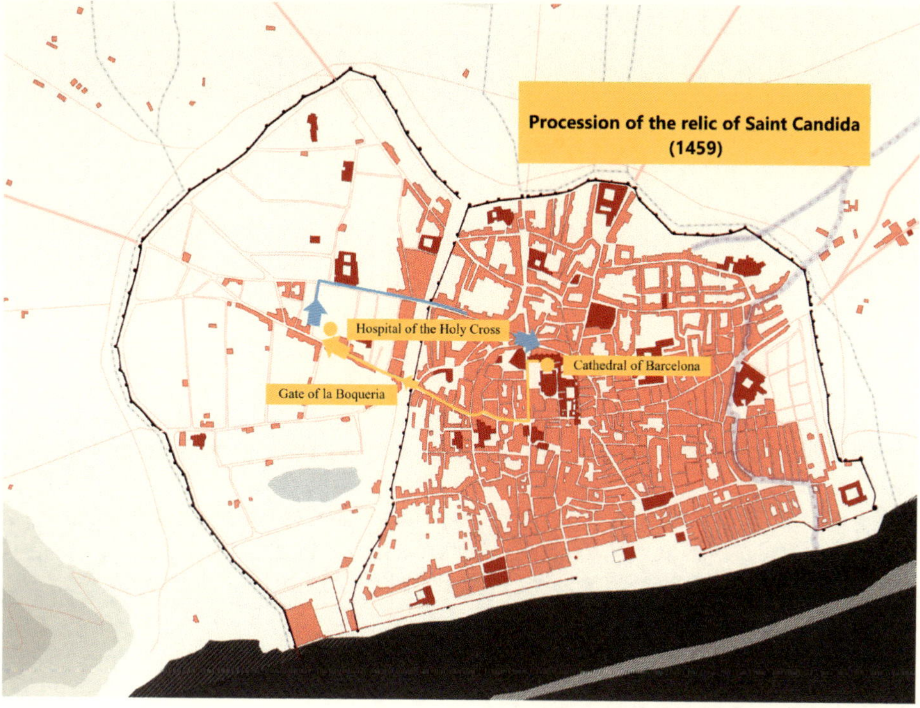


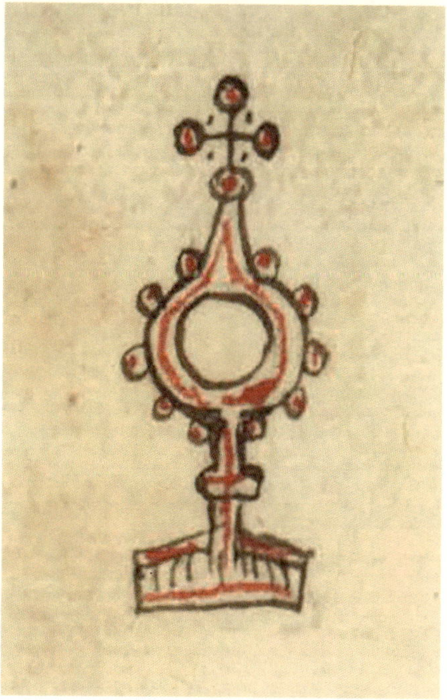

Fig. 3. The procession of Saint Candida. Map based on the *Carta Històrica de Barcelona* (Barcelona: Arxiu Històric de la Ciutat de Barcelona).
Fig. 4. Reliquary of Saints Comas and Damian as depicted by notary Jaume Safont in his dietary (Barcelona: Biblioteca de Catalunya, Biblioteca de Catalunya, ms. 978, *Dietari de las turbacions de Catallunya,* f. 56v).

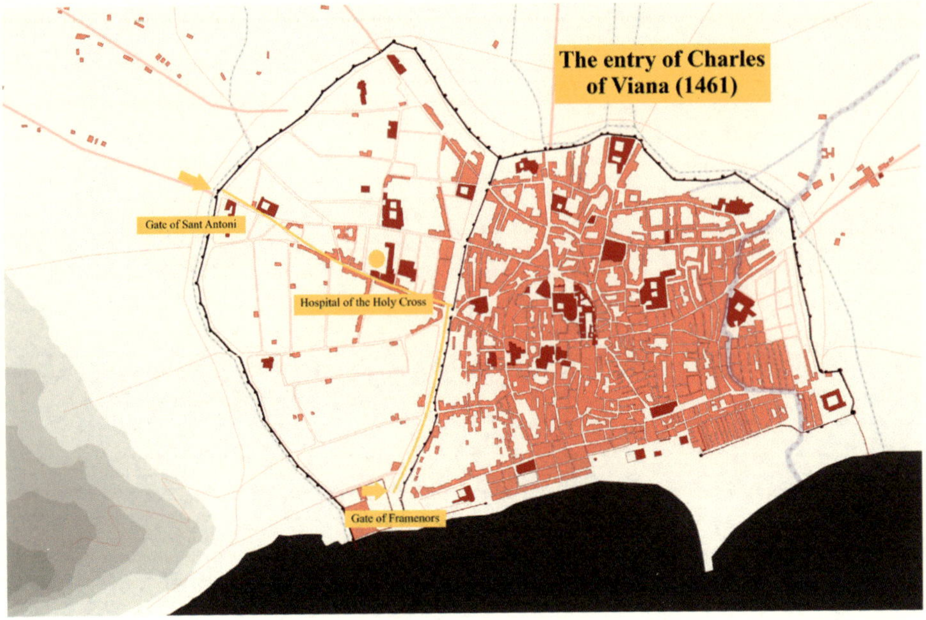


Fig. 5. The entry of Charles of Viana in Barcelona. Map based on the *Carta Històrica de Barcelona* (Barcelona: Arxiu Històric de la Ciutat de Barcelona).

Jaume Marcé Sánchez

# Emfiteusi i transformació urbana. Els efectes de la unificació hospitalària en la Barcelona del Quatre-cents*

## 1. *Introducció*

L'obra de Francesc Carreras Candi sempre és un recurs habitual i amable. Els seus treballs són curulls de dades que abasten àmplies cronologies i territoris, alhora que inclouen reflexions que, amb el temps i l'esforç de noves fornades d'investigadors, s'han demostrat més o menys encertades. Un d'aquests estudis el va dedicar a l'origen de l'emfiteusi, a fi d'analitzar-ne l'evolució durant els segles medievals i les seves característiques més essencials (Carreras Candi 1910). Entre moltes altres qüestions, l'historiador i polític barceloní va apuntar dues idees que ara val la pena assenyalar. En primer lloc, Carreras Candi indicava que l'emfiteusi era un element que havia ajudat a confirmar i consolidar els fonaments de la societat feudal, en tant que s'havia emmotllat fàcilment als interessos que tenien els senyors sobre els seus dominis. En segon lloc, i posant el focus en la realitat barcelonina, l'autor afirmava que l'emfiteusi no va ser mai un component creador de nous espais urbans.

Amb els anys, les idees plantejades per Carreras Candi no han rebut la mateixa atenció. Si bé la relació entre el feudalisme i l'emfiteusi ha estat matèria de debat (Serra 1989; Benito 2003: 615-624), la seva importància com a eina per entendre el desenvolupament urbà no ha gaudit de la mateixa gratitud. Així ho apuntava fa trenta anys José R. Juliá Viñamata (1991), qui destacava el valor i les oportunitats que oferien l'estudi de l'emfiteusi urbana i els contractes d'establiment, ja que podien aportar noves dades sobre determinats aspectes urbanístics, arquitectònics i econòmics de les ciutats baixmedievals. A continuació, posarem el focus sobre una famosa institució hospitalària per veure les possibilitats que ofereix el plantejament adés esmentat.

Situem-nos en el mes d'abril de 1401, quan el Consell de Cent i el capítol de la catedral van materialitzar la fusió de quatre hospitals que estaven sota el seu control per fundar-ne un de nou, l'hospital de la Santa Creu. Mesos després, s'afegirien a la unificació el de Santa Eulàlia del Camp, que pertanyia a l'homònim monestir, i el de Santa Margarida o dels mesells, que estava en mans del

* Aquest treball forma part del projecte *El notariado público en el Mediterráneo Occidental. Escritura, instituciones, sociedad y economía (siglos XIII-XV)* (Ministerio de Ciencia e Innovación, PID2019-105072GB-I00).

bisbe i del dit capítol. Segons l'escriptura fundacional, tots els béns mobles i immobles dels antics centres van conformar la dotació de la flamant institució.[1] Això incloïa, també, els edificis i els horts on els hospitals havien acomplert la seva funció assistencial durant segles.

Fruit de les necessitats econòmiques que va tenir la Santa Creu durant els primers anys, els seus administradors van cercar la manera de rendibilitzar el patrimoni amb què l'hospital havia estat dotat. I una part de l'estratègia seguida va tenir un efecte directe sobre les antigues estructures hospitalàries, algunes de les quals van ser desmantellades per ser establertes en emfiteusi i, posteriorment, vendre'n el domini directe. Així doncs, podem dir que la fundació i construcció de l'hospital de la Santa Creu no només va tenir un impacte sobre la zona en què es va projectar, el Raval de la ciutat, sinó, també, en els espais que eren ocupats pels hospitals que havien pres part de la fusió.

De manera breu, per copsar els efectes de la unificació ens podem fixar en l'esdevenir de l'hospital d'en Bernat Marcús, un centre que havia estat fundat a mitjan segle XII al peu de la via que connectava la ciutat amb el Vallès. Durant el mes d'agost de 1401, els administradors de la Santa Creu van establir en emfiteusi les dependències de l'antiga institució, exceptuant la capella que li era annexa i que encara segueix dempeus (Dalmases 1994). Entre els dies 11 i 17 d'aquell mes, el notari Pere Bruguera va autoritzar cinc establiments emfitèutics que tingueren per objecte les cambres del centre.[2] Els nous tinents haurien de pagar un cens anual que oscil·laria entre 9 i 12 morabatins[3] i, a més, lliurar l'entrada de l'establiment. Una vegada resolts els pagaments, els administradors de la Santa Creu van vendre el domini directe que tenien sobre aquelles possessions. De l'operació resultant, els administradors van reportar un ingrés de 3.035 sous[4] per raó de les entrades i de 22.400 sous per la venda del domini.[5]

Les gestions que van dur a terme els administradors de la Santa Creu sobre hospital d'en Marcús no van ser pas excepcionals, si bé van ser reproduïdes en la majoria dels edificis i horts de la resta d'hospitals. Entre tots, però, el cas més destacable és el de l'hospital d'en Pere Desvilar. Primer, perquè és el més ben documentat. Dins dels protocols notarials de Joan Torró es poden trobar els establiments emfitèutics que van tenir per objecte totes les dependències del centre. En segon lloc, perquè les intervencions que s'hi van realitzar van aportar una important suma de diners a les arques del nou hospital. Un tercer motiu respon a la rica informació que aporten els contractes emfitèutics signats i les condicions en ells incloses, ja que permeten copsar la transformació que

1. Arxiu Capitular de Barcelona (a partir d'ara ACB), Diversorum B, 1-2-1775, editat per: Castejón 2007: 143-152.

2. Arxiu Històric de la Santa Creu i Sant Pau (a partir d'ara AHSCP), Capbreus, vol. VI, inv. 4, Llibres [2], f. 68r-73v; Arxiu Històric de Protocols de Barcelona (a partir d'ara AHPB), Pere de Bruguera, 64/4, f. 65r-68v i 77r-78r.

3. El cost del morabatí equivalia a 9 sous (Benito 2003: 703).

4. Si no s'indica el contrari, sempre ens referirem a sous barcelonins.

5. AHSCP, Capbreus, vol. VI, inv. 4, Llibres [2], f. 68r-73v.

va patir el què era conegut com l'Hospital de la Ciutat, així com el seu entorn. I finalment, perquè l'espai que havia ocupat el centre, amb el temps, va quedar completament esvaït.

El present treball té per objectiu estudiar la intervenció que els administradors de la Santa Creu van dur a terme sobre l'hospital d'en Pere Desvilar, analitzant els procediments seguits, destacant les reformes materialitzades i reivindicant, encara que sigui subtilment, la rellevància dels establiments emfitèutics com una eina per conèixer la transformació d'un petit espai de la Barcelona baixmedieval. Abans d'entrar en matèria, però, convé explicar breument quins van ser els orígens de la institució que ara ens ocupa.

## 2. *La fundació de l'hospital d'en Pere Desvilar*

L'any 1308 Pere Desvilar i la seva muller Blanca van fundar una institució assistencial que seria coneguda pel nom del primer en la vilanova de Barcelona. Desvilar era un navilier d'origen badaloní molt proper al rei i plenament inserit en l'activitat política barcelonina (HUGUET 2013: 380-381; BRIDGEWATER 2020: 162). Al costat del pont de Sant Daniel i relativament a prop del monestir de clarisses, Desvilar va construir un edifici amb una capella annexa, els quals va oferir al Consell de Cent el 20 d'abril d'aquell mateix any (ROCA 1920: 15).

Tradicionalment, la fundació de Pere Desvilar ha estat identificada com a hospital. Això no obstant, autors com Antoni Conejo o Teresa Huguet han apuntat que el funcionament de la casa, sobretot durant els primers anys, hauria estat més proper al d'una almoina (CONEJO 2002: 290; HUGUET 2013: 375-378). En efecte, Desvilar va indicar que la institució per ell fundada havia de servir per repartir menjar a quatre persones pobres, amb les quals hi mantingués alguna relació de parentela. En un inici, la seva fundació no contemplava l'opció d'oferir-les-hi allotjament de forma contínua. Val a dir, però, que a finals de juliol de 1311, quan el mercader va decidir augmentar el nombre de pobres beneficiaris fins a dotze en el seu testament, Desvilar va demanar que s'hi habilités un dormitori que seria ofert a qualsevol que no tingués un lloc a on sojornar (ROCA 1920: 16-17; BATLLE, CASAS 1980: 178-180).

Pere Desvilar va deixar indicat en el seu testament que, un cop morís, el govern del centre passaria a mans del seu germà Jaume i, a la mort d'aquest, l'hospital seria administrat pels consellers de Barcelona, els cònsols de la mar o els prohoms de la ciutat. És important apuntar que Desvilar mai va voler que l'administració de l'hospital estigués «in regimine alicuius diocesani vel alterius ecclesiastice persone» (ROCA 1920: 16). I aquest és un factor que caldrà tenir en compte quan més endavant sigui tractada la fusió hospitalària de 1401.

En el moment en què el Consell en va prendre les regnes, l'hospital va quedar plenament integrat en la política ciutadana. La primera evidència que tenim de l'exercici de l'autoritat del municipi data de 1325, quan Pere de Vilafranca i Ferrer de Moià van ser escollits administradors. A partir d'aquest moment, tal com Pol Bridgewater (2020: 164-169) ha demostrat recentment, els càrrecs de govern s'articularien a imatge i semblança de la resta d'oficis municipals; la gestió hospitalària es tecnificaria en la mateixa mesura que ho faria l'estructura del Consell.

La principal missió assistencial de l'hospital era el repartiment de porcions alimentàries a un selecte grup de pobres. Encara que l'any 1311 Pere Desvilar n'havia designat dotze, el seu nombre va anar en augment durant la centúria (Roca 1920: 16). Bona part dels nous beneficiaris seguirien mantenint algun lligam de parentela amb el llinatge d'en Desvilar, però d'altres serien triats a discreció del Consell de Cent, a fi de donar resposta a les eventuals emergències que tinguessin alguns oficials del municipi que, per raó de malaltia o vellesa, no poguessin seguir desenvolupant les seves funcions (Bridgewater 2020: 170-171).

Al llarg de la centúria, l'activitat assistencial que acomplia l'hospital d'en Pere Desvilar es va consolidar i va ser necessari millorar-ne les instal·lacions. Un canvi important en les seves funcions es va produir a partir de 1370, quan el Consell de Cent va resoldre que la institució s'especialitzaria en l'acollida de pobres malalts. Es tractava d'una ampliació dels seus serveis, que no va tenir cap mena de repercussió sobre les disposicions originals del promotor, però que requeria disposar de més espai per als malalts i els seus cuidadors. Malauradament, les notícies pervingudes sobre les intervencions que s'hi van dur a terme són més aviat vagues. Si bé alguns pagaments fets pel Consell de Cent permeten intuir un canvi en la fesomia i les funcions del complex, és realment difícil concretar com es van materialitzar aquestes reformes.[6]

Un cop es va consumar la unificació hospitalària el 1401, el d'en Pere Desvilar va ser l'únic hospital que, tot i participar de la fusió, va seguir funcionant de forma autònoma. El centre va restar al marge del govern de la Santa Creu i es va mantenir sota la supervisió i vigilància del Consell de Cent. La raó que explicaria aquest fet era la clàusula del seu fundador mencionada a l'inici de l'article: l'administració de l'hospital mai podria estar controlada per una autoritat eclesiàstica. Tot i això, el procés esdevingut l'any 1401 va acabar provocant certs canvis en l'estructura del centre i el seu funcionament.

Arran de la fusió, la Santa Creu va ser dotada amb gairebé tot el patrimoni dels antics hospitals. I el matís adverbial és important, ja que justament la contribució que va fer el d'en Pere Desvilar sembla que no va ser completa. Encara que aquesta és una qüestió que mereix ser tractada àmpliament en un altre estudi, ara voldria apuntar que l'aportació patrimonial que va fer únicament es va concretar en l'edifici del mateix hospital, sense incloure, doncs, cap altra de les possessions que formaven part del seu bast domini.[7] Així doncs, les úniques accions que des de la Santa Creu es van (poder) dur a terme sobre el patrimoni de l'hospital d'en

6. Arxiu Històric de la Ciutat de Barcelona (a partir d'ara AHCB), *Clavaria*, 1370, vol. 9, f. 118v; citat per Bridgewater 2020: 173-174.

7. L'any 1388 l'hospital de Pere Desvilar posseïa el domini directe de 133 immobles que es trobaven tan dins com fora de Barcelona (Bridgewater 2020: 437-444).

Pere Desvilar es van centrar en les seves dependències, les quals van ser fragmentades en unitats menors, establertes en emfiteusi i, posteriorment, en alguns casos, se'n va vendre el domini directe.

### 3. *El desmantellament de l'hospital de la ciutat*

L'estructura que tenia l'hospital d'en Pere Desvilar l'any 1401 la coneixem per l'acció que els administradors de la Santa Creu van dur a terme sobre l'edifici. Un cop es va materialitzar la unificació, l'hospital va ser desarmat completament (CONEJO 2002: 321-322; CASTEJÓN 2007: 29-30; CONEJO 2020: 23-24). Sabem que comptava amb una cambra per als malalts, una segona per a les dones i una cuina. La primera, que devia ser una llarga sala longitudinal de quatre trams articulats per arcs probablement ogivals i del tipus diafragma, es va poder dividir fàcilment en quatre ambients homogenis. El mateix mètode va ser emprat en la cambra de les dones, que va ser compartimentada en dues estances. Finalment, la cuina també va ser fragmentada en dues meitats. A banda dels espais esmentats, l'hospital en disposava d'altres. Concretament, un celler, una torre i l'habitació «in qua datur elemosina sive caritas Petri de Vilario»[8] que també van ser establerts en emfiteusi però que no van ser dividits en dependències més petites.

Totes les estances de l'hospital de Pere Desvilar s'agrupaven a l'interior d'un edifici en forma de L. El seu segment més curt, que s'annexava a la capella de Santa Marta, disposava de dues botigues i de la cambra de Pere Desvilar. Per altra banda, la crugia més llarga consistia en una nau disposada longitudinalment en sentit est-oest, on s'aplegaven la resta d'espais suara esmentats i als quals s'hi podia accedir a través d'un pòrtic interior que els vorejava.

El 10 de desembre de 1401 es van signar els primers establiments emfitèutics que tenien per objecte les dependències de l'antic hospital. Eren un total de vuit contractes, pels quals els administradors de la Santa Creu van transferir l'usdefruit dels béns a diversos menestrals i mercaders que es comprometien a pagar anualment un cens determinat i una entrada, que era el preu per accedir o percebre l'ús d'un immoble (BENITO 2003: 639). A més a més, els nous tinents haurien d'acomplir amb tot un seguit d'obligacions que van quedar registrades en les clàusules dels instruments i que analitzarem a continuació. Anys després, es van acabar signant quatre contractes més, pels quals els administradors de la Santa Creu van establir les dependències restants (taula 1).

La compartimentació de l'edifici va requerir una sèrie de reformes per fer efectiva la divisió de les dependències i, alhora, garantir cobertura jurídica sobre els drets lligats a l'ús dels immobles que se'n van derivar. En primer lloc, en els establiments es recordava que la construcció de les mitgeres havia de ser coste-

8. AHSCP, Capbreus, vol. VI, inv. 4, Llibres [1], f. 141r-144v.

TAULA 1. Establiments fets sobre les antigues dependències de l'hospital de Pere Desvilar.

| Data | Nom | Ofici | Bé | Cens | |
|---|---|---|---|---|---|
| 10/12/1401 | Pere Miró | Corder | Hospici amb dues botigues, amb les dependències del pis superior on repartia almoina Pere Desvilar i amb la cambra que es troba sobre la volta | 8 | 3.200 |
| 10/12/1401 | Pere Joan | Peller | Primera arcada de la cambra dels malalts | 6 | 1.205 |
| 10/12/1401 | Ramon Degà | Barber | Segona arcada de la cambra dels malalts | 5 | 740 |
| 28/11/1404 | Pere Miró | Cultor | Tercera arcada de la cambra dels malalts | 5 | 400 |
| 10/12/1401 | Pere Cuchó | Cultor | Quarta arcada de la cambra dels malalts | 5 | 615 |
| 16/03/1406 | Pere Miró | Corder | Primera arcada de la cambra de les dones | 4 | 22 |
| 10/12/1401 | Ramon Degà | Barber | Segona arcada de la cambra de les dones | 4 | 365 |
| 10/12/1401 | Pere Guerau | Fabrer | Meitat de la cuina | 3 | 380 |
| 10/12/1401 | Pere Guerau | Fabrer | Meitat de la cuina | 3 | 380 |
| 10/12/1401 | Jaume Salvador | Mercader | *Lo Seller* | 3 | 620 |
| 10/05/1402 | Esteve Terrer i Clara | Mariner | *La Torra* | 3 | 600 |

jada pels tinents que havien rebut en emfiteusi les estances de l'hospital.[9] Així mateix, en els casos que va ser necessari, alguns emfiteutes van ser autoritzats a obrir nous portals per poder entrar i sortir de les cases. És el cas, per exemple, de la primera arcada (tram) de la cambra dels malalts, que havia estat establerta a Pere Joan i no tenia cap sortida, car era una secció de la sala dels homes a la qual només s'hi accedia per la porta que hi havia en el segon tram. A Pere se li va permetre construir dos accessos: l'un en el carrer que menava al monestir de Santa Clara i l'altre pel nou carrer que dividia els terrenys situats entre l'hospital i el Rec Comtal.[10]

9. «Et sub pacto etiam et condicione quod vestris missionibus et expensis habeatis vos claudere sive miganare cum vicinos vestros» (AHSCP, Capbreus, vol. VI, inv. 4, Llibres [1], f. 149r-152v).

10. «Et etiam quod possitis facere portale in pariete dicte domus sive prime archade versus dictum vicum per quod itur ad dictum monasterium Sancte Clare, vel etiam in pariete qui est iuxta dictam voltam» (AHSCP, Capbreus, vol. VI, inv. 4, Llibres [1], f. 126r). La mateixa autorització va ser concedida a Pere Cuchó, qui va rebre en emfiteusi la quarta arcada de la mateixa cambra: AHSCP, Capbreus, vol. VI, inv. 4, Llibres [1], f. 137r-140v.

La circulació de les aigües pluvials també va quedar regulada en els contractes. En diversos establiments els administradors de la Santa Creu van obligar als tinents a reformar les teulades amb l'objectiu de modificar l'orientació dels vessants. En avant, les aigües de les cases haurien de discórrer vers el nou *vic* creat, alliberant, així, l'androna o carreró del seu darrere.[11] Una mostra d'això l'ofereix el contracte d'establiment de la quarta arcada o tram de la cambra dels homes, on s'especificà que Pere Cuchó havia de «dare operam cum effectu quod aque pluviales discurrentes [...] versus vicum de na Larda discurrant et discurrere habeant versus dictum vicum».[12] Més evidents són les reformes que s'haurien de dur a terme sobre les teulades de la cuina i del celler, on les aigües haurien de discórrer «ad dictum vicum novum [...] et non versus dictam endronam».[13]

Finalment, la darrera reforma que es va emprendre va ser la divisió efectiva del terrat de l'hospici de Pere Desvilar respecte de la capella de Santa Marta. Era una intervenció necessària tal com ho indicaven les ordinacions d'en Santacília, car eren dos edificis adjacents que ja no formaven part del mateix conjunt.[14] Per aquest motiu, els administradors de la Santa Creu van obligar a Pere Miró, el nou tinent d'aquell espai, que ell mateix «de propriis missionibus et expensis habeat claudere taliter quod non possit habere aspectum in terramine capelle Sancte Marte que ibi est, nec in tegulata ipsius capelle».[15]

Al marge de les reformes estructurals que s'havien de dur a terme, en els establiments signats va ser inclosa una clàusula d'immissió que pretenia regular l'exercici dels drets de propietat dels nous establerts (RIBALTA 2001: 125-154; 2005: 19-23). La disposició en qüestió fixava els límits per a la construcció de taules o envans fixes sobre el nou *vic*, les quals podrien tenir, a tot estirar, fins a sis pams d'amplada «prout alii vicini habentis hospicia sive domos in eodem vico facere possunt».[16]

La transformació de les dependències de l'hospital en cases i obradors requeria tota una sèrie de regulacions que, en tant que va ser necessari, van ser incloses en els establiments emfitèutics respectius. Les mesures responien a una estratègia patrimonial ben definida, que tenia com a objectiu últim obtenir nous ingressos que ajudessin a la construcció de la Santa Creu. És per aquest motiu que, un cop cadascuna de les cambres va ser establerta en emfiteusi i s'havien cobrat les respectives entrades (un total de 8.527 sous), els administradors de l'hospital en van vendre el domini directe. Exceptuant l'hospici adjacent a la capella de Santa

11. Quan parlem de *vic* (del llatí, *vicus*) ens referim a l'eix que és fruit d'una reforma viària esdevinguda en una àrea determinada de la ciutat (SABATÉ 1997: 158-159).

12. AHSCP, Capbreus, vol. VI, inv. 4, Llibres [1], f. 137r-140v. La mateixa obligació la trobem també en la segona arcada de la cambra de les dones (AHSCP, Capbreus, vol. VI, inv. 4, Llibres [1], f. 149r-152v).

13. AHSCP, Capbreus, vol. VI, inv. 4, Llibres [1], f. 153r-164v.

14. «[...] encara que si dos vehins són eguals en terrat, que abdosos se han a tancar miges que passatge ne vista no sia del hu a l'altre» (BOSCÀ 1977: 168).

15. AHSCP, Capbreus, vol. VI, inv. 4, Llibres [1], f. 141r-144v.

16. AHSCP, Capbreus, vol. VI, inv. 4, Llibres [2], f. 87r-90v.

Marta, l'hospital es va desprendre de tots aquells béns. No obstant això, és difícil indicar el valor total del conjunt. Si bé per les arcades de les cambres dels malalts i de les dones es van cobrar 12.010 sous,[17] no és possible saber quant es va percebre per la cuina, el celler i la torre. El domini sobre aquests espais va ser venut juntament amb d'altres possessions per un total de 14.400 sous als marmessors de Joan Aldomar. Malauradament, en el contracte de compra-venda no es va indicar el preu que es va pagar per cadascun dels béns de forma individualitzada.[18]

L'estratègia patrimonial iniciada amb les dependències de l'hospital de Pere Desvilar va ser reproduïda, mesos més tard, en els terrenys que hi havia al voltant. Així doncs, per acabar d'entendre l'impacte que aquesta va tenir sobre l'antic conjunt hospitalari, passem a veure com va ser la intervenció dels administradors en aquest segon espai.

## 4. *Una arrencada complicada*

Per explorar les intervencions que es van dur a terme sobre els terrenys que es trobaven entre l'hospital i el Rec Comtal, convé retrocedir fins el 7 d'octubre de 1401, quan Joan Desvall arribà a Altura per trobar-se amb el rei.[19] El Consell de Cent el va enviar en qualitat de missatger per transmetre diverses demandes a Martí l'Humà, entre les quals es trobava la petició per edificar en el gran solar que hi havia rere l'hospital de Pere Desvilar i que era limítrof al Rec Comtal.

Unes setmanes més tard, el 25 d'octubre, l'Humà va respondre favorablement a la sol·licitud. El rei va delegar a Bernat Serra, batlle general de Catalunya i conseller seu, totes les gestions que fossin necessàries. Bernat hauria de supervisar la construcció d'arcs, pilars, porxos i altres edificis en el dit solar, els quals, posteriorment, es podrien establir en emfiteusi i/o vendre. Tanmateix, i atenent el rerefons econòmic de la petició, els ingressos generats per la venda, pel valor de les entrades, per morabatins i per qualsevol altre cens els hauria de concedir i assignar a perpetuïtat a l'hospital de la Santa Creu (Castejón 2007: 166-169).

La petició que es va fer al monarca no era pas excepcional. Qualsevol qüestió en matèria urbanística era competència seva o del batlle per delegació. Ampliar o fer més estrets els carrers, obrir voltes sobre algunes vies, construir en les antigues muralles de la ciutat o fer caure alguns envans i parets són al-

17. La primera arcada de la cambra dels homes va ser comprada per Bartomeua, muller de Guillem de Vallseca (AHSCP, Capbreus, vol. VI, inv. 4, Llibres [3], f. 6v-9v). La segona se la van quedar els marmessors de Jaume Blanquer (AHSCP, Capbreus, vol. VI, inv. 4, Llibres [3], f. 39v-42v). La tercera, la quarta i les dues arcades de la cambra de les dones van ser adquirides pels marmessors de Jaume Nicolau (AHSCP, Protocols, vol. V, inv. 3, Protocol [2], f. 83r-83v).

18. AHSCP, Capbreus, vol. VI, inv. 4, Llibres [4], f. 71v-79r.

19. «Divendres, a VII dies del dit mes [octubre] lo dit senyor en lo loch d'Altura. Aquest dia vench en Johan dez Vall, fill d'en Pere dez Vall, per missatger de la ciutat de Barchinona al senyor rei» (Arxiu de la Corona d'Aragó [ACA], Reial Patrimoni, Mestre Racional, vol. 927, *Manual-diario del escribano de ración Ramón Fivaller*, f. 109v).

gunes de les competències que li eren atribuïdes (CARRERAS CANDI 1918: 532). Podem citar un cas documentat per Josefina Mutgé (1987: 200) que recorda vivament la petició d'Altura. L'any 1330 Guillem Fermas, comprador de l'infant Pere, comte de Ribagorça i Empúries, va fer una petició a Alfons el Benigne. Fermas, que posseïa uns immobles a tocar de l'abeurador del rei, va demanar permís per construir un pont que li facilités l'accés a les seves cases, el qual entenem que havia de passar per damunt del Rec Comtal. Un cop Alfons va estudiar-ne la sol·licitud, el 18 de juny d'aquell mateix any va ordenar al batlle que n'aprovés la construcció.

Retornem ara al cas que ens ocupa. I és que pocs mesos després d'aquell 25 d'octubre, el batlle va posar fil a l'agulla. El 4 de febrer de 1402 Bernat Serra va establir en emfiteusi a Miquel Roure aquell gran espai, concedint-li, també, llicència per edificar-hi.[20] Gràcies al contracte sabem que es disposava d'un solar que mesurava 63 canes i mitja de llargària[21] –entre el Pont de Santa Marta i el pont de fusta que estava prop de la muralla nova i que anava al carrer de na Larda– i 6 canes i mitja d'amplària –entre les propietats de l'hospital de Pere Desvilar i el Rec Comtal–.[22] Parlem d'una superfície més o menys rectangular, al tombant dels 960 m$^2$ i que es trobava a tocar de l'estructura hídrica més important de la Barcelona medieval: el Rec Comtal.

En l'establiment emfitèutic es van incloure tot un seguit de mesures per a protegir el Rec. En primer lloc, s'indicà que qualsevol estructura hauria de sobrepassar 3 canes per damunt del mateix. En segona instància, s'ordenava que els edificis no podrien tenir ni entrada ni sortida per la part de la plaça, és a dir, per on creuava el Rec; la tindrien per un nou *vic* que rebria el nom de la Santa Creu, que partia els terrenys que es trobaven rere l'hospital en dos sectors i que es disposava en un sentit paral·lel al Rec Comtal. A l'últim, es feia explícit que no es podria torbar ni bloquejar el curs de les seves aigües.[23] Una vegada es van definir les precaucions adés esmentades, s'establí que Miquel hauria de pagar un cens anual d'1 morabatí i lliurar una entrada de 100 sous.

20. AHSCP, Capbreus, vol. VI, inv. 4, Llibres [1], f. 174v-176v.

21. Les mesures de longitud indicades difereixen en els contractes registrats en el protocol i en el llibre de Joan Torró. Mentre el primer indica que foren 63 canes, el segon diu que van ser 63 canes i mitja. Prenc com a vàlides les dades del llibre, ja que corresponen a una redacció pretesament més detallada i extensa.

22. «Et terminatur predicta ab oriente, partem in capella predicta Sancte Marte, et partem in proprietatibus seu edificiis dicti hospitalis d'en Vilar, àlies de la Ciutat, et partem in quadam magna domo Berengarii Giberti, mercatoris civis dicte civitatis, que tenetur sub dominio et alodio dicti hospitalis Sancte Crucis [...], a meridie, partem in dicto ponte fusteo et partem in patuo qui ibi est, ab occidente, in quodam magno patuo sive magna platea qui ibidem est, et a circio, in dicto ponte Sancte Marte» (AHSCP, Capbreus, vol. VI, inv. 4, Llibres [1], f. 175v).

23. La protecció jurídica del Rec apareix codificada en l'usatge 31: «Cequiam aque molendinorum que fluit ad Barchinonam mandamus esse intactam omni tempore. Et qui eam presumptive fregerit, componat principi centum uncias auri Valencie per unamquamque vicem; et qui in absconso hoc ad rigandum fecerit, componat principi per singulas vices ternas uncias auri predicti» (ABADAL, VALLS I TABERNER 1913: 74).

Tal com s'havia indicat des d'Altura, Miquel va haver d'entregar els diners de l'entrada al prior de l'hospital.[24] Posteriorment, Bernat Serra va transferir als administradors de la Santa Creu els drets que tenia sobre aquell terreny.[25] En avant, Miquel Roure, que tenia l'usdefruit, seria l'encarregat d'emprendre l'activitat constructiva sobre el solar. Convé recordar, però, que els acords registrats en el privilegi d'Altura encara seguien vigents. Això vol dir que la Santa Creu hauria de rebre tots els ingressos que es generessin a raó de la venda o l'establiment de qualsevol bé parcel·lat sobre aquell espai. I en aquest punt el contracte signat entre Bernat Serra i Miquel Roure és, com a mínim, desconcertant. En efecte, els beneficis que li hagués reportat qualsevol explotació immobiliària eren pràcticament nuls. I costa de creure que Miquel ho desconegués en el moment previ a la signatura de l'instrument, car les condicions estaven clarament descrites en l'establiment. Sigui com vulgui, però, un mes després de la rúbrica del contracte, Miquel Roure va renunciar i transferir al prior de la Santa Creu tots els drets que tenia sobre aquell gran solar. La seva acció la va justificar dient que «michi fore dampnosum et inutile propter condiciones et retenciones in eodem instrumento stabilimenti apositas et contentas».[26] Així, va ser a partir d'aquest moment –i no abans–[27] que els administradors de l'hospital van poder parcel·lar i establir en emfiteusi aquell espai, supervisant, indirectament, les obres que en ell havien de ser executades.

Abans de tractar com es va dur a terme l'edificació del solar, queda una pregunta per respondre. Atenent que els beneficis econòmics que Miquel podria extreure de l'operació eren mínims, quina fou la raó de ser de l'establiment signat entre ell i Bernat? Dels possibles vincles que hi poguessin haver entre l'un i l'altre poca cosa puc aportar.[28] Ara bé, és ben cert que l'establiment deixava en mans de Miquel emprendre immediatament –o retardar– el procés constructiu sobre el solar. En el contracte no s'havia inclòs cap clàusula relativa a l'obligatorietat de construir-hi ni tampoc de fer-ho en un termini concret. No obstant això, es tractava d'una operació que podia reportar importants beneficis econòmics a la Santa Creu, els quals es podrien invertir en cobrir part del deute que la construcció de l'hospital estava generant.

Com a hipòtesi, doncs, podem plantejar que el fet que va permetre desencallar l'afer va ser l'accés de Miquel Roure a l'administració de l'hospital de la Santa Creu.[29] I l'ordre dels fets sembla apuntar en aquesta direcció. Si el 4 de

24. AHSCP, Capbreus, vol. VI, inv. 4, Llibres [2], f. 11r-11v.

25. AHSCP, Capbreus, vol. VI, inv. 4, Llibres [2], f. 11v-13v.

26. AHSCP, Capbreus, vol. VI, inv. 4, Llibres [2], f. 26r-27v.

27. La interpretació que van fer Josep M. Roca (1920: 20-21) i Nativitat Castejón (2007: 30) sobre aquest episodi és errònia. Bernat Serra no havia establert el dit solar a Miquel Roure com a administrador de l'hospital, sinó a títol personal «als seus i als qui ell volgués», respectant, evidentment, els drets que el monarca havia concedit a l'hospital. De fet, en el moment de la signatura del contracte Miquel Roure encara no era administrador del centre.

28. Ambdós van coincidir treballant al servei de la Cancelleria Reial en les darreres dècades del segle XIV. Miquel Roure ocupava el càrrec d'escrivà del tresorer i Bernat el d'escrivà del racional. Com a mostra, vegeu ACA, Reial Patrimoni, Mestre Racional, vol. 384, f. 159r i f. 170v.

29. Juntament amb Ramon Desvalls, Ferrer de Marimon, Antoni Bussot i Lluís de Gualbes, Miquel Roure fou un dels cinc consellers presents en la reunió de l'1 de febrer de 1401, en la qual

març de 1402 Miquel havia renunciat als drets d'ús sobre el dit solar a favor de l'hospital, el 5 de maig d'aquell mateix any era escollit administrador de la Santa Creu en substitució de Guillem Colom. Finalment, cinc dies més tard de l'elecció, els administradors de la Santa Creu van feixurar aquell gran solar en diferents patis per a ser establerts en emfiteusi.

## 5. *Cases, hospicis i obradors al voltant d'un nou "vic"*

El 10 de maig de 1402 es van signar dinou establiments emfitèutics.[30] Així, podem dir que, per fi, l'edificació d'aquell gran pati ja es podia endegar. Els administradors de l'hospital es volien assegurar que les intervencions es realitzarien en un període de temps relativament curt. Per aquest motiu, en tots els establiments es va incloure l'obligació de construir-hi cases o hospicis en un lapse de temps inferior a dos anys; els tinents en serien els responsables i haurien de costejar-ne les despeses.[31] Tots els contractes van incloure la clàusula d'immissió que limitava la construcció de taules o envans en el nou *vic*. A més, en els contractes signats sobre les parcel·les tocants al Rec Comtal s'hi van afegir, també, les regulacions que el protegien i prohibien torbar les seves aigües.

Seguint els apunts d'Etienne Hubert (1993: 185) sobre les estratègies patrimonials empreses per algunes institucions religioses, podríem plantejar que la divisió del solar en múltiples unitats d'habitació (i potser, també, la de les dependències de l'hospital) responia a una voluntat de fer més rentable o assequible l'oferta dels establiments. Sigui com vulgui, però, les coses no van procedir tal com els administradors de la Santa Creu desitjaven; la nota «fuit restitutum dicto hospitali ex post stabilitum» escrita al marge d'alguns establiments així ho sembla demostrar.[32] Fins a deu emfiteutes van acabar renunciant als contractes signats el maig de 1402. La urgència i les despeses que els tinents havien d'assumir possiblement van ser els motius que van provocar que molts acabessin retornant els drets d'ús adquirits sobre les parcel·les. Davant d'aquesta situació, entre els mesos de novembre de 1404 i març de 1406, els administradors de la Santa Creu van reparcel·lar els béns que havien estat restituïts i els van establir altra vegada,

es van ponderar diverses qüestions relatives a la fusió hospitalària venidora (ACB, Diversorum B, 1-2-1775, editat per CASTEJÓN 2007: 143-152).

30. AHSCP, Capbreus, vol. VI, inv. 4, Llibres [2], f. 87r-90v, 91r-94v, 95r-98v, 99r-102v, 103r-106v, 123r-126v, 127r-130v, 138r-141r, 141v-144v, 145r-148v, 149r-152r i 152v-155v; AHSCP, Protocols, vol. V, inv. 3, Protocol [1], f. 43r i 43v; AHSCP, Protocols, vol. V, inv. 3, Protocol [1], f. 45v.

31. «Et sub pacto etiam et condicione quod infra duos annos a presente die in antea numerandos, vos et vestri successores in hiis habeatis in dicto solo sive patuo terre construere sive construi et fieri facere vestres et eorum missionibus et expensis hospicium sive domus» (AHSCP, Capbreus, vol. VI, inv. 4, Llibres [2], f. 87v).

32. La nota marginal es pot trobar a AHSCP, Protocols, vol. V, inv. 3, Protocol [1], f. 43r, 43v i 45v; AHSCP, Capbreus, vol. VI, inv. 4, Llibres [2], f. 123r-126v; 127r-130v i 138r-141r. Algunes renúncies van ser registrades en el protocols de Joan Torró: AHSCP, Protocols, vol. V, inv. 3, Protocol [2], f. 53v-54r.

reconsiderant, però, les quantitats que els nous tinents haurien de pagar, tant pel cens anual com per l'entrada. En total parlem de cinc establiments nous,[33] quatre dels quals sabem que van quedar exempts del pagament del cens durant dos anys, a fi de facilitar un poc més l'edificació d'aquells solars.[34]

Per raó de les entrades pagades, la Santa Creu va ingressar un total de 808 sous, una suma que certament contrasta amb els 8.527 sous corresponents a les entrades per l'establiment de les antigues dependències de l'hospital. La diferència entre un valor i l'altre s'explicaria pels atributs o les condicions en què es trobaven els béns i les obligacions imposades en els contractes. Així, mentre uns tinents tan sols havien de dur a terme unes intervencions mínimes, com l'obertura de portals o la construcció de mitgeres, a uns altres se'ls va obligar a construir cases i hospicis des de zero.

Una vegada els contractes d'establiment van ser firmats, els administradors de la Santa Creu van vendre el domini directe d'alguns béns. És el cas de les parcel·les que van ser establertes a Pere Guerau, a Antònia i a Berenguer Carreres, les quals van ser comprades pels marmessors de Jaume Aldomar el 20 de febrer de 1405.[35] Però aquest no va ser el destí de totes les possessions. Exceptuant els béns establerts a Nicolau Boxet i Miquel Quadres, dels quals no he trobat cap més referència, la resta va romandre dins del domini de l'hospital com a mínim vint anys més.

Gràcies al capbreu començat l'any 1421 és possible observar les millores que es van dur a terme sobre els patis que havien estat establerts a Pere Rovira,[36] Ramon Degà,[37] Joan Cabirol,[38] Bartomeu Sala[39] i Joan Franc.[40] A l'hora de confessar els béns que tenien pel domini de la Santa Creu, ells mateixos o d'altres que, per una via o altra, n'havien adquirit l'ús, van indicar què contenien aquelles

33. AHSCP, Capbreus, vol. VI, inv. 4, Llibres [4], f. 8v-11r; AHSCP, Protocols, vol. V, inv. 3, Protocols [2], f. 69r-70r; 70r; 70v i 81r-v.

34. Al marge de cadascun dels contractes s'indicà que «fuit conventuum quod iste [...] non solvat censum II annorum venturum, ratione operis faciendi».

35. AHSCP, Capbreus, vol. VI, inv. 4, Llibres [4], f. 71v-79r.

36. AHSCP, Capbreus, vol. VI, inv. 4, Llibres [16], f. 60r. El 4 de gener de 1407 Pere Rovira va vendre l'usdefruit sobre les dues propietats que tenia al calderer Antoni Marquès. AHPB, Joan Nadal, 54/57, f. 65r-67r i 67r-69r. Antoni deia que tenia «quodam staticum domorum cum duobus portalibus cum envano» i «quodam alium staticum domorum cum envano».

37. AHSCP, Capbreus, vol. VI, inv. 4, Llibres [16], f. 12r. La confessió la va fer Sansa, vídua de Ramon Degà, que va indicar que tenia «quendam solum sive patium terre in quo fuerunt constructe et hedificate domus cum envanis et tabulis» i un altre que li era adjacent.

38. La propietat establerta a Joan Cabirol es va dividir l'any 1416, quan Joan en va vendre una part al mestre d'aixa Bartomeu Puig. Així, en el capbreu de 1421 una la va confessar el dit Bartomeu i l'altra Rafaela, muller del dit Joan, ja mort (AHSCP, Capbreus, vol. VI, inv. 4, Llibres [16], f. 52r i 85v). Bartomeu va confessar tenir «quodam patium sive solum terre sive partem patui quod fuit de pertinenciis illius patui quod fuit stabilitum Johanni Cabirol» i Rafaela «quasdam domos per dictum quondam maritum suum ibi noviter constructas».

39. AHSCP, Capbreus, vol. VI, inv. 4, Llibres [16], f. 46v. Bartomeu Sala va confessar «duo staria que solebant esse solum sive patuum terre».

40. AHSCP, Capbreus, vol. VI, inv. 4, Llibres [16], f. 48r. Joan Franc va confessar «quatuor staria que solebant esse solum sive patuum terre» i també «quodam staticum domorum cum envano».

possessions. Així, dues dècades més tard ja s'apreciaven canvis importants. En l'antic solar que vorejava l'hospital de Pere Desvilar hi trobem una illa formada per una sèrie de *domos* i estatges que s'articulaven al llarg d'un nou eix que ja es coneixia com el nou *vic* de la Santa Creu (fig. 1).

En poc més de deu anys, els administradors de l'hospital de la Santa Creu havien donat un canvi d'imatge radical a un espai que, just abans de la unificació, era exclusivament ocupat per l'hospital de Pere Desvilar i la capella de Santa Marta. D'aleshores ençà la fesomia de l'antic centre era diferent i al seu voltant s'hi havien construït un nombre divers de cases on hi vivien artistes, menestrals, mercaders i mariners de la Barcelona baixmedieval. Aquell solar prenia vida i s'urbanitzava, i l'hospital de la Santa Creu n'era el responsable i promotor. I no només això. El *vic* sobre el qual havia estat articulat aquell conjunt de cases va prendre, no per casualitat, el nom de la Santa Creu. Una decisió gens baladí i que s'entén com una marca de promoció i poder, que si bé recordava una advocació multisecular barcelonina, sobretot evocava la nova institució hospitalària que s'havia aixecat a l'altre extrem de la ciutat.

## 6. *La dissort de l'hospital d'en Pere Desvilar*

Les intervencions que es van dur a terme sobre l'hospital d'en Pere Desvilar van repercutir sobre la seva activitat assistencial. La reforma que havia estat impulsada durant els anys setanta del segle XIV, per la qual l'hospital s'havia compromès, també, a l'acolliment de pobres malalts, va quedar en no-res. A causa de les reformes esdevingudes a partir de 1401 l'immoble es va quedar sense els espais necessaris per poder desenvolupar tal funció. A partir d'aleshores, l'hospital fundat per Desvilar retornaria al compliment de les tasques que el seu promotor havia disposat en el seu testament i que, durant més de mig segle, havia servit, també, als interessos del Consell de Cent.

Les accions que es van executar sobre les antigues dependències de l'hospital van provocar un canvi evident en aquella illa de la vilanova de Barcelona. Els administradors de la Santa Creu van desmantellar una institució que era i es donava a conèixer com l'Hospital de la Ciutat. El centre va ser dividit en unitats menors i els tinents que van rebre en emfiteusi les seves cambres van ser els executors de les reformes. Però de les estructures que havien format part d'aquell conjunt no n'ha quedat res. L'any 1715 Felip V va arrasar el barri de la Ribera, allà on es trobava l'hospital, amb l'objectiu de materialitzar el projecte de la Ciutadella ideat per Verboom (TORRAS 2005: 265-283).[41] Afortunadament, a l'Arxiu Històric de la Ciutat de Barcelona es conserva un plànol anterior a l'enderrocament que ajuda a tenir una idea aproximada de com era l'indret: la *Planta de la ciutat de*

41. Anys després, el 1734, l'Ajuntament de Barcelona va adquirir uns nous terrenys en què reedificaria l'hospital fundat per Desvilar en el carrer de la riera de Sant Joan (CONEJO 2002: 292).

*Barcelona y Moniuic y Moll y Atachos*.[42] És un document gràfic que probablement sigui de factura municipal i que es va elaborar en el context del setge dirigit pel duc Vendôme l'any 1697 (Pujades, Soberón, Cubeles 2020: 81-83). En ell s'hi pot veure la zona que va ocupar l'hospital i un conjunt de cases que van ser construïdes i disposades a banda i banda del *vic* de la Santa Creu (fig. 2).

Per concloure, aquest article pretén evidenciar les possibilitats que ofereix l'anàlisi dels establiments emfitèutics, en general, i de les clàusules que s'hi inclouen, en particular. No només ha estat possible identificar l'estratègia patrimonial que els administradors de la Santa Creu van dur a terme durant els primers anys del segle XV, sinó que també s'han pogut recuperar les intervencions que aquests van impulsar sobre les cambres de l'Hospital de la Ciutat i el seu entorn. Així, gràcies al seu estudi, ha estat possible entendre el desenvolupament sobre un espai molt delimitat de la ciutat comtal.

Les accions que es van dur a terme a inicis del quatre-cents van significar un punt i a part en la història de l'antic hospital. Però encara que les mides de la institució van ser reduïdes, la seva tasca original continuaria uns quants segles més. Per descobrir-la, tan sols falta capbussar-se en el riquíssim fons de l'Arxiu històric de l'Hospital de la Santa Creu i Sant Pau, on es conserva molta de la documentació administrativa i notarial de l'hospital fundat per Pere Desvilar i Blanca.

## *Bibliografia*

Abadal de Vinyals, Ramon; Valls i Taberner, Ferran (ed.), 1913. *Usatges de Barcelona,* Barcelona, Patronat de la Diputació Provincial.

Batlle Gallart, Carme; Casas i Nadal, Montserrat, 1980. "La caritat privada i les institucions benèfiques de Barcelona (segle XIII)", Manuel Riu (ed.), *La pobreza y la asistencia a los pobres en la Cataluña medieval. Volumen misceláneo de estudios y documentos*, Barcelona, CSIC: I, 118-190.

Benito Monclús, Pere, 2003. *Senyoria de la terra i tinença pagesa al comtat de Barcelona (segles XI-XIII)*, Barcelona, IMF-CSIC.

Boscà, Joan Francesc, 1977. *Memorial històric*, Barcelona, Associació de Bibliòfils de Barcelona.

Bridgewater Mateu, Pol, 2020. *"Car vosaltres havets a veure sobre hospitals": El Consell de Cent i la construcció de la primera política hospitalària a la Barcelona baixmedieval*, Tesi doctoral, Universitat de Barcelona.

Carreras Candi, Francesc, 1910. Notes *sobre los orígens de la enfiteusis en lo territori de Barcelona*, Barcelona, Fills de Jaume Jepús Impressors.

Castejón Domènech, Nativitat, 2007. *Aproximació a l'estudi de l'Hospital de la Santa Creu de Barcelona: repertori documental del segle XV*, Barcelona, Fundació Noguera.

Conejo da Pena, Antoni, 2002. *Assistència i hospitalitat a l'edat mitjana. L'arquitectura dels hospitals catalans: del gòtic al primer renaixement*, Tesi doctoral, Universitat de Barcelona.

Conejo da Pena, Antoni, 2020. "«La present casa, molt Illustre y magnífica per la grandeza de son edifici». L'hospital de la Santa Creu de Barcelona: 1401-1417", *Lambard. Estudis d'Art Medieval*, 28: 9-56.

42. AHCB, núm. reg. 20096, olim 17932.

DALMASES I PONS, David, 1994. "La capella d'en Marcús, els antecedents del seu fundador i l'advocació a la Mare de Déu de la Guia", *Lambard. Estudis d'Art Medieval*, 6: 113-58.

HUBERT, Etienne, 1993. "Economie de la propriété immobilière: les établissements religieux et leurs patrimoines au XIVe siècle" *Rome aux XIIIe et XIVe siècles. Cinq études réunies par Etienne Hubert*, Roma, École Française de Rome & Viella: 233-247.

JULIÁ VIÑAMATA, José Ramón, 1991. "La enfiteusis como factor transformador del paisaje en la Barcelona de principios de siglo XV", *Universitas Tarraconensis*, 10: 129-150.

MUTGÉ VIVES, Josefina, 1987. *La ciudad de Barcelona durante el reinado de Alfonso el Benigno (1327-1336)*, Barcelona, IMF-CSIC.

PUJADES BATALLER, Ramon; SOBERÓN RODRÍGUEZ, Mikel; CUBELES BONET, Albert, 2020. "Entre el realisme i la idealització: la façana marítima de Barcelona i les vistes urbanes", Ramon Grau, Carme Muntaner (ed.), *Vistes panoràmiques, cartes militars i plànols urbanístics a Barcelona del segle XVI al XIX*, Barcelona, Ajuntament de Barcelona & Institut Cartogràfic i Geològic de Catalunya: 76-103.

RIBALTA HARO, Jaume, 2001. "Immissions i acció negatòria a Catalunya: una lectura històrica i comparativa d'una modernització legislativa", *Revista de Dret Històric Català*, 1: 125-154.

RIBALTA HARO, Jaume, 2005. *Dret urbanístic medieval de la Mediterrània*, Barcelona, Universitat Pompeu Fabra i Institut d'Estudis Catalans.

ROCA, Josep Maria (ed.), 1920. *Ordinacions del Hospital General de la Santa Creu de Barcelona (any MCCCCXVII)*, Barcelona, Fidel Giró.

SABATÉ CURULL, Flocel, 1997. *El territori de la Catalunya medieval. Percepció de l'espai i divisió territorial al llarg de l'Edat Mitjana,* Barcelona, Fundació Salvador Vives i Casajuana.

SERRA PUIG, Eva, 1989. "Notes sobre els orígens i l'evolució de l'emfiteusi a Catalunya", *Estudis d'Història Agrària*, 7: 126-138.

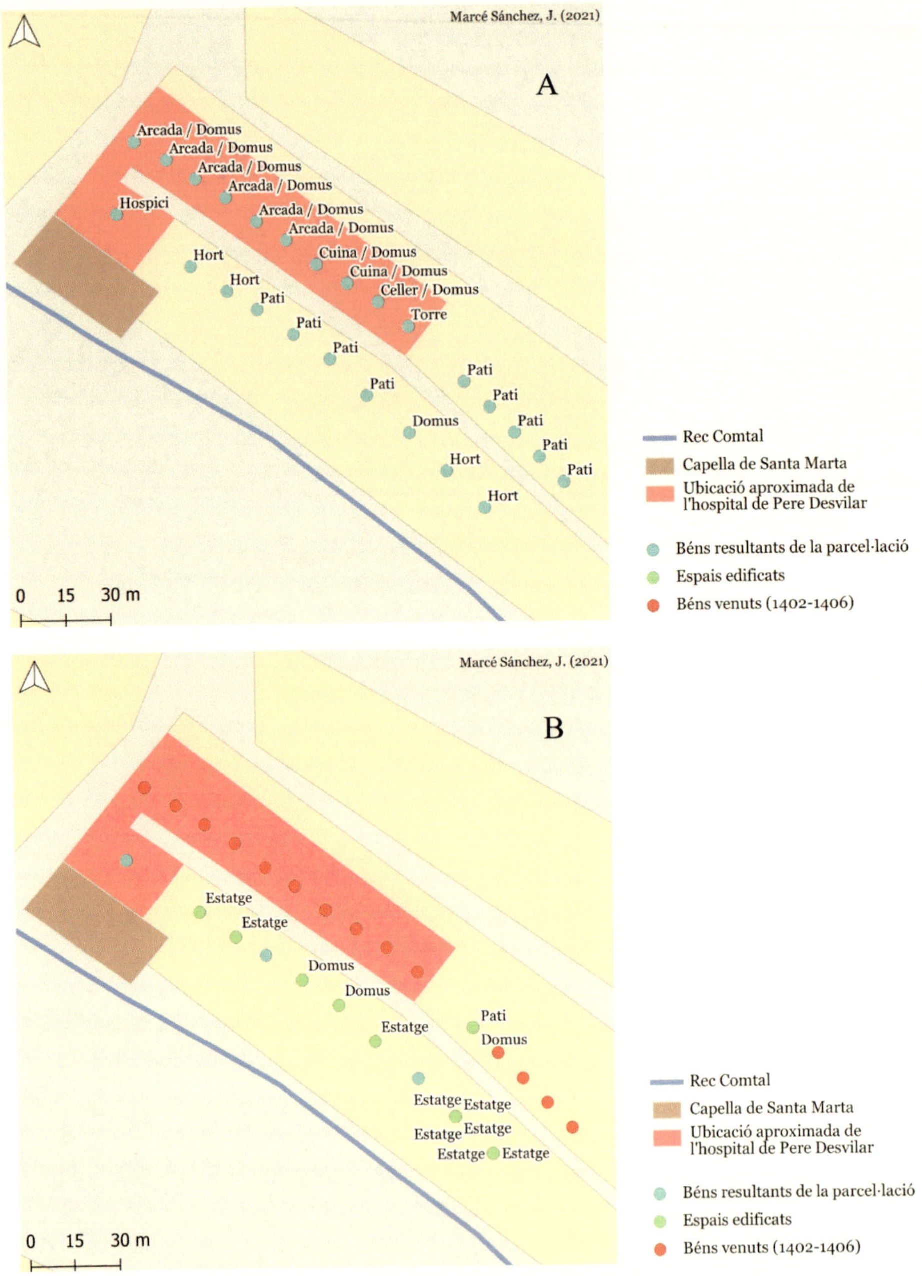


Fig. 1. Proposta de reconstrucció de les parcel·lacions fetes en l'hospital de Pere Desvilar (A) i canvis duts a terme sobre les dependències del mateix hospital (B). Elaboració de l'autor.

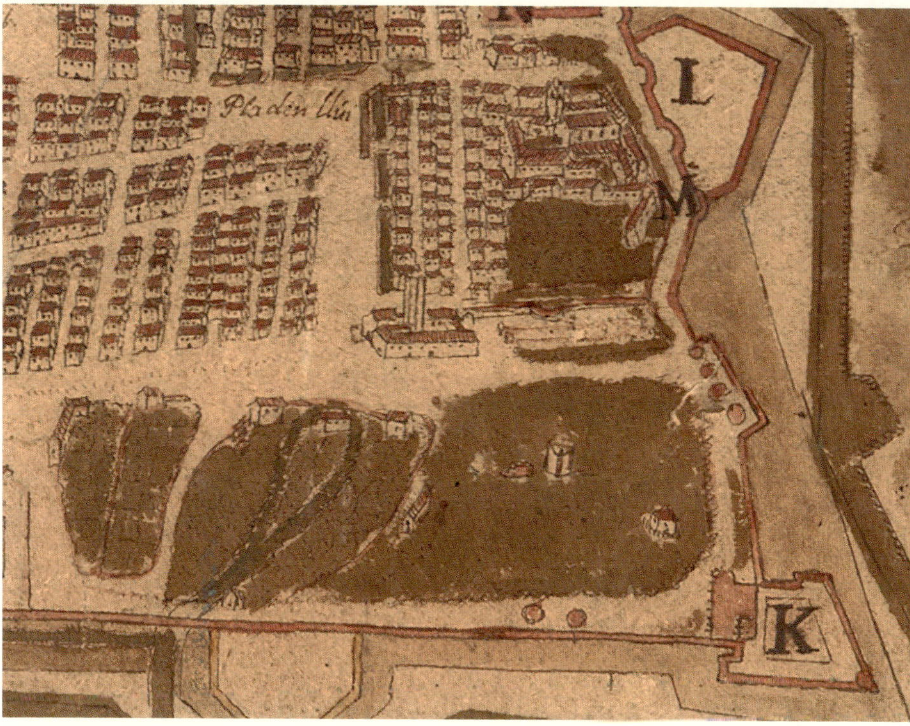


Fig. 2. *Planta de la ciutat de Barcelona y Moniuic y Moll y Atachos*, detall, 1697. Al centre es pot veure el tram final del Rec Comtal i, a la dreta, un conjunt de cases construïdes a banda i banda del *vic* de la Santa Creu (Barcelona: AHCB, C0202_20096). © AHCB. Imatge obtinguda de https://bit.ly/3Nxr6vS.

Fabio Gabbrielli

# L'ospedale di Santa Maria della Scala a Siena: funzioni, sviluppo architettonico e immagine pubblica (XII-metà XIV secolo)

L'ospedale di Santa Maria della Scala a Siena, come è noto, è stato uno dei maggiori complessi a carattere assistenziale, per dimensioni, organizzazione e funzioni, dell'Europa del basso Medioevo. Le sue origini risalgono alla fine dell'XI secolo, quale emanazione della canonica del Duomo, ma già alla fine del secolo seguente il Capitolo amministrava in autonomia i beni patrimoniali ed eleggeva il proprio rettore. Fra il XIII e il XV secolo avvenne il progressivo passaggio da un'istituzione a carattere religioso, con ampi margini di autonomia, a un ente laico sotto l'egida pubblica, pienamente integrato nell'apparato istituzionale del Comune.[1]

La fortuna del Santa Maria della Scala, quello straordinario successo che gli valse, già alla fine del Trecento, una tale fama da essere preso a modello per la fondazione di grandi ospedali europei,[2] viaggiò in parallelo con la fortuna stessa della città. Figli della strada sono stati definiti entrambi,[3] ovvero figli di quella via Francigena che per secoli costituì uno dei motori dello sviluppo urbanistico ed economico della città e, al tempo stesso, garantì al Santa Maria un rivolo costante di pellegrini e mercanti in viaggio verso Roma. Di questa umanità, variegata e cosmopolita, ne abbiamo una viva testimonianza documentaria nel *Libro del pellegrino*, un eccezionale registro nel quale furono annotati, tra la fine del XIV e i primi del XV secolo, più di quattrocento tra uomini e donne che, diretti a Roma, avevano lasciato in deposito i loro denari nei forzieri dell'ospedale e che, per ragioni ignote, non vi avevano fatto ritorno (Piccinni, Travaini 2003). Le loro località di provenienza coprono quasi ogni parte d'Europa, offrendoci uno spaccato impressionante tanto del ruolo fondamentale del viaggio nella società medievale quanto della fama di luogo affidabile e sicuro che il Santa Maria si era conquistata nel tempo. Il pellegrino riceveva vino e pane al momento dell'arrivo, vino, pane e cibi cotti ogni sera, un letto nel pellegrinaio e, per tutelarsi dai furti,

1. Per un inquadramento generale delle vicende istituzionali e dei rapporti tra l'Ospedale, il Comune e l'Episcopato: Pellegrini 2003; Lugarini 2011: 17-30; Pellegrini 2016; Piccinni 2016a; Sordini 2010.

2. Piccinni 2016b.

3. Per Siena: Sestan 1961. Per il Santa Maria della Scala: Piccinni 1995: 13.

poteva depositare denaro e piccoli oggetti preziosi per poi riprenderli nel viaggio di ritorno.

Ma l'aspetto più qualificante del Santa Maria della Scala, analogamente ad altri grandi ospedali urbani, fu la polifunzionalità. Tra il Due e il Trecento, senza che venisse meno l'originaria funzione di ospitalità, l'ospedale elargiva quotidianamente elemosine in pane, garantiva la cura dei malati e dei feriti (con tanto di presenza fissa di un medico e di un chirurgo), accoglieva i bambini abbandonati (per i quali alla fine del Duecento fu realizzata nella piazza del Duomo un'apposita struttura), istruendoli e accompagnandoli fino alla maggiore età (Piccinni 1995; Sordini 2010). Attività tutte mirabilmente descritte in quella sorta di "Buongoverno ospedaliero"[4] che è il ciclo quattrocentesco di affreschi del Pellegrinaio "di mezzo" (Gabbrielli 2014). Era insomma la principale istituzione di riferimento per arginare le tante e diversificate forme di disagio, povertà e malattia che gravavano sulla società. In più l'ospedale gestiva un'enorme proprietà terriera e immobiliare (Epstein 1986), elargiva prestiti allo Stato e svolgeva anche un'attività di tipo bancario, accettando depositi di denaro in cambio di interessi (Piccinni 2012). Nei suoi locali, inoltre, venivano immagazzinati i prodotti agricoli provenienti dalle grance, si preparavano le medicine e non mancavano attività artigianali e di trasformazione di materie prime funzionali alla vita dell'ospedale stesso.

Il carattere polifunzionale è alla base della straordinaria complessità e varietà delle strutture che tutt'oggi ne compongono il tessuto edilizio, assimilabile più ad un pezzo di città che ad singolo edificio, articolato in numerosi corpi di fabbrica, cortili e vicoli, una strada interna, chiese ed oratori di compagnie laicali, distribuiti, per cinque, sei o sette livelli, lungo tutto il versante sud-occidentale del colle del Duomo (Siena 1986; Sordini 2010; Gabbrielli 2021).

L'attuale complesso edilizio non è nato da un progetto unitario, da un preciso disegno, ma da un lungo processo di ampliamenti, annessioni e trasformazioni, strettamente connesse alle necessità ricettive, alle disponibilità finanziarie e al crescente ruolo economico e sociale che l'ospedale venne ad acquisire nella città e nel territorio tra il XII e il XV secolo.

Per circa un secolo dalla prima attestazione, dell'anno 1090,[5] l'ospedale fu pienamente integrato con la canonica, sul piano amministrativo e forse anche su quello topografico essendo plausibile l'ipotesi di un'ubicazione diversa da quella attuale, sempre nella piazza del Duomo ma a fianco e non di fronte alla cattedrale, dove appunto risiedeva la sede dei canonici. Il distacco topografico dalla sede originaria sarebbe avvenuto alla fine del XII secolo, in concomitanza con le prime espressioni di una propria organizzazione interna e di un'autonomia amministrativa nella gestione del patrimonio. Nel 1186, infatti, l'ospedale è per la prima

4. L'espressione è di Gabriella Piccinni.

5. Archivio di Stato di Siena (da ora in poi ASS), *Ospedale, Diplomatico,* 1090, marzo 29 (Sordini 2010: 17).

volta attestato *ante gradus,* vale a dire davanti alla scalinata del Duomo, nel sito dove ancora oggi si trova.[6]

Le indagini di stratigrafia degli elevati hanno individuato nella muratura in pietra situata al centro dell'attuale facciata sulla piazza del Duomo, esclusi i due portali a sesto acuto, inseriti posteriormente, il più antico edificio ad oggi riconoscibile.[7] È assai probabile, come è stato di recente ipotizzato, che si tratti dell'antico pellegrinaio, qui eretto a seguito del trasferimento di sito, preceduto da un portico duecentesco in pietra e mattoni.[8] Il portico, attestato dalle fonti scritte nel 1248, è ancora esistente sebbene tamponato nelle tre arcate e più volte trasformato al suo interno.[9] Si tratta degli unici edifici, dell'attuale facciata di Santa Maria della Scala, che hanno conservato strutture anteriori alla grande fase edilizia di fine XIII-primo XIV secolo, i soli, pertanto, che ci permettono qualche valutazione sulle scelte architettoniche operate prima del periodo "novesco".[10] Nel caso del pellegrinaio, poi chiesa, non possiamo altro che notare, data l'assenza di elementi architettonici e ornamentali riconducibili alla fase originaria, l'impiego di un'accurata tecnica litotomica per la muratura esterna, a corsi orizzontali e paralleli di conci di "pietra da torre" squadrati e spianati, comunemente utilizzata nell'edilizia monumentale, soprattutto religiosa, di XII-XIII secolo. Caratteri diversi presenta il portico (fig. 1), evidentemente realizzato a distanza di tempo rispetto al pellegrinaio: tre archi a sesto acuto su pilastri a spigoli arrotondati, costituiti da filari regolarmente alternati di laterizi e di "pietra da torre". L'alternanza di pietre e mattoni a fini ornamentali è presente in alcuni edifici civili senesi di XII-XIII secolo (Fonte di Follonica, Porte di Campansi e San Maurizio, Palazzo Malavolti, ecc.) ma è soprattutto in ambito religioso che tale soluzione ha le più rilevanti attestazioni, coinvolgendo un notevole numero di edifici situati in una fascia territoriale per lo più compresa tra Siena e Volterra, tra i quali si annoverano la celebre chiesa di San Galgano a Montesiepi e i locali monastici, duecenteschi, della omonima abbazia cistercense (MORETTI 1982: 62-71; GABBRIELLI 2010: 144-145). Il riferimento ai monaci di San Galgano, che dalla metà del Duecento iniziarono a gravitare sulla città di Siena, anche con l'acquisizione di importanti incarichi (operai della fabbrica del duomo e camerlenghi della Biccherna), potrebbe non essere un caso.[11]

6. L'ipotesi di due diverse ubicazioni è stata formulata da SORDINI 2010: 19-25.

7. PARENTI 1991: 30-33, il quale interpreta l'edificio, fin dall'origine, come chiesa dell'ospedale.

8. SORDINI 2010: 26-29. Sui caratteri architettonici dei pellegrinai: MORETTI 2014.

9. «In porticu extra peregrinarium dicti hospitalis» (ASS, *Ospedale, Diplomatico,* 1248 maggio 12; SORDINI 2010: 28-29). Sulle trasformazioni interne e sugli apparati decorativi: GAVAZZI, MONTEVECCHI, SBARDELLATI 2014.

10. Sul governo dei Nove (1287-1355): BOWSKY 1986.

11. Di quanto il Santa Maria della Scala possa essere stato debitore dei cistercensi di San Galgano, è un campo di ricerca tutto da esplorare. Ricordiamo, ad esempio, che la presenza, nelle infermerie dell'abbazia, di un medico fisico e di un medico chirurgo è documentata fin dal 1255 (CANESTRELLI 1993: p. 70 n. 3), e che le vaste proprietà terriere dei monaci erano organizzate in aziende agricole denominate grance (o grange).

Nel 1257 fu concesso all'ospedale di erigere una propria chiesa.[12] Si trattò di un atto importante poiché all'autonomia della gestione patrimoniale si aggiungeva, ora, quella della cura d'anime. Probabilmente il pellegrinaio del XII secolo, a seguito di questo atto, fu trasformato in chiesa, dotata del preesistente portico (Sordini 2010: 28-29, 36-37). La trasformazione del pellegrinaio in chiesa, entro il 1272, anno in cui quest'ultima risultava già funzionante, determinò un'espansione degli edifici verso la zona retrostante, dove una nuova struttura, a due navate, corrispondente alle attuali sale di San Galgano e di Sant'Ansano, destinata ad accogliere poveri, malati e pellegrini, fu realizzata modificando due ambienti preesistenti, come è stato documentato da uno scavo archeologico del 2005.[13] Questi si sviluppavano per almeno due piani e si affacciavano su una strada pubblica retrostante al nucleo originario dell'ospedale, la via di Vallepiatta, poi nota come "strada interna" del Santa Maria della Scala. Il nuovo pellegrinaio, suddiviso in due navate da grandi arcate semicircolari, si attestò al di sopra delle due strutture, sfruttando il forte dislivello naturale che caratterizza l'area retrostante alla piazza del Duomo. Fu la fase iniziale della grande espansione dell'ospedale sul versante sud-occidentale della collina, attestata, dalla metà del Duecento, da un gran numero di atti inerenti all'acquisto di case, palazzi, orti e terreni, collocati lungo la via di Vallepiatta o nelle sue vicinanze, fino alla completa acquisizione, da parte del Santa Maria della Scala, della strada stessa (Giorgi, Moscadelli 2005: 82-91; Sordini 2010: 38-43, 51-52, 61-62).

Atti testamentari, donazioni e lasciti di facoltosi oblati incrementarono la ricchezza dell'ospedale, mentre si fece più forte il legame con il Comune, il quale si pose a tutela del Santa Maria offrendo sostegno economico, politico e giudiziario. Nell'anno 1257, lo stesso in cui la sede apostolica concesse l'edificazione della chiesa, il Comune decise di spostare il tracciato della cinta muraria della città, predisponendo l'abbandono del tratto situato a valle della "strada interna". Ciò consentì all'ospedale, tra il Due e il Trecento, di ampliarsi fino alle vecchie mura, attestandosi su di esse con le sue strutture, quale limite sud-occidentale dell'intero complesso.[14]

Dalla fine del Duecento il Santa Maria della Scala divenne uno dei principali strumenti attraverso i quali i membri delle grandi famiglie magnatizie, dal 1277 escluse dalla partecipazione al governo della città, potevano esprimere la loro azione politica e sociale, oltre che umana e cristiana. Personaggi come Bernardino d'Alamanno Piccolomini, Ristoro di Giunta Menghi o Scozia di Rinaldo Tolomei, membri a vario titolo, tra il Due e il Trecento, del Santa Maria, erano cittadini di spicco del tessuto sociale, magnati, già attivissimi protagonisti della finanza e della politica senese.[15]

12. ASS, *Ospedale, Diplomatico*, 1257, giugno 27 (Sordini 2010: 28).

13. I due ambienti sono stati interpretati, alle quote interessate dallo scavo, come case (Sordini 2010: 35-389; Causarano et al. 2011).

14. Sordini 2010: 38-43. Tale limite sarà scavalcato nel XV secolo.

15. Pellegrini 2012: 999; Pellegrini 2014: 282-283; Pellegrini 2016: 293; Mucciarelli 2001: 70-80.

La stessa figura del rettore, eletto tra i più influenti membri della città, aveva una marcata fisionomia aristocratica, prerogativa che fu normalizzata con lo Statuto del 1318 (STATUTI SENESI 1877: 14). La sua azione non era più limitata al governo di un'esperienza religioso-assistenziale ma assumeva prerogative di carattere politico, fino a costituire un punto di riferimento essenziale nella vita sociale ed economica della città (PELLEGRINI 2012: 1003; 2016: 295-296).

D'altra parte, se la carica di rettore era riservata all'aristocrazia, il variegato mondo dei *fratres* di Santa Maria della Scala contemplava al suo interno tutte le espressioni sociali, dai magnati ai membri di casati meno noti e agli esponenti del ceto medio, vale a dire quella *mezzana gente* a cui era riservato, per legge, il governo della città. Insomma, dalla fine del Duecento, il Santa Maria si configurò sempre più, a pieno titolo, come l'ospedale della città, quale espressione dell'intero corpo sociale (PELLEGRINI 2016: 290-295). Era giocoforza che il referente principale non fosse più l'Episcopato ma il Comune, con il quale ebbe a tessere un rapporto interlocutorio e non privo di contrasti.

Tutto ciò si riflette nello stile e nel carattere degli interventi architettonici che sul finire del secolo cambiarono il volto dell'ospedale sulla piazza del Duomo, vale a dire la sua dimensione pubblica e rappresentativa. Intorno al 1290 fu infatti costruito, a fianco della chiesa, il Palazzo del Rettore (fig. 2), e nel 1298 fu edificata, sul lato opposto, la Casa dei Gettatelli (o delle Balie; PARENTI 1991: 33-39). Entrambi gli edifici sono in laterizi, a due piani, con portali e bifore a sesto acuto e cornici orizzontali alle quote dei davanzali delle finestre e delle imposte degli archi, secondo i più aggiornati canoni stilistici dei maggiori palazzi, pubblici e privati, della città. Anzi, se guardiamo alla cronologia, il Palazzo del Rettore, anticipando di otto anni l'inizio del cantiere del Palazzo del Comune, rappresenta un episodio di avanguardia stilistica nella formulazione del gotico civile senese o gotico "novesco".[16] E la Casa dei Gettatelli (fig. 3), in parte ripristinata nei primi del XX secolo, non è da meno: insieme agli stilemi del gotico senese, ormai maturi, la facciata originaria ostentava una raffinata cortina muraria in laterizi accuratamente foggiati, arrotati e rifiniti con una graffiatura estesa all'intero prospetto, come nei più importanti edifici di fine Duecento e primi Trecento.[17]

Il Palazzo del Rettore e la Casa dei Gettatelli rientrano in quel processo di progressiva specializzazione delle funzioni e degli ambienti che tra il Due e il Trecento ha caratterizzato l'evoluzione del Santa Maria della Scala. Ma sono anche l'espressione più evidente, con il loro linguaggio architettonico, di quella lenta metamorfosi istituzionale che dall'originaria dimensione religiosa stava trasformando il maggiore ospedale cittadino in "un'impresa della pubblica carità".[18]

16. Sul gotico di età "novesca": GABBRIELLI 2010: 111-256. Sul Palazzo del Rettore ivi: 138-139 fig. 105-106, 141-142.

17. Ora limitata a pochi lacerti concentrati per lo più negli archi. GABBRIELLI 1991b: 140-144, 151; GABBRIELLI 2010: 157.

18. L'espressione è di Gabriella Piccinni (2012). La "laicizzazione" delle forme e delle tipologie architettoniche degli ospedali, legata al processo di municipalizzazione dell'assistenza, è

In entrambe le facciate l'eccezionalità dei cantieri è sottolineata da due epigrafi. Quella del 1298 (fig. 4) specifica la funzione a cui era destinato il rispettivo edificio: «Hec domus facta e(st) p(ro) gittatellis i(n) an(n)o D(omi)ni MCCLXXXXVIII i(n) quo t(em)p(o)re sunt i(n) numero CCC gitatelli et plus», e quella del 1290 (fig. 5) riporta anche il nome del rettore, Orlando di Guglielmo da Chiusure (1286-1294), che ne dovette promuovere l'iniziativa: «Ann(o) D(omini) MCCLXXXX factu(m) e(st) istud palatç(i)u(m) t(em)p(o)r(e) d(omi)ni Orlandi d(e) Kisure rectoris c(!)ospital(is) S(ancte) M(a)rie d(e) pecunia hospitalis».[19] Il rettore viveva e operava all'interno del complesso di Santa Maria della Scala, ma in un *palatçium*, appunto, in un edificio all'altezza del suo ruolo e del ceto di provenienza, per nulla distinguibile dai caratteri dell'architettura civile di elevato rango, che per altro a Siena, tra fine Duecento e prima metà Trecento, accomunava nello stile, come nei materiali e nelle finiture, il pubblico e il privato. Solo l'accentuato sviluppo in senso orizzontale, a sei assi di aperture che si aggiungono alle tre preesistenti, cui seguirà più tardi, fra Tre e Quattrocento, la soprelevazione di un piano e la realizzazione di un coronamento merlato, tradisce l'appartenenza all'edilizia pubblica anziché privata, così come, del resto, la Casa dei Gettatelli, ad esso speculare, a due piani e otto assi di bifore in seguito ampliate a dieci (Gabbrielli 2010: 232-234).

Per tutta la prima metà del Trecento, periodo in cui la dimensione europea dell'economia finanziaria della città entrò in crisi, con il ritiro delle compagnie bancarie dai mercati internazionali, il Santa Maria della Scala divenne un rifugio ideale per le grandi ricchezze prodotte nel secolo precedente (Piccinni 2012). Fu il presupposto per un'ulteriore, poderosa espansione del complesso ospedaliero.

Protagonista di questa straordinaria stagione fu Giovanni di Tese Tolomei, altro personaggio di spicco della società senese, magnate, bene inserito nel sistema politico comunale quale membro del Consiglio Generale, podestà di comunità e console di Mercanzia, infine rettore di Santa Maria della Scala dal 1314 al 1339. Sotto il suo rettorato vide la luce lo Statuto del 1318, con il quale l'ospedale ebbe un assetto organizzativo all'altezza delle molteplici attività che era chiamato a svolgere, ed ebbe un ulteriore, potente impulso l'attività edilizia, volta in particolare all'ampliamento e alla riorganizzazione delle strutture assistenziali.[20]

Nel 1327-1328 fu costruito un nuovo pellegrinaio degli uomini, quello che nel Quattrocento sarà affrescato da Lorenzo di Pietro e Domenico di Bartolo. Ad esso si accedeva, dalla piazza del Duomo, tramite l'attuale portale, forse realizzato in tale occasione, in asse con il pellegrinaio stesso e un tempo condiviso con la chiesa. Il portale (fig. 6) presenta un arco a sesto acuto che, nella combinazione

stata evidenziata, con tempi e modalità diverse, anche in altri contesti europei, come in Germania (Leistikow 1967, p. 53) e in Catalogna (Conejo 2002: 121-122, 447-595).

19. Sulle due epigrafi: Gabbrielli 1991a: 103-105. Sul rettore Orlando di Guglielmo: Statuti senesi 1877: 158-161. La Casa dei Gettatelli, invece, fu realizzata al tempo di Ristoro di Giunta Menghi (1294-1313), sotto il cui rettorato fu compilato lo Statuto del 1305 (Statuti senesi 1877: 161-172; Pellegrini 2005).

20. Su Giovanni di Tese: Pellegrini 2012.

dei cunei in pietra calcarea chiara e delle cornici in serpentinite scura, riproduce i colori araldici della città come nei portali del Palazzo del Comune (GABBRIELLI 1991b: 151-153). Negli anni Trenta fu edificato un altro pellegrinaio maschile, con assetto ortogonale al precedente e con uno dei lati maggiori prospiciente la via di Vallepiatta. E nel 1336-38 fu la volta di un terzo pellegrinaio, riservato alle donne, il più grande di tutto l'ospedale, situato tra la piazza del Duomo, all'angolo con via del Capitano, e la strada interna.[21] In tutti i casi si tratta di moduli parallelepipedi, fortemente sviluppati in senso longitudinale e in altezza, a cinque o a sei piani, con il pellegrinaio vero e proprio sempre collocato al livello della piazza del Duomo, mentre ai piani inferiori sono riservate le più svariate funzioni: cantine e stalle nel caso del Pellegrinaio delle Donne, magazzini e abitazioni nel pellegrinaio su Vallepiatta dove sono ancora riconoscibili numerose finestre affacciate sulla strada, ora tamponate e inglobate in posteriori strutture.

La costruzione di nuovi e grandi pellegrinai nella prima metà del Trecento era giustificata dall'aumento della popolazione, dall'abbassamento dei livelli di vita, che per la prima volta coinvolse anche numerosi artigiani e bottegai, e dalla vistosa crescita del numero dei pellegrini in viaggio verso Roma a seguito dell'istituzione del giubileo da parte di Bonifacio VIII.

L'edificazione del Pellegrinaio delle Donne divenne l'occasione per una generale riorganizzazione dell'intero settore femminile, dove erano ospitati anche i bambini abbandonati, ormai in larga parte autonomo da quello maschile, con un proprio ingresso, un pellegrinaio, una cappella, una corte interna, un pozzo e un'abitazione destinata alle *Sopradonne*, due figure sottoposte al rettore ma con funzioni di responsabilità (SORDINI 2010: 209-218). Come l'accesso al pellegrinaio del settore maschile avveniva attraverso la chiesa dell'ospedale, l'accesso al pellegrinaio femminile avveniva tramite una cappella, anch'essa affacciata sulla piazza del Duomo e separata dalla corsia vera e propria per mezzo di una transenna lignea, come in altri ospedali europei del basso Medioevo (GABBRIELLI 2020: 214-215). Con la costruzione del Pellegrinaio delle Donne, inoltre, proseguì l'opera di monumentalizzazione e di ridefinizione architettonica del fronte dell'ospedale sulla piazza del duomo avviata nel 1290. Fu prolungata la Casa dei Gettatelli con altre due bifore e fu occupato l'angolo tra piazza del Duomo e via del Capitano con l'estremità nord-est del nuovo pellegrinaio (fig. 7). Le scelte formali, in età moderna parzialmente alterate, furono analoghe a quelle impiegate, qualche decennio prima, nel Palazzo del Rettore e nella Casa dei Gettatelli, vale a dire lo stile in uso nella più aulica architettura civile della città, al punto che fino a qualche anno fa, sulla scorta di un'errata interpretazione di Girolamo Macchi (1649-1734), era diffusa la convinzione, poi rivelatasi errata, che si trattasse di un palazzo privato, in seguito acquisito e ristrutturato dal Santa Maria (TULIANI 2005). Nella facciata dell'ospedale anche la sala-corsia (o pellegrinaio), grande protagonista di tutta l'architettura ospedaliera d'Europa (GABBRIELLI 2020), perse gli originari connotati di ascendenza religiosa per assumere quelli di un palazzo.

21. Sui pellegrinai di Santa Maria della Scala: SORDINI 2010: 59-76; SORDINI 2014.

Ancora una volta la ridefinizione del volto pubblico di Santa Maria della Scala si manifestò nelle forme inconfondibili del gotico "novesco" (bifore e portali a sesto acuto, archi ricassati, doppie cornici orizzontali, ecc.), ed anche le finiture furono aggiornate sulle tecniche più costose e all'avanguardia: il fronte su via del Capitano, l'unico che abbia conservato, insieme ad alcuni tratti del primo piano dell'ampliamento della Casa dei Gettatelli, il trattamento originale, ostenta, sull'intera superficie, una finitura a laterizi accuratamente arrotati e graffiati a spina di pesce (fig. 8), in linea con i principali monumenti in cotto della città.[22]

Immancabile, anche in questo caso, l'epigrafe (fig. 9), collocata non al centro della facciata, in asse col portale di ingresso al settore femminile, come ci saremmo potuti aspettare, ma all'estremità del pellegrinaio, proprio all'angolo tra piazza del Duomo e via del Capitano, e molto in alto, quasi a voler estendere il suo contenuto a tutto il fronte dell'ospedale e non ad uno specifico settore come nel caso delle precedenti iscrizioni, in sintonia con il tenore omnicomprensivo del contenuto stesso: «Anno Do(mi)ni MCCCXXXVIII questo spedale è facto a uso de povari (et) delli (i)nfermi (et) d(e) gittatelli al tempo di messere Giovann(i) di Tese de Talomei rectore del decto spedale».[23] In effetti l'epigrafe si data a soli tre-quattro anni di distanza da un'altra fondamentale opera che, collocata al di sopra dell'ingresso principale del Santa Maria, di fronte alla cattedrale, davvero irradiava l'operato del Tolomei, per la centralità e per la forza delle immagini, sull'intero fronte dell'ospedale. Ci riferiamo, naturalmente, al celeberrimo ciclo pittorico con le *Storie della Vergine*, ora perduto, dipinto da Simone Martini e dai fratelli Lorenzetti intorno al 1334-35. In una delle mensole della tettoia trecentesca a protezione delle *storie*, stando ad una testimonianza di Girolamo Macchi, campeggiava l'arme del rettore, al quale probabilmente era spettato un ruolo importante nella stessa genesi del programma iconografico.[24]

Tra fine Duecento e primi Trecento si assiste, nel fronte sulla piazza del duomo, ad un poderoso investimento in immagine da parte del Santa Maria della Scala, sia con la costruzione di edifici dal tono aulico e monumentale, sia con la realizzazione del ciclo pittorico mariano per il quale si ricorre ai più quotati pittori del tempo, nell'ottica di un ruolo quanto più possibile paritetico con il Comune e la Cattedrale. Il tutto suggellato da una concentrazione di epigrafi inerenti fatti costruttivi che non ha equali in altri complessi edilizi della città, segno di autoconsapevolezza del proprio ruolo da parte della comunità ospedaliera (in particolare dei rettori) ma anche della necessità di affermazione e di difesa dei propri margini di autonomia amministrativa e istituzionale rispetto al potere politico. Non a caso, forse, la prima delle tre epigrafi, quella del 1290, si conclude, un po'

22. Gabbrielli 1991b: 140-145; cf. Gabbrielli 2005.

23. Dubbi sull'originalità dell'attuale collocazione dell'epigrafe a causa dell'eccessiva altezza in Gabbrielli 1991a: 105-109.

24. Macchi, 1662-1724: 100v-101r; Macchi 1709-1720: c. 281v. In corrispondenza di due delle quattro scene era la seguente iscrizione: «Hoc opus fecit Petrus Laurentii et Ambrosius eius frater 1335» (Ugurgieri Azzolini 1649, II: 338). Sugli affreschi si veda la recente scheda di Caffio 2017.

insolitamente, sottolineando che la costruzione del Palazzo del Rettore è avvenuta *de pecunia hospitalis* (GALLAVOTTI 1985: 63). Negli anni precedenti il rettorato di Giovanni di Tese, del resto, si era consumato un duro scontro tra l'Ospedale e il Comune, a seguito del disegno politico dei Nove volto ad esercitare un più incisivo e stretto controllo sui principali ospedali della città, primo tra tutti il Santa Maria della Scala. Si trattava, in particolare, dell'obbligo della registrazione in *Biccherna* delle proprietà donate agli ospedali e dell'imposizione, per norma, della nomina di ufficiali comunali nella gestione economica e contabile. A riprova del nuovo rapporto istituzionale che il Comune intendeva configurare fu la ripetuta richiesta, negli anni 1305-1309, di apporre la propria insegna sulla facciata dell'ospedale. Più precisamente si trattava di due armi in pietra da collocare ai lati dell'ingresso principale, come a sottolineare l'appartenenza al Comune stesso. Il Santa Maria della Scala, dinanzi ad una richiesta di tale impatto comunicativo, reagì immediatamente opponendosi in nome della *libertas ecclesiastica*. In seguito, tuttavia, forse per evitare il protrarsi di uno scontro con il Comune controproducente anche per l'Ospedale stesso, i frati apposero gli stemmi (fig. 10) di loro iniziativa, pur non mancando di sottolineare che ciò non era un segno di sottomissione e che non andava inteso come una rinuncia alle prerogative di autonomia dell'istituzione.[25]

Solo tra fine Trecento e Quattrocento il Comune ottenne il pieno controllo amministrativo e politico sull'Ospedale, arrivando a nominare anche il rettore (PELLEGRINI 2003: 37-42), ma già durante il periodo "novesco" i rapporti tra i due enti erano diventati strettissimi e soprattutto si era definitivamente affermata l'idea del carattere pubblico, e pertanto "comunale", degli ospedali urbani, *in primis* del Santa Maria della Scala, da tempo percepito come ospedale "della città", stante «la relazione profonda che la comunità ospedaliera intratteneva con l'intera *civitas*» (PELLEGRINI 2016: 294). E ciò malgrado i tentativi di resistenza da parte della comunità dei *fratres* alle richieste del governo.

Gli interventi nella facciata sulla piazza del Duomo, con il ciclo mariano, le epigrafi, le armi del Comune e il ricorso al più aggiornato gotico "novesco", attestano la volontà, da parte dell'istituzione ospedaliera, di accrescere il proprio ruolo e prestigio tramite la realizzazione di opere portatrici di una forte identità civica e, allo stesso tempo, riflettono il processo di laicizzazione e di municipalizzazione delle attività assistenziali ormai in atto.[26]

25. Sulla questione, che si trascinò fino al 1339-40, si vedano: NARDI 2003; PELLEGRINI 2003: 33-35; PELLEGRINI 2014: 279-294.

26. Per un quadro generale: PICCINNI 2020.

## *Bibliografia*

Bowsky, William M., 1986. *Un Comune italiano nel medioevo. Siena sotto il regime dei Nove, 1287-1355*, Bologna, Il Mulino.

Caffio, Alessandra, 2017. "I perduti affreschi della facciata dell'ospedale di Santa Maria della Scala a Siena", Alessandro Bagnoli, Roberto Bartalini, Max Seidel (a cura di), *Ambrogio Lorenzetti*, Milano, Silvana: 363-373.

Canestrelli, Antonio, 1993. *L'abbazia di San Galgano*, Firenze 1895, rist. anast. Pistoia, Tellini.

Causarano, Marie A.; Salvadori, Frank; Sordini, Beatrice; Tixier, Benjamin, 2011. "Nuova definizione di spazi abitativi all'interno del Santa Maria della Scala di Siena tra '300 e '400: storia e archeologia", Fabio Gabbrielli (a cura di), *Ospedale di Santa Maria della Scala: ricerche storiche, archeologiche e storico-artistiche*, Siena, Protagon: 55-76.

Conejo, Antoni, 2002. *Assistència i hospitalitat a l'edat mitjana. L'arquitectura dels hospitals catalans: del gòtic al primer renaixement*, Tesi di dottorato, Universitat de Barcelona.

Epstein, Stephan R., 1986. *Alle origini della fattoria Toscana. Lo spedale di Santa Maria della Scala in Siena e le sue terre (metà '200-metà '400),* Firenze, Salimbeni.

Gabbrielli, Fabio, 1991a. "Gli indicatori cronologici utilizzati nello studio degli elevati del Santa Maria", Enrica Boldrini, Roberto Parenti (a cura di), *Santa Maria della Scala, Archeologia e edilizia sulla piazza dello Spedale*, Firenze, All'Insegna del Giglio: 97-112.

Gabbrielli, Fabio, 1991b. "Osservazioni di cronotipologia sulle aperture a sesto acuto della facciata dello Spedale", Enrica Boldrini e Roberto Parenti (a cura di), *Santa Maria della Scala, Archeologia e edilizia sulla piazza dello Spedale*, Firenze, All'Insegna del Giglio: 138-160.

Gabbrielli, Fabio, 2005. "Finishing Techniques for Exposed Brickwork in 12th to 15th-century Tuscan Architecture", Johannes Cramer, Dorothée Sack (a cura di), *Technik des Backsteinbaus im Europa des Mittelalters,* Petersberg, Michael Imhof Verlag: 50-56.

Gabbrielli, Fabio, 2010. *Siena medievale. L'architettura civile*, Siena, Protagon.

Gabbrielli, Fabio (a cura di), 2014. *Il Pellegrinaio dell'ospedale di Santa Maria della Scala*, Grosseto, Effigi.

Gabbrielli, Fabio, 2020. "Modelli di architettura ospedaliera tra XII e XV secolo", Gabriella Piccinni (a cura di), *Alle origini del welfare. Radici medievali e moderne della cultura europea dell'assistenza,* Roma, Viella: 203-223.

Gabbrielli, Fabio, 2021. "La 'strada interna' e gli spazi confraternali", Fabio Gabbrielli, Michele Pellegrini (a cura di), *La via delle confraternite, Ospedale e gruppi confraternali lungo la 'strada interna' di Santa Maria della Scala: documenti, immagini e strutture materiali*, Grosseto, Effigi: 133-142.

Gallavotti Cavallero, Daniela, 1985. *Lo Spedale di Santa Maria della Scala in Siena. Vicenda di una committenza artistica*, Pisa, Pacini.

Gavazzi, Massimo; Montevecchi, Nadia; Sbardellati, Andrea, 2014. "Indagini sull'architettura e sulle decorazioni della cappella del Manto. Lo sviluppo costruttivo dalla fase originaria all'assetto documentato da Domenico di Bartolo", Fabio Gabbrielli (a cura di), *Il pellegrinaio dell'ospedale di Santa Maria della Scala*, Grosseto, Effigi: 197-207.

Giorgi, Andrea, Moscadelli, Stefano, 2005. *Costruire una cattedrale. L'Opera di Santa Maria di Siena tra XII e XIV secolo*, Monaco di Baviera, Deutscher Kunstverlag.

Leistikow, Dankwart, 1967. *Dieci secoli di storia degli edifici ospedalieri in Europa. Una storia dell'architettura ospedaliera*, Ingelheim am Rhein, C. H. Boehringer Sohn.

Lugarini, Renato, 2011. *Il Capitolo dell'ospedale di Santa Maria della Scala, Aspetti istituzionali e riflessi documentari (Siena, fine XII.XIV secolo)*, Siena, Protagon.

Macchi, Girolamo, 1662-1724. *Diario*, Biblioteca Comunale degli Intronati di Siena, ms. A.XI.23.

Macchi, Girolamo, 1709-1720. *Memorie*, Archivio di Stato di Siena, ms. D 108.

Moretti, Italo, 1982. "Bicromia 'struttiva' nell'architettura romanica volterrana-senese", *Prospettiva*, 29: 62-71.

MORETTI, Italo, 2014. "I pellegrinai nell'architettura ospedaliera del Medioevo", Fabio Gabbrielli (a cura di), *Il pellegrinaio dell'ospedale di Santa Maria della Scala*, Grosseto, Effigi: 23-39.

MUCCIARELLI, Roberta, 2001. *La terra contesa. I Piccolomini contro Santa Maria della Scala (1277-1280),* Firenze, Olschki.

NARDI, Paolo, 2003. "Un *consilium* di Paolo Liazari a favore dell'ospedale senese di Santa Maria della Scala", Antonio Padoa, Maria G. di Renzo, Gian Paolo Massetto (a cura di), *Amicitiae Pignus, Studi in ricordo di Adriano Cavanna*, II, Milano, Giuffrè: 1609-1621.

PARENTI, Roberto, 1991. "Una parte per il tutto. Le vicende costruttive della facciata dello Spedale e della piazza antistante", Enrica Boldrini, Roberto Parenti (a cura di), *Santa Maria della Scala, Archeologia e edilizia sulla piazza dello Spedale*, Firenze, All'Insegna del Giglio: 20-94.

PELLEGRINI, Michele, 2003. "L'ospedale e il Comune, immagini di una relazione privilegiata", *Arte e assistenza a Siena, le copertine dipinte dell'Ospedale di Santa Maria della Scala*, Pisa, Pacini: 29-45.

PELLEGRINI, Michele, 2005. *La comunità ospedaliera di Santa Maria della Scala e il suo più antico Statuto (Siena, 1305)*, Pisa, Pacini.

PELLEGRINI, Michele, 2012. "Le «limosine di messer Giovanni», Società, demografia e religione in una fonte senese del Trecento", Duccio Balestracci et al. (a cura di), *Uomini paesaggi storie. Studi di storia medievale per Giovanni Cherubini,* II, Siena, Salvietti e Barabuffi: 997-1013.

PELLEGRINI, Michele, 2014. "La norma della pubblica pietà. Istituzioni comunali, religione e pia loca nella normativa statutaria senese fino al Costituto volgare del 1309", Gabriella Piccinni, Nora Giordano (a cura di), *Siena nello specchio del suo Costituto in volgare del 1309-1310*, Pisa, Pacini: 249-294.

PELLEGRINI, Michele, 2016. "L'esperienza religiosa dei "fratres" e delle "sorores" di Santa Maria della Scala: una "comunità estesa" nella società senese fra Due e Trecento", Anna Benvenuti, Pierantonio Piatti (a cura di), *Beata civitas, Pubblica pietà e devozioni private nella Siena del '300*, Firenze, Sismel-Galluzzo: 275-296.

PICCINNI, Gabriella, 1995. "Linee di storia dell'ospedale di Santa Maria della Scala e dell'area circostante", *Santa Maria della Scala, Dall'ospedale al museo*, Siena, Alsaba: 11- 21.

PICCINNI, Gabriella, 2012. *Il banco dell'ospedale di Santa Maria della Scala e il mercato del denaro nella Siena del Trecento*, Pisa, Pacini.

PICCINNI, Gabriella, 2016a. "Il contesto politico-sociale del Santa Maria della Scala", Anna Benvenuti, Pierantonio Piatti (a cura di), *Beata civitas, Pubblica pietà e devozioni private nella Siena del '300*, Firenze, Sismel-Galluzzo: 229-249.

PICCINNI, Gabriella, 2016b. "I modelli ospedalieri e la loro circolazione dall'Italia all'Europa alla fine del Medioevo", Gregoria Cavero (a cura di), *Civitas Bendita: encrucijada de las relaciones sociales y de poder en la ciudad medieval*, León, Universidad de León: 8-26.

PICCINNI, Gabriella (a cura di) 2020. *Alle origini del welfare. Radici medievali e moderne della cultura europea dell'assistenza*, Roma, Viella

PICCINNI, Gabriella; TRAVAINI, Lucia, 2003. *Il Libro del pellegrino (Siena 1382-1446). Affari, uomini, monete nell'Ospedale di S. Maria della Scala*, Napoli, Liguori.

SESTAN, Ernesto, 1961. "Siena avanti Montaperti", *Bullettino Senese di Storia Patria*, 58: 28-74.

SIENA, 1986. "Siena, La fabbrica di Santa Maria della Scala", *Bollettino d'Arte*, Volume speciale.

SORDINI, Beatrice, 2010. *Dentro l'antico Ospedale. Santa Maria della Scala, uomini, cose e spazi di vita nella Siena medievale*, Siena, Protagon.

SORDINI, Beatrice, 2014. "Il Pellegrinaio e i pellegrinai di Santa Maria della Scala. Evoluzione dell'assistenza tra spazi e persone (metà XIII-metà XV secolo)", Fabio Gabbrielli (a cura di), *Il pellegrinaio dell'ospedale di Santa Maria della Scala*, Grosseto, Effigi: 41-57.

STATUTI SENESI, 1877. *Statuti senesi scritti in volgare ne' secoli XIII e XIV, Volume III. Statuto dello Spedale di Siena*, Luciano Banchi (a cura di), Bologna.

TULIANI, Maurizio, 2005. "A proposito del palazzo detto degli Squarcialupi: un'attribuzione errata", *Bullettino Senese di Storia Patria*, 112: 463-469.

UGURGIERI AZZOLINI, Isidoro, 1649. *Le Pompe Sanesi, o' vero Relazione delli huomini, e donne illustri di Siena, e suo Stato*, Pistoia, Nella stamperia di Pier Antonio Fortunati.

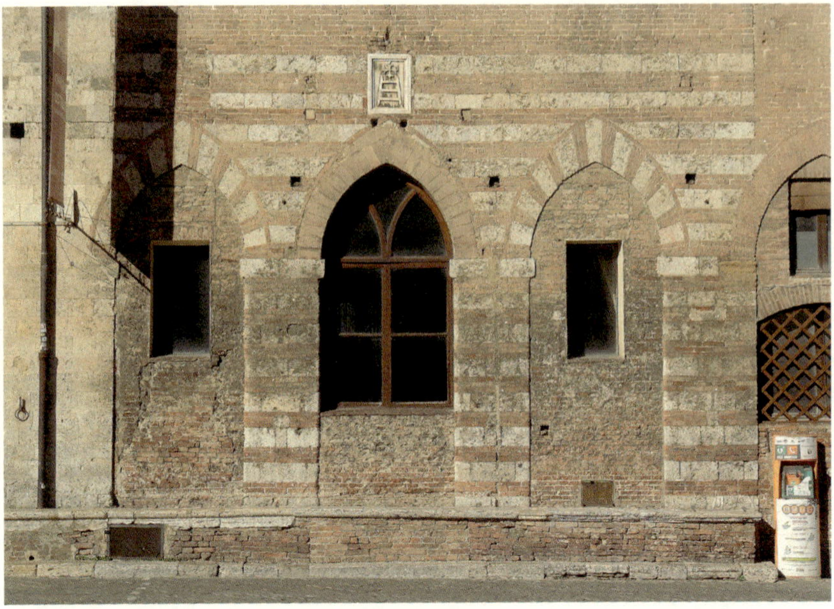

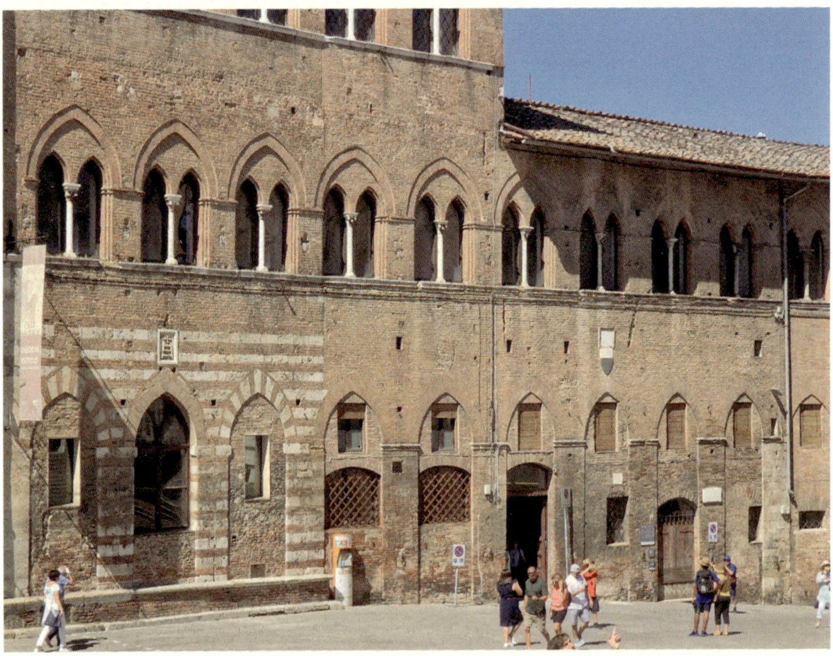

Fig. 1. Siena, ospedale di Santa Maria della Scala. Portico della chiesa (già pellegrinaio), ante 1248. Foto: Fabio Gabbrielli.
Fig. 2. Siena, ospedale di Santa Maria della Scala. Palazzo del Rettore, 1290. Foto: Fabio Gabbrielli.

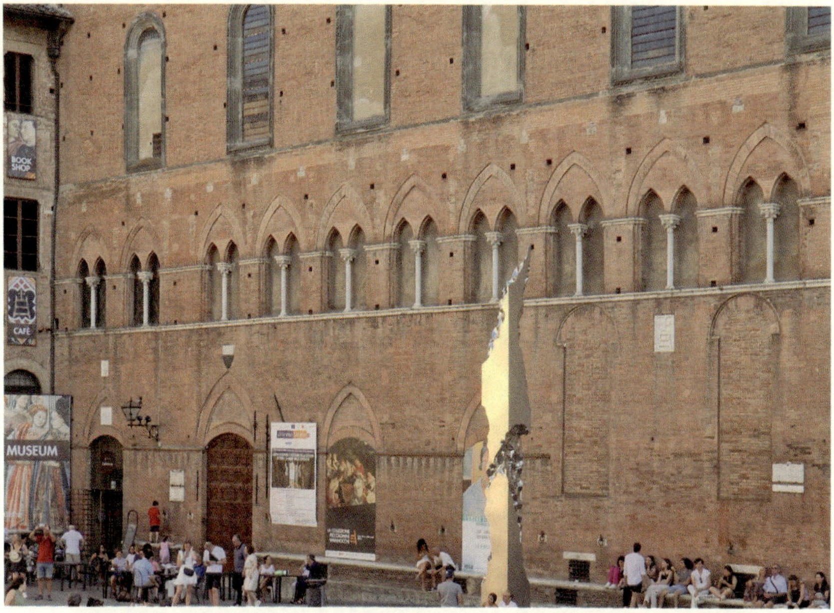


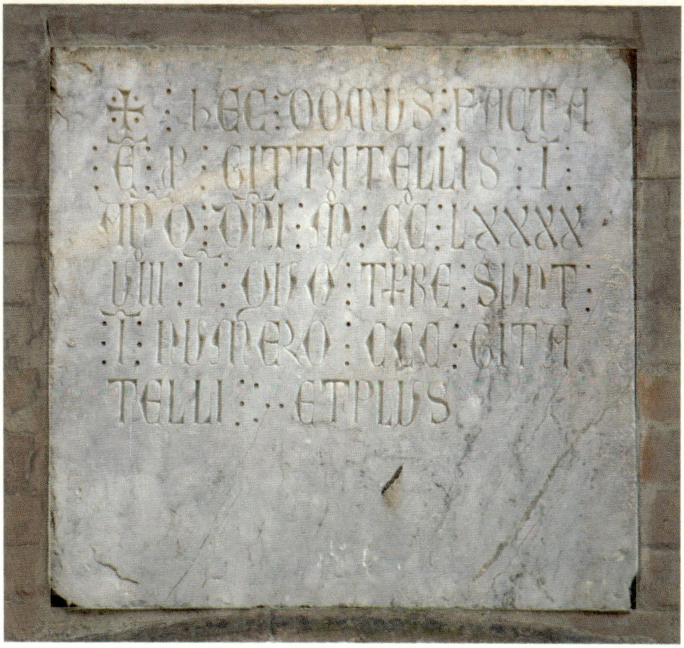

Fig. 3. Siena, ospedale di Santa Maria della Scala. Casa dei Gettatelli, 1298. Foto: Fabio Gabbrielli.

Fig. 4. Siena, ospedale di Santa Maria della Scala. Casa dei Gettatelli, epigrafe del 1298. Foto: Jacopo Bruttini.

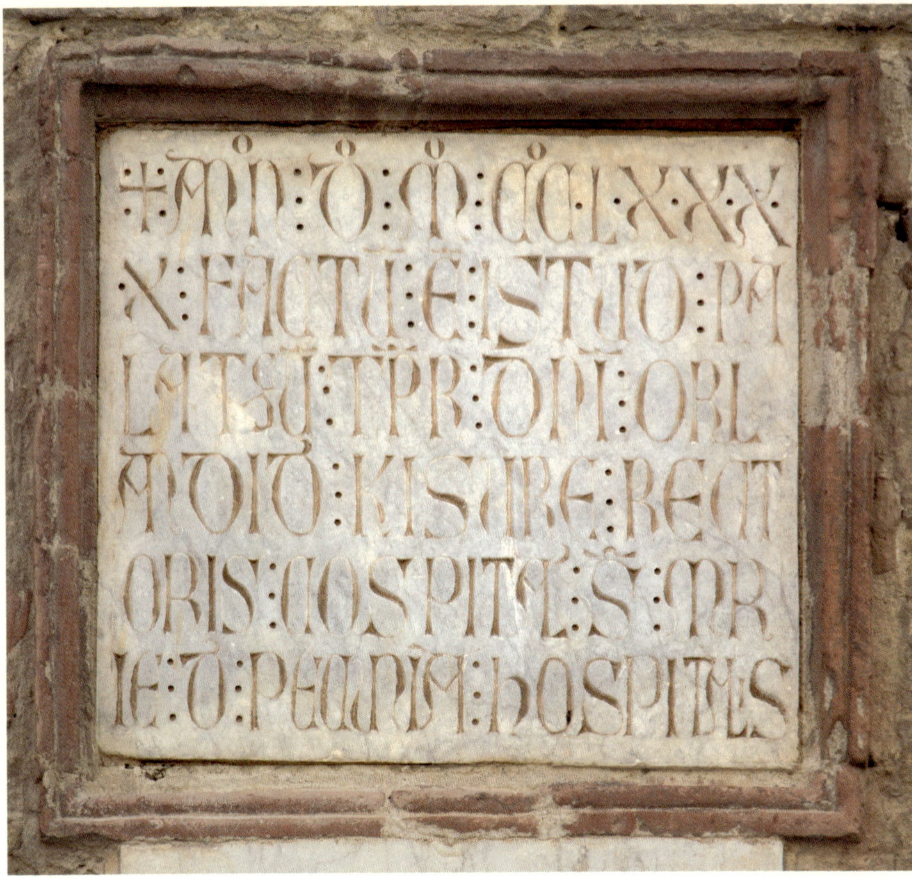

Fig. 5. Siena, ospedale di Santa Maria della Scala. Palazzo del Rettore, epigrafe del 1290. Foto: Jacopo Bruttini.

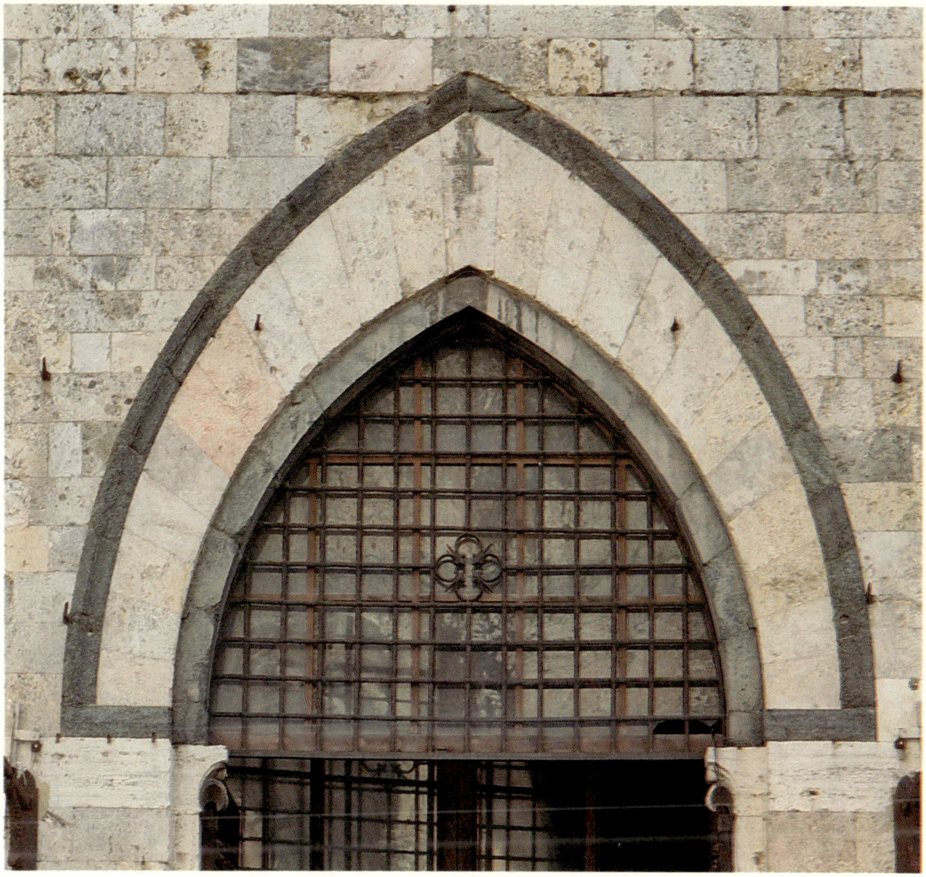

Fig. 6. Siena, ospedale di Santa Maria della Scala. Portale principale, primi XIV secolo circa. Foto: Fabio Gabbrielli.

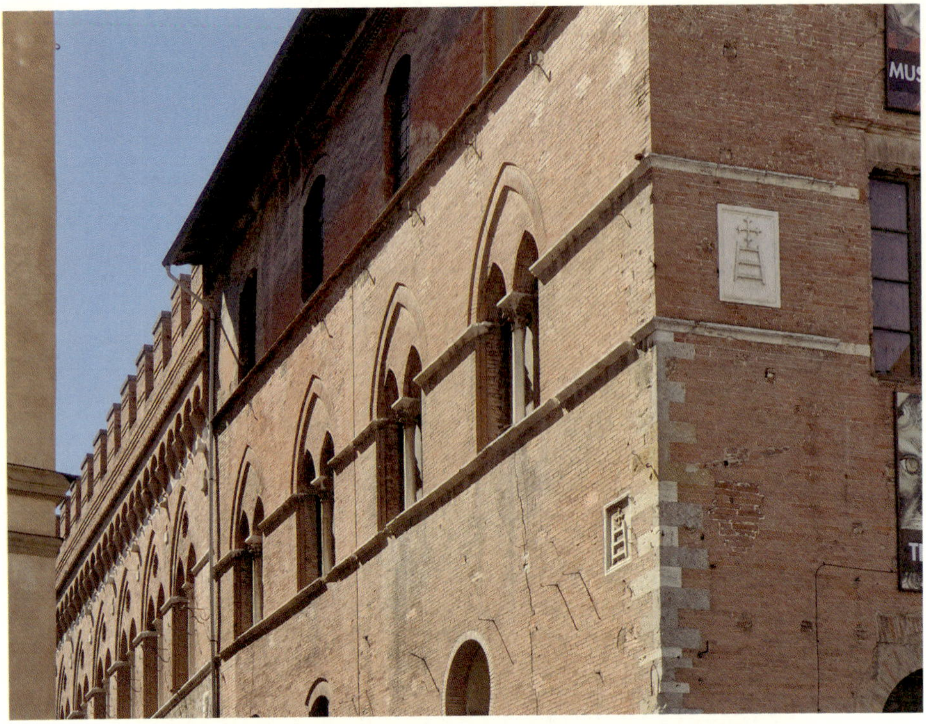


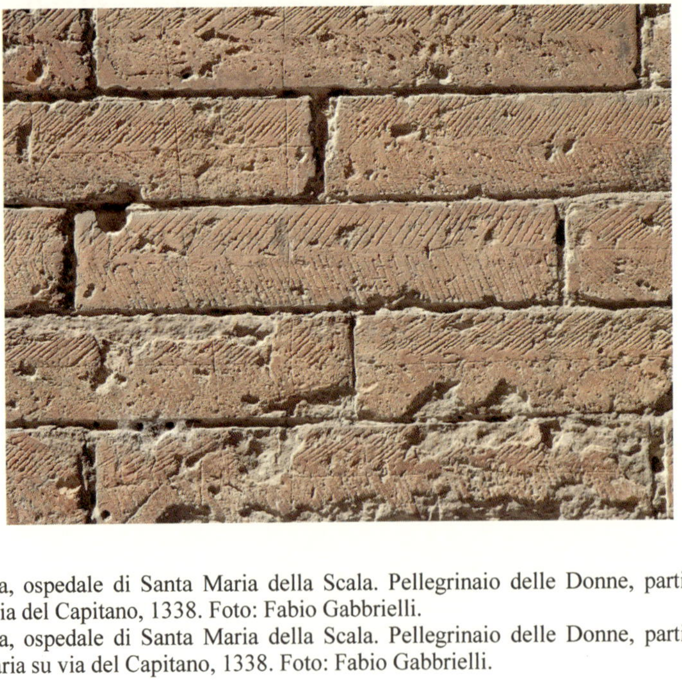

Fig. 7. Siena, ospedale di Santa Maria della Scala. Pellegrinaio delle Donne, particolare della facciata su via del Capitano, 1338. Foto: Fabio Gabbrielli.
Fig. 8. Siena, ospedale di Santa Maria della Scala. Pellegrinaio delle Donne, particolare della cortina muraria su via del Capitano, 1338. Foto: Fabio Gabbrielli.

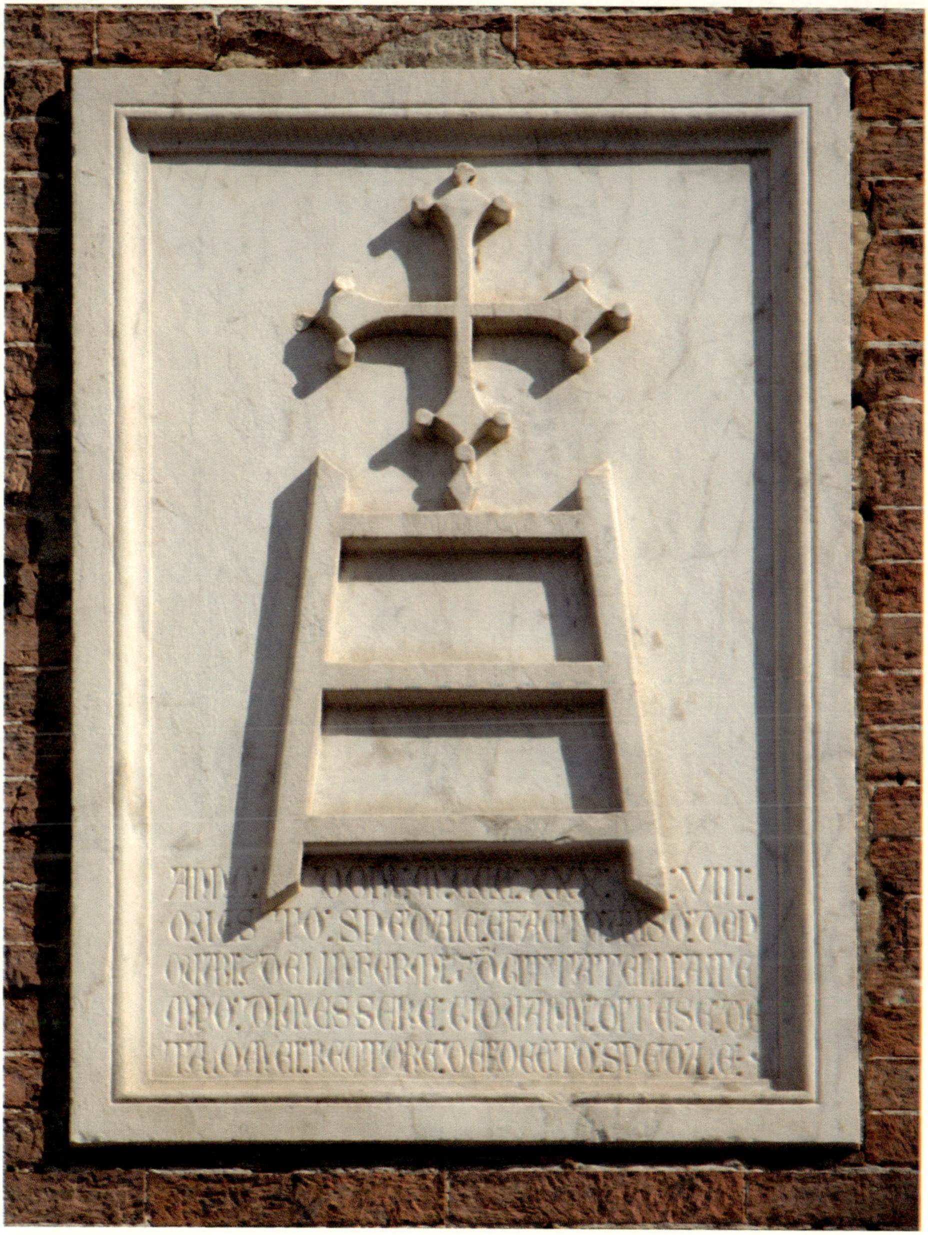

Fig. 9. Siena, ospedale di Santa Maria della Scala. Pellegrinaio delle Donne, arme dell'ospedale con epigrafe del 1338. Foto: Jacopo Bruttini.

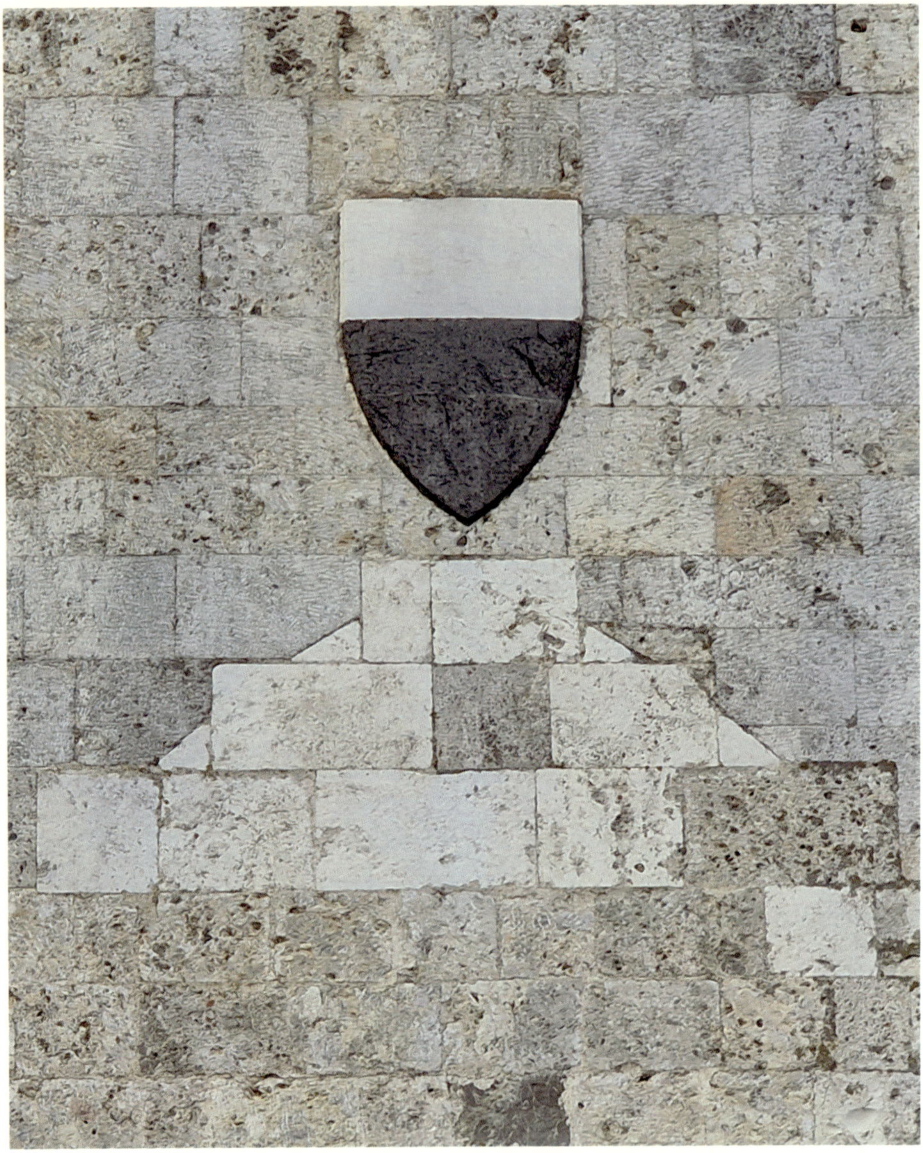

Fig. 10. Siena, ospedale di Santa Maria della Scala. Arme del Comune di Siena. Foto: Fabio Gabbrielli.

Salvatore Marino

# The Urban Impact of Hospitals in Medieval Naples

Medieval historians studying the origins of Naples as a kingdom capital have paid little attention to the role of the city's welfare system. Historians seeking to understand the origins of this urban community, which aspired to become the capital of a kingdom, have focused on various aspects: the maritime port, the relationship with the hinterland and surrounding countryside, the development of a trade surplus and the growth of foreign markets, its favorable geographic position, and its vicinity to Rome (Feniello 2012: 567-584; Patroni Griffi, Leone 1984). In addition to these factors, I argue that at least three more should be added: the existence of a lay university, the development of a strong network of monastic houses, both male and female, and the emergence of a social-medical system that, as we will see, was built on the foundation of fourteen hospitals established between the 12th and 13th centuries (Bertini, Colesanti, Soler 2020, 56-60). The totality of these various elements conditioned the urban development of a city that, as is well known, by the end of the 13th century became a royal capital on the way to becoming one of the most important cities in the Mediterranean.

The primary goal of this essay is not to examine the reasons why Naples was chosen as the royal capital but to reconstruct the origins of its urban welfare network, identify key developments in its urban and economic impact on the city, and demonstrate how the buildings and charitable activities fostered growth and expansion in new urban areas that were usually outside the city walls. The role of hospital buildings and spaces in the development of medieval cities has only recently been the subject of scholarly attention (Keyvanian 2015). The case of Naples is woefully understudied because of the lack of documentation and because surviving medieval structures do not allow to easily locate the various welfare institutions. Furthermore, the continuity and influence of medieval institutions are difficult to quantify because many hospitals changed names, others only functioned for a few decades, and many were incorporated into larger welfare institutions. The few studies we do have of medieval hospitals mostly focus on individual institutions with a forced discussion of the larger urban context or examine the architecture of churches associated with hospitals.[1]

1. Giovanni Vitolo is one of the few scholars to have at least discussed in his history of the hospital of St. Eligio and the Mercato the development of the earliest hospital system in Naples (Vitolo 2003, 71-86); Rosalba Di Meglio has studied 14th century Corregge and the hospitals in that

This essay will explore the evolution of the Neapolitan hospital network with a chronological approach: from the early welfare network established in the Swabian-Norman period, its growth under the Angevins, and the reforms and consolidation of a more modern urban welfare system. The hospital foundations will be considered in relation to their urban context, demonstrating their profound impact on the areas outside the city walls: St. Giovanni a Mare and St. Eligio in the Mercato, l'Annunziata in the area called Malpasso, St. Antonio di Vienne in Carbonara, St. Nicola al Molo, and the Incoronata in the Corregge. The map (fig. 1)[2] clearly shows the dynamics of urban development in Naples and the relationship between the expansion of the city's walls to encompass the most important civic buildings and medieval hospital structures.

## 1. *Origins of the Hospital Network in the Norman-Swabian Period*

Before the arrival of the Angevin dynasty in the Kingdom of Sicily (1266), Naples had a well-established network of small charitable institutions, some of which dated back to the first centuries of Christianity. Most were small hospitals that were dependent, directly or indirectly, on the Neapolitan Church or monastic houses; other institutions were administered by hospital orders or established by noble houses.

The oldest charitable organization was the *Diakonía* of San Gennaro all'Olmo, founded around 680 by Bishop Agnello on the site of a fifth-century bathhouse.[3] Nearby, in the atrium of the cathedral, at the current site of the chapel of the Tesoro of San Gennaro, Bishop Atanasio (876-898) established the hospital of *Sanctae Neapolitanae Ecclesiae*, dedicated to St. Andrea, but commonly known as St. Atanasio after its founder. This hospital was the most important charitable institution governed by the Neapolitan church. It was active throughout the Middle Ages and was eventually incorporated into the Casa Santa dell'Annunziata in 1440. In the 13$^{th}$ century, it had twelve beds, housed pilgrims, and distributed bread and money to the laity and clergy on the main feast days of the year (Mazzocchi 1751: 274; D'Addosio 1883: 240; Marino 2015: 119). Other episcopal hospitals were those of St. Severo and St. Andrea a Nido, both scarcely documented. St. Severo, which existed at least since 1134, was annexed to the church

area of the city (Di Meglio 2003, 172-179, 185-191). For the architectural history of the churches of S. Eligio and the Incoronata, see, respectively: Bruzellius 2004; Vitolo 2008.

2. Figure 1 does not indicate all the hospitals that existed in medieval Naples; the map highlights the hospitals at the center of this essay.

3. In medieval Naples and Rome, a *diakonia* was a charitable institution, usually founded next to a church building, dedicated to the care of the poor and the distribution of alms. The diaconate-hospital of San Gennaro all'Olmo, located at the crossroad of via St. Gregorio Armeno and via St. Biagio dei Librai, was incorporated into the ancient bath built by Bishop Nostriano (452-465) and enlarged by Bishop Paolo about 766. It remained active throughout the Middle Ages (Capasso 1895: 87-89; Celano 1858, 3: 752-754; Feniello 2002: 77-78).

of S. Giorgio (CAPASSO 1892, 2/1: 413; VETERE 2000: 163). St. Andrea a Nido, documented from 1139 to 1404, was located near the historic diaconate of the same name in the neighborhood of Nido (presently Via Paladino; CAPASSO 1895: 87-88; PILONE 1996: 198).

There were at least three monastic hospitals that cared for monks, nuns, and pilgrims: St. Agnello Maggiore, St. Gregorio Armeno, and St. Severino. The first, documented already in 1168, was overseen by the monastery of St. Agnello and was located on the northwestern part of the city (VETERE 2000: 38). The second, with a more autonomous administration, is amply documented from 1207 to the end of the 14th century (PILONE 1989: 66, 76, 81-87, 98, 129-133; VITOLO 2001: 140-141). The hospital of San Severino, most probably founded in the first half of the 12th century, was part of the massive monastery of St. Severino. According to Giovanni Vitolo, the charitable institution obtained its autonomy from the monastery between the 12th and 13th centuries and grew its real estate patrimony within the city through numerous donations and bequests. The hospital also increased its charitable activities, expanding its services from the care of sick monks and the housing of pilgrims to the assistance and care of the poor (VITOLO 2003: 77-79).

In addition to episcopal and monastic hospitals, the city was served by hospitals established by noble families and confraternities. One such example is the hospital of St. Michele Arcangelo, established in the eleventh century by the Morfisa family and active until at least the beginning of the 14th century. The hospital of St. Maria *ad Campanianum* was built on the initiative of a lay confraternity at the beginning of the 13th century. This hospital, located around the Mercato nuovo (present day piazza Mercato), probably ceased its activity when it was incorporated at the end of the century into the nearby church of St. Eligio, which will be discussed below.

The hospital of San Giovanni a Mare was founded in the area called Campo Moricino,[4] which was the medieval manufacturing and commercial center of the city. The hospital was administered by the Knights Hospitaller, and its first document, a bequest of four *tarì* given by Tufia Iuppari, dates from 10 March 1186. The origins of the hospital date to the reign of King William II of Sicily (1166-1189), as evidenced by a document from 1231 in which Emperor Frederick II confirmed a piece of land for the *Hospitali Sancti Iohannis Hierosolimitani Neapolis* in perpetuity (RADOGNA 1873: 15). The original purpose of the hospital was to care for ships returning from the crusades in the Holy Land, a fact that explains its location, close to the shore. Around the middle of the 13th century, the building was enclosed within the city walls and became the heart of the neighborhood that grew around it, and the chapels of its church became the headquarters of five lay

4. The name "Campo Moricino" (*Muricinum*) probably derives from the presence of a low wall built between the tenth and eleventh centuries that was later replaced by a more substantive wall between the 12th and 13th centuries. The toponym was used until the middle of the 14th century (CAPASSO 1895: 31; VITOLO 2003: 56-58).

confraternities (fig. 2).[5] Despite being hidden today among buildings constructed through the centuries, the church is still visible thanks to a series of restorations. The original church plan was a basilica with three naves covered in ribbed vaults subdivided by Roman columns, a transept, and a semi-circular apse. Between the 13th and 14th centuries, the church was transformed and expanded with the construction of lateral chapels, a new transept, and three apses (fig. 3). The hospital was placed behind the apse, with a great vaulted hall and a room that connected the hospital to the church. The top floor, corresponding to the first transept, served as the prior's house (De Martino 2008: 25-50; Ricciardi 1999: 229-252).

Finally, another charitable institution connected to a hospital order was the hospital of St. Antonio di Vienne, dedicated to caring for those afflicted with ergotism, the so-called "sacred fire" or Saint Anthony's fire. The date of its foundation is uncertain. It could possibly date back to the reign of Frederick II (1198-1250), or possibly to the time of Joanna I (1343-1382).[6] The reasons for this uncertainty are the lack of a foundational document and the fact that the hospital was eventually rebuilt in a different location. Mario Gaglione has clarified that the church and hospital of St. Antonio were founded in the first two decades of the 13th century outside of the northern walls of the city, for obvious health reasons, in the area of Carbonara. In 1303, King Charles II placed the charitable institutions under royal protection. The church was later rebuilt outside the gate of Porta Capuana, where today stands the Angevin church of St. Antonio Abate, which gave its name to the surrounding neighborhood (around the present-day piazza Carlo III). The church was not yet completed in 1308, but in 1335 we find documents that make a distinction between an old hospital and church and the new hospital and church (Gaglione 2007: 94-95, 101).

In addition to these eleven hospitals active in Naples, during the first half of the 13th century we can document the existence of another three, of which we know little, probably because of their brief existence. The first of these, documented in 1231, was the hospital of St. Maria *ad Balneum*, located in present-day via San Gregorio Armeno, next to the church that took its name from one of the many baths that existed in the ancient city center.[7] The second hospital, St. Giovanni Maggiore, was planned in 1248 by the governors of the confraternity of the Holy Cross, but whether or not the plan came to fruition is unknown.[8] Finally,

5. The extension of the walls dates to the years between 1245 and 1263 (Vitolo 2003: 57-59). For the attribution of the Gerosolimitani in Naples between the 13th and 14th centuries, see: Vetere 2000: 103 and Pilone 1989: 76, 119, 130. A complete overview of the sources and bibliography for the study of San Giovanni a Mare can be found in Vitolo 2003: 85-86, notes 117-120. On the Knights Hospitaller in southern Italy, see Salerno 2001 and Salerno 2010: 127-137.

6. Camera 1841-1860: 148; Celano 1856, 5: 530; D'Engenio Caracciolo 1623: 639; Galante 1872: 426-429; Sigismondo 1788, vol. 3: 23; Venditti 1969: 800-801.

7. The hospital is cited in the will of Ranieri Praxiccio (Vetere 2000: 168). The bath was known as the new bath and since the ducal period had given its name to the entire neighborhood: la *Regio Balnei Novi* (Feniello 2002: 74).

8. The term "Staurita" (from Greek *Stauros*) was a place where the cross is exposed; it refers to a secular-ecclesiastical administrative system and expresses the ability of a community to ad-

far from the city's walls, the hospital of St. Maria Piedigrotta was active in 1230. The hospital, then an important landmark for those traveling between Naples and Pozzuoli, was still in operation in 1370, when it was administered by Tommaso Brancaccio Casillo, the future archbishop of Chieti.[9]

As we have seen, this first hospital network was composed of fourteen small charitable institutions: ten were located inside the city walls; one (the hospital of Santa Maria di Piedigrotta) was located far from the city center; another (St. Antonio Abate or di Vienne) was located outside the northern walls of the city; and finally, two hospitals (St. Maria *ad Campanianum* and St. Giovanni a Mare) were located against the southern walls, in the area of Campo Moricino that, between 1258 and 1263, would be enclosed by a first expansion of the city walls to the southeast (along the present day Via Duca di San Donato) with the creation of Porta Nova. This expansion would encompass warehouses, buildings, shops, houses, and the hospital of the Knights Hospitaller, the center of social, charitable, and religious life in that area of the city (fig. 2).

## 2. *The Expansion of the Hospital Network: The Areas of Mercato and Malpasso*

On 2 July 1270, King Charles I of Anjou (1266-1285) granted the request of a confraternity of French merchants living in Naples to build a hospital and church dedicated to Saints Eligio, Dionisio, and Martino on a piece of land located next to the walls of the Mercato square.[10] Nine days later, the confraternity obtained approval from the Archbishop of Naples, Aiglerio, for the construction of the church, which would have a cemetery and a right of burial limited to the sick poor and foreigners who were not living in the city (VITOLO 2003: 44-47, 64-68). The following November, the Angevin king gave the hospital eight ounces of gold that his son, Charles (the future King Charles II, 1285-1309) wanted to donate to the charitable institution to facilitate its opening.[11] In 1272, the church was still under construction, but the hospital was probably functioning thanks to the support of its confraternity, governed by four *magistri* and three counselors, all French lay residents in Naples (VITOLO 2003: 123-128). This fact demonstrates that the hospital was established with the goal to provide care and burials to the French brethren of the new king, even if in time the hospital would lose

minister itself independently. The governors, Marino di Gennaro and Stefano Manco, sold on 29 November 1248 a piece of land to fund the construction of a hospital («pro fabricanda una domo [...] in qua facere debemus hospitale»: RADOGNA 1894: 715).

9. In November 1230, the hospital received from Pandolfo Siginolfo a monetary bequest to buy matresses, and in 1246-1250 the hospital owned land in Piedigrotta (VETERE 2000: 164; PILONE 1999: 553).

10. By the 14th century, the church and hospital were referred to in documents as St. Eligio.

11. REGISTRI 1955, vol. 7: 194, n. 51 (22 November 1271): «Mandat ut Hospitali beati Eligii, quod fundatur extramuros Neapolis, solvat unc[ias] auri VIII [...] quas Karolus primogenitus noster dicte ecclesie vo[l]vit solvere».

this particular focus. In September 1276, the same archbishop approved the new statutes of the hospital, which stated that the administrators of the confraternity could use for the benefit of the institution the personal effects of those who died in the hospital and that one of the three priests assigned to the church would provide for the spiritual needs of the sick (Volpicella 1877: 716-717).

The success of this new institution required an expansion of the hospital building, the church, and the cemetery. The king once again gave support to the charitable association. On 17 March 1279, he donated a large tract of land in the Campo Moricino, located northeast of the existing structure toward the Mercato and near the walls (fig. 2).[12] According to Caroline Bruzellius, the work to expand the church to the west, with the construction of a new transept and three apses, concluded at the end of the century (Bruzellius 2004: 17-18). A later expansion of the cemetery and hospital complex occurred in 1304-1305, when King Charles II of Anjou gave the hospital of St. Eligio a nearby space for wounded veterans, donating 30 ounces for its construction. In these years, the new charitable institution was already inserted into the social and religious fabric of the city, as seen by the bequests and donations on the part of various exponents of the Neapolitan nobility, in addition to the royal family, and French merchants and nobles. As demonstrated by Giovanni Vitolo, «its success was naturally rendered possible above all thanks to the spirit of sacrifice on the part of the brothers, who often lived with the sick or volunteered their time in the institution» (Vitolo 2003: 71).

Until 1350, the church, hospital, and cemetery of St. Eligio were outside the urban walls. After 1350, they were integrated, together with the entire area of the Mercato, within the new walls that extended to the stream called Lavinaio (the present via Lavinaio), structured around the Mercato gate (fig. 2; Vitolo 2003: 56-62). Regarding the complex, the church, which has been considered the first example of French Gothic in Naples (fig. 4), has received considerable attention.[13] The configuration of the original hospital, however, remains to be properly understood. One thing we know for sure is that it was located on the left side of the church, where in the 16th century the new hospital and the later *Educandato femminile* (women's educational institute) were constructed. What remains uncertain is the function of the space, divided into four naves, that was located between the church and hospital. It is possible that this space housed the first nucleus of

12. Registri 1967, vol. 21: 39, n. 140 (17 March 1279): «[…] de solo vacuo in campo Moricini dicte civitatis Neapolis contiguo ipsi ecclesie pro ampliando hedificio domus infirmorum et cimiterii defunctorum et corpore ipsius ecclesie dicti hospitalis in larg. can. III et in long. can. XLI, incipientes a cruce lapidea fixa prope ipsum hospitale in loco ubi fit forum et finientes quantum superius protenduntur ex recta linea mensure descendentes versus septentrionem et iuxta menia civitatis predicte […]».

13. The complex architectural history of the church and hospital of St. Eligio has been examined by Caroline Bruzellius (2004) in her authoritative study. For the church, see also the volume by De Feo 2017; for the surviving frescoes in the church, see Lucherini 2012, 181-192. Giovanni Vitolo (2003) has pieced together the earliest decades of the charitable association and its development in the social, religious, and economic life of the urban center, particularly the area of Campo Moricino, later the piazza Mercato.

the hospital, which was expanded northward at the end of the 14th century on the land donated by King Charles II to the confraternity. The 14th century fourth nave, which still has some original frescoes, probably functioned as an entrance to the hospital and later a passageway to the church (fig. 5-6).[14]

In 1300, the city had a solid and diverse system of charitable institutions that were strengthened in the last decades of the 13th century, not only by the foundation of the hospital of St. Eligio, but also by three other bastions of care. Two of these were within the walls, in the heart of the city: the hospitals of St. Maria "de Bella", in the parish of St. Maria Maggiore alla Pietrasanta, and the hospital of St. Cataldo, in the parish of St. Paolo Maggiore, but affiliated with the hospital of St. Giovanni a Mare. The third hospital, a hospice for wounded soldiers, was outside the southern walls of the city and was incorporated in 1305 with the hospital of St. Eligio.[15] The total number of hospitals active in Naples during the reign of Charles II of Anjou (1285-1309) had grown to eighteen: thirteen inside the walls and five outside. In addition to increasing the number of charitable institutions in the center of the ancient city, a significant development was the economic, social, and religious impact on the urban landscape that two lay hospitals (St. Giovanni a Mare and St. Eligio) had in the area of Mercato Nuovo, the principal manufacturing area of the city, crowded with houses, merchants, and artisan workshops that, as we will see, would be called to administer the most important charitable associations in the capital (fig. 2).

In the first decades of the 14th century, the kingdom's capital saw a dramatic increase in population, and new residential and work areas developed outside the city walls. The expansion of the port, the paving of city streets, the creation of a new city market, and the urbanization of Chiaia and the hills of St. Erasmo were evidence of the rise of a city that by 1320 had grown to 35,000 inhabitants.[16] Coinciding with this urban growth, there was a considerable consolidation of the social and welfare system with the establishment of new charitable associations, many dedicated to specific needs of urban society, such as catering to foreigners, travelers, priests, monks, students, prostitutes, and the poor. Other institutions,

14. I would like to thank Stefano D'Ovidio, who posited this plausible theory in need of further research during his presentation at the Conference of the Society for the Medieval Mediterranean in Crete (July 2022).

15. The hospital of St. Maria "de Bella" is mentioned in the will of Stefania Carandente, 15 April 1287 (VITOLO 2003: 82). The hospital of S. Cataldo was active before 1299, when it was in possession of several shops donated by Charles II of Anjou; over the 14th century the hospital was one of the most prestigious charitable institutions in the city with numerous donations from some of the leading Neapolitan families. For the sources and bibliography of this understudied hospital, see: VITOLO 2003: 85-86.

16. The population inside the city of Naples during the reign of Charles I of Anjou (1266-1285) was between 25,000 and 28,000 people (VENDITTI 1969: 667-829). About 1320, the population increased to 35,000 inhabitants (SAKELLARIOU 2012: 446), but probably another 10,000 people lived in the suburbs outside the city walls and came into the city daily for work. For a comparison of Naples with other Italian cities at the beginning of the 14th century, see PINTO 2014: 41-42.

such as the Annunziata, were able to provide a wide range of charitable services, thus becoming the most important charitable institutions in the capital.

Fifty years after the foundation of the hospital of St. Eligio, on 15 December 1318, a lay confraternity dedicated to St. Maria Annunziata successfully petitioned the Angevin court for a garden next to the eastern walls of the city, with the aim of building a hospital and church. On 8 March 1320, work on the *Domus Annunciate* began, and the project was placed under royal protection (Marino 2014: 3-11). The new hospital gave medical care to the sick, offered hospice and donations for the poor, accepted abandoned children, and distributed dowries to the *exposite*, poor girls with no means of support. The institution, which served at the same time as a hospital, orphanage, and school, provided from its very foundation a multiplicity of social services for the entire population of the capital and kingdom (Camera 1860, vol. II: 106. D'Addosio 1883: 13). The hospital did not stay long on the site where it was founded. In 1343, Sancha of Majorca, wife of King Robert of Anjou (1309-1343), offered to the officials who administered the association a larger piece of land only a short distance away from the garden in which the first hospital was built (D'Engenio Caracciolo 1623: 397; Imperato 1629: 27-28; Celano 1792: 236).

The new church and hospital were built in the same location where they stand today, in accordance with the wishes of the queen, who had a personal income of 5000 ounces of gold given to her by her husband Robert to support good works. Nothing remains of the 14th century structure: the hospital was rebuilt *ex novo* by Queen Joanna II d'Angiò Durazzo (1414-1435) in 1433, and the church was rebuilt at the beginning of the 16th century.[17] One of its few artistic remnants from the late Middle Ages is the wood statue of Madonna dei Repentiti (Madonna of the Repentant Sinners), displayed in a side chapel of the church. According to Stefano D'Ovidio, the sculpture dates to the beginning of the 15th century and probably represents the confraternity that promoted the hospital (fig. 7; D'Ovidio 2022: 60). The most noteworthy aspect of the Casa Santa dell'Annunziata (which is how the hospital was known in the following centuries) is the fact it was built in an infamous, crime-ridden part of the city called Malpasso (literally, Bad Walk) located outside the city walls between the two principal gates of the city. Notwithstanding its location, the hospital fostered the development of numerous shops and businesses to support its operation. As with St. Eligio in the Piazza del Mercato, the hospital triggered the urban and commercial development of a new area that would eventually be enclosed within the city's walls.

During the reign of Robert d'Angiò (1309-1343), the capital's hospital network continued to grow and consolidate with the foundation of six other charitable institutions, three within the walls and three located outside. The three hospitals inside the walls were founded by noteworthy individuals close to the

17. The actual building complex, designed by Luigi Vanvitelli, was built in the 18th century following a devastating fire in January 1757. For the remnants of the 14th century church, see Bertaux 1895: 50; for evidence of the 16th century church, see D'Addosio 1883: 59-60.

king, thus reinforcing the relationship between the Neapolitan elite and the neighborhoods where the new institutions were established. In the center of the Regione or Seggio di Nido, Bartolomeo di Capua, royal protonotary, founded in 1314 the twelve-bed hospital of S. Maria di Alto Spirito, located next to the church of Monteverginella (on via Palladino). We know little about this hospital, which probably did not function for long (Vitolo 2003: 83-84). Nearby, in the piazza di St. Maria della Rotonda, between the piazza St. Domenico and the convent of St. Chiara, the Spaniard Giovanni de Haya, lawyer and counselor to King Robert, founded around 1330 the hospital of St. Caterina dei Celani for the sick poor. In a privilege from Pope Innocent IV, 15 April 1360, the hospital was described as being under royal patronage (Camera 1860, vol. 2: 420. Ceva Grimaldi 1857: 249). Near the church of S. Giovanni Maggiore, Ingheranno Stella, Archbishop of Capua and Grand Chancellor of the Kingdom, established in 1338 the hospital of St. Ludovico di Tolosa to care for university students and poor clergymen (*Studentibus in Studio Neapolitano de hospitali pauperum clericorum studentium*: Camera 1860, vol. 2: 68).

Three other hospitals were built outside the city walls during the reign of Robert of Anjou. In 1326, around Porta St. Gennaro, the Carmignano family patronized a church and hospital dedicated to St. Maria dei Vergini, located outside the northern walls of the city. Eight years later, the church and hospital were entrusted to the Order of the Crociferi, which governed the small charitable institution until the middle of the 16th century.[18] Outside the western walls, in the area of Chiaia, the hospital of St. Caterina was established around 1320. During the first decades of its existence, the hospital cared for priests and clergymen.[19] Finally, a group of citizens founded the hospital and church of St. Maria Maddalena, located outside the Porta del Mercato around Ponte Guizzardo (or Ricciardo, later called *della Maddalena*), adjacent to the ancient River Sebeto, a marshy area far from the urban center. The hospital, which existed since the beginning of the 14th century, was established by Charles II of Anjou, a devotee of Mary Magdalene. The new institution underwent several difficulties during its first few decades because of its lack of financial resources and the absence of a charitable organization to support it. In 1324, the three masters that governed the church and hospital, unable to continue, left the administration of the pious institution to the Dominican convent of S. Pietro a Castello (Di Meglio 2003: 179). The hospital's

18. The church still exists and is located on via dei Vergini in front of the Palazzo dello Spagnolo. The Carmignano family had a vast landed patrimony in the area outside Porta St. Gennaro and had an entire neighborhood called Porta St. Gennaro or dei Carmignano, one of the seven minor quarters of the city that was later included in the Sedile or Seggio di Montagna. According to Neapolitan tradition it was this family that in 1334 entrusted the hospital to the Order of the Crociferi. See D'Engenio Caracciolo 1623: 607-608; Celano 1860, 5: 394-395.

19. The hospital was built on land donated on 27 June 1320 by Maddalena Dentice, prioress of the Dominican convent of S. Pietro a Castello (Ambrosio 2003: 16). We know little about this convent that is mentioned in an Angevine register from 1339-1340 and dated from 1362 (Tutini 1644: 180; Vitolo 2003: 82).

circumstances changed, however, in 1330, when a few of the hospital's founders joined with other members of the military, administrative, and business elite of the city and established a confraternity dedicated to overseeing and growing the endowment and services of the new institution. In a few years, the area around the hospital saw the development of new buildings, gardens, and a cemetery (Di Meglio 2013: 153-154; D'Engenio Caracciolo 1623: 651-652; Vitale 1999: 93-103). Once again, a charitable institution had a significant impact in the underdeveloped areas of the city and expanded its social, economic, and religious fabric. The institution of the Maddalena is a good example of a hospital located near a bridge, where travelers, foreigners, and prostitutes congregated (Albini 2001: 205-251; Gazzini 2002: 1-12).

## 3. *The Reign of Joanna I (1343-1381) and the Area of Corregge*

During the reign of Joanna I, Naples was afflicted by the plague and a series of wars that would last around a century and caused immense suffering among the people. The monarchy and local institutions responded to this increased need with the foundation of new hospitals and the maintenance of existing hospitals with concessions and privileges. Rosalba Di Meglio has proven the importance of the efforts of Queen Joanna I, who promoted the foundation of three hospitals, forming a semi-circle around Castel Nuovo, where she resided, as if «she wanted to surround the symbolic center of royal power with a sort of spiritual bastion, made up of those hospitals, considered the best charitable institutions» (Di Meglio 2003: 187). The three new hospitals (St. Elisabetta, St. Nicola al Molo and l'Incoronata) were established around the Largo delle Corregge, immediately outside the western walls of the city, an important political and urban center since the 13th century. Beginning in 1279, the area around Castel Nuovo saw the construction of several public buildings, such as the Admiralty and the Tribunale della Vicaria, and a number of sumptuous noble palaces with parks and gardens, including the Taranto palace, home to barons and royal officials. Completing the urban development of the area were a number of charitable institutions.

Of the three hospitals promoted by Joanna I in Largo delle Corregge, the first was dedicated to St. Elisabetta. Work began on 15 January 1344, in the area that today houses the Palazzo della Prefettura in the piazza Plebiscito. The hospital was founded to care for the members of fallen noble families.[20] The second hospital was that of St. Nicolo al Molo (St. Nicholas at the Pier), which by the late Mid-

20. The hospital of St. Elisabetta (later St. Spirito) was in reality financed by Robert of Anjou, who left funds in his will to finance its construction. The name of the hospital was later changed to St. Spirito and was still active in the 15th century. Camera 1860, vol. II: 500: «Regis Roberti, mandatum pro constructione unius hospitalis in territorio prope ecclesiam S. Spiritus de Neapoli iuxta Castrum novum, in quo pauperes familiares regii repagulum inveniant, suscipiantur, nutriantur et sustententur sub vocabulo S. Elisabet ad Dei honorem ac pro salute animae dicti Regis Roberti, iuxta eius ordinationem in suo testamento».

dle Ages would become one of the leading charitable organizations in the capital. On 25 October 1345, the queen granted to the leaders of the confraternity of St. Nicola al Molo a piece of land in perpetuity for the construction of a hospital that would remain *opus manum nostram*, that is, established by royal decree and therefore placed under her direct protection (MONTI 1936: 12-13). If the new institution at first cared for the needy poor by the beginning of the 15th century they also began to care for abandoned children, as evidenced by a document from 1403, a bequest that was expressly for «le spese delli infermi e per allevar li figlioli se buctavano in S. Nicola». More difficult to date is exactly when the hospital began to care exclusively for sailors. By the beginning of the 16th century, the hospital provided care exclusively for sailors, but its focus on those who lived by and of the sea probably dates to the first half of the 15th century. Giuliana Boccadamo has demonstrated that the hospital's unique location made it the center and symbol of the community of the Porto (Harbor) and, between 1376 and 1500, received more than fifty donations from the inhabitants of the area (BOCCADAMO 2019: 5, 13). In the 14th century, the administration of the institution was in the hands of the confraternity, but during the reign of Joanna II (1414-1435) it passed to five governors periodically elected by the eight *piazze* (squares) near the Porto.[21]

The third hospital founded by Queen Joanna I in the Corregge was l'Incoronata, financed by her directly and endowed with significant feudal incomes from Naples and Aversa. In 1365, the queen began to purchase expensive private properties to be used for the construction of the hospital and church. About the same time, she also requested from the French court a relic from the Holy Crown of Thorns, previously housed in the Sainte-Chapelle of Paris. This is the reason the church and hospital were first dedicated to Santa Maria Spina Corona and Santa Maria dell'Incoronata. A series of documents between 1368-1376 demonstrate that the queen closely followed the construction of the hospital and church. On 8 October 1372, the administration of the institution was handed over to the Carthusian monastery of St. Martino. The following year, the queen approved the statutes of the hospital, which had about fifty personnel, most of whom lived on the hospital grounds. The procurator, doctor, surgeon, apothecary, barber, and launderer came on a daily basis. The hospital was large and flourishing in the 14th century, but gradually began to decline in the 15th century, so much so that by 1525 the hospital spaces were rented to private citizens and the administrative spaces housed clergy for church services. The charitable institution consisted of a large hall with a room for one or two nobles, a series of rooms for priests and servants, a garden, and warehouses (ENDERLEIN 1996: 17-46; VITOLO 2008: 31-

21. Joanna II granted its administration solely and exclusively to the eight *piazze* closest to the Porto: Nobile, Porto, Rua Catalana, Orefici, Selice, Loggia dei Genovesi, St. Giovanni Maggiore, St. Caterina Spina Corona. Every year the Seggio of Porto elected two governors; every six months the Piazza degli Orefici elected two governors and the remaining Piazze elected one. The governors had to be at least 40 years old, know how to read and write, and had not served in the position in the last five years (BOCCADAMO 2019: 12-13).

37). The only visible evidence of the hospital today is one portico on via Medina (fig. 8).

The hospital of St. Marta was close to the Incoronata. This small hospital was run by the Neapolitan confraternity of the same name and supported by Emperor Phillip II of Constantinople, brother of Louis di Taranto, the second husband of Joanna I. In his will, Phillip II di Taranto gave to abbot Marco Francone the task of supervising the construction of the hospital, which from 1373 housed the confraternity of St. Marta, a brotherhood that grouped small businessmen, merchants, artisans, and families from the Amalfi coast. The hospital was not long-lived. Shortly after 1426, the brothers abandoned the church and hospital because of the damage that the structures had suffered during the Angevin-Aragonese war and transferred their seat to a church in front of the bell tower of St. Chiara (Di Meglio 2003: 156-158, 173-174, 178-179). Although of modest size, the hospital of St. Marta once again shows the role played by common people (bankers, merchants, and artisans) in the administration of charitable organizations, as was the case with St. Eligio in Piazza Mercato, the Annunziata in Malpasso, and St. Nicola in the city port area.

## 4. *Towards a Modern Urban Welfare System*

At the end of the 14th century, the capital enjoyed a vast and well-established hospital network composed of about thirty charitable institutions, some of which were small and would eventually cease functioning, while others, such as St. Eligio, the Annunzaita, and St. Nicolo al Molo, would become the main hospitals of the city, serving as models for the rest of the kingdom and benefiting from bequests and donations on behalf of monarchs, nobles, and the people more generally (Vitolo 2003: 96; Marino 2015: 84-91; Boccadamo 2019: 13). Between the 14th and 15th centuries, this network was enhanced by two new foundations. In 1383, the recently enthroned Charles III of Anjou-Durazzo founded the hospital of St. Maria della Pietà, called Pietatella a Carbonara, because it was located at the bottom of the stairs of the church of St. Giovanni a Carbonara, outside the city's walls. To support its construction, the king designated it royal land and by December 1385 the hospital was already functioning, governed by five lay leaders, one appointed by the nobles of the Seggio di Capuana, and the other four by the popular *piazze*, all confirmed by the king. This hospital cared for people wounded in tournaments and jousts that took place in the area of the Carbonara, outside Porta Capuana. Like several hospitals in the city, it was eventually attached to the Annunziata, which later suppressed it (D'Addosio 1883: 241-242).

The other hospital established during this period was that of St. Angelo a Nido, founded by Cardinal Rinaldo Brancaccio at the beginning of the 15th century, near the church of the same name, and under the patronage of the Brancaccio family, which also appointed the rectors who ran the institution (Vitale 1993: 39 and Russo 1991). The foundation of the hospital of St. Angelo a Nido ended the period of medieval hospital construction during which monarchs, nobles, ecclesiastical authorities, and the people were engaged in supporting these institutions, both big and small. Groups across Neapolitan society almost competed against each other to create a vast welfare system capable of responding to the community's varied needs: the poor and sick, fallen noble houses, the poor clergy, sailors, university students, abandoned children, widows, and wounded soldiers. These institutions would serve Naples until the next wave of charitable foundations in the 16th century, when the city saw a dramatic population increase and the need arose for an expanded welfare system with new specialized hospitals, such as the Incurabili, aimed at treating infective diseases, or the Real Casa di St. Giacomo for the Spanish community (Novi 2020).

In the course of the 15th century, the charitable institutions of Naples, as in other cities throughout Europe, went through their unique process of welfare reform. In Barcelona, Milan, and Palermo, for example, 15th century reform resulted in the creation of one large new hospital complex that incorporated many smaller hospitals. In Naples, however, the reforms led to the growth and strengthening of existing hospitals, such as the Casa Santa dell'Annunziata (Marino 2020: 183-187). The process of consolidation and centralization was slow, beginning in the first decades of the 15th century and ending in the middle of the 16th century. Its first step was the reform of the administration of small institutions, such as the hospitals of St. Atanasio, St. Antonio di Vienne, the Maddalena for reformed prostitutes, and five similar institutions in Pozzuoli. These institutions were later completely incorporated into the Annunziata, along with two other hospitals, St. Maria della Pietà (1542) and St. Angelo a Nido (1560) (Marino 2014: 20-21, 35, 56). At the same time, the Angevine and Aragonese monarchies dramatically increased the financial resources of the Casa Santa dell'Annunziata through grants, donations, and privileges. The Annunziata also benefited from donations and bequests *ad pias causas* from nobles and commoners in Naples and throughout the kingdom. In the second half of the 15th century, the hospital of the Annunziata had the capacity to care for one thousand sick and seven hundred children, and was one of the most important welfare institutions in the Kingdom of Naples.[22]

Another common aspect of welfare reform was the increasing role of the laity in the administration of hospitals. In Naples, the process had already begun by the end of the 14th century, with lay confraternities establishing and running hospitals and appointing administrators and governors. The management of these institutions fell to the local elites, both of the noble Seggi and more popular districts, as seen with the hospitals of St. Eligio, the Annunziata, St. Nicola al Molo, and St. Maria della Pietà. The Annunziata was, from its very beginning (1318-1338), governed by the brothers of the confraternity that promoted its foundation.

22. In 1474 Pope Sistus IV granted indulgences to those who visited and gave alms to the Annunziata, where «*multique alie persone necessarie in eodem hospitali commorentur ad eo quod numerum millesimum ascendant [...] plures septingentes infantes expositi*» (Archivio Municipale di Napoli, Sezione Real Casa Santa dell'Annunziata, Pergamene, n. 302). For the finances of the Annunziata, see Colesanti, Marino 2016: 314-325.

From 1339, the confraternity held annual elections of the governors, usually five in total: the *magnificus magister*, who represented the noble Seggio di Capuana; and four *magistri yconomi*, who oversaw expenditures, and were elected by the Seggio of the Popolo (of the People). The government of the institution was an expression of both the influence of the patrician families in the Seggio di Capuana and the rising class of wealthy merchants and professionals in the Seggio del Popolo, who quickly understood that the office of governor of the Annunziata could serve as an opportunity to climb the social and political ladder in the neighborhood, city, and kingdom.

In the late Middle Ages, there were more than two hundred families that participated in the governance of the Annunziata and competed for the prestigious position of hospital governor. Of them, about a fifth were from the noble Seggio di Capuana; the rest came from the Seggio del Popolo. Members of some of these families were also administrators in other Neapolitan welfare institutions, such as the confraternity of S. Marta and the hospital of St. Eligio. The administration of the large financial patrimonies of many of these institutions increasingly required a certain egree of expertise, and a small number of Neapolitan families were developing these competencies.[23] Not surprisingly, the administrators of the Annunziata came from families of merchants, artisans, bankers, businessmen, and tax collectors, who were trained and skilled in the increasingly complex financial management of these institutions. The administration of hospitals also required the skills of other professionals, namely notaries, medical professionals, and apothecaries. The families often worked together to establish financial agreements and partnerships that guaranteed the support of the king and the seggio, and ensured that important public offices, such as the *magister yconomus Annunciate*, would stay in their hands.[24]

By the middle of the 15$^{th}$ century, the Annunziata was one of the wealthiest institutions in the city and kingdom, with a vast patrimony of estates and property. Most of its property was located within the city walls. In the area between Porta Capuana and Porta Nolana, and the Lavinaio, the Annunziata owned about twenty buildings; in the area of Mercato it owned about forty, some located in the strip of land along the southern walls of the city, some near the Scalesia, the Rua Francesca, and the Rua Novella, but also in the area of Porto and Portanova (fig. 9).[25] The hospital thus became the center of social life and urban development in the entire southeastern area of the city. Not only did the sick, poor, pilgrims, children, and widows benefit from the institution, but the entire community, espe-

23. Vitolo 2003: 107-116; Di Meglio 2003: 236-246; Feniello 2003: 41-42 e 69; Colesanti, Marino 2016: 312-314. For a comparison with Milan, see Albini 1993: 212-220.

24. On families from the Amalfi coast who concentrated in the area of the Scalesia, see Capone, Leone 1996: 173-186 and Feniello 2003: 15-88; on the Coppola family, see Schiappoli 1972: 155-269.

25. Of the 330 properties identified (houses, shops, ovens, taverns, warehouses, mills, furnaces, etc.) 175 were within or near the city walls. The list is elaborated in: Colesanti, Marino 2016: 322-325.

cially those in the Mercato, gained an enormous financial boon from the hospital, which required a constant supply of specialized services from doctors, surgeons, and apothecaries. The hospital also encouraged an entire economy of merchants and artisans: weavers, shoemakers, carpenters, ironsmiths, gardeners, etc. (fig. 10). The entire community interacted at some level with the hospital and benefited from direct payment for services, small loans, or simple charity (MARINO 2018: 171-205).

## *Bibliography*


ALBINI, Giuliana, 1993. *Città e ospedali nella Lombardia medievale*, Bologna, Clueb.

ALBINI, Giuliana, 2001. "Strade e ospitalità, ponti e ospedali di ponte nell'Emilia occidentale (secc. XII-XIV)", Roberto Greci (ed.), *Studi sull'Emilia occidentale nel Medioevo: società e istituzioni*, Bologna, Clueb: 205-251.

AMBROSIO, Antonella, 2003. *Il monastero domenicano femminile dei SS. Pietro e Sebastiano. Regesti dei documenti dei secoli XIV-XV*, Salerno, Carlone.

BERTAUX, Émile, 1895. "Gli affreschi dell'antica chiesa di Santa Maria Annunziata, *Napoli Nobilissima*, 4: 49-52.

BERTINI Antonio; COLESANTI Gemma T.; SOLER SALA, Maria, 2020. "La rete monastica nel tessuto urbano di Napoli (secc. XII-XVI)", *Svmma. Revista de Cultures Medievals*, 15: 55-73.

BOCCADAMO, Giuliana, 2019. *La malattia della vita. Ospedali e assistenza a Napoli in età moderna*, Naples, Liguori.

BRUZELLIUS, Caroline, 2004. *The Stone of Naples. Church Building in Angevin Italy. 1266-1343*, New Haven, London, Yale University Press.

CÂMERA, Matteo, 1841-1860. *Annali delle due Sicilie dall'origine e fondazione della monarchia fino a tutto il regno dell'augusto sovrano Carlo III di Borbone*, vol. 1-2, Naples, Stamperie e Cartiere del Fibreno.

CAPASSO, Bartolomeo, 1880. "La fontana dei quattro del Molo di Napoli. Ricordi storici", *Archivio Storico per le Province Napoletane*, 5: 158-194.

CAPASSO, Bartolomeo, 1895. *Topografia della città di Napoli*, Naples, Forni.

CAPONE, Gabriele; LEONE, Alfonso, 1996. "La colonia scalese dal XIII al XV secolo", Alfonso Leone (ed.), *Ricerche sul Medioevo napoletano. Aspetti e momenti della vita economica e sociale a Napoli tra decimo e quindicesimo secolo*, Naples, Athena: 173-186.

Casiello, Stella, 2005. *San Giovanni a Mare: storia e restauri*, Naples, Arte Tipografica.

CELANO, Carlo, 1792-1860. *Notizie del bello, dell'antico e del curioso della città di Napoli*, vol. 1-5, Naples, Stamperia De Pascale.

CEVA GRIMALDI, Francesco, 1857. *Memorie storiche della città di Napoli*, Naples, Forni.

COLESANTI, Gemma Teresa, MARINO, Salvatore, 2016. "L'economia dell'assistenza a Napoli nel tardo medioevo". *Reti Medievali Rivista*, 17-1: 309-344, https://doi.org/10.6092/1593-2214/503.

D'ADDOSIO, Giovan Battista, 1883. *Origini, vicende storiche e progressi della Real S. Casa dell'Annunziata di Napoli*, Naples, Tip. Antonio Cons.

D'ANDREA, David; MARINO, Salvatore (ed.), 2022. *Confraternities in Southern Italy. Art, Politics, and Religion (1100-1800)*, Toronto, Centre for Renaissance and Reformation Studies-University of Toronto.

DE FEO, Emanuela, 2017. *La chiesa di Sant'Eligio al Mercato a Napoli. Storia, indagini documentarie, rilievi, analisi critica*, Fisciano, Cua.

DE MARTINO, Gianluigi, 2008. "Il restauro della chiesa di San Giovanni a mare in Napoli", Giovanni Carbonara (ed.), *Trattato di Restauro Architettonico*, vol. 10, Turin, UTET: 25-50.

D'Engenio Caracciolo, Cesare, 1623. *Napoli sacra*, Naples, Beltano.

Di Meglio, Rosalba, 2003. "La Disciplina di S. Marta: mito e realtà di una confraternita popolare", Giovanni Vitolo, Rosalba Di Meglio (ed.), *Napoli angioino-aragonese. Confraternite, ospedali, dinamiche político-sociali*, Salerno, Carlone: 147-234.

Di Meglio, Rosalba, 2013. *Ordini mendicanti. Monarchia e dinamiche político-sociali nella Napoli dei secoli XIII-XV*, Raleigh, Aonia.

D'Ovidio, Stefano, 2022. "Sacred Imagery, Confraternities, and Urban Space in Medieval Naples", David D'Andre, Salvatore Marino (ed.), *Confraternities in Southern Italy. Art, Politics, and Religion (1100-1800)*, Toronto, Centre for Renaissance and Reformation Studies, University of Toronto: 43-102.

Enderlein, Lorenz, 1997. "Die Gründungsgeschichte der Incoronata in Neapel", *Römisches Jahrbuch der Biblioteca Hertziana*, 31: 15-46.

Feniello, Amedeo, 2002. "Un aspect du paysage napolitain au Moyen Âge: les bains dans la ville du Xe au XIIIe siècle", *Médiévales*, 43: 71-82.

Feniello, Amedeo, 2003. "Mercanzie e cariche pubbliche: la fortuna dei D'Afflitto, uomini d'affari italiani del XV secolo", Alfonso Leone (ed.), *Il commercio a Napoli e in Italia meridionale nel XV secolo*, Naples, Athena: 15-88.

Feniello, Amedeo, 2012. "Alle origini di Napoli capitale", *Mélanges de l'École Française de Rome. Moyen Âge*, 124-2: 567-584.

Gaglione, Mario, 2007. "Sulla fondazione della chiesa e dell'ospedale di S. Antonio Abate in Napoli", *Scrinia. Rivista di Archivistica, Paleografia, Diplomatica e Scienze storiche*, 4: 89-104.

Galante, Gennaro Aspreno 1872. *Guida sacra della città di Napoli*, Naples, Stamperia del Fibreno.

Gazzini, Marina, 2002. "Gli utenti della strada. Mercanti, pellegrini, militari", *Reti Medievali Rivista*, 3: 1-12.

Imperato, Ferrante, 1629. *Discorsi intorno all'origine, regimento e stato della gran Casa della Santissima Annuntiata di Napoli*, Naples, Egidio Longo.

Keyvanian, Carla, 2015. *Hospitals and Urbanism in Rome, 1200-1500*, Leiden-Boston, Brill.

Lucherini, Vinni 2012. "Un papa francese a Napoli: un'immagine trecentesca di Urbano V identificata e le effigi dei fondatori di Sant'Eligio", *Le plaisir de l'art du Moyen Age. Commande, production et reception de l'oeuvre d'art. Melanges en hommage a Xavier Barral i Altet*, Paris, Picard: 181-192

Marino, Salvatore, 2014. *Ospedali e città nel Regno di Napoli. Le Annunziate: istituzioni, archivi e fonti*, Florence, Olschki.

Marino, Salvatore, 2015. *L'Archivio dell'Annunziata di Napoli. Inventari e documenti (secoli XII-XIX)*, Battipaglia, Laveglia e Carlone.

Marino, Salvatore, 2018. "Trabajo y aprendizaje en los hospitals de la Baja Edad Media. Aproximación comparativa entre Barcelona, Milán, Nápoles y Siena", *Reti Medievali Rivista*, 19-2: 171-205, https://doi.org/10.6092/1593-2214/5955.

Marino, Salvatore, 2020. "Riforme del welfare e modelli ospedalieri nella Corona d'Aragona", Gabriella Piccinni (ed.), *Alle origini del welfare. Radici medievali e moderna della cultura europea dell'assistenza*, Rome, Viella: 183-202.

Mazzocchi, Alessio Simmaco, 1751. *Dissertatio historica de cathedralis ecclesiae Neapolitanae*, Naples, Excudentibus Novello de Bonis Tipografia.

Monti, Gennaro Maria, 1936. *Da Carlo I a Roberto d'Angiò: ricerche e documenti*, Trani, Vecchi.

Novi Chavarria, Elisa, 1936. *Accogliere e curare. Ospedali e culture delle nazioni nella Monarchia ispanica (secc. XVI-XVII)*, Rome, Viella.

Patroni Griffi, Filena; Leone, Alfonso, 1984. *Le origini di Napoli capitale*, Altavilla Silentina, 1984.

Pilone, Rosaria, 1989. *Il Diplomatico di S. Gregorio Armeno conservato nell'Archivio di Stato di Napoli*, Naples, Laurenziana.

PILONE, Rosaria, 1999. *L'antico inventario delle pergamene del monastero dei SS. Severino e Sossio*, Rome, Istituto Storico Italiano per il Medioevo.

PINTO, Giuliano, 2014. "Tra demografia, economia e politica: la rete urbana italiana (XIII-inizio XVI secolo)", *Edad Media*, 15: 37-57.

RADOGNA, Michele, 1873. *Monografia di S. Giovanni a Mare, baliaggio del S. M. O. Gerosolimitano in Napoli,* Naples, Tipografia dell'Industria.

RADOGNA, Michele, 1894. "Di una vetusta icona di Cristo crocifisso, scultura in legno serbata dal sodalizio dei 66 sacerdoti in S. Giovanni Maggiore", *Archivio Storico per le Province Napoletane*, 19: 711-717.

REGISTRI, 1955, 1967. *I registri della cancelleria angioina ricostruiti da Riccardo Filangieri*, Naples, Accademia Pontaniana, vol. 7/21.

RICCIARDI, Emilio, 1999. "La chiesa di S. Giovanni a Mare in Napoli. Documenti, descrizioni e antiche planimetrie", *Campania Sacra*, 30/1-2: 229-252.

RUSSO, Francesco, 1991. *Regesti delle pergamene di S. Angelo a Nilo. La cappella Brancaccio dei Frati minori conventuali*, Naples, Laurenziana.

SAKELLARIOU, Eleni, 2012. *Southern Italy in the Late Middle Ages. Demographic, Institucional and Economic Change in the Kingdom of Naples, c. 1400-c. 1530*, Boston, Brill.

SALERNO, Mariarosaria, 2001. *Gli Ospedalieri di San Giovanni di Gerusalemme nel Mezzogiorno d'Italia (secc.* XII-XV*)*, Taranto, Centro Studi Melitensi.

SALERNO, Mariarosaria, 2010. "Legami familiari e rapporti con il potere nel Mezzogiorno angioino. Gli ospedalieri di San Giovanni di Gerusalemme tra monarchia e papato", *Mélanges de l'École Française de Rome – Moyen Âge*, 122/1: 127-137.

SCHIAPPOLI, Irma, 1972. *Napoli aragonese: traffici e attività marinare*, Naples, Giannini.

SIGISMONDO, Giuseppe, 1788. *Descrizione della città di Napoli e suoi borghi*, vol. 3, Naples, Terres.

TUTINI, Camillo, 1644. *Dell'origine e fundation de' seggi di Napoli*, Naples, Beltrano.

VENDITTI, Arnaldo, 1969. "Urbanistica e architettura angioina", Ernesto Pontieri (ed.), *Storia di Napoli. Cultura e letteratura*, vol. 3, Naples, SESN: 667-888.

VETERE, Carla, 2000. *Le pergamene di San Gregorio Armeno*, Salerno, Carlone.

VITALE, Giuliana, 1993. "Uffici, militia e nobiltà. Processi di formazione della nobiltà di seggio a Napoli: il casato dei Brancaccio fra XIV e XV secolo", *Dimensioni e problemi della ricerca storica*, 2: 22-42.

VITALE, Giuliana, 1999. "I santi del re: potere economico e pratiche devozionali nella Napoliangioina e aragonese", Giovanni Vitolo (ed.), *Pellegrinaggi e itinerari dei santi nel Mezzogiorno medievale*, Naples, GISEM-Liguori: 93-128.

VITOLO, Giovanni, 2001. *Tra Napoli e Salerno. La costruzione dell'identità cittadina nel Mezzogiorno medievale*, Salerno, Carlone.

VITOLO, Giovanni, 2003. "L'ospedale di S. Eligio e la Piazza del Mercato", Giovanni Vitolo, Rosalba Di Meglio (ed.), *Napoli angioino-aragonese. Confraternite, ospedali, dinamiche politico-sociali*, Salerno, Carlone: 39-146.

VITOLO, Paola, 2008. *La Chiesa della regina. L'Incoronata di Napoli, Giovanna I d'Angiò e Roberto di Oderisio*, Rome, Viella.

VOLPICELLA, Scipione, 1877. "S. Eligio Maggiore di Napoli al 1582", *Archivio Storico per le Province Napoletane*, 2: 713-724.

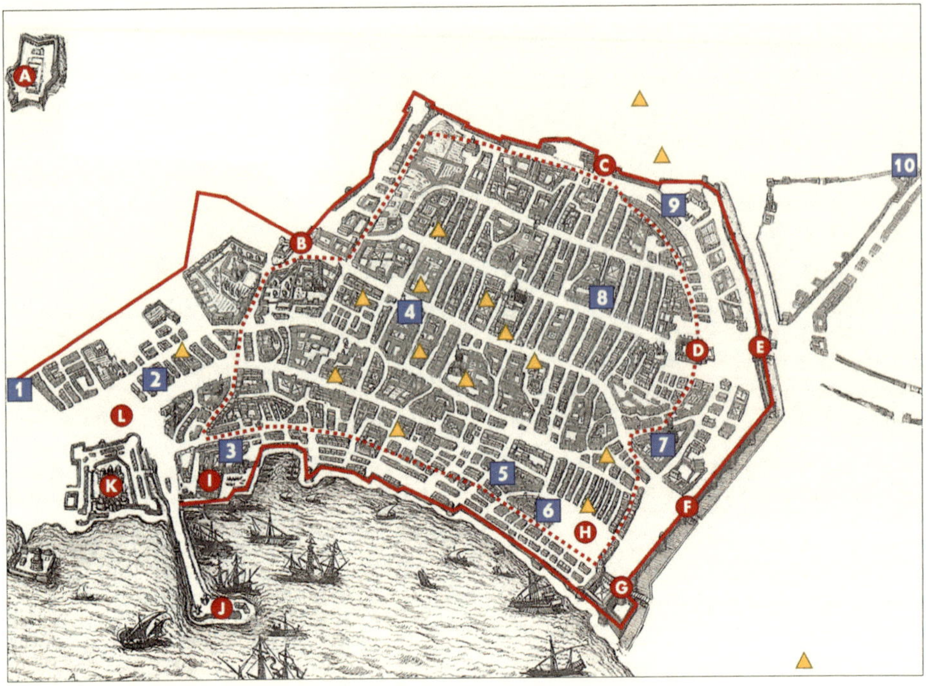

• = Main urban areas and civic buildings

A = Castel Sant'Elmo
B = Porta Reale
C = Porta San Gennaro
D = Castel Capuano
E = Porta Capuana
F = Porta Nolana
G = Porta del Carmine
H = Piazza Mercato
I = Arsenale
J = Molo grande
K = Castel Nuovo
L = Largo delle Corregge

······ = Angevin city walls (around 1350)
—— = Aragonese city walls (1484-1500)

□ = Main hospitals

1 = S. Elisabetta (then S. Spirito)
2 = Incoronata
3 = S. Nicola al Molo (Sailors)
4 = S. Angelo a Nido
5 = S. Giovanni a Mare (Gerosolimitano)
6 = S. Eligio
7 = Annunziata
8 = S. Atanasio
9 = S. Maria della Pietà
10 = S. Antonio di Vienne

△= Smaller hospitals and hospices

Fig. 1. Distribution of the hospitals in the medieval Naples. From the map by Antoine Lafréry. 1566, Naples: Museo di San Martino. Map customized by Salvatore Marino.

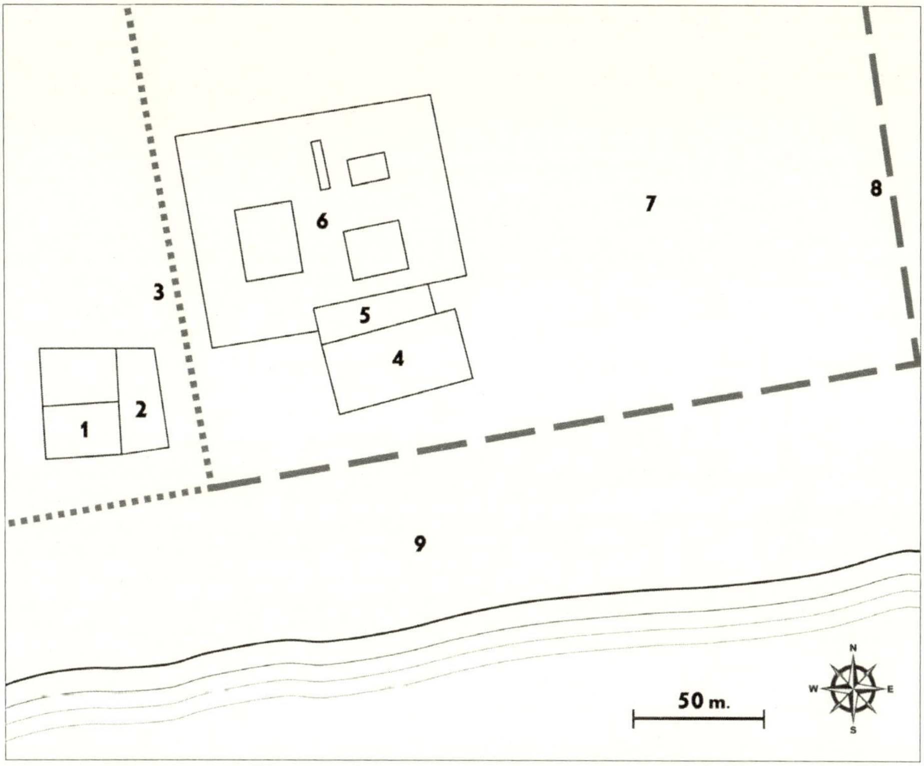


1 = Church of S. Giovanni a Mare
2 = Hospital of S. Giovanni Gerosolimitano
3 = Porta Nova
4 = Church of S. Eligio
5 = The "Forth Nave"

6 = Hospital of S. Eligio (c. 15th - 18th)
7 = Marker Square
8 = Porta del Mercato
9 = Seaside

· · · · · = City walls (1258-1263)
- - - - - = City walls (around 1350)

Fig. 2. The area of Moricino or Market Square between the 13th and 14th century. Map customized by Salvatore Marino on partial hypothesis in VITOLO 2003: 57.

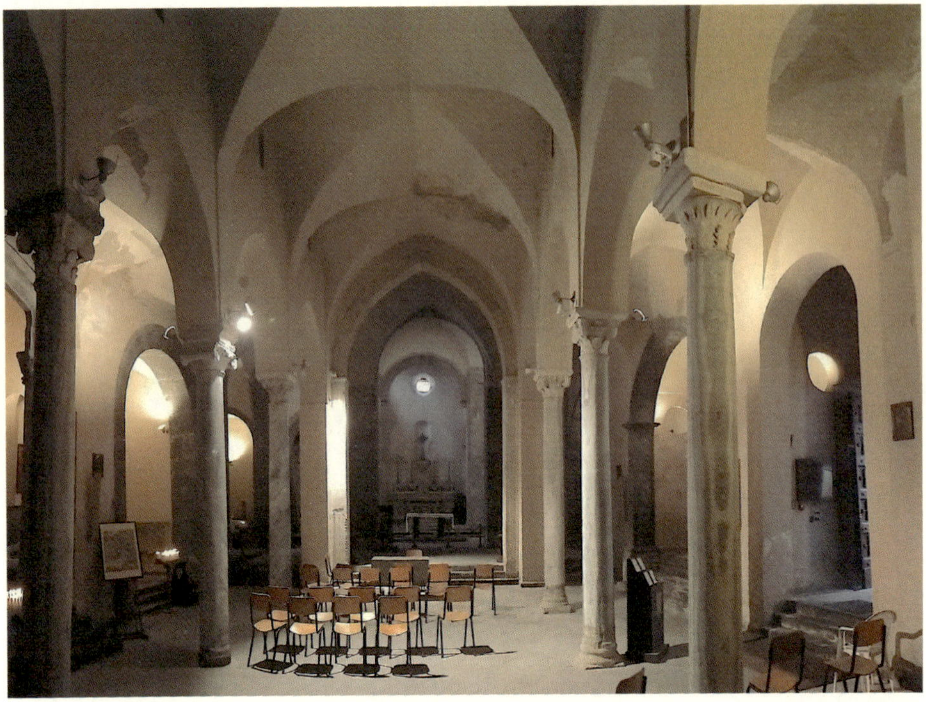

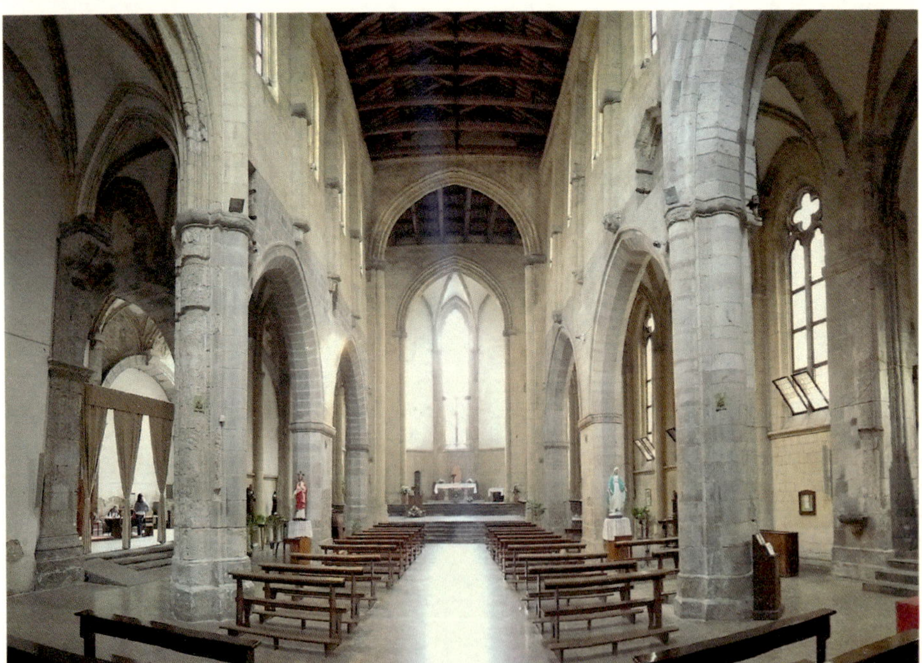

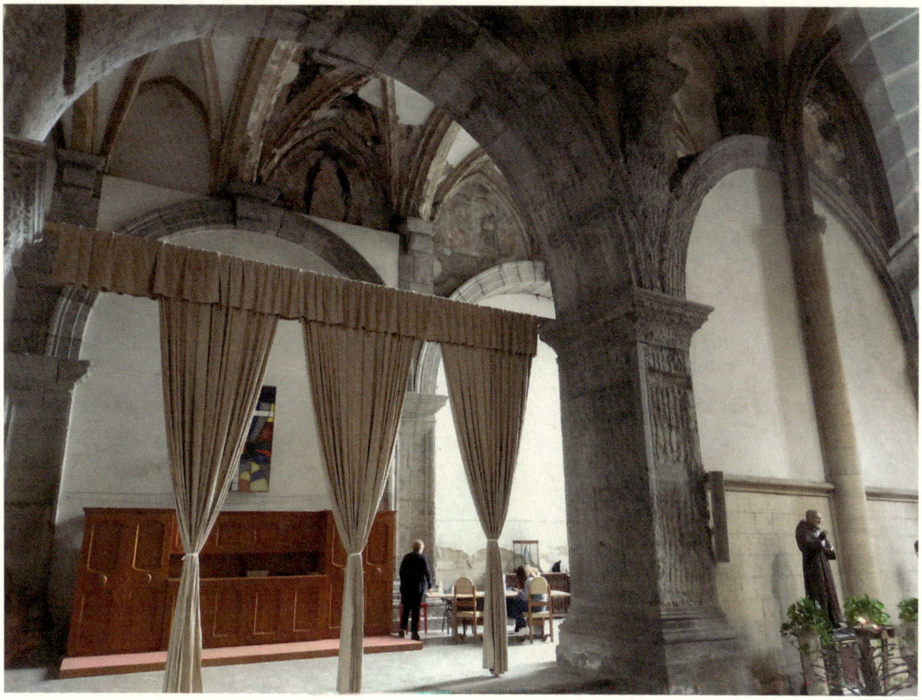

Fig. 3 (*on the other page*). Naples, church of S. Giovanni a Mare. Central nave, c. 12th. Photograph: Salvatore Marino.
Fig. 4 (*on the other page*). Naples, church of S. Eligio. Central nave, c. 14th. Photograph: Salvatore Marino.
Fig. 5. Naples, church of S. Eligio. Fourth aisle, c. 14th. Photograph: Salvatore Marino.

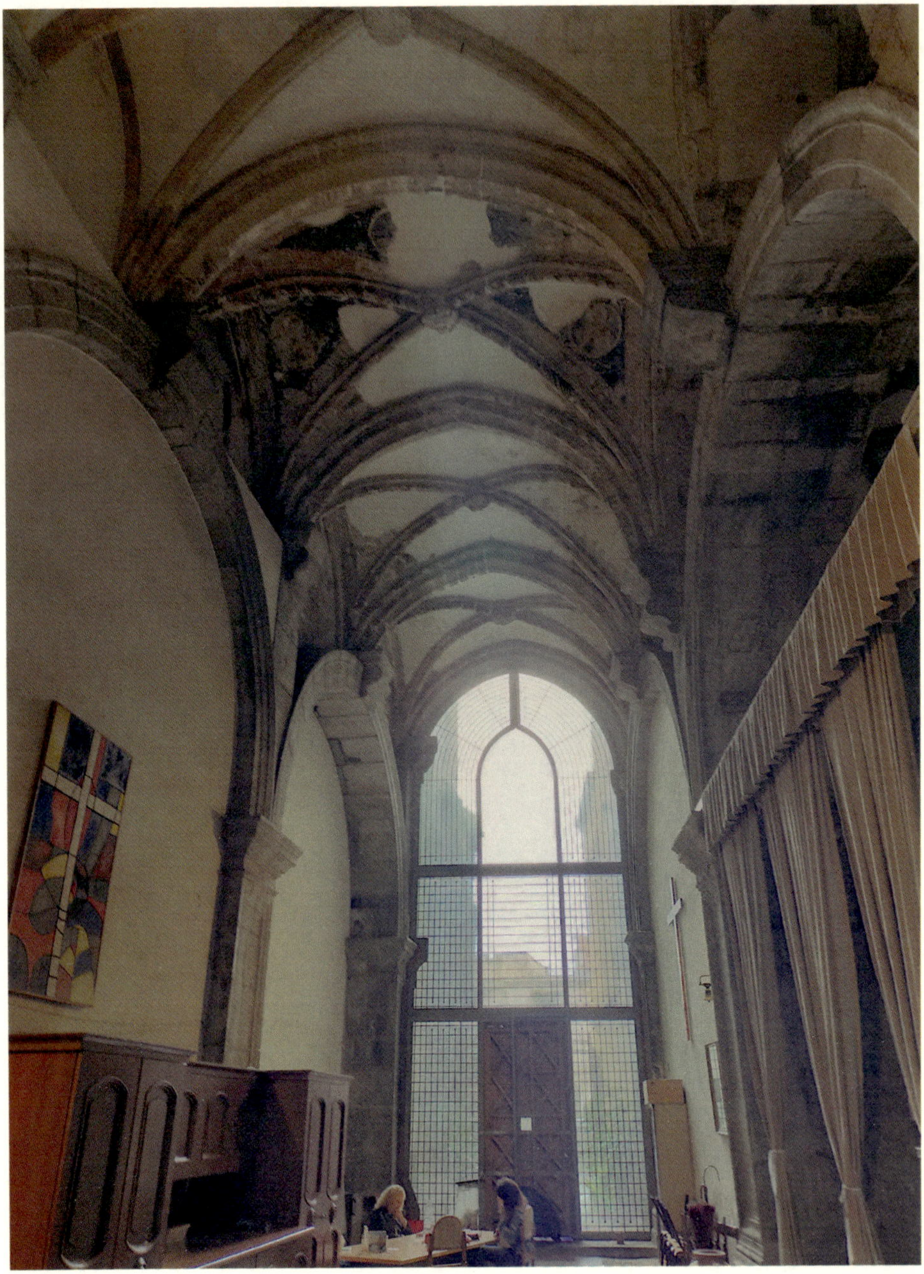

Fig. 6. Naples, church of S. Eligio. Fourth aisle with the entrance to the medieval hospital, c. 14th. Photograph: Salvatore Marino.

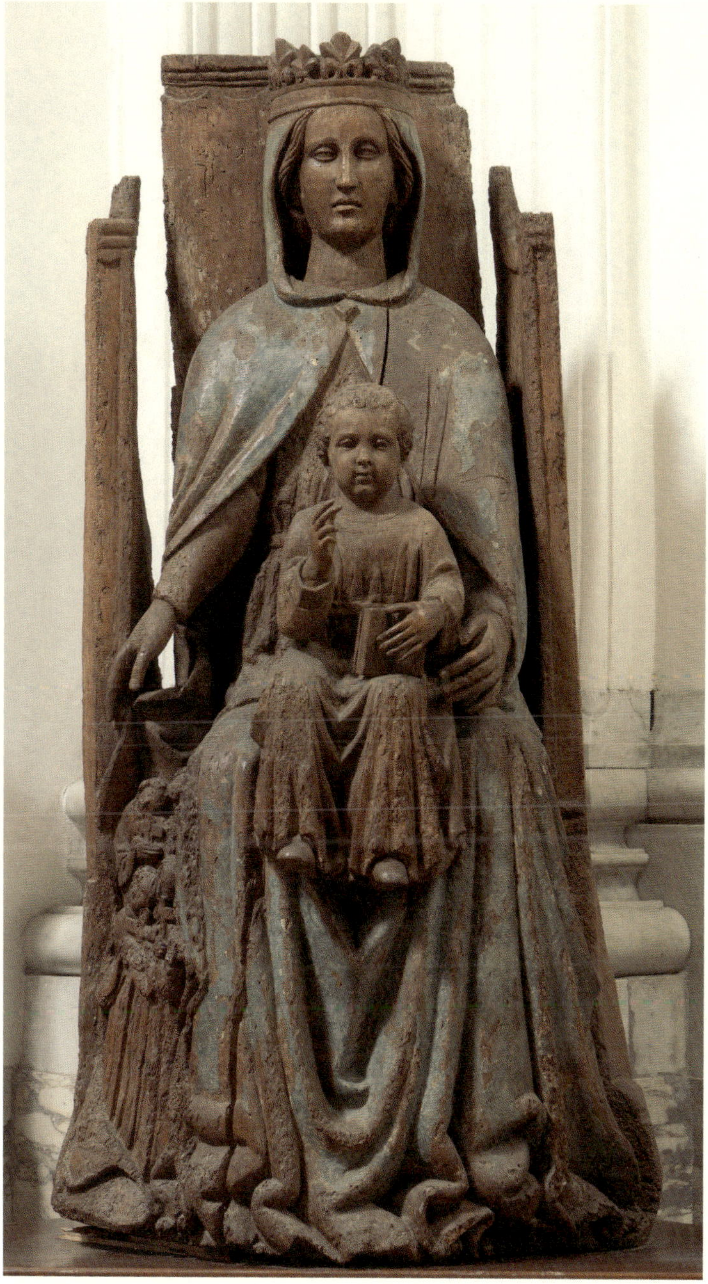

Fig. 7. Naples, church of Annunziata, *Madonna dei Repentiti,* c. 15th. Photograph: Marco and Luciano Pedicini, published in D'OVIDIO 2022: 91.

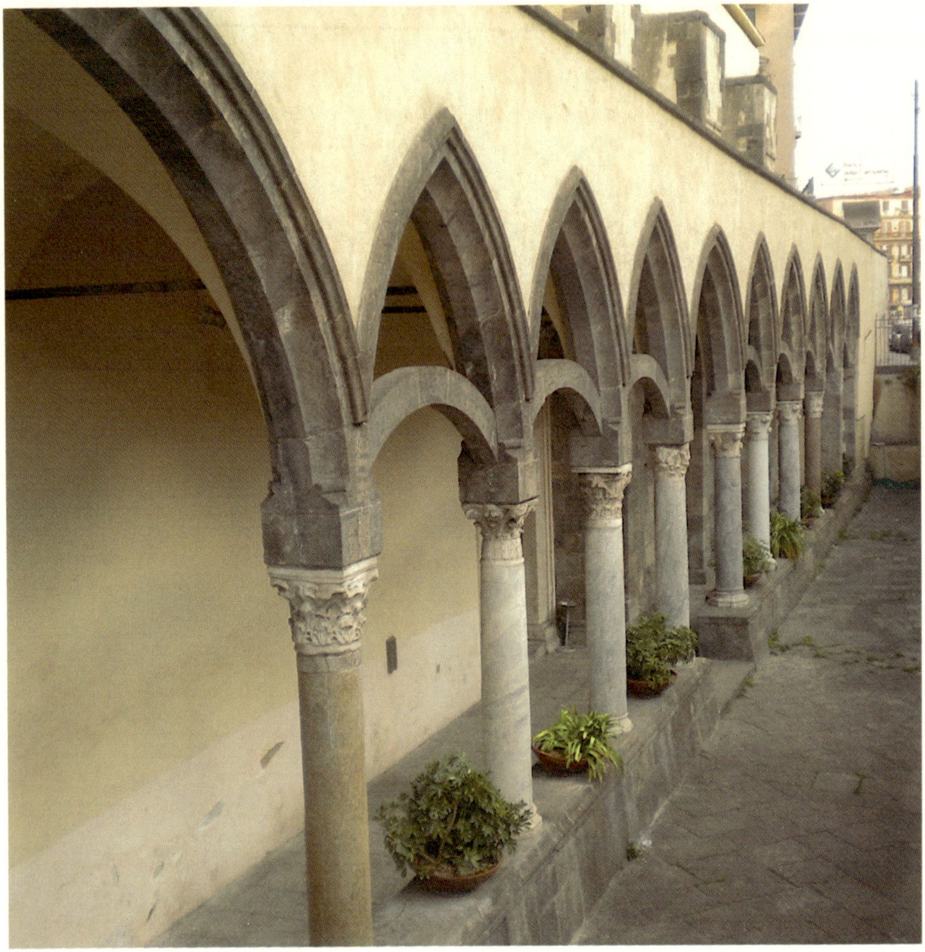

Fig. 8. Naples. Portico between the medieval hospital and church of the Incoronata, c. 14t[h]. Image obtained from https://cosedinapoli.com/chiese-e-monumenti/chiesa-di-santa-maria-dellincoronata (public domain).

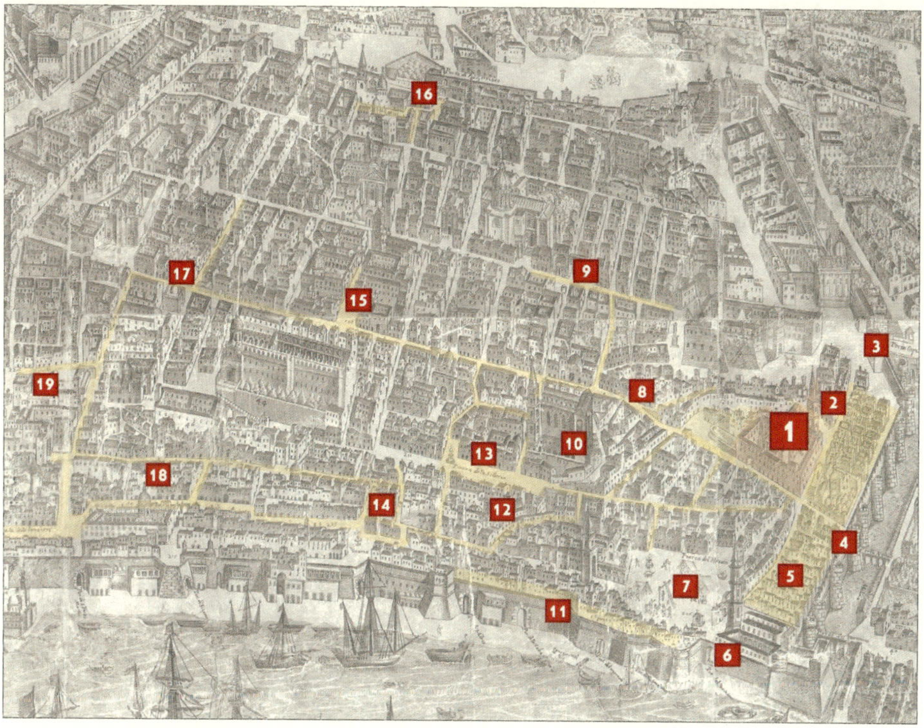


1 = Casa Santa dell'Annunziata
2 = La Maddalena
3 = Porta Capuana
4 = Porta Nolana
5 = Lavinaio
6 = S. Maria del Carmine Maggiore
7 = Piazza Mercato
8 = Forcella
9 = Capuana
10 = Sant'Agostino
11 = Mura meridionali
12 = Rua Francesca
13 = Selleria e Seggio del Popolo
14 = Rua Novella
15 = San Biagio dei Librai
16 = Porta San Gennaro
17 = Via Nilo
18 = Portanuova
19 = Banchi Nuovi

Fig. 9. Alessandro Baratta: *Fidelissimae Urbis Neapolitanae,* 1627 and 1629. Detail with the distribution of Annunziata real estate in the city of Naples, c. 15th (Naples, Collezione Banca Intesa-San Paolo, on loan at Museo di San Martino). Map customized by Salvatore Marino.

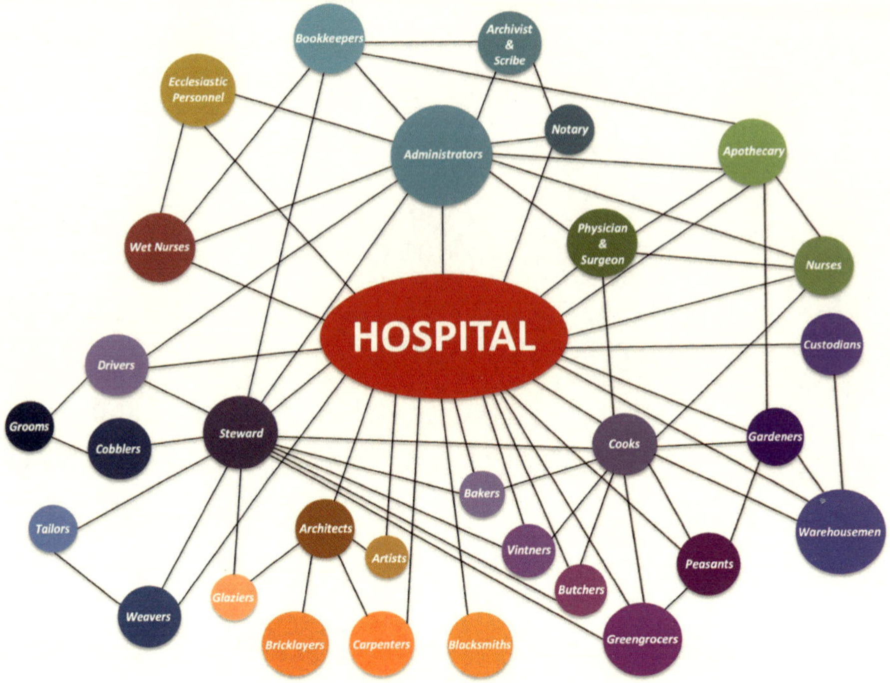


Fig. 10. Graph on the world of work connected to the Annunziata in Naples. Graphic elaborated by Salvatore Marino.

Raúl Villagrasa-Elías

# El loco, el niño y el hospital: la inclusión del pobre verdadero en el espacio urbano renacentista*

Cuando el personaje literario del Lazarillo de Tormes abandonó sus chanzas, penurias y vagabundeos, ejerció el oficio de pregonero. Su trabajo consistía en publicar en voz alta y a los cuatro vientos información útil para sus vecinos. Anunciaba el precio de los vinos, las cosas extraviadas y los tránsfugas huidos de la ley (Rico 2005: 129); suponía un nexo de unión entre el poder y la ciudadanía. Para la Zaragoza de los siglos XV y XVI se conservan los textos[1] que los pregoneros divulgaban por calles y plazas. A fecha de 7 de enero de 1486 notificaron lo siguiente:

> […] manyana domingo fazer processión general al spital de Senyora sancta María de Gracia de la dita ciudat, la qual cada un anyo se acostumbra fazer al dicho spital por la festividat de los Innocentes.

Llama la atención una palabra en concreto: "Innocentes". He aquí el porqué. El hospital mencionado no es otro que Santa María de Gracia de la ciudad de Zaragoza, fundado por María de Castilla y Alfonso el Magnánimo en 1425. Como otros muchos nosocomios europeos de la época, pero especialmente de la corona

* Este capítulo se ha desarrollado gracias a un contrato predoctoral de Formación de Personal Investigador (FPI) (BES-2017-081778) del Ministerio de Economía, Industria y Competitividad del Gobierno de España, y está enmarcado en el proyecto de investigación «Scripta manent III. De registros privados a textos públicos. Un archivo medieval en la red» (PID2020-116104RB-I00), dirigido por Cristina Jular Pérez-Alfaro y financiado por el programa estatal de I+D+i, Convocatoria Orientada a los Retos de la Sociedad, del Ministerio de Ciencia e Innovación del Gobierno de España, con plataforma digital en www.scriptamanent.info. A su vez, se inserta en la Red de Excelencia «Cultura escrita medieval hispánica: del manuscrito al soporte digital (CEMH)» (RED2018-102330-T) de la Agencia Estatal de Investigación del Ministerio de Ciencia e Innovación del Gobierno de España, con plataforma digital en www.libromedievalhispanico.net.

1. La materia prima de este capítulo se basa en las secciones de Libros de Actas (LA) y Libros de Pregones (Preg.) o cridas del Archivo Municipal de Zaragoza (AMZ) debido, en gran medida, a la ausencia de fuentes propias del hospital de Nuestra Señora de Gracia. Los LA recogen las reuniones anuales del concejo y sus oficiales. El más antiguo abarca la anualidad de dic. de 1439 a dic. de 1440. No hay series completas hasta el volumen de 1489. He revisado desde el volumen más antiguo hasta 1523, un total de 21 ejemplares. Por otro lado, los pregones comienzan en 1406. Siguiendo las signaturas archivísticas he analizado Pre. 1, 2, 3 y 4 que suman 47 cuadernillos de 1406 a 1514. Una primera aproximación a estos fondos diplomáticos: Falcón 1988; 2006.

de Aragón, este se situó bajo el amparo de la Virgen María.[2] Concretamente, la advocación hacía referencia a la Virgen de Gracia, cuyo origen proviene de la visita del arcángel san Gabriel a la futura madre de Jesús y sus palabras: «Dios te salve, María, llena eres de gracia» (Lc 1,28). Por tanto, si el sanatorio de referencia para Zaragoza y el reino de Aragón estuvo bajo el amparo de santa María de Gracia, ¿por qué no se celebró la procesión del hospital en sintonía con la adoración de la Virgen?

En la práctica era imposible porque durante el día de la Encarnación, cercano al de la Asunción, ya se celebraba una procesión a Santa María del Portillo, parroquia de esta misma ciudad. Por tanto, el objetivo del presente ensayo es dar respuesta a esta pregunta: ¿por qué se eligió el día de los Santos Inocentes para celebrar la procesión de este hospital? A modo de respuesta, la hipótesis que manejo es que los administradores del centro, miembros de la elite política y eclesiástica de la ciudad, utilizaron lo lúdico y lo festivo para promocionar el establecimiento y, a la vez, definieron quiénes eran los verdaderos merecedores de su atención: los inocentes, es decir, los niños y dementes. A través de este proceso, diferentes partes del hospital –tanto la institucional como la humana– superaron los muros del establecimiento para ocupar, aunque fuera por un día, un espacio que les era ajeno –la ciudad– creando al mismo tiempo dinámicas de segregación e integración.

## 1. *¿Quiénes fueron los inocentes?*

Según la tradición hagiográfica cristiana, los Santos Inocentes fueron los niños de Belén menores de dos años masacrados por las tropas del rey Herodes en un intento de acabar con el niño Jesús (Mt 2,13-18). Pese a la inexistencia de datos históricos que evidencien aquel suceso, el culto por los pequeños asesinados se difundió por la cristiandad tanto artística (García García 2011) como literariamente. Con el tiempo, y para la época que nos atañe, aquella inocencia se hizo extensible a la infancia.[3]

Entre las filas del pauperismo de las ciudades bajomedievales y modernas se encontraban en gran número criaturas de pocos días, meses o años, abandonadas principalmente por el fallecimiento de los progenitores, su miseria o nacimiento ilegítimo.[4] Las autoridades respondieron principalmente haciendo uso de dos instituciones: por un lado, dándoles cabida en centros hospitalarios donde los

2. Recordemos la extensa red de las *Annunziate* a nivel italiano y, especialmente, al sur de la península (Marino 2014). Sobre la figura artística de la Madre de Dios (Conejo 2015: 110-115).

3. Dos estudios de la infancia para el norte de Castellón y sur de Aragón: Aparici, Navarro 2010; Aparici, Villanueva, 2021.

4. García Herrero (2006, I, 70) nos informa del caso de Gaspar Eli, quien argumentó «que cómo se avía de casar» con Catalina Cunchillos de Alcorisa si «le avían dicho que tenía dos o tres fillos [*abandonados*] en el espital de Caragoça» (1493). Más allá de la anécdota, véanse las reflexiones de la autora sobre la infancia abandonada en pp. 62-71. Por el contrario, también conocemos

alimentaban y contrataban nodrizas, por otro, controlando e insertando a los muchachos en familias para el aprendizaje de un oficio, especialmente a través del Padre de Huérfanos. Esta figura ya se documenta en el reino de Valencia durante el siglo XIV.[5] Con este entramado institucional se buscó que los más pequeños no engrosaran círculos marginales, mendicantes y delictivos. En Zaragoza la iniciativa es más tardía (1475).

La capital aragonesa disponía del hospital de Santa María de Gracia para cuidar de los niños y niñas de menor edad. Los estatutos del Padre de Huérfanos de 1487 así lo manifiestan: «Mientras no les halle amo, llevarlos al Hospital de Nuestra Señora de Gracia, que les ha de dar de comer» (SAN VICENTE 1965). En las ordinaciones del centro de 1508 se expresaban claramente las tareas de la «mujer que tiene cargo de los ninyos».[6] Como intermediario entre esta casa y el exterior, un «corredor de nodriças» se dedicaba a su contratación, al menos en 1508 (GARCÍA HERRERO 2006, v. I: 90). Sabemos que en 1489 el hospital zaragozano solicitó más recursos para financiar el salario de estas trabajadoras (GARCÍA HERRERO 2005: 59). A partir de 1543 se fundaron los «hospitalicos» de niños y niñas huérfanos, ocupándose propiamente de esta tarea para descargar la presión asistencial del hospital general (ROYO 1994).[7]

Por lo que parece evidenciar la historiografía para la corona de Aragón –en ambas penínsulas y las islas–, y aun a riesgo de generalizar para tan amplios territorios, los grandes hospitales cívicos de los siglos XV-XVI tendieron a ocuparse de la asistencia de huérfanos y dementes.[8] En el caso del reino de Aragón, ese primer impulso institucional se complementó con nuevos establecimientos especializados en el cuidado de los más pequeños creados durante el quinientos. Así, la ciudad de Barbastro también contó con un hospicio para los infantes a partir de 1575, complementando los esfuerzos del hospital principal de San Julián y Santa

casos de adopción como el de la pequeña Isabel en 1481: p. 81. El documento en vol. II, pp. 276-277.

5. Véase RUBIO VELA (1990). Para el Padre de Huérfanos acúdase a pp. 128-133 y para la limosna para casar huérfanas, intentando evitar así su caída en la prostitución, pp. 120-128. Precisamente la metrópoli valenciana funcionó como foco de atracción de migrantes desde el siglo XIV, muchos de ellos huérfanos que aparecen en contratos de *afermament*. Así lo contempla la legislación municipal (NARBONA 2012: 177). Los registros del Padre de Huérfanos durante la segunda mitad del cuatrocientos ratifican la importancia de la industria textil (NAVARRO 1993).

6. Se trata de un cargo diferente de la «mujer enfermera», responsable de las enfermas. La «mujer que tiene cargo de los ninyos» se ocupaba de su higiene y coordinaba el trabajo de nodrizas y sirvientas. Estas últimas podían hilar para vender el producto y beneficiar a la institución. La descripción de su oficio en MONTERDE 2008: 518.

7. Compleméntese con el estudio más reciente de M.ª Ángeles Montanel (2018).

8. El caso de la *santa Creu* de Barcelona sobresale gracias a la conservación de varios registros de los niños huérfanos: para la multitud de situaciones relacionados con los más pequeños y con algunos casos de (cuasi)adopción véase: VINYOLES, ILLANES 2015. Para conocer dicho registro acúdase a MARINO 2019. El cuidado de los más pequeños se complementa con la asistencia de dementes: HUGUET-TERMES, ARRIZABALAGA 2010. Para los reinos de Nápoles y Sicilia: MARINO 2015. Compleméntese con: VILLAGRASA-ELÍAS 2016.

Lucía (Arcarazo, Lorén 2000: 76-77).[9] Se trataba de un sistema diferente al florentino, tendente a la especialización, representado para el caso que nos concierne por el *ospedale degli Innocenti* diseñado por Filippo Brunelleschi (1419).

La formulación de afirmaciones generalistas conlleva el riesgo de encontrar excepciones, como el caso valenciano, el cual evidencia la utilización del término "inocente" más allá de la infancia. En 1409 nació el hospital de *Innocents, folls e orats*, es decir, un lugar dedicado al cuidado de los dementes.[10] Esta expresión se utilizó de forma cotidiana, como cuando en los procesos inquisitoriales de finales del siglo XV de la ciudad de Daroca la atribución de locura servía para desprestigiar la declaración de determinadas personas:

> [...] si por ventura avrá deposado Joan Gil, moço, habitante en Mofort, ni a su deposición no se le deve dar fe ni crédito alguno, por quanto es ignocent y loco, que merecería estar en el espital con los ygnocentes y locos, que demás cuerdos tienen por locos en el dicho espital [...].[11]

De hecho, ambos grupos, niños y dementes, fueron objeto del transporte sanitario. En estos siglos de reformas hospitalarias, determinados municipios centralizaron la asistencia de estos colectivos. Las autoridades de Daroca enviaban los recién nacidos a Maluenda, Calatayud o Zaragoza (Rodrigo 1995: 303-307). Igualmente, el concejo de Ateca encomendó una «moçuela que echaron en el spital» a Pascual Guillén y su mujer para asearla y llevarla a la localidad castellana de Embid (Rubio, Martínez 2019: 209).

El caso de los dementes guarda una gran diferencia, ya que buena parte de estos transportes fueron forzosos debido a la desestabilización de la paz social de la comunidad. Algunos ejemplos: en 1417 los prohombres de Villarreal enviaron a Valencia «un home foll, o orat, qui avien amenat a la dita vila dos hòmens de Borriol, ab ses cormes en les mans, e lo qual ere stat remès de un loch en altre per amenar aquell al hespital dels ignocents» (Doñate 1980: 809); a mediados de la centuria las autoridades zaragozanas confirmaron que Jaime Pezonada, "insensado", había sido remitido también al hospital valenciano por herir al abad de Santa Fe;[12] en 1476 el concejo de Murcia ordenó a Juan Serrano que ingresara a la mujer de Guillén, armero, en este mismo establecimiento (Asensi 1992: 82); en 1479 Argel de Lanuza recorrió más de cien kilómetros para dejar a su hija, «ignocenta clamada Honoreta», en el hospital de santa María de Gracia de Zaragoza (Pallarés 2008: 592); en 1481 Marica de Andorra, loca y ladrona de Huesca, «bistas sus locuras e de la forma que faze los ditos furtos», fue encomendada a su hermano para «que

9. La solicitud ya se envió a Roma en 1501.

10. Resulta fundamental la monografía de Hélène Tropé (1994). Véase la extensión del término «inocente» a mediados del siglo XVI en Valencia para referirse a niños moriscos: Franco, Moreno 2019.

11. Otro ejemplo: «a la deposición de uno llamado Anthón Estevan, que bive en Armiella, si abrá deposado, por quanto es hombre vario, ygnocent, que quantas vezes lo interrueguen cada vez dirá y deposará de su manera [...]» (Motis, García Marco, Rodrigo 1995: 503-504, 517 y 521).

12. AMZ, LA, 1 (1439 dic.-1440 dic.), f. 128v (17/09/1440).

la saque de la ciudad e que nunca torne, e si no la quiere sacar su ermano, que la ciudad la faga leuar a Caragoca, al spital, e que la fagan poner en una caseta do los locos stán» (PÉREZ GALÁN 2013: 304); y, finalmente, los jurados de Daroca hicieron lo propio con varios pacientes entre 1485 y 1506, entre ellos Pedro el Inocente que «apedreava los retablos de la ciudat» (RODRIGO 1995: 316).

Por supuesto, las categorías de la locura fueron múltiples y diferentes de las nuestras. Hélène Tropé (1994: 79-80) ha explicado las diferencias entre loco, mentecato y furioso, tres de las denominaciones más usuales, y cada una con variable responsabilidad legal.[13] Por último, es posible que expresiones como "insensado" o similares encajaran tanto en categorías actuales de discapacidad intelectual como trastorno mental. Lo que sí resultó evidente es el esfuerzo de las autoridades por auxiliar/controlar a estos sujetos, no importa si fue en hospitales centralizadores como el de Zaragoza o especializados como el de Valencia.[14]

El doble significado de "inocente" y la preocupación de los gobiernos por el colectivo se sumaron al contexto devocional, cultural y festivo propio del invierno, una época con fuerte componente transgresor donde el niño y el demente adquirieron un mayor protagonismo. Más allá de la fiesta de carnaval, celebración por antonomasia en esta época del año, Ladero Quesada (2004: 38-40) pone de manifiesto el papel de estos dos grupos en fiestas similares en diciembre y enero adaptadas a cada región. Uno de los mejores ejemplos es la fiesta del obispillo, en la que un muchacho del coro de la catedral era investido obispo y había que obedecerle en todo momento. Normalmente se elegía al pequeño mitrado para el 6 de diciembre, fiesta de san Nicolás de Bari,[15] patrón de los niños, y su autoridad no terminaba hasta el día de los Santos Inocentes, fecha del sermón. Con similar objetivo la ciudad de Venecia erigía esta vez a un obispo *dei pazzi*.

La fiesta del asno, celebrada el 4 de enero especialmente en Francia, rememoraba la huida a Egipto de la sagrada familia. Justamente en Valencia algunos inocentes del hospital pedían por la ciudad, siempre acompañados de este animal. En Francia se documenta desde el siglo XII la *fête des fous* o *fête de l'âne*, por la cual se introducía un asno en el interior de la iglesia. La fiesta duraba quince días, desde Navidad hasta la Epifanía. En el interior del templo nombraban al *pape des fous* o al *évêque des innocents* el 28 de diciembre. Los niños del coro oficiaban la misa que dirigía el *episcopum puerorum*. Las máscaras, los juglares y los disfraces eran comunes, como *le fou* o el *joker* de las cartas, también popularizado por el cómic y el cine en las últimas décadas como el personaje antagonista de Batman. En el fondo, estas fiestas y personajes enraízan en las saturnales romanas y se convirtieron en tema común de la literatura medieval (TRAVIESO 2001) y, después, de la dramaturgia moderna (GARCÍA LORENZO 1988). Cuando los ino-

13. Para comprender el tratamiento y la consideración de la locura véase también: HUGUET-TERMES, ARRIZABALAGA, 2010.

14. En este mismo volumen, el capítulo *The Hospitals of the City of Valencia during the Middle Ages and the Renaissance: Academic Knowledge and Ideological Instrumentalisation,* de María Luz López Terrada y Carmel Ferragud trata específicamente el caso valenciano.

15. Recordemos que este obispo fue el precedente de Santa Claus.

centes, especialmente los dementes, desfilaban por Zaragoza en época moderna, como ahora veremos, vestían paños de colores llamativos, contrapuestos, como muestra de su locura.[16] A modo ilustrativo, remito a las siguientes imágenes que apuntan en esta dirección: por un lado, las múltiples representaciones del *fou* en iniciales y márgenes de códices (fig. 1), por otro, ciertos personajes de *El combate entre don Carnal y doña Cuaresma* (1559) de Pieter Brueghel el Viejo (fig. 2). En esta última obra es posible encontrar figuras contrapuestas: primero, las que componen el cortejo del carnaval, enmascaradas, con instrumentos, sombreros y utensilios pintorescos, o el bufón de colores llamativos que ilumina la escena con su antorcha en el centro, y segundo, los pobres y tullidos mendigando que visten con colores grises y marrones.[17]

Recientemente, Miquel Raufast (2014) ha puesto de manifiesto que durante múltiples ceremonias cívicas los pobres y marginados participaron la mayor de las veces como actores pasivos en la recepción de la limosna. De hecho, en la época moderna y con el aumento del pauperismo y los conflictos sociales, los pobres se quejaron por los rituales humillantes en este tipo de desfiles (Federici 2019: 133). En la ciudad de Zaragoza el Padre de Huérfanos era consciente de la utilidad de enviar a los niños a comitivas, entierros y procesiones para la recolección de limosnas (San Vicente 1965: 188). La presencia de niños y locos, y por extensión también de pobres, estaba perfectamente normalizada en las ceremonias públicas, siempre y cuando cumplieran su papel: despertar la piedad de sus vecinos.

En cambio, en los casos que enumeraré a continuación, la pasividad se sustituyó por un efímero protagonismo, un papel semiactivo, contenido y guiado por gestos determinados. Según Asunción Fernández (2000: 284-285), los dementes del hospital general de Zaragoza en el siglo XVIII acudían a las procesiones de la ciudad portando pendones, el escudo de la institución y tocando flautas y tambores. Esa imagen fue idéntica a la que percibió Felipe II a su llegada a la capital aragonesa en 1585, tal y como manifestó su acompañante Henri Cock (1876: 155-156). Una procesión salió a recibirlos…

> […] primeramente iban los mentecautos, ansí hombres como mujeres, con su cruz adelante, los cuales tienen su sustento en el hospital de la Annonciata (*sic*).[18] Los hombres iban todos con sus tamborilillos vestidos con paños de dos colores. Después destos seguían los huérfanos que por toda España se llaman los niños de la doctrina.[19]

16. La contraposición de colores y su percepción es distinta ayer y hoy, siendo en algunos casos sinónimo de locura, transgresión e influencia diabólica (Pastoureau 2006).

17. Además de la imagen adjunta a este texto, otros ejemplos de *fou* pueden ser consultados en la base de datos *Enluminures* que incluye un sinfín de miniaturas: http://www.enluminures.culture.fr/documentation/enlumine/fr/ [29/09/2022].

18. Henri Cock escribe «hospital de la *Annunziata*» cuando el nombre real era santa María de Gracia. Pudiera parecer un error; sin embargo, en realidad, la Virgen de Gracia remite al momento de la Anunciación.

19. Describe con mayor detalle esta entrada real Teófilo Ruiz (2001: 157-160), y concluye destacando la progresiva «ritualización del poder» por parte de las autoridades. A modo de com-

En 1489 este mismo hospital recibió una bula del papa Clemente VII. En el último cuarto del siglo XVI, la célebre *Historia* de Diego de Espés (2019: 686) nos cuenta que la recepción de dicho privilegio corrió a cargo de Juan de Lanuza, lugarteniente general del reino, junto al obispo Conchillos, mitrado ilerdense y comisario de la bula, y «muchos del ospital» que salieron «a reçivirla a la puerta de la puente de piedra con un cruçefixo de madera». Idénticos elementos fueron reproducidos también en las celebraciones valencianas por el casamiento de Felipe III en 1599, tal y como describió Felipe de Gauna:

> Como fue que de los primeros y delanteros de todos yvan más de quinze pares de locos mansos del Hospital General, de dos en dos, hazidos de las manos, haziendose visaxes con sus rostros, mirando a todos riéndose, y puestos en horden de proseción por el hombre y padre dellos que los rexía, los quales locos yvan vestidos con sus ropas largas de dos colores quarteados, de paño amarillo y assul, con las caperussas o monteras de lo mismo, los cuales seguían en proseción a un crusifixo que traya delante dellos un otro loco más manso con otros dos de la misma suerte vestidos, que le yvan al lado del que llevava la crus, con sus candeleros grandes con sirios escondidos en ellos alumbrando el sobredicho crusifixo, y estos locos son los que no tienen el seso del todo perdido sino que se andan con su simplisidad y locura sirviendo al Hospital en lo que puede (TROPÉ 1994: 324).

Pese a todas las disputas que se sucedieron entre instituciones y corporaciones en las procesiones cívicas –a fin de cuentas, la linealidad del desfile implicaba jerarquía–, los jurados zaragozanos y valencianos no dudaron en situar en la cabecera a los niños y dementes. Querían mostrar, sin duda, la labor social del hospital.

Teresa Huguet-Termes y Jon Arrizabalaga (2010: 89-90) han documentado este mismo proceso de ambigüedad, comedia, carnaval y metáfora para la Barcelona coetánea. En un cadalso situaron las autoridades a niños, nodrizas y enfermos psiquiátricos con motivo de la entrada de la reina Isabel: «sia fet cadeffal de lo Spital, hon steran les dides dels infants del Spital e tots los ignoscents». Y con la llegada del primogénito Carlos en 1461 se permitió que «orats e ignoscents» se pintaran las caras y enmascararan: «ab les cares pintades de almàngara e de mascara, armats ab lances velles e cervalleres rovallades, e ab mitres de paper blanch sobre lur cap, a forme de bisbes».[20]

## 2. *Devoción y festividad*

Las procesiones fueron un elemento muy común como muestra de devoción colectiva. Representaron un modo de sociabilidad urbana adscrito a la religio-

plemento véase también su cap. 5, "Las fiestas y el poder: espacios de inclusión y exclusión" (pp. 133-154).

20. En uno de estos actos, aunque de 1589, un criado francés del hospital de Barcelona salió a la calle desnudo de cintura para abajo durante una procesión para evitar la peste y, arrebatando el crucifijo que llevaba un muchacho, se lo puso en el culo (THOMAS 2001: 381).

sidad oficial. Su componente piadoso no las remite directamente a la jerarquía eclesiástica, sino que, como apunta María Isabel Falcón (2003: 62-63), dependían de las autoridades municipales. Los jurados disponían el itinerario, las multas, las prohibiciones, el protocolo, etc. "Religión cívica" es el concepto que mejor resume esta hibridación entre el fervor y los gobiernos urbanos,[21] una parte del universo lúdico y festivo (Rodrigo 2008) en el que cofradías (Tello 2013: 125-141) y hospitales participaron.

Domingo Buesa (1987) ha sido de los primeros en establecer una tipología de las procesiones de la Zaragoza del siglo XV. Distingue tres tipos: devocionales, penitenciales y en agradecimiento por las campañas militares contra el reino de Granada. Entre las primeras encontramos las principales fiestas religiosas, como el culto a la Virgen, los santos, los mártires y los patronos de la ciudad, en las que numerosas reliquias salían de los templos. En segundo lugar, Buesa sitúa las procesiones penitenciales, cuyo objetivo era la restitución de la normalidad ante calamidades: plagas de langostas,[22] falta de lluvia, escasez de las cosechas, el hambre y la peste. Por último, la guerra contra el infiel granadino fue un acontecimiento de notoria relevancia. Cada uno de los avances militares fueron vividos con regocijo por la ciudad.

María Isabel Falcón (2011) ha realizado un ejercicio similar centrándose en el culto a los santos, sus fiestas, procesiones e imágenes. La autora plantea que las festividades religiosas y sus expresiones externas crearon un ciclo que organizaba la mentalidad bajomedieval urbana. La Navidad daba inicio al ciclo festivo para después continuar con la Cuaresma, la Pascua, la Ascensión, el Pentecostés y el Corpus Christi, todo esto complementado con los diferentes santos y patrones particulares, bien fueran municipales, parroquiales o de cofradías. Dos cultos importantes en Zaragoza fueron los de san Valero y el Ángel Custodio; sin embargo, en el otoño medieval el protagonismo se lo llevaba santa Engracia, quien en 1480 se convirtió en patrona de la ciudad. Otras devociones algo menos relevantes fueron Dominguito de Val desde mediados del siglo XIII, san Fabián y san Sebastián, san Cristóbal, san Pedro Mártir, santa Catalina y san Jorge, entre otros.

Jean P. Barraqué (2008) también ha analizado la documentación municipal zaragozana y esta temática, especialmente los libros de cridas. Según él, en la ciudad de Zaragoza coexistieron dos tipos de cultos, una «religión real» –en referencia a la monarquía–, comparable con las ciudades del sur de Italia, y una «religión cívica», más cercana a la Italia septentrional. En este fenómeno, las procesiones y los actos públicos tuvieron especial importancia. El culto a la persona del rey[23] se llevó a cabo con comitivas y festejos que pedían por su salud o celebraban la victoria contra el musulmán, con las entradas de los miembros de la familia real,

21. Para la definición del concepto de «religión cívica», ya utilizado por André Vauchez y Bernard Chevalier en los años 1980 y 1990, véase su más reciente aplicación para la capital aragonesa: Melón 2017.

22. Este mismo problema en García, Torreblanca 1993.

23. En la misma línea, véase Serrano 2011.

exequias y celebraciones por bodas y bautizos. Y, de forma similar, la religión urbana también se benefició de los festejos y las procesiones, como la que ya hemos comentado de santa Engracia. Esta fidelidad al monarca y esa exaltación de lo propio desarrollaron en Zaragoza un sentimiento de identidad aragonesa como cabecera del reino.[24]

## 2.1. *La procesión del hospital*

El binomio procesión-hospital para nada es propiedad exclusiva del caso zaragozano, ni siquiera de las principales urbes.[25] El hospital de San Leonardo de la localidad inglesa de York manifestó un enorme interés en la promoción de la institución a través de los actos representados durante la festividad del Corpus Christi, siendo en el siglo XIV una manifestación vinculada al papel de la mujer y el ciclo mariano (RICE 2019). Pedro Fernández de Híjar, uno de los señores más notables en Aragón, fundó a principios del siglo XIV el hospital de la Santa Cruz en la localidad homónima. Parece ser que un pedazo de la Vera Cruz se encontraba en la iglesia parroquial de Híjar, la cual era exhibida mediante procesión, tal como recoge el programa devocional articulado en torno a este hospital. A fin de cuentas, caridad y piedad no dejaban de ser parte de la propaganda señorial que apuntalaba el poder y la memoria del linaje (IRANZO 1997: 110 y 122). Las hermandades, activas protagonistas en la religiosidad popular bajomedieval, también actuaron como promotoras de instituciones y eventos (NAVARRO 2000).[26]

El comienzo de la construcción de un hospital o su posterior inauguración fueron momentos oportunos para su puesta en valor a través de procesiones, misas y colocación de primeras piedras, como ocurriera en la Barcelona de 1401 o la Lérida de mediados de siglo (CONEJO 2002: I, 386 y 512-517; II, 79-80 y 120). En Brescia, con motivo de la construcción del gran hospital cívico, los pobres enfermos fueron trasladados en compañía del resto de la población. Se representó así la afirmación del proceso secularizador con la erección de un edificio emblemático (ALBINI 2013: 387). En Tivoli se documenta la procesión de la *inchinata* desde al menos el siglo XV, y en ella el hospital de San Juan fue un escenario central de la teatralidad. Allí, los creyentes imitaban los gestos de Cristo lavando los pies del caminante (PERRY 2017). El dramatismo barroco no hizo más que reafirmar estos eventos demostrativos de la ideología gubernamental (RODRÍGUEZ DE LA FLOR 1989: 17-56).

Parece que la procesión del hospital zaragozano fue discontinua durante décadas o, al menos, pudo variar su momento de celebración y su número. Los

24. Conocemos en mayor medida ejemplos urbanos, por tanto, véase un caso rural: TELLO 2012.

25. A propósito de las procesiones hospitalarias en la Lombardía medieval, véase la aportación de Marina Gazzini, *Quando l'ospedale è la meta del viaggio. Processioni e pellegrinaggi nella Lombardia medievale* en este mismo volumen.

26. En Teruel, a finales del siglo XVI, la procesión al hospital general se realizaba el día de santa Catalina: MUÑOZ 1999: 1163.

registros de pagos del concejo muestran que en 1440 hubo un desfile el martes de Pascua (Cisneros 1986: 14)[27] y, por ejemplo, en 1492 se prepararon dos procesiones: la del 22 de enero (*ibidem*: 56)[28] y la del 28 de diciembre (*ibidem*: 67).[29] En cambio, en 1486 se desarrolló el 8 de enero, tal como he citado al inicio de este capítulo. A este baile de fechas se suma el hecho de que el día de los Santos Inocentes difiera entre ayer y hoy. En la actualidad se ha asentado la celebración el 28 de diciembre, sin embargo, según el Evangelio de Mateo, la persecución de las criaturas comenzó pocos días después de la visita de los Reyes Magos.

El historiador del quinientos Diego de Espés (2019: 615-616) ya apuntó los problemas derivados de la convocatoria de la procesión del hospital de 1486. Además de la recién mencionada fecha del 8 de enero, data por entonces ya ortodoxa, los jurados decidieron celebrar otra el 28 de marzo, el tercer día de Pascua, parece que con carácter extraordinario. Así lo notificaron al prior del Cabildo de la Seo y, sin esperar respuesta, publicaron la convocatoria el día de antes. La catedral zaragozana se opuso «porque en la Paschua no se savía ni entiende se ha hecho jamás proçessión general sino la particular de la Seo a Sancta María» y «porque en aquel día aun está ocupado el pueblo en cumplir el precepto de la confessión y comunión». Añadió el Cabildo –recordemos que también era administrador del hospital zaragozano– que hacerlo de esta manera «sería innovar y añadir a la concordia que tienen con la ciudad y hospital assentada de en cada un año a haçer proçessión general al hospital el primer domingo inmediate siguiente después de la fiesta de los Santos Innocentes». En conclusión, el Cabildo eclesiástico zaragozano, aunque a través de la pluma de Diego de Espés, nos está indicando que la procesión ordinaria el día de los Inocentes ya estaba asentada en 1486.

La procesión en sí misma no parece diferenciarse del resto de romerías zaragozanas, variando el itinerario y los espacios para la teatralidad. El desfile comenzaba y acababa en la catedral de la Seo, siendo el punto intermedio el hospital. Como era costumbre, los jurados ordenaban la limpieza de fachadas y calles bajo pena de multa.[30] En ocasiones, se cubría el suelo con juncos para evitar que el polvo y el barro dificultaran su paso. Al final de la celebración, el mayordomo o el tesorero repartían limosnas entre los pobres.[31] Se prohibía trabajar ese día, así como la utilización de cohetes, máscaras y la práctica de juegos de azar. Los hombres iban separados de las mujeres y al menos una persona de cada casa debía acudir.[32] La jerarquía urbana se plasmaba en el orden del desfile, del cual estaban

27. AMZ, LA, 1 (1439 dic.-1440 dic.), f. 63v (13/04/1440).

28. AMZ, LA, 1492, f. 119v.

29. *Ibidem*, f. 310r.

30. Tomo como referencia para la descripción el pregón de 1486 (AMZ, Preg., 1486, f. 7v-8r). Disponemos de otros similares para los años 1500 (f. 8r-v) y 1513 (f. 3r-v).

31. En las procesiones darocenses las autoridades municipales también aprovechaban para distribuir limosna al final de las procesiones (Rodrigo 1995: 296).

32. Una advertencia similar se da en 1517 en la ciudad de Lérida. Las autoridades municipales imponían una pena al cabeza de familia que no acudiera a la procesión del hospital (Conejo 2002: 538).

excluidos musulmanes y judíos. Encabezaban la marcha los jurados y los cargos municipales

> [...] con sus trajes de gala y con brandones de cera ornados con escudetes de Aragón o de Zaragoza y astas de diversos colores con enseñas bordadas, junto a ellos el arzobispo y el cabildo con las vestiduras litúrgicas apropiadas. Todo el mundo guardaba un riguroso orden protocolario, según la dignidad de cada uno (FALCÓN 2003: 63).

Es posible documentar los diferentes pagos relacionados con esta y otras procesiones en los libros de actas de los jurados. Para la de 1440 el concejo contrató a un astero para la confección de doce varas por ocho sueldos jaqueses (CISNEROS 1986: 14).[33] La música era también importante: trompeteros y tamborileros acompañaban el cortejo, así lo refleja un pago de 48 sueldos.[34] Posiblemente, el maestro de canto pudo estar presente en ese interludio en el que se oficiaba el sermón en la iglesia del hospital,[35] ya que su salario aparece entre las cuentas municipales de 1492. Desconocemos si existió un coro con los niños a cargo del hospital.[36] Por último, el consistorio presupuestó la compra «de candelas, XXXIIII libras».[37]

## 3. *El contexto: la caridad zaragozana a finales del siglo XV*

Santa María de Gracia había nacido en 1425 con el lema «*Domus infirmorum urbis et orbis*», una proclama ambiciosa que pasadas unas décadas se resquebrajaba ante el proletariado urbano empobrecido. Desde 1450 a 1515 observamos una progresiva maduración institucional que engrandecería la fama del nosocomio durante la época moderna; sin embargo, el proceso no estuvo exento de dificultades. Zaragoza se asentaba como capital del reino, crecía demográficamente –3.983 fuegos en 1495–[38] y, por ende, aumentaba el pauperismo. En este doble contexto, un hospital cada vez más fortalecido y una ciudad en expansión, se entiende que terminara por cristalizar la división entre los verdaderos y falsos pobres. Algunos hitos en estos años:

- En 1455 la cofradía de San Cosme, San Damián y San Valentín de barberos y cirujanos zaragozanos prestaba apoyo laboral al hospital, hermandad que en

33. AMZ, LA, 1 (1439 dic.-1440 dic.), f. 63v (13/04/1440). Un pago similar al astero Johan de las Borjas por varas para las procesiones de la ciudad (CISNEROS 1986: 67): AMZ, LA, 11 (1491 dic.-1492 dic.), f. 310r). De las varas encargadas una docena fueron para la procesión del hospital de ese año.

34. AMZ, LA, 9 (1489 nov.-1490 dic.), f. 49v-50r (31/03/1490) (CISNEROS 1986: 46).

35. Pudo oficiar sermones el obispo auxiliar Juan Crespo en 1492: «Item el dicho capitol y consello deliberó que el sermonador de l[a] ciudat que era el reuerendo maese Crespo, obispo de Castro, (*tachado*) sermone la quaresma en el spital de Senyora santa Maria de Gracia»: AMZ, LA, 11 (1491 dic.-1492 dic.), f. 81v (11/02/1492).

36. AMZ, LA, 11 (1491 dic.-1492 dic.), f. 232r) (CISNEROS 1986: 64).

37. *Ibidem*, f. 119v (CISNEROS 1986: 56).

38. El dato en SERRANO MONSALVO 1995, vol. I.

1488 había incorporado también a los médicos (Fernández Doctor 2003: 21-22).

- En noviembre de 1471 una crisis financiera afectó al hospital. Las elites urbanas tuvieron que rescatar a la institución habiendo comprobado «[...] que por la mucha pobreza de aquella van muchos de los dichos pobres, criaturas menores ya fuera de leche, e otros incensados, quasi despullados e descalços e stán en punto de perecer de frio, e los lechos assí de los enfermos como de los otros stán depauperados de ropas» (Falcón 1980: 217).

A la vez que se ayudaba al pobre verdadero, las autoridades municipales acordaron crear unos estatutos contra los culpables de aquella situación: «muchos e infinitos gallofos e echacuervos que andan en ciudat por casas e tabernas, gastando la sustancia de los pobres que no pueden treballar e senyaladamente de los del dito Spital» (Falcón 1980: 200-201 y 217-219).[39] También a finales de 1471 se denunciaron los destrozos cometidos por egipciacos (gitanos) llegados a la ciudad (Falcón 2006: 212). Sin duda, sujetos ajenos a la caridad de la «*domus infirmorum urbis et orbis*».

- En 1475 se establecía en Zaragoza la figura del Padre de Huérfanos con estatutos de 1487.
- José Á. Sesma (1977: 165 y 242) advierte que a finales del siglo XV y principios del XVI la Diputación afianzó la ayuda al hospital zaragozano. De hecho, cuando en 1492 los diputados suplicaron al rey que auxiliara al establecimiento, estos buscaron la empatía del monarca, «pues tiene el nombre de Spital del Rey». En mayo de 1501 los diputados solicitaron que las ayudas esporádicas se conviertan en limosna anual (5.000 ss.). En las Cortes de 1512 se concedió la facultad de entregar un máximo de 1.000 florines al año en función de la hacienda del reino.[40]
- El cuerpo normativo del centro fue renovado en estas décadas. Las primitivas ordenanzas, de las que nada ha quedado, sufrieron las modificaciones de Fernando el Católico de 1496 y 1503 (Falcón 1980: 222-226.) En 1508 fueron sustituidas por las de Alfonso de Aragón, arzobispo de Zaragoza e

39. En este contexto de necesidad económica se documentan varios casos de pleitos relacionados con rentas, como la que mantuvo la institución con el mercader Yusuf Xama (Abella 2005: 202-204). Seis años después, en 1477, el hospital obtenía cierta liquidez vendiendo los lugares de Pueyo y Lierta: Archivo Histórico Nacional, Clero, C. 590, N. 5. Imágenes disponibles en PARES: http://pares.mcu.es/ParesBusquedas20/catalogo/description/2320192?nm [consultado *online* 21/11/2021].

40. La embajada enviada en 1491 para solicitar ayuda al monarca está transcrita en p. 446. Comienza así: «Item, suplicaran los dichos embaxadores a su alteza, se quiera acordar de una tan insigne e tan notable e santa casa como es el spital suyo, entre todos sus reynos tan principal, como es la Virgen María de Gracia de Caragoça, en donde tanta anima recibe refección temporal ayudando al cuerpo et al alma con lo spiritual, en donde de todas las naciones del mundo se acullen».

hijo de este monarca, y, para el caso que nos ocupa, lugarteniente general del reino (MONTERDE 2008).[41]

## 4. *Intensificación económica de la implicación municipal*

De forma progresiva, esta institución trató de afianzar sus finanzas superando los muros de la ciudad de Zaragoza. Lo vemos en los censales que vendió a entidades como el ducado de Híjar o la Comunidad de Aldeas de Daroca (VILLAGRASA-ELÍAS 2016: 77-78), la recaudación de limosnas dentro y fuera de Aragón –gracias a la licencia de 1503 de Isabel la Católica para hacerlo por todos sus reinos–,[42] las mandas testamentarias otorgadas fuera de Zaragoza,[43] el ganado que pacía en el Pirineo[44] o la asunción de rentas de otras casas de caridad, como es el caso del hospital de Alquézar.[45]

En este sentido, los libros de actas del consistorio zaragozano recogen pasajes relacionados con la supervisión del centro, como la revisión de la contabilidad (1442),[46] la necesidad de aumentar la inversión en nodrizas (1490)[47] o la petición de los regidores a los jurados para que visitaran el centro cuatro veces al año (1492).[48] A todo ello se sumaban decisiones relacionadas con la economía hospitalaria (sin ánimo de exhaustividad): permiso para vender una serie de casas y tierras propiedad del hospital, muchas en Zaragoza, pero otras en Pina, Zuera e incluso Teruel (1490);[49] intervención en pleitos de la institución (el caso

41. Según Maiso (1978) las ordenanzas de 1508 supusieron un aumento del control de la casa por parte de la monarquía.

42. Archivo General de Simancas, CCA, CED, 6, 99, 4. Documento digitalizado disponible en PARES: <http://pares.mcu.es/ParesBusquedas20/catalogo/description/2313710?nm> [consultado *online* 21/11/2021].

43. Como Fernando de Borja, de la localidad homónima, que en 1479 dejaba donaciones para el hospital borjano y el zaragozano (VILLAGRASA-ELÍAS 2016: 107); o el mercader alemán Pascual Bude de Metali que en 1478 se acordaba del «Espital de Sant Spirit de Rabenespuch [Ravensburg] del Imperio de Alamanya dos mil sueldos, et en el Spital del Rey de Caragoca» (PALLARÉS 2006: 104-106).

44. En 1480 el hospital mantuvo pleito contra la Val de Tena y la localidad de Hoz de Jaca por los daños contra la cabaña ganadera de la institución (FERNÁNDEZ 1983: 105). Sabemos que en 1484 Lope de Lara era su «ganadero mayoral» (PALLARÉS 2008: 594). Proceso contra Jayme Boray por haber robado cierto ganado del hospital y de Martín Moya (AMZ, LA, 4 (1468 dic.-1469 dic.), f. 117r-v (06/06/1469; documentado por Falcón [2006]). Sobre las cabezas de ganado del centro y las carnicerías zaragozanas: AMZ, LA, 12 (1495 dic.-1496 dic.), f. 311r-312v (21/11/1496).

45. En 1439 el clérigo Martín de Pan y Vino, en calidad de patrono del hospital de Alquézar, instituyó como administradores a dos mercaderes zaragozanos. Las rentas censales de dicho centro pasaron en ese momento a engrosar las arcas de santa María de Gracia (VILLAGRASA-ELÍAS 2016: 50).

46. AMZ, LA, 2 (1442 feb.-dic.), f. 89r (22/10/1442).

47. AMZ, LA, 9 (1489 nov.-1490 dic.), f. 135r (29/10/1490). Documento transcrito por GARCÍA HERRERO 2006: II, 292-293.

48. AMZ, LA, 11 (1491 dic.-1492 dic.), f. 123v (4/05/1492).

49. AMZ, LA, 9 (1489 nov.-1490 dic.), f. 132r-v (26/10/1490).

de una viña en 1490);[50] licencia para vender el treudo y una propiedad situados en Sarvisé, localidad en el valle pirenaico de Broto, debido a la tardanza en cobrar las rentas y la lejanía con la institución (1500).[51]

A la explotación de propiedades agrícolas y urbanas dentro y fuera de Zaragoza, la capacidad como censualista y la caridad público-privada se sumó una fuente de financiación extra que coincidió con la instauración de la procesión de los inocentes: las multas.

### 4.1. *Análisis lexicométrico de los pregones*

Los libros de cridas o pregones guardan repetidamente menciones relacionadas con el hospital de Santa María de Gracia. El nosocomio aparece principalmente de tres formas en estos textos: primero, como elemento publicitado con su propia procesión; segundo, como parte del recorrido en otras romerías debido a su importancia urbanística, y, tercero, como beneficiario de la mitad o el tercio de las multas que recaudaba el consistorio.[52]

He realizado un ejercicio estadístico que creo proporciona resultados significativos, aunque, como es lógico, hemos de interpretarlos con precaución, al situarnos en un periodo pre-estadístico con una fuente –los pregones– que ni se han conservado al completo ni tienen como objetivo el registro sistemático de datos numéricos. He contabilizado manualmente las veces que aparece el término "hospital" en relación con Santa María de Gracia.[53] Lógicamente, he incorporado sus variantes morfológicas: hespital, espital, ospital, spital. He aplicado esta metodología sobre los pregones zaragozanos conservados –47 cuadernillos entre 1406 y 1514–.[54]

Los resultados de este análisis lexicométrico se pueden apreciar en la gráfica 1. Si bien el libro de cridas más antiguo que conservamos es de 1406 y la fundación del hospital data de 1425, no es hasta 1441 cuando la institución aparece mencionada por primera vez. Recuérdese que en 1440 ya documentamos una procesión dedicada al hospital, según los libros de actas, una comitiva que no estaba vinculada con los Santos Inocentes. Entre 1440 y 1477 las referencias en los pregones son mínimas, aun cuando la crisis financiera más grave se dio en 1471. A partir de 1478 la dinámica varía levemente. A finales de la década de 1480, las menciones aumentan considerablemente hasta 1513, viviendo una

50. AMZ, LA, 9 (1489 nov.-1490 dic.), f. 112v-113r (22/09//1490) y f. 116. (07/10/1490).

51. AMZ, LA, 13 (1500 mar.-nov.), f. 33r-v (23/04/1500). Este mismo volumen contiene más ejemplos de licencias para la venta de propiedades.

52. Algunas de las multas: por contradecir la normativa en la venta de fruta y otros comestibles (1488); por cometer fraude en el peso de paja y leña (1494); por vender los carniceros carne en mal estado (1494); por entorpecer el paso en la plaza del mercado (1500), y por no denunciar el juego y a los rufianes por parte de cualquier mesonero (1502) (San Vicente 1988: 42, 54, 62-63, 71, 75).

53. Podrían aparecer como antropónimos casos que no han sido contabilizados: ej. Jaime del Hospital.

54. Más información sobre la fuente en nota 1.

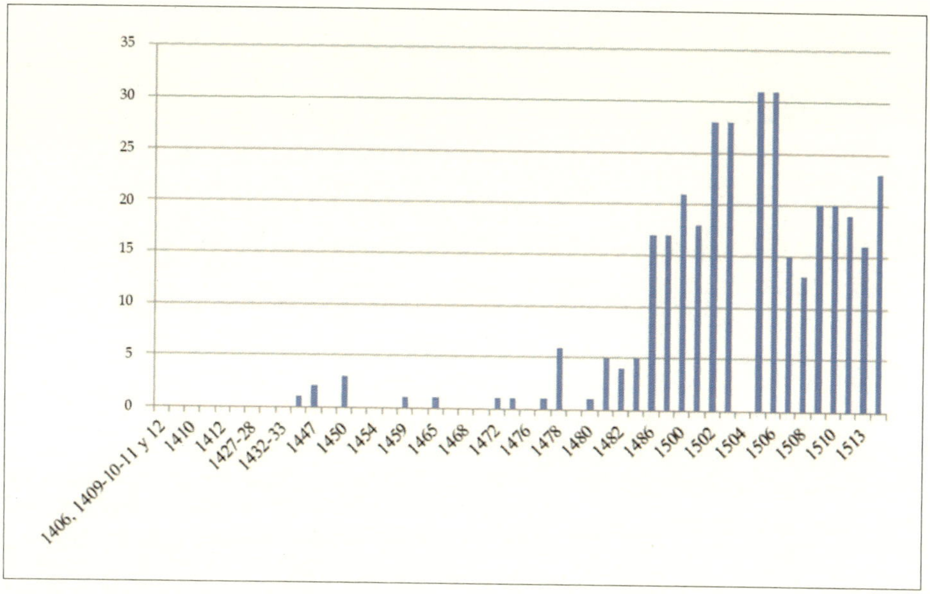


Gráfica 1. Menciones de la palabra "hospital" en los libros de pregones del Archivo Municipal de Zaragoza entre 1406 y 1514.

intensificación significativa en los primeros años del siglo XVI –31 alusiones en 1506–.

Este ejercicio me permite afirmar que existió una mayor preocupación por parte del consistorio zaragozano a finales del siglo XV y principios del XVI, lo que refuerza su inclusión en la vida urbana y la dotación de recursos económicos extras.

## 5. *Conclusiones*

Si bien es cierto que la diferenciación entre el verdadero y el falso pobre hunde sus raíces en el siglo XIV, es evidente que la mayor expresión del fenómeno se dio en Zaragoza entre 1470 y 1510. En este proceso convergieron aspectos relacionados con la historia social, económica y de las mentalidades:

1. Pese a la inexistencia de documentación contable y registros de enfermos del hospital, es palpable la preocupación por determinados colectivos: los incapacitados para trabajar, los enfermos, los huérfanos y los dementes.
2. La caridad con respecto a ciertos grupos se complementó con la represión de otros, aquellos que atacaban a la moralidad cristiana, representaban lastres para la sociedad y se salían de los canales laborales establecidos por

las autoridades: la prostituta, el rufián, el vago, el maleante, el gitano y el sodomita (Navarro, Villagrasa-Elías 2018).

3. El hospital de Santa María de Gracia ya no era únicamente referente de una ciudad, sino de un reino –más tarde incluso de regiones adyacentes–, con tentáculos económicos extendidos por un amplio territorio y el soporte estatal de la Diputación y las Cortes.
4. Todo este apoyo institucional y su crecimiento situaron al hospital como uno de los centros más influyentes a lo largo del siglo XVI, siendo emulado por nosocomios de la península ibérica, América y Centroeuropa.
5. Las autoridades municipales visitaron la institución y controlaron la contabilidad, aunque no pudieron evitar crisis económicas como la de 1471. El análisis lexicométrico de los pregones evidencia una mayor preocupación por sostener financieramente a santa María de Gracia, haciendo uso de multas, a partir de la década de 1480.
6. El gobierno urbano utilizó la fiesta para publicitar ante la ciudadanía el papel del nosocomio y, de forma deliberada, eligió en las últimas décadas del cuatrocientos la festividad de los Inocentes como fecha ordinaria. Determinados sujetos fueron expuestos e "invadieron", aunque de forma contenida, el espacio urbano.
7. El poder municipal y eclesiástico utilizó la figura del inocente en su doble vertiente como parte de su ejercicio propagandístico, apropiándose de un ciclo festivo tradicionalmente trasgresor y, en este caso, llamativo por las máscaras y los colores, pero reglado en sus formas.
8. Los pregones –escritos convertidos en oralidad– anunciaban la ideología de la elite ciudadana, personificada en las reuniones del concejo zaragozano, para llenar las calles de devoción, luz y color en un ejercicio de publicidad representativa y alteridad dentro de la comunidad cristiana. Todo ello en esa transición entre "la piedad y la horca" si aplicamos la expresión de Bronisław Geremek (1989).

## *Bibliografía*

Abella Samitier, Juan, 2005. "Una familia de mudéjares aragoneses en el tránsito de la Edad Media a la Moderna: los Xama de Zaragoza", *En la España Medieval*, 28: 197-212.

Albini, Giuliana, 2013. "Ospedali e società urbana: Italia centro-settentrionale, secoli XIII-XVI", ed. F. Ammannati. *Assistenza e solidarietà in Europa Secc. XIII-XVIII, Atti della Quarantaquattresima Settimana di Studi, 22-26 aprile 2012*, Florencia, Firenze University Press: 384-398.

Aparici Martí, Joaquín; Navarro Espinach, Germán, 2010. "*Considerada encara la pocha edat e ignocència*… Los primeros años de vida para los niños del siglo XV", *Millars: Espai i Història*, 33: 55-74.

Aparici Martí, Joaquín; Villanueva Morte, Concepción, 2021. "Jóvenes huérfanos en el Maestrazgo medieval: aproximación a su vida a través de los documentos de tutela", *Revista de Humanidades*, 42: 107-132.

Arcarazo García, Luis A.; Lorén Trasobares, M. Pilar, 2000. *El santo hospital de San Julián Mártir y Santa Lucía y otros hospitales de Barbastro*, Barbastro, CESB.

Asensi Artiga, Viviana, 1992. *Tratamiento documental de la sanidad municipal en Murcia a finales del siglo XV*, Murcia, Universidad de Murcia.

Barraqué, Jean P., 2008. "Entre religión real y religión urbana", *En la España Medieval*, 31: 249-274.

Benali, Abdelkader *et al.*, 2019, *Conversation Pieces: The World of Bruegel*, Brujas, Hannibal.

Buesa Conde, Domingo, 1987. "Manifestaciones de la religiosidad popular en la Zaragoza del siglo XV. Las procesiones devocionales, penitenciales y en acción de gracias por la toma de Granada", *Aragonia Sacra*, 2: 49-58.

Cisneros Coarasa, Javier (coord.), 1986. *Actos comunes de los jurados de Zaragoza (1440-1496)*, Zaragoza, IFC.

Cock, Henri, 1876. *Relación del viaje hecho por Felipe II, en 1585, a Zaragoza, Barcelona y Valencia,* Madrid.

Conejo da Pena, Antoni, 2002. *Assistència i hospitalitat a l'edat mitjana. L'arquitectura dels hospitals catalans: del gòtic al primer renaixement*, Tesis doctoral Universitat de Barcelona.

Conejo da Pena, Antoni, 2015. "La disseminació d'hospitals al bisbat de Tortosa durant l'edat mitjana", *Recerca*, 16: 91-120.

De Espés, Diego, 2019. *Historia ecclesiastica de la ciudad de Çaragoça desde la venida de Jesuchristo, señor y redemptor nuestro, hasta el año de 1575*, Asunción Blasco Martínez, Pilar Pueyo Colomina (ed.), Zaragoza, IFC.

Doñate Sebastiá, José M.ª, 1980. "Saludadores y médicos en la baja edad media", *Primer Congreso de Historia del País Valenciano. Celebrado en Valencia del 14 al 18 de abril de 1971*, vol. II, Valencia, Universidad de Valencia: 803-810.

Falcón Pérez, M.ª Isabel, 1980. "Sanidad y beneficencia en Zaragoza en el siglo XV", *Aragón en la Edad Media*, 1980: 183-226.

Falcón Pérez, M.ª Isabel, 1988. "Las 'actas municipales medievales' como fuente de investigación", en *Metodología de la investigación científica sobre fuentes aragonesas, Actas de las III Jornadas*, Zaragoza, ICE-UZ: 279-319.

Falcón Pérez, M.ª Isabel, 2003. "Gobierno y poder municipal en las ciudades de Aragón en la Baja Edad Media", *El món urbà a la Corona d'Aragó del 1137 als decrets de Nova Planta, XVII Congrés d'Història de la Corona d'Aragó, Barcelona. Poblet. Lleida, 7 al 12 de desembre de 2000*, vol. 1, Barcelona, Universidad de Barcelona: 59-100.

Falcón Pérez, M.ª. Isabel, 2006. *El municipio de Zaragoza entre 1468 y 1472 según los Libros de Actos Comunes de sus Jurados*, Zaragoza, Ayuntamiento de Zaragoza.

Falcón Pérez, M.ª Isabel, 2011. "Devociones populares, procesiones e imágenes de santos en la Zaragoza del siglo XV", *Aragonia Sacra*, 21: 171-200.

Federici, Silvia, 2019. *Calibán y la bruja. Mujeres, cuerpo y acumulación originaria*, Madrid, Traficantes de Sueños.

Fernández Doctor, Asunción, 2000. *El Hospital Real y General de Nuestra Señora de Gracia de Zaragoza en el Siglo XVIII*, Zaragoza, IFC.

Fernández Doctor, Asunción, 2003. *Documentos para la historia de las profesiones sanitarias: el Colegio de Médicos y Cirujanos de Zaragoza (siglos XV-XVIII)*, Zaragoza, Colegio Oficial de Médicos de Zaragoza.

Fernández Otal, José A., 1983. *La Casa de Ganaderos de Zaragoza: derecho y trashumancia a fines del siglo XV*, Zaragoza, IFC.

Franco Llopis, Borja; Moreno Díaz del Campo, Francisco J., 2019. "El morisco oculto. La pintura de encubrimiento en momentos de crisis", Borja Franco, Francisco J. Moreno (ed.), *Pintando al converso. La imagen del morisco en la península ibérica (1492-1614)*, Madrid, Cátedra: 413-445.

García García, Francisco de Asís, 2011. "La matanza de los Inocentes", *Revista Digital de Iconografía Medieval*, 3, 5: 23-37.

García Herrero, M.ª Carmen, 2005. *Del nacer y el vivir: fragmentos para una historia de la vida en la Baja Edad Media*, Zaragoza, IFC.

García Herrero, M.ª Carmen, 2006. *Las mujeres en Zaragoza en el siglo XV*, 2 vols., Zaragoza, PUZ.

García Herrero, M.ª Carmen; Torreblanca Gaspar, M.ª Jesús, 1993. "San Miguel y la plaga de langosta (claves para la interpretación del voto taustano de 1421)", *Aragón en la Edad Media*, 10-11: 281-306.

García Lorenzo, Luciano, 1988. "Locos e inocentes: 'El Misteri del Rey Herodes' y la tradición teatral", *Revista de dialectología y tradiciones populares*, 43: 279-290.

Geremek, Bronisław, 1989. *La piedad y la horca*, Madrid, Alianza Editorial.

Huguet-Termes, Teresa; Arrizabalaga, Jon, 2010. "Hospital Care for the Insane in Barcelona, 1400-1700", *Bulletin of Spanish Studies*, 87/8: 81-104.

Iranzo Muñío, M.ª Teresa, 1997. "Pobreza, enfermedades y símbolos del poder señorial en Híjar. El Hospital de la Santa Cruz, 1300-1312", *Aragón en la Edad Media*, 13: 105-124.

Ladero Quesada, M. Ángel, 2004. *Las fiestas en la cultura medieval*, Barcelona, Areté.

Maiso González, Jesús, 1978. "Aspectos del hospital de Gracia de Aragón bajo los Austrias", *Estudios del Departamento de Historia Moderna*, Zaragoza, Universidad de Zaragoza: 267-322.

Marino, Salvatore, 2014. *Ospedali e città nel Regno di Napoli. Le Annunziate: istituzioni, archivi e fonti (secc. XIV-XIX)*, Florencia, Olschki.

Marino, Salvatore, 2015. "The 'Children of the Soul' in Naples between the Medieval and Early Modern Period", Maria C. Rossi, Marina Garbellotti (ed.), *Adoption and Fosterage Practices in the Late Medieval and Modern Age*, Roma, Viella: 173-188.

Marino, Salvatore, 2019. *El Memorial dels infants. Edició crítica d'una font per a l'estudi de la infància a la Barcelona del segle XV*, Barcelona, Fundació Noguera.

Melón Juncosa, Inmaculada, 2017. "Procesiones y religión cívica en Zaragoza. Los pregones del concejo entre 1450 y 1500", *Aragón en la Edad Media*, 28: 91-140.

Montanel Marcuello, M.ª Ángeles, 2018. "Marginalidad y asistencia social: huérfanos en la Zaragoza moderna", María de los Ángeles Pérez, José Luis Betrán (ed.), *Nuevas perspectivas de investigación en Historia Moderna: economía, sociedad, política y cultura en el mundo hispánico*, Madrid, Fundación Española de Historia Moderna: 446-455.

Monterde Albiac, Cristina. 2008. "Las ordinaciones del Hospital de Nuestra Señora de Gracia de Zaragoza establecidas por don Alfonso de Aragón, arzobispo de Zaragoza y lugarteniente general del reino", *Aragón en la Edad Media*, 20: 505-528.

Motis Dolader, Miguel Á.; García Marco, Javier; Rodrigo Estevan, M.ª Luz, 1995. *Procesos inquisitoriales de Daroca y su comunidad*, Daroca, Centro de Estudios Darocenses.

Muñoz Garrido, Vidal, 1999. "Asentamiento del patrimonio del capítulo general de racioneros de Teruel en la Baja Edad Media", *Aragón en la Edad Media*, 14-15/2: 1151-1166.

Narbona Vizcaíno, Rafael, 2012. "Las leyes de pobres en la metrópolis: mendigos, miserables, trabajadores en Valencia, 1306-1462", *Clío & Crimen*, 9: 165-284.

Navarro Espinach, Germán, 1993. "Aprendices textiles en Valencia medieval. Los contratos del padre de huérfanos Tomàs Oller (1461-1468)", *II Congreso de Jóvenes Historiadores y Geógrafos,* Valencia, CSIC: 141-147.

Navarro Espinach, Germán, 2000. "El Hospital de Santa María de Villaespesa y de San Juan Bautista en la ciudad de Teruel a través de los actos notariales de Alfonso Jiménez (1481-1518)", *Aragón en la Edad Media*, 16: 565-590.

Navarro Espinach, Germán; Villagrasa-Elías, Raúl, 2018. "Sodomía y abusos sexuales en los hospitales zaragozanos del Quinientos", Concepción Villanueva, Antoni Conejo, Raúl Villagrasa-Elías (ed.), *Redes hospitalarias: historia, economía y sociología de la sanidad*, Zaragoza, IFC: 191-200.

Pallarés Jiménez, Miguel Á., 2006. *Las Cuevas de Cañart a finales de la Edad Media*, Cuevas de Cañart, Asociación Cultural "El Morrón".

Pallarés Jiménez, Miguel Á., 2008. "Veinticinco documentos medievales aragoneses de desamor", *Aragón en la Edad Media*, 20: 579-600.

PASTOUREAU, Michel, 2006. "Ver los colores de la Edad Media. ¿Es posible una historia de los colores?", Michel Pastoureau. *Una historia simbólica de la Edad Media occidental* (ed.), Buenos Aires, Katz: 125-145.

PÉREZ GALÁN, Cristina, 2013. "Los grandes hospitales urbanos en Aragón en el siglo XV: Nuestra Señora de la Esperanza en Huesca y Nuestra Señora de Gracia en Zaragoza", ed. Francesco Ammannati. *Assistenza e solidarietà in Europa Secc. XIII-XVIII, Atti della Quarantaquattresima Settimana di Studi, 22-26 abril 2012*, Florencia, Firenze University Press: 291-305.

PERRY, Rebekah, 2017. "Procession and the Evolving Allegorical Landscape of the Late Medieval City", Diana B. Presciutti (ed.), *Space, Place and Motion. Locating Confraternities in the Late Medieval and Early Modern City*, Leiden-Boston, Brill: 127-154.

RAUFAST CHICO, Miquel, 2014. "Las ceremonias de la caridad: asistencia, marginación y pobreza en el escenario urbano bajomedieval", Teresa Huguet-Termes et al. (ed.), *Ciudad y hospital en el Occidente europeo (1300-1700)*, Lérida, Milenio: 401-414.

RICE, Nicole R., 2019. "The Feminine Prehistory of the York Purification: St. Leonard's Hospital, Civic Drama, and Women's Devotion", *Speculum*, 94/3: 704-738.

RICO, Francisco (ed.), 2005. *Lazarillo de Tormes*, Madrid, Cátedra.

RODRIGO ESTEVAN, M.ª Luz, 1995. "Poder municipal y acción benéfico-asistencial: el concejo de Daroca, 1400-1526", *Aragón en la Edad Media*, 12: 287-318.

RODRIGO ESTEVAN, M.ª Luz, 2008. "Lo lúdico y lo festivo en el Aragón medieval: fuentes documentales para su estudio", *Aragón en la Edad Media*, 20: 661-676.

RODRÍGUEZ DE LA FLOR, Fernando, 1989. "La urbe y su metáfora: el espacio sagrado de la fiesta", *Atenas castellana. Ensayos sobre cultura simbólica y fiestas en la Salamanca del Antiguo Régimen*, Salamanca, Junta de Castilla León: 17-56.

ROYO GARCÍA, Juan R., 1994. "Los hospitalicos de niños y de niñas de Zaragoza en 1605 según la visita del arzobispo Tomás de Borja", *Revista de Historia Jerónimo Zurita*, 69-70: 115-128.

RUBIO SEMPER, Agustín; MARTÍNEZ GARCÍA, Francisco J., 2019. *Libro de la Pecha de la villa de Ateca. II. Años 1474 a 1492*, Zaragoza, IFC.

RUBIO VELA, Agustín, 1990. "Infancia y marginación. En torno a las instituciones trecentistas valencianas para el socorro de los huérfanos", *Revista d'Història Medieval*, 1: 111-153.

RUIZ, Teófilo F., 2001. *Historia social de España, 1400-1600*, Barcelona, Crítica.

SAN VICENTE PINO, Ángel, 1965. *El oficio de Padre de Huérfanos en Zaragoza*, Zaragoza, Cátedra de Zaragoza.

SAN VICENTE PINO, Ángel, 1988. *Instrumentos para una historia social y económica del trabajo en Zaragoza en los siglos XV a XVIII*, vol. 1, Zaragoza, Real Sociedad Económica Aragonesa de Amigos del País.

SERRANO MARTÍN, Eliseo, 2011. "Imágenes del rey e identidad del reino en los rituales y celebraciones públicas en Aragón en el siglo XVI", *Obradoiro de historia moderna*, 20: 43-71.

SERRANO MONSALVO, Antonio, 1995. *La población de Aragón según el fogaje de 1495*, vol. I, Zaragoza, IFC.

SESMA MUÑOZ, José Á., 1977. *La Diputación del Reino de Aragón en la época de Fernando II*, Zaragoza, IFC.

TELLO HERNÁNDEZ, Esther, 2012. "La religiosidad popular en las tierras de frontera. Entre Aragón y Valencia: las romerías al santuario de la Balma de Zorita", Francisco García, Juan F. Jiménez (ed.), *La historia peninsular en los espacios de frontera: las "extremaduras históricas" y la "transierra" (siglos XI-XV)*, Cáceres-Murcia, SEEM: 559-570.

TELLO HERNÁNDEZ, Esther, 2013. *Aportación al estudio de las cofradías medievales y sus devociones en el reino de Aragón*, Zaragoza, IFC.

THOMAS, Werner, 2001. *Los protestantes y la Inquisición en España en tiempos de Reforma y Contrarreforma*, Lovaina, Leuven University Press.

TRAVIESO GANAZA, Mercedes, 2001. "La fiesta del loco en el *Jeu de la Feuillée*", coord. Domingo Pujante et al. *Écrire, traduire et représenter la fête*, Valencia, Universitat de València: 19-32.

TROPÉ, Hélène, 1994. *Locura y sociedad en la Valencia de los siglos XV al XVII*, Valencia, Diputació de València.

Villagrasa-Elías, Raúl, 2016. "'Recollir los pobres et tener hospitalitat'. Asistencia hospitalaria en el Somontano de Barbastro (ss. XII-XVI)", *Revista de la CECEL*, 16: 37-60.

Villagrasa-Elías, Raúl, 2016. "Política hospitalaria en los concejos aragoneses del Cuatrocientos", ed. Paulino Iradiel et al. *Identidades urbanas Corona de Aragón-Italia. Redes económicas, estructuras institucionales, funciones políticas (siglos XIV-XV)*, Zaragoza, PUZ: 163-176.

Villagrasa-Elías, Raúl, 2016. *La red de hospitales en el Aragón medieval (ss. XII-XV)*, Zaragoza, IFC.

Vinyoles Vidal, Teresa, Illanes Zubieta, Ximena, 2015. "Treated As Sons and Daugthers", ed. Maria C. Rossi & Marina Garbellotti. *Adoption and Fosterage Practices in the Late Medieval and Modern Age*, Roma, Viella: 127-142.

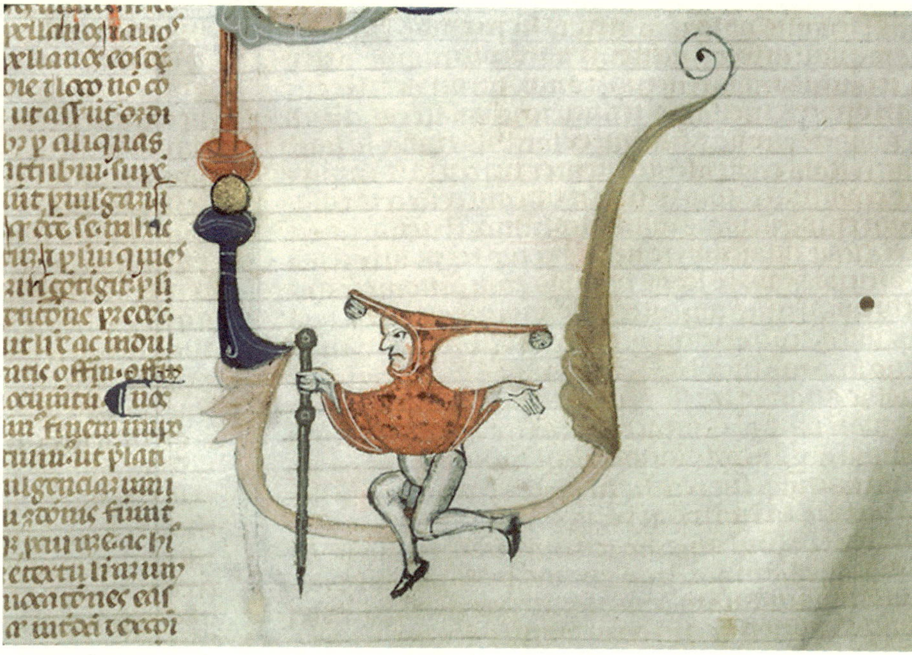

Fig. 1. Músico/hombre armado/*fou*, detalle. *Recueil de droit canonique*, siglo XIII. (Tours: Bibliothèque municipale, Ms. 568, f. 332). Imagen: © Bibliothèque municipale de Tours.

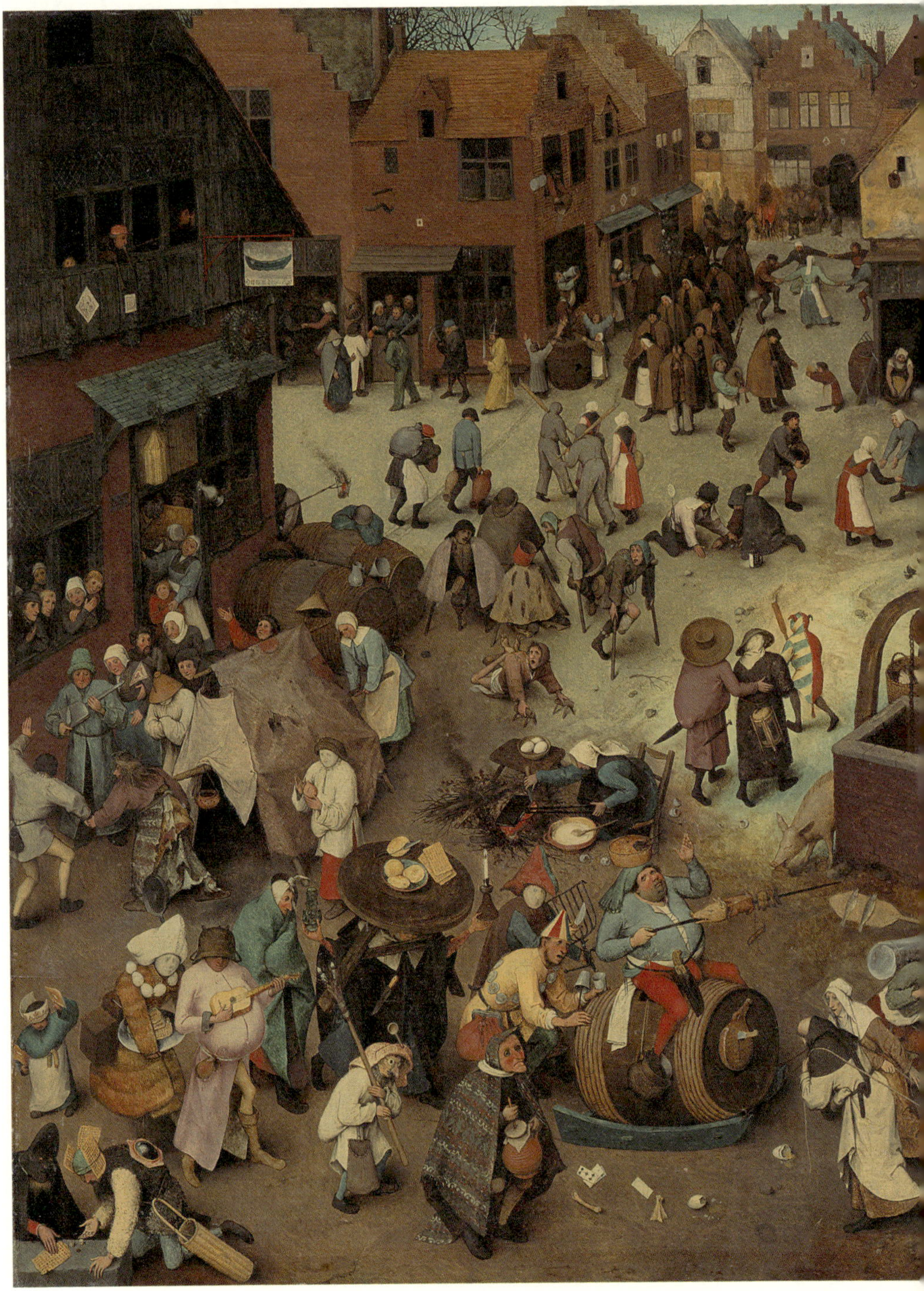

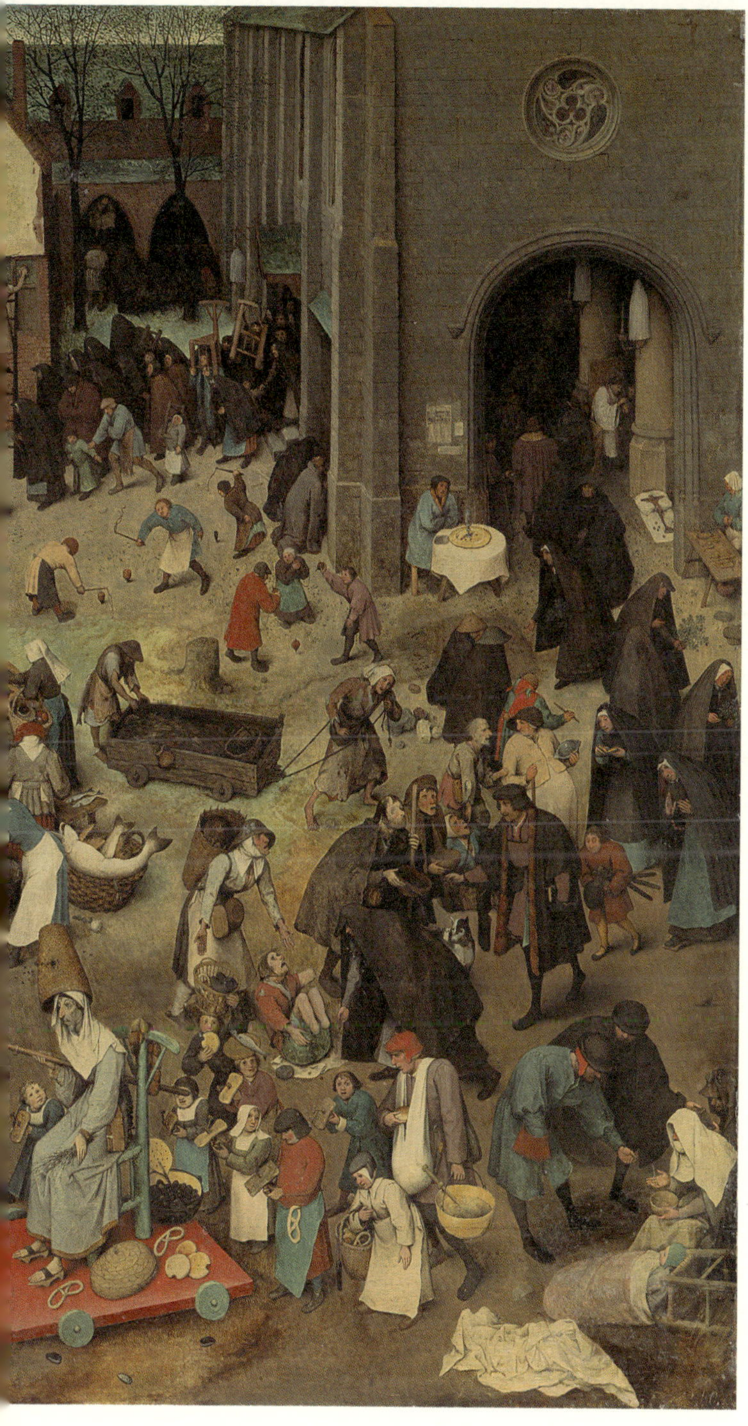

Fig. 2. Pieter Brueghel el Viejo: *El combate entre don Carnal y doña Cuaresma*, 1559. (Viena: Kunsthistorisches Museum). Imagen: © Wikimedia Commons.

Pere Manel Marquès i Carreras

# The Architecture of the *Māristān* of Granada. Models, Memory and History of a Building in Recovery

## 1. *Introduction*

This study on the *Māristān* of Granada arises from our particular interest in the convergence between art, medicine, and religion in certain spaces, such as, for example, a hospital. From a practical point of view, this convergence between religion and medicine in the Middle Ages appears in a determined space, such as in hospitals and other spaces of care. Therefore, we can say that, beyond the theoretical conceptions that underlined this confluence, philanthropic foundations were driven by the exercise of charity on behalf of the powerful. Antoni Conejo (2011: 19) notes that the first European hospitals we know of were born under the concepts of *caritas* and *hospitalitas*. Their goal was to provide shelter to passers-by, the poor, and pilgrims, whether they were sick or not. In Christian terms, the exercise of the virtue of charity was understood as a vehicle for divine love, and hospitality was one of the seven works of mercy.

This was found not only in Europe, but also in the Muslim world. In relation to this, Olivia R. Constable (2003: 2) discusses the Middle Ages centres of assistance to travellers and identifies a line of continuity that is critical to understanding the *Māristān* of Granada. This is the line of continuity and familiarity between *pandocheia*, *funduqs* and *fondacos*, institutions that were found along the Mediterranean coasts and functioned similarly to modern day hostels, even if they also had other purposes. According to Constable, «these protean institutions had common ties, yet they took many forms, serving not only as hostelries, but also as commercial depots, warehouses, emporia, taxation offices, taverns, prisons, and brothels». They evolved depending on the different conquests, «as when Byzantine Syria came under Umayyad rule in the seventh century and the Arabic *funduq* replaces the *pandocheion,* or when Christian armies conquered Muslim cities in Spain and local *funduqs* became known as *alhóndigas* or *fondechs*» (Constable 2003: 4). The *Funduq*, *khān*, *ribāt* and *wakāla* were different welfare institutions that appeared in the Muslim East, along with the *bīmāristān* (a Persian term that means "place of the sick" and which in the Iberian Peninsula adopted the name of *māristān* by contraction). Francisco Franco Sánchez (1999: 142) comments that these were absent in Umayyad times and were brought in by the Abbasid dynasty, heirs of Sassanid culture. He concludes that Persian culture and administration became useful tools for a state still under construction and in need of urgent solutions. Going back to the display of charity in these centres, Constable (2003: 42) explains:

At the same time, *funduqs* also became instruments of religious charity in the medieval Muslim world. Many were established as *waqfs,* inalienable pious endowments intended to provide revenues for a good purpose. *Funduqs* and other hostels were frequently founded by men of wealth and power, often Muslim rulers or amirs, who saw them as tools to serve the ends of philanthropy, profit, and propaganda. Their religious and philanthropic aspects were much more pronounced than for *pandocheion* in the late antique Christian context, where these functions had normally been assigned to *xenodocheions.* Not every *funduq* served both commercial and charitable functions equally, and there was scope for wide variation across the distance of the Islamic world. Yet this striking mélange of commercial and philanthropic purpose remained fundamentally characteristic of the medieval Islamic *funduq* from Damascus to Córdoba.

We do not intend to fall into an idealised mythification of the hospital in medieval times as an idyllic place where religious orthopraxis was perfectly practiced. In fact, apart from what we have said above, we must understand how, from the thirteenth and fourteenth centuries on, hospitals became more socially focused, leading to an increased role for the civil authorities. The hospital thus became a tool of regulation and control over extreme poverty and marginalization, acting as an indispensable social tension reliever on behalf of governments. Municipal governments promoted, protected, and maintained the hospitals under the guise of performing a work of mercy and a moral obligation (Fontanals 2014: 50-51). However, their objective was eminently practical, even if it was dressed up as religious.

This new development is in keeping with the *Māristān* of Granada. In the Islamic world, the concept of *caritas* did not apply, but the concept of *ihsān* held great importance. In the *Qur'an*, in Sura An-Nahl, God commands to do justice and *ihsān,* which can be translated into English as follows: «Indeed, Allah commands justice, grace, as well as courtesy to close relatives. He forbids indecency, wickedness, and aggression. He instructs you so perhaps you will be mindful» (An-Nahl 16,90). Franco Sánchez takes up the definition given by Ibn Taymīya between the 13th and 14th centuries, who speaks of *ihsān* as virtuous conduct, which is to perform "good deeds", that is, what God commands. As for what God commands, it is that which He has instituted, that which is in accordance with God's Sunnah and that of His Prophet.[1] Hence, *ihsān* is to act for the good of others, doing good deeds because of the divine will, or rather, by extension of it. Answering the call for good with good deeds, knowing that

1. Taqī l-Dīn Ahmad Ibn 'Abd al-Halīm Ibn Taymīya (661-728/1263-1328), ed. ar. and trans. fr. of Laoust, H. *Ibn Taymiyya. Al-Hisba fil-Islam,* Paris, 1986, ed. ar. p. 92, trans. fr. p. 107 [quoted in Franco 1999: 138].

it comes from God (FRANCO 1999: 138), we could say that it is more a naturally human action than a spiritual necessity in order to be rewarded in the afterlife. It is treating mankind properly as a way to show respect to the divine creation. We could even use a final commentary from the Qur'an to illustrate this *ihsān*: «Worship Allah alone and associate none with Him. And be kind to parents, relatives, orphans, the poor, near and distant neighbours, close friends, ⌜needy⌝ travellers, and those ⌜bondspeople⌝ in your possession. Surely Allah does not like whoever is arrogant, boastful» (An-Nissà 4,36). Virtues reflected in what Constable explains about *funduqs,* and which we will see later in the founding text of the *Māristān* of Granada.

With all of that, and without distorting theoretical and religious intentions, we must understand a similar practical motivation in both the Christian and Muslim worlds: both used religion to camouflage a set of political practices aimed at controlling social tension among poor people. This does not modify the precedent consideration, but it is a matter to keep in mind.

The firsts *bīmāristānat*[2] are to be found in the East. In pre-Islamic times, in Yundishapur, present-day Iran, we find a 3rd century AD reference of a health care centre that survived the Arab-Muslim attacks of 638 and evolved into a public hospital. The *bīmāristān* of Damascus, founded during the caliphate of Walid Ibn Abdelmálek in the early eighth century, is also mentioned as one of the earliest of these hospitals (GARRIGA 2010: 39-40).

According to Carles G. Bárcena (2001: 7), the first *bīmāristān* in the Islamic world was established in Baghdad during the reign of Caliph Harin ar-Rashid (786-809). Its most immediate predecessor was probably the hospital in the city of Gundeshapur, in the southwest of present-day Iran, which was built under the Sassanid dynasty. The hospital was an important intellectual centre that brought together the most renowned doctors of the time. Some of them, at least twenty-four of whom are known to us, went on to practice their profession in Baghdad's *bīmāristān* and teach their knowledge to disciples.

The history of the *bīmāristān,* though, goes back a long way. From the 4th century onwards, the Byzantine Empire saw the development of *xenodocheia*, «véritables institutions charitables chrétiennes, elles connaissent un essor important sous Jutinien (525-565). Ces infirmeries monastiques, à la fois sorte d'hospices, hôpitaux, auberges ont peut-être servi de modèle aux bîmâristâns»[3] (CLOAREC 1998: 23). In the 6th century, these *xenodocheia* increasingly specialised in the accommodation of sick people, and the institution evolved into a hospital proper. Constable explains what the fundamental differences between the *xenodocheia* and the *pandocheia* are:

2. Plural of the word *bīmāristān* (GARRIGA 2010: 40).

3. English translation: «True Christian charitable institutions, they experienced a major expansion under Justinian (525-565). These monastic infirmaries, which served as a hospice, hospital, and inn all at the same time, may have served as a model for the *bīmāristān*».

The differential trajectories of the *pandocheion* and the *xenodocheion* in late antiquity, one into an Islamic context and the other into Christian settings (both European and Byzantine), suggest intriguing correlations between functions, religious associations, and cross-cultural transferability. Put in its most simple form: commercial and secular institutions are more apt to cross boundaries created by faith than ones with a greater religious valency. Thus, while the ubiquitous *pandocheion* transferred easily from pagan and Jewish setting, to a Christian, then Muslim, context, the strongly Christian *xenodocheion* could not make the transition to Islam. The open-door policy of the *pandocheion* (its tradition of "accepting all comers") was an important factor in allowing the fluid transfer of this institution into an Islamic setting after the seventh century (Constable 2003: 38).

Contrary to what happened in the Christian world, we can affirm that the *bīmāristān*'s secular character was an important aspect of the institution. However, this does not mean that it was detached from the religious factor, as we have already seen.

Between the 9th and 11th centuries, Baghdad saw the number of *bīmāristānat* multiply, and in the 11th century the institution spread to cities such as Aleppo and Antioch, but it was in the 12th century when we find a great increase in the number of these centres for the care of the sick, to which the most prestigious medical schools were linked (Bárcena 2001: 8). In Damascus a famous *bīmāristān* was built by order of Nûr al- Din, who reigned in Syria between 1146 and 1174. A great architectural promoter, he built ramparts, consolidated citadels and multiplied mosques and schools. The hospital he commissioned in 1154 housed the most important medical school in the entire Muslim East (Cloarec 1998: 83-86). Ibn Jubayr (1998: 332), a geographer who travelled throughout the Near East between 1183 and 1185, explains that this *bīmāristān* had a daily assignment of fifteen *dinars*. It had a few administrators, who were in charge of the registers where the names of the sick were recorded, together with the expenses related to their medicines, their meals, and many other things. The doctors visited the hospital every day in the morning, examined the sick, and ordered the preparation of suitable remedies and food, according to the needs of each person.

Other *bīmāristān* of importance in the Muslim East included the *bīmāristān* Arghûn of Aleppo and the *bīmāristān* Qaymari of Damascus, both from the 13th century. The arrival of these institutions in the Muslim West, according to the specific bibliography, happened at a later date, with examples such as the hospitals of Fez and Granada. However, this does not mean that there were no earlier care centres in cities such as Cordoba and Granada or in North Africa. The so-called Corral del Carbón of Granada, built in the 14th-century, is a good example of an *alhóndiga* (*funduq al-jadd*), not a hospital, that was built before the city's *Māristān* (Constable 2003: 249).

## 2. *The Māristān of Granada: Foundation, Architecture*

The construction of what is thought to be the first Islamic hospital in the Iberian Peninsula[4] is the result of a process that began in the East, in cities such as Damascus, Cairo, and Tunisia in the 9th and 10th centuries. These institutions arrived in the West later, particularly in Al-Andalus, with the 14th-century *bīmāristān* of Granada being the first in the Iberian Peninsula. However, as Alfonso Fernández and Rubén Maña (2016: 57-58) point out, this hypothesis is not necessarily true: the *bīmāristān* of Granada is the first we can document reliably, at a time when the scarcity of data on welfare institutions in Al-Andalus contrasts with the abundance of hospitals and monasteries in the north of the peninsula, as well as in the eastern Islamic world.

What is true, as Franco Sánchez (1999: 150)[5] emphasizes, is that welfare institutions, in all their complexities, existed in al-Andalus from an earlier time. A very important document related to the foundation of the hospital is the inscription written on a slab (fig. 1) in the form of a pointed horseshoe arch made up of two pieces of marble containing twenty-six lines of cursive writing, which is preserved in the Alhambra Museum. According to Francisco Enríquez's 19th-century drawings (fig. 2), this stone was placed above the pier of the Nasrid *Māristān*'s main façade. Likewise, Juan de Dios de la Rada y Delgado also places this memorial stone at this same site (fig. 3).

The aforementioned drawing by Enríquez, together with similar pieces from the same period, is a visual document of great importance for our knowledge of the building.

Nonetheless, as it has been previously stated (GARCÍA, GIRÓN, SALVATIERRA 1989: 14), these drawings were significantly embellished as a response to the City Council of Granada, who had allowed the destruction of the *Māristān*, under the pretence that «ha desaparecido ya casi todo lo que constituía su mérito y el resto no se puede sostener»[6] (*El Grito de Granada*, 6/8/1843). The destruction of the building caused a great social controversy in Granada in the summer of 1843.

In addition to informing us of the dates of the construction of the building, from October 1365 to June 1367, i.e., a mere twenty months, the inscription also informs us that this type of foundation (i.e., a *bīmāristān*) had no precedents since the introduction of Islam in the country, something that could be understood as surprising, given that we know of the existence of welfare institutions in Cordoba, Seville, and Algeciras. Some scholars point to the possibility that Muhammad V was only stating the building's extraordinary magnificence, unparalleled

4. A statement that, as Lampérez Romea (1922: 302) says, it is not correct. We know of one in Cordoba in the 8th century and of another one in Algeciras in the 12th century.

5. The author states as well that «no tenemos noticias fehacientes de otros hospitales de origen islámico en el reino de Granada. Ni los viajeros árabes Ibn Battuta […] Abd al Basīt […], ni al-Qalasādī […], ni al-Hayārī […], ni Luis de Marmol, ni Andrea Navaggiero» (FRANCO 1999: 160).

6. English translation: «almost everything that constituted its merit has disappeared and the rest cannot be sustained».

by any other pious works carried out to date (García, Girón, Salvatierra 1989: 98). And, even more interestingly, the inscription claims that the foundation of the building on behalf of Muhammad V of Granada was an «embroidery of glory added to the excellent cape of holy war».

This is an observation to bear in mind, because the construction of the building must be framed during the second reign of Abu ‘Abd Allah Muhammad V. Because public works of beneficence demonstrated the ruler’s virtuousness, the monarch may have sought to reinforce his image as a politico-religious authority through the *bīmāristān* of Granada (Fernández, Maña 2016: 59), a type of institution which he might have encountered during his exile to Morocco, in the city of Fez, after he was dethroned in 1359 due to internal riots. In his second reign after the exile, propagandistic architecture became one of Muhammad’s most powerful allies. Franco Sánchez (1999: 156) concludes that, in imitating the prestigious capital of Fez, Muhammad V wished to endow the people of Granada with a benefit hitherto unheard of in Al-Andalus (as the text of the foundation stone emphasises).

It is also noteworthy that the inscription makes use of the specific term “*māristān*”, instead of “*bīmāristān*”, which shows how what had started as a colloquialism was, by then, a concrete and accepted term in Granada, used in an official context. Regarding the nomenclature, Torres Balbás (1944: 482) writes that the word *māristān* was a popular contraction of *bīmāristān*, and that the word passed from Persian into Arabic with its meaning of “home for the sick”, that is, a hospital or a building in which mentally ill people were locked up. In the late Middle Ages, most Islamic hospitals catered mostly to the insane and, therefore, the term *māristān* was almost always used to refer to asylums for the mentally ill, especially in Morocco.

This explains what Hyeronimus Münzer wrote in his *Travels through Spain and Portugal (1494-1495),* published in 1920 under the title *Itinerarium Hispanicum.* All the specific literature accepts that when Muntzer talks about the *casa de locos* of Granada, he is referring to the *Māristān*. In this regard, Münzer (2002: 135) mentions that King Ferdinand granted a tenth of the total revenue of Granada to build temples, to support the poor in the hospitals and to the mental asylum –the *Māristān*–, which was built by the Moors, and that he increased its revenue and did not reduce it in any way. Juan Antonio García and Mariano Martín mention the possibility that Münzer did not refer to the *Māristān*, despite the general acceptance of the specific literature.

Beyond these aspects regarding the institution’s foundation and terminology, another important factor in the building’s history is its location. Mariano Martín and Juan Antonio García (1984) delimit the contours of the building, reminding us that the exact location of the complex was not known until the discovery of its archaeological remains in the late 1970s. On the site of the former hospital there was a neighbours’ corral and its characteristics and layout led to the suspicion that the remains of the Muslim building, such as pillars, walls, or beams, might have been used in its construction. It was not until July 1978 that it could be determined with certainty that the remains of the *Māristān* were located there. The remains that could be observed consisted essentially of part of the southern body of the old building, which was preserved up to the eaves, as well as at least the eastern perimeter wall, which was never demolished (GARCÍA, GIRÓN, SALVATIERRA 1989: 16). From then on, it could be stated that the side boundaries of the *Māristān* were two parallel streets that went down to the Carrera del Darro, which can only be the present-day Bañuelo and Concepción streets, the latter of which is called Casa de la Moneda in Dalmáu's plan, and was adjacent to the Convent of Zafra. Therefore, the main façade of the *Māristān* faced the doorway of the church of the Convent of the Immaculate Conception (MARTÍN, GARCÍA 1984: 8).

Thus, the site on which the hospital is located is on the southern slope of the Albaicín hill, right next to the river Darro, in the Coracha neighbourhood, near the well-known Puente del Cadí or Puerta de los Tableros, which guarded the fluvial way into the city. It is, together with the Baño del Nogal (on Bañuelo street) and the Casa nazarí of Zafra, the main Muslim remain in the area. Antonio Almagro and Antonio Orihuela (2003: 82) comment that this neighbourhood on the banks of the Darro was one of the most popular in the city because of its good climate, especially in summer, which may explain the suitability of the site for the construction of a place for the sick.

However, the *Māristān* was not the first structure to be built on that site. Archaeological excavations have shown that it was preceded by several other buildings in the area, the floors of which cannot be reconstructed because of the impact of the construction of the courtyard *alberca* (a pool-like structure; GARCÍA, GIRÓN, SALVATIERRA 1989: 26). What has been confirmed is that the *Māristān* is the result of the "rehabilitation" of an old building, which may have been built by a predecessor of Muhammad V, perhaps by the other major developer of the building, Yūsuf I. The *pre-Māristān* building would have occupied the entire site of the present-day *Māristān* and would have established the layout of four sections around a courtyard. The internal layout of these sections is not known at this stage. The existing gates were clearly built at a later stage, so the interior had to be different. The purpose of this building is also unknown, but its public character can be deduced from the history of the area and its subsequent use. Experts have commented on the possibility that it was an *alhóndiga* (*fanādīq,* meaning a place where everyone is welcome) which functioned as public grain market where the city's cereal was stored, and which served as a support for people in times of hardship. Juan Antonio García and Vicente Salvatierra say that the plan of the early building corresponds to this type of building (GARCÍA, GIRÓN, SALVATIERRA 1989: 27-29). On the other hand, Pedro Salmerón and other authors, in addition to comparing the *Māristān*'s plant to the *fanādīq*, note its resemblance to *ribats* (monasteries) and *madrazas* (Islamic schools). The similarities in plan and elevation with the Corral del Carbón in Granada have also been continuously noted (SALMERÓN et al. 2020: 73).

It seems that the alterations carried out on the pre-existing building consisted of the raising of an extra floor above the original first floor, which entailed the modification of the accesses to the rooms and their probable internal reform (García, Girón, Salvatierra 1989: 29), and the construction of a large *alberca* in the middle of the courtyard. All these reforms were carried at the same time as the parallel embellishment of the building. In addition, an 11th century well was recently discovered under the *alberca* of the *Māristān*, build way before the construction of the hospital (Pastor 2021).

From a perspective rooted in the history of art, the artistic value of the hospital cannot be separated from its practical conception. And when we talk about the building's artistic value, we cannot leave out the drawings that, following the demolition plan of the *Māristān*, were made in the 19th century. These graphic representations may have been idealised, but they also form part of the aesthetic conception of the building as a whole. We will not dedicate a specific subsection to talk about the representations by Enríquez or Juan de Dios de Rada y Delgado, but we will use the drawings for our explanation, at the same time that we will contrast what the experts say about them with the references that the restorers and conservators use today to carry out their work.

If we begin with the ground plan (fig. 4), which gives us a more or less historically reliable overview of the complex, we see that Enríquez proposes a porticoed architectural model, enclosed on all four sides, rectangular, with a courtyard in the middle, in which we find the famous *alberca* with the two lion fountains on each of its longitudinal sides. It is a rather large *alberca*, measuring 4.5 m on the short sides, 16.20 on the long sides, and with a depth of 1.10 m (Salmerón et al. 2020: 72). There is an important matter related to the *alberca* that must be taken into account at a functional level: the *Māristān* was located in a strategic point of the routes that men and animals used to transport water into the city before the construction of the *Acequia Real* of the Alhambra. This explains the suitability of the site and its links to primitive water-related structures. Water had a strong ritualistic component, as we see in spaces such as the mosque's *sahn*, where we find the *sabil,* the fountain where the ritual ablutions are made before entering the *haram.* A ritual component that we surely also find here, beyond the therapeutic component of water.

The different rooms communicate with the peristyle on the ground floor and the gallery on the first floor. We see four stairwells on the sides, although it has also been speculated that these were in the middle of the lateral bodies. The dimensions of the entire plot occupied by the *Māristān* where of 37.30 x 25.15 m, while the courtyard measures 26.16 x 15.00 m (Salmerón et al. 2020: 77).

The digital reconstructions of the building made by Pedro Salmerón (fig. 5), which were commissioned as part of the restoration project of the hospital, show that the *Māristān* is situated on irregular terrain, that slopes down towards the Carrera del Darro, so that the building has to overcome the unevenness of the slope. Commenting on the architecture of the building, Salmerón (2020: 78) says:

> Se puede afirmar que se trata de una estructura dotada de un magnetismo especial, de un atractivo sutil, si se piensa como objeto arquitectónico con una geometría decidida

en el entramado urbano medieval, poseedora de una fuga de tipo perspectivo que señala a la fortificación de la Alhambra, cuyos bastiones se alzan en picado en una bellísima vista que crea un fondo dominante.[7]

He also notes that the famous *Patio de los leones* at the Alhambra is almost contemporaneous with the *Māristān*, and that they share the same concept of a porticoed courtyard on all four sides and the symbolic presence of lion-shaped sculptures. The lions symbolise guardianship and strength, as they were the conductors of the most precious commodity, water, which is not only vital for sustenance but also aesthetic and sonorous.

At the same time, this digital reconstruction is very useful for guessing what the building looked like volumetrically. The aesthetics of the complex must have been more austere than ornate, although there was no lack of sculptural decoration on the doors and windows, especially on the main gate, as we have seen in the drawing by Juan de Dios de Rada y Delgado (fig. 3). There were four two-story buildings topped by a gable roof, with a large courtyard in the middle, which reveals a regular rhythm of the pillars on both the first and second floors.

Regarding the façade of the *Māristān* presented by Enríquez (fig. 2), those currently responsible for the restoration project, probably guided by archaeological evidence, dismiss the existence of horseshoe arch windows, purportedly placed symmetrically to the tombstone containing the foundation inscription. Enríquez's drawing shows three windows on each side of the main door: two twin windows and one at each end. In addition, the walls have two small openings, one on either side of the main door, but lower down. This rendition of the façade does not reflect the unevenness shown by the reproductions linked to the restoration project, since the façade had to adapt to the slope of the street that separates the *Māristān* from the Convento de la Concepción that is just in front of it. The two corners of the main façade were chamfered at the bottom, resolving the agreement with the meeting edge of the walls by turning a sharp horseshoe half-arch on each of them, resulting in a small cylindrical surface (MARTÍN, GARCÍA 1984: 20). Something that we see in Enríquez's drawing, as Martín and García point out.

Francisco Enríquez also made a drawing of the section (fig. 6) of the hospital in which we see one of its long sides, made up of nine horseshoe arches and the openings of the stairwells, which the artist is unsure about how to depict. In the central opening, we can see the lion sculpture that was on one side of the *alberca*. The *alberca* is also reflected in its depth in this drawing. The upper floor has an open gallery with a single horseshoe arch in the centre, smaller than those below, and a single horseshoe arch at the end. The three openings between the pillars have twin horseshoe-arched windows. As we can see in the digital reconstruction, and as we will try to explain below, the section presented by Enríquez does not

7. English translation: «It can be said that this is a structure endowed with a special magnetism, a subtle attraction, if it is thought of as an architectural object with a decisive geometry in the medieval urban fabric, possessing an escape of a perspectival type that points to the fortification of the Alhambra, whose bastions rise steeply in a beautiful view that creates a dominant backdrop».

correspond to the original appearance of the courtyard, since –as García, Girón and Salvatierra (1989: 28) comment– it is likely that he created the entire elevation from an idealisation of other models. These could be, for example, those illustrated by al-Harīrī al-Basrī in his *Maqāmāt,* in the 13th century, where we find curious representations of the *khān* of Wasit (fig. 7 and 8), a place of assistance to travellers where al-Harīth spent the night. Olivia R. Constable (2003: 90) says of this building:

On arrival in Wasit, al-Harīth found that this *khan* was tidy and inexpensive, and although there were many other guests, he was given his own room [...]. The two manuscripts show remarkably similar views of the courtyard of this *khan,* illustrating storage rooms on the first floor, a second level with a carved wooden balcony-rail, columns, and smaller guest chambers (though a number of patrons are shown asleep in the courtyard), and above a roof and attic space with windows.

These two floors of rooms appear in the same way as the *Māristān* of Granada, with the upper ones individually accessible through a balcony or gallery overlooking the courtyard. The layout is also similar. It remains to be seen whether the hospital of Granada also shared an attic with windows, which Enríquez's drawings do not show. Instead, they do show us a first floor above the stairwells, as if it were an attic. When it is said that Enríquez idealised a series of models for his drawings, perhaps it is not in terms of spatial distribution, but in terms of decoration, for example with the use of the horseshoe arch, typically Muslim, although not exclusively so. In installations that were used by merchants, such as the *khan,* security was a matter of vital importance, as can be seen in the detail that these illustrators of the *Maqāmāt* put into the doors and locks. Enríquez has no need for this, as his illustrations are for a hospital. Nevertheless, we can see that the distribution of space in Islamic care centres is similar regardless of their specific function. Constable (2003: 93) notes that the central courtyard of the *khān* [8] of Wasit is typical: «Although there were many regional variations in the style of hostelries, *khāns* and *funduqs* in the medieval Muslims world normally had an internal courtyard (sometimes covered) surrounded by porticoes, with rooms for storage and stabling on the ground floor». This model can also be used to explain the courtyard of the *Māristān* of Granada.

Returning to Enríquez's section, the horseshoe arches on the first floor would not be rooted in reality, while Juan Antonio García and Mariano Martín consider this solution to be correct for the upper floor. In this regard, we can compare Enríquez's plan (left) with a more realistic representation of the section, that of Juan Antonio García and Mariano Martín (right) (fig. 9). However, we must bear in mind that the current restoration project does not contemplate the presence of horseshoe arches on the upper floor, but rectangular openings (fig. 10). Martín

8. Cloarec (1998: 150) tells us that *Khâns* facilitated trade across the Muslim world. They were staging posts for caravans or built in commercial centres to accommodate merchants and goods.

and García (1984: 21) consider that there were galleries on brick pillars on all four sides of the courtyard, which gave access to other long, narrow naves by means of slightly pointed horseshoe arches. There were nine of these arches on the larger sides and five on the smaller ones. Enríquez depicts these naves continuously in his plans, but, according to Mariano Martín and Juan Antonio García (1984), they were probably divided into small rooms, similar to those found in the Corral del Carbón, also in the city of Granada. In the front nave, there were four small chambers on each side of the vestibule, on the inside of the façade wall.

If we compare, therefore, the section of the *Māristān* made by Enríquez with the proposal of Mariano Martín and Juan Antonio García and the appearance that the current curators intend to give to the complex, based on archaeological criteria, we can observe the evolutionary process that the idyllic image of the *Māristān* has undergone since the 19th century.

The layout of the porticoed courtyard with this arrangement of rectangular openings and quadrangular pillars, according to the experts, bears a strong resemblance to what is known as the Corral del Carbón (fig. 11 and 12), which was a *funduq* or *alhóndiga*.[9] It relates to the utilitarian and distributive organisation of the *Māristān*, with rooms connected to circulation rings at two heights (SALMERÓN et al. 2020: 80). A similarity that becomes clear when we compare the images of the Corral del Carbón with the virtual reconstructions associated with the restoration project of the hospital building.

We have already mentioned that the oldest description of the *Māristān* of Granada is that of Ibn al-Jatib, the vizier of Muhammad V, who, retelling the life of the sultan, and referring to his second period of rule after returning from the city of Fez, describes the *Māristān* of Granada. We have added Ibn al-Jatīb's description here in order to highlight his references to the architecture, or rather to its spatial organisation, but also because of its usefulness in defining it welfare mission. We have used a translation by Franco Sánchez (1999: 170), who complements his translation with the following footnote: «Hemos preferido ser fieles al ampuloso lenguaje de este panegírico que escribe Ibn al-Jatīb a Muhammad V (uno de sus mentores en el poder) a riesgo de restar belleza a la traducción. El lenguaje es un reflejo más, entre la multitud de hechos y circunstancias que caracterizan una época».[10] Ibn al-Jatīb describes the Māristān of Granada as follows:

Among the attitudes of sincerity and beneficence (*al-ihsan*) of the extraordinary "spiritual struggle" there is the construction of the supreme hospital (*al-māristān al-a'tam*), a good deed established until the end of time and the privilege of the best of cities. It is not achieved without the main of conquests, which is regarding to the abundance of poverty and the appearance of need, which pro-

9. For futher information about this attendance centres and this one in particular, see CONSTABLE 2003: 249.

10. English translation: «We have preferred to be faithful to the bombastic language of this panegyric written by Ibn al-Jatīb to Muhammad V (one of his mentors in power) at the risk of detracting from the beauty of the translation. The language is just one more reflection, among the multitude of facts and circumstances that characterise an era».

vokes in him the magnanimity of devotion (*al-'dīn*) and a strengthened spirit; therefore, it manifests the attitude of companionship of close friends, and the goal is al-Andalus. It is a compendium of beauties and a sumptuous building. It has numerous rooms (*masākin*), a large courtyard (*sāha*), flowing waters and a healthy atmosphere, it has numerous storerooms and places for ablutions. It is well maintained and well organised. It surpasses the hospital of Egypt in its large courtyard, in the healthfulness of its air, and in its waters, which gush over the sandstone and black rock, rippling as if in the sea and flowing into the trees. Anyone who is feeble is allowed to enter, only if he agrees. Its stewards are kind-souled, in imitation of the spirituality of the madrasa or the *zāwiya*, and with the determination of one who knows he is destined for the grave –quite the opposite of the purposes of kings–. On it there is an inscription with his good name of the sultan at the end, immortalised on the walls for the memory; it is an unusual preservation in the face of oblivion of the tomb –in the very centre of the city of private chambers and reserved chambers!– and it is like a slow chanting of the Qur'an, day and night. All this comes only from his alms (*sadaqītihi*), and from the greatness of his intentions.[11]

We must highlight some aspects of the definition given by Ibn al-Jatīb. Regarding the architecture of the building, which is the subject that concerns us, al-Jatīb comments that the hospital has numerous rooms, a large courtyard, many storerooms and places for ablutions. This is related to the adjective that the writer attributes to the *Māristān*, which he calls the "supreme" hospital, the most important (*al-māristān al-a'tam*). This fact could, as we have already mentioned, explain why the founding inscription of the building describes it as unprecedented since the introduction of Islam into the country. This does not necessarily mean that there were no other hospitals in Al-Andalus (which is highly unlikely), but rather that until that time there were none of such importance and magnitude. At the same time, this definition would disprove the attribution of the *Māristān* of Granada as a psychiatric hospital that arises from the commentary of Hieronymus Münzer, who speaks of the *Māristān* as a "madhouse", since Ibn al-Jatīb states that «anyone who is weak is allowed to enter». Therefore, it would not have been founded on the premise of being a psychiatric hospital, although there may have been patients who could be defined as insane.

The *Māristān* of Granada constitutes the most complete example of a Muslim hospital in the Iberian Peninsula. It was a seat of Islamic medicine, outstanding for its efficiency and success during the Middle Ages. At the architectural level, we have tried to refer to its models and to give a general view of what, as far as we know, was the form and function of this building complex. The Nasrid *Māristān* can be studied from different perspectives: the history of the building, its functionality, its artistic value (i.e., studying its architecture from an aesthetic point of view, as well as the decorative arts and sculpture in it), regarding the polemic about the conservation of

11. Ibn al-Jatib. *Ihāta*, vol II, p. 48 i 50-51. Translation from the Spanish version by Franco 1999: 156.

the building, the current and past restoration projects, or the graphic representations of the building. Here, we simply wanted to focus on its architecture and its uses by outlining a brief text on the subject, but we could not fail to place our contribution in a more general context to which it is indebted. Founded by Muhammad V in the mid-14th century, after his exile in Fez, the *Māristān* of Granada functioned for some 150 years as the hospital of the capital of the Kingdom of Granada, constituting a link in this process of hospital formation which, through Byzantium and later the Muslim world, was the seat of medieval medical knowledge. A building of evident decorative sobriety, which nevertheless contained a beautiful example of Hispano-Muslim decorative art, especially around the door and with the lion fountains in the *alberca*. With the subsequent Christian conquest of the city, it was used as a mint, wine warehouse, convent, neighbours' corral, etc., and was finally demolished in 1843, leaving us with a not inconsiderable quantity of drawings and illustrations. It was the subject of various archaeological excavations at the end of the 20th century, and once again regained prominence in the cultural debate in the city of Granada and is currently the subject of a restoration project which we hope will be carried out in the next few years.

## *Bibliography*

ALMAGRO, Antonio; ORIHUELA, Antonio, 2003. "El Maristán nazarí de Granada. Análisis del edificio y una propuesta para su recuperación", *Boletín de la Real Academia de Bellas Artes Nuestra Señora de las Angustias*, 10: 80-109.

BÁRCENA, Carles G., 2001. "El bimaristan, un modelo de hospital islámico. Historia de los primeros centros psiquiátricos del mundo", *Natura Medicatrix*, 62: 6-11.

CLOAREC, Françoise, 1998. *Bîmâristâns, lieux de folie et de sagesse. La folie et ses traitements dans les hôpitaux médiévaux au Moyen-Orient*, Paris, Harmattan.

CONEJO DA PENA, Antoni, 2011. *«Domus seu hospitale». Espais d'assistència i de salut a l'edat mitjana*, Barcelona, Universitat de Barcelona.

CONSTABLE, Olivia Remie, 2003. *Housing the Stranger in the Mediterranean World*, Cambridge, Cambridge University Press.

CLAYE, J., GIDE, J., GAILHABAUD, J. (ed.) 1858. *L'architecture du V^me au XVII^me siècle et les arts qui en dépendent: la sculpture, la peinture murale, la peinture sur verre, la mosaïque, la ferronerie, etc. / publiés d'après les travaux inédits des principaux architectes français et étrangers par Jules Gailhabaud*, Paris, Gide, T. 3. https://catalog.hathitrust.org/Record/009268277.

FERNÁNDEZ VÁZQUEZ, Alfonso; MAÑA ARES, Rubén, 2016. "El legado islámico en los cuidados psiquiátricos. El Maristán de Granada", *Cultura de los cuidados*, 45: 52-63.

FRANCO SÁNCHEZ, Francisco, 1999. "La asistencia al enfermo en Al-Andalus. Los hospitales hispanomusulmanes", *La medicina en Al-Andalus*, Granada, Junta de Andalucía: 135-165.

FONTANALS JAUMÀ, Reis, 2014. "Asistencia y municipio a través de las fuentes medievales y modernes: el caso del Hospital de la Santa Creu de Barcelona", Teresa Huguet, Pere Verdés, Jon Arrizabalaga, Manuel Sánchez (ed.), *Ciudad y hospital en el Occidente europeo. 1300-1700*, Lleida, Milenio: 49-75.

GARCÍA GRANADOS, Juan Antonio; SALVATIERRA CUENCA, Vicente, 1984. "El Maristán de Granada: entre la fantasía romántica i la realidad arqueológica", *Revista de Arqueología*, 42: 16-25.

GARCÍA GRANADOS, Juan Antonio; GIRÓN IRUESTE, Fernando; SALVATIERRA CUENCA, Vicente, 1989. *El Maristan de Granada. Un hospital islámico*, Madrid, Asociación Española de Neuropsiquiatría/Asociación Mundial de Psiquiatría.

García Granados, Juan Antonio; Salvatierra de Cuenca, Vicente, 1986. "El Maristán de Granada: Urbanismo y funciones", *Arqueologia Espacial*, 10: 311-326.

Garriga Guitart, David, 2010. *Del bimaristán al hospital psiquiátrico: historia de la enfermería y la salud mental en el Islam,* Madrid, Asociación Nacional de Enfermería de Salud Mental.

Lbn Yubayr, 1988. *A través del Oriente. El siglo XII ante los ojos*, Barcelona, Serbal.

Lampérez Romea, Vicente, 1922. *Arquitectura civil española de los siglos I al XVIII,* Madrid, Saturnino Calleja, vol. II.

Martín García, Mariano; García Granados, Juan Antonio, 1984. "El Maristan de Granada tres el hallazgo de sus restos", *Cuadernos de Arte de la Universidad de Granada,* 16: 7-41.

Münzer, Jerónimo, 2002. *Viaje por España y Portugal (1494-1495),* Madrid, Polifemo.

Salmerón Escobar, Pedro, et al., 2020 "El Maristán nazarí de Granada. Recuperación de un monumento en una difícil encrucijada", *Cuadernos de la Alhambra,* 49: 71-91.

Torres Balbás, Leopoldo, 1944. "El Maristán de Granada", *Al-Andalus,* 9: 481-498.

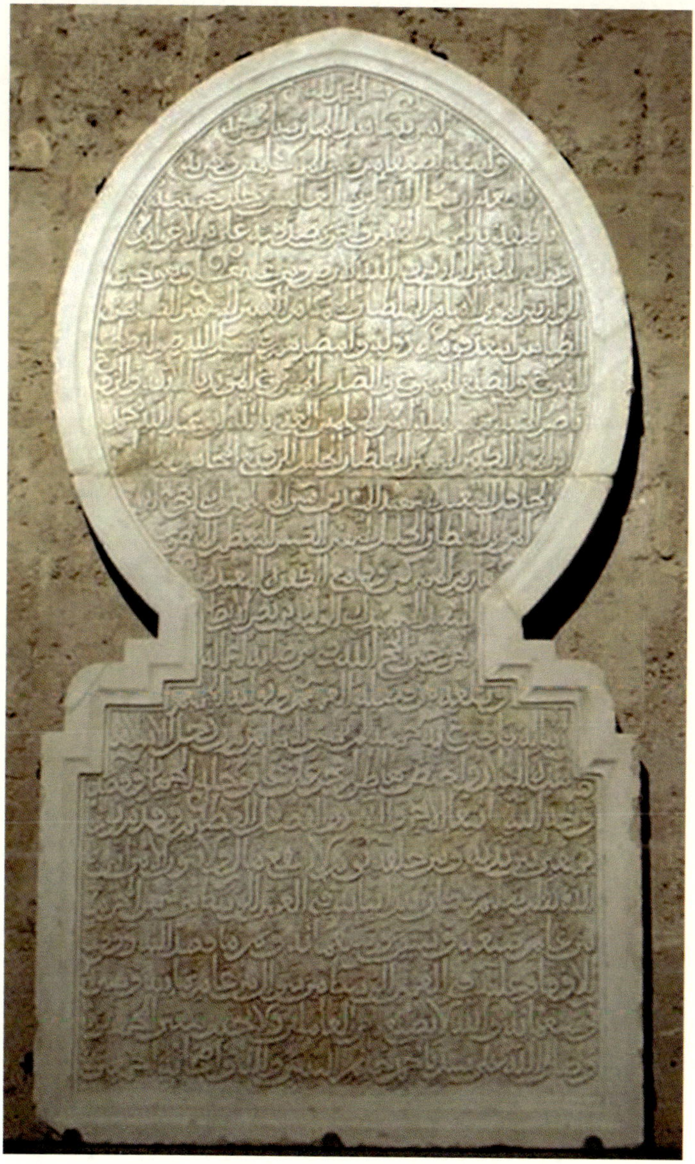

Fig. 1. Foundational inscription of the *Māristān* of Granada, 1367 (Granada: Museo de la Alhambra). Image obtained from bit.ly/3mKTH7t.

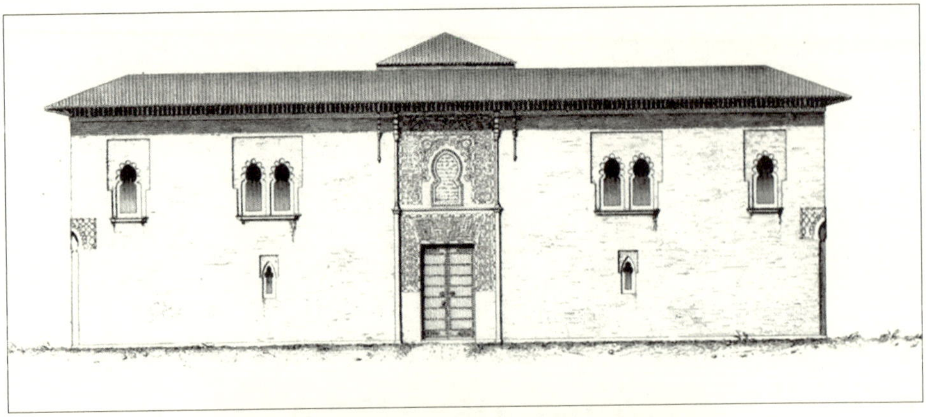

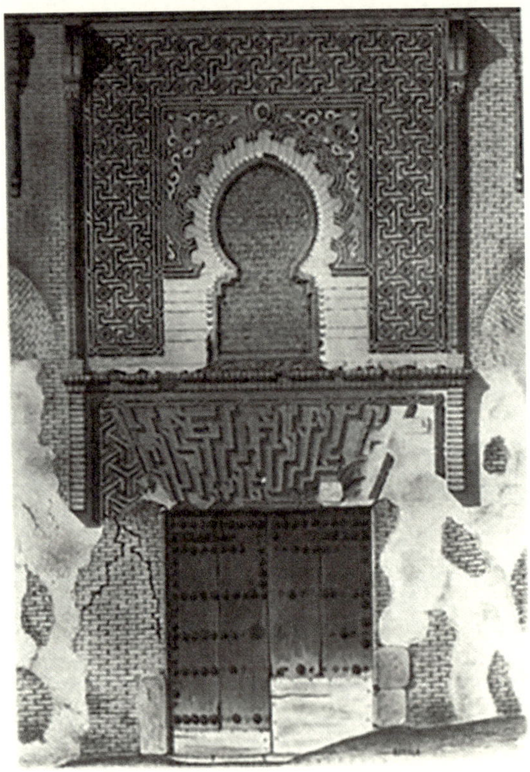

Fig. 2. Drawing of the façade of the *Māristān* by Francisco Enríquez, from Claye, Gide, Gailhabaud 1858: 148.
Fig.3. Drawing of the main door of the *Māristān* of Juan de Dios de Rada y Delgado. Image obtained from Martín, García 1984.

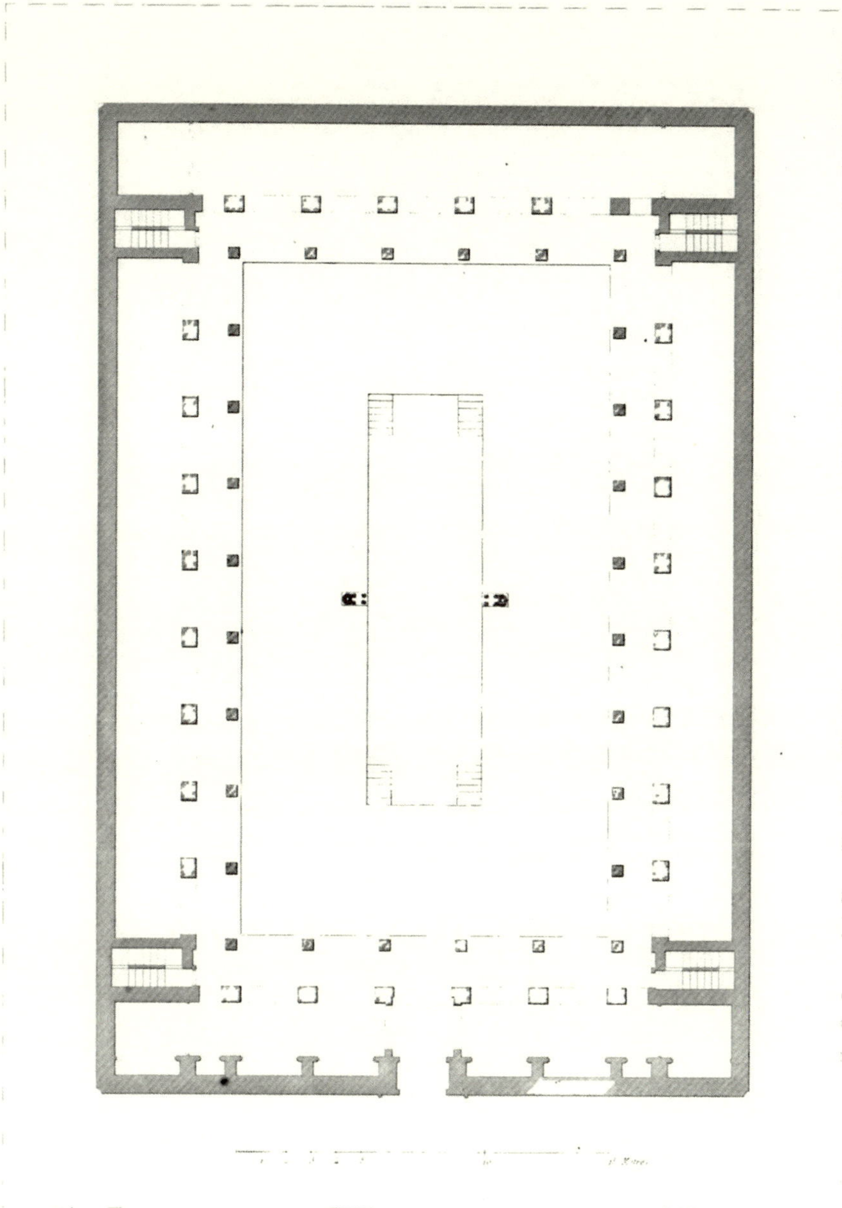

Fig. 4. Plan of the *Māristān* by Francisco Enríquez, from CLAYE, GIDE, GAILHABAUD 1858: 148.

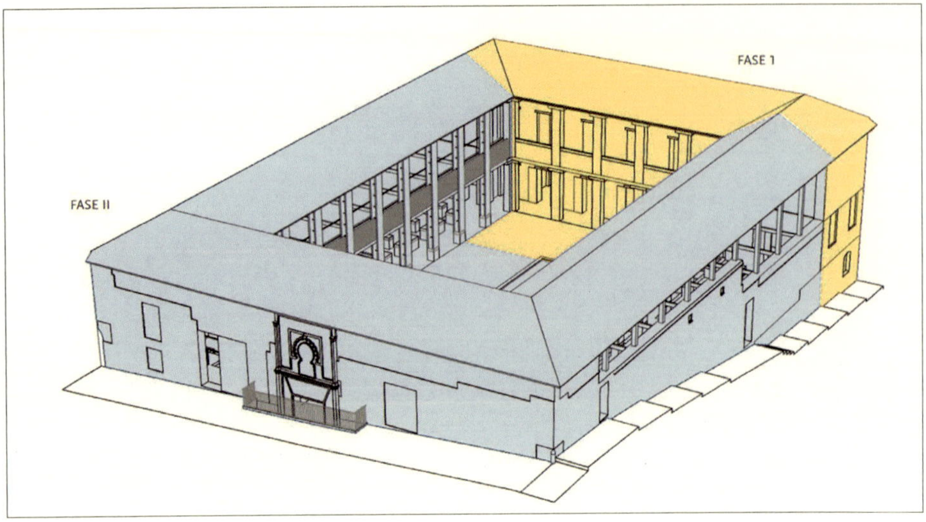


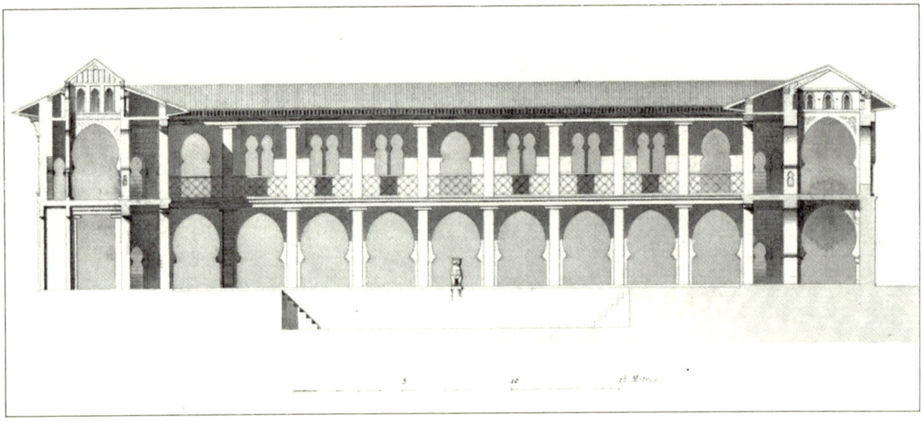

Fig. 5. Plans and perspective of the *Māristān* with an indication of the phases of action, Image obtained from SALMERÓN et al. 2020: il. 11.
Fig. 6. Drawing of the *Māristān's* section by Francisco Enríquez, from CLAYE, GIDE, GAILHABAUD 1858: 148.

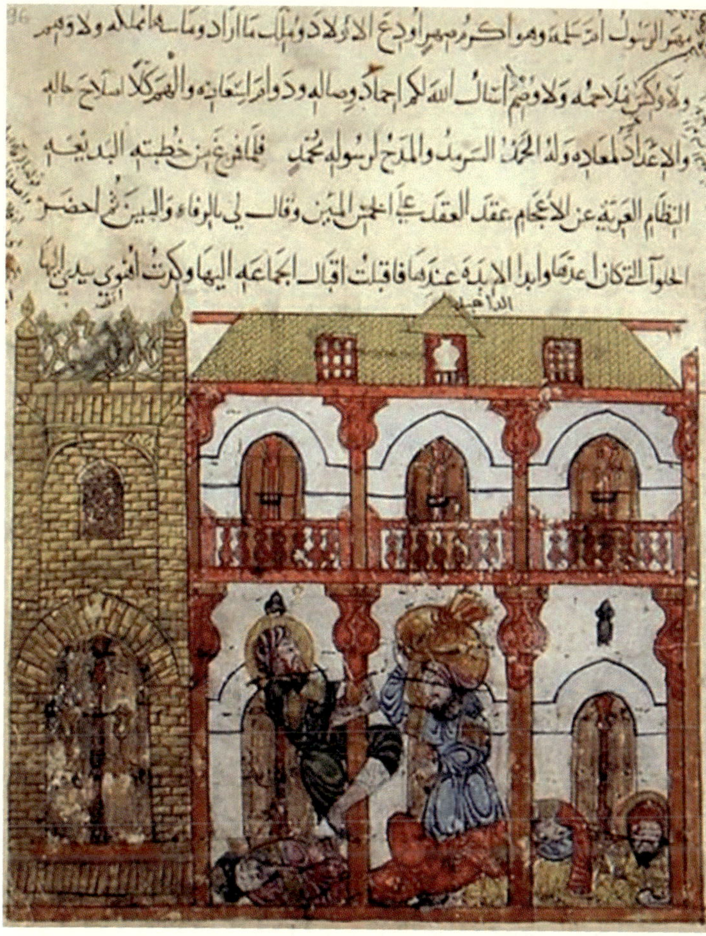

Fig. 7. Illustrations of the *khān* of Wasit in *Maqāmāt* de al-Harīrī al-Basrī, c. 1240 (St. Peresburg: Russian Academy of Sciences, Institute for Oriental Studies, MS C-23, f. 99r).

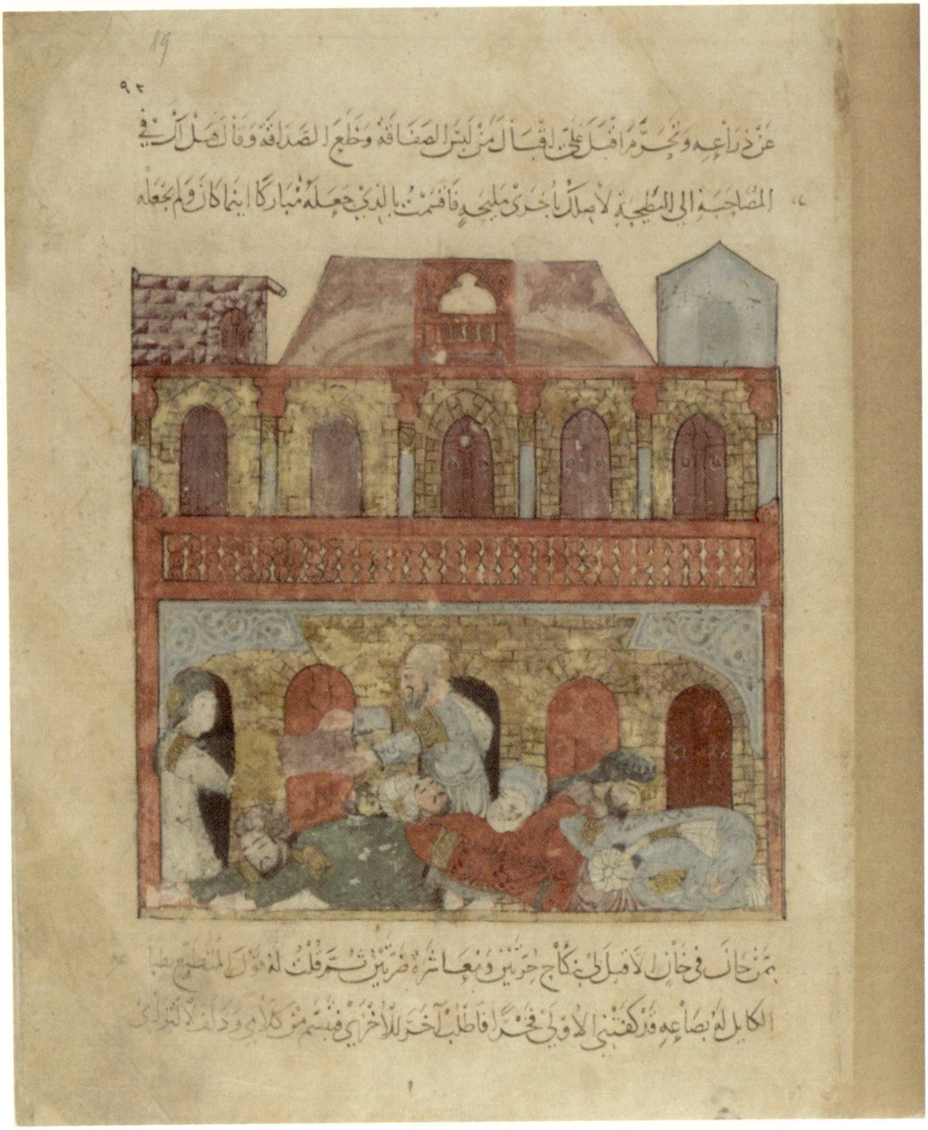

Fig. 8. Illustrations of the *khān* of Wasit in *Maqāmāt* de al-Harīrī al-Basrī. Abou Mohammad al-Qāsim ibn ʿAli ibn Mohammad ibn ʿAli al-Hariri al-Basri: *Les Makamat de Hariri ; exemplaire orné de peintures exécutées par Yahya ibn Mahmoud ibn Yahya ibn Aboul-Hasan ibn Kouvarriha al-Wasiti*, 1237 (Paris: BNF, MS arabe 5847, f. 89r).

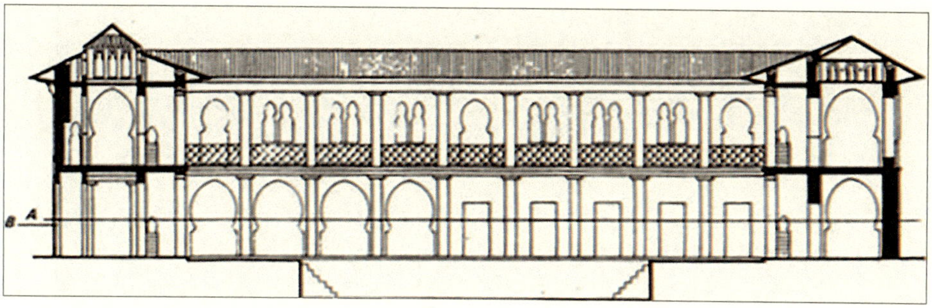


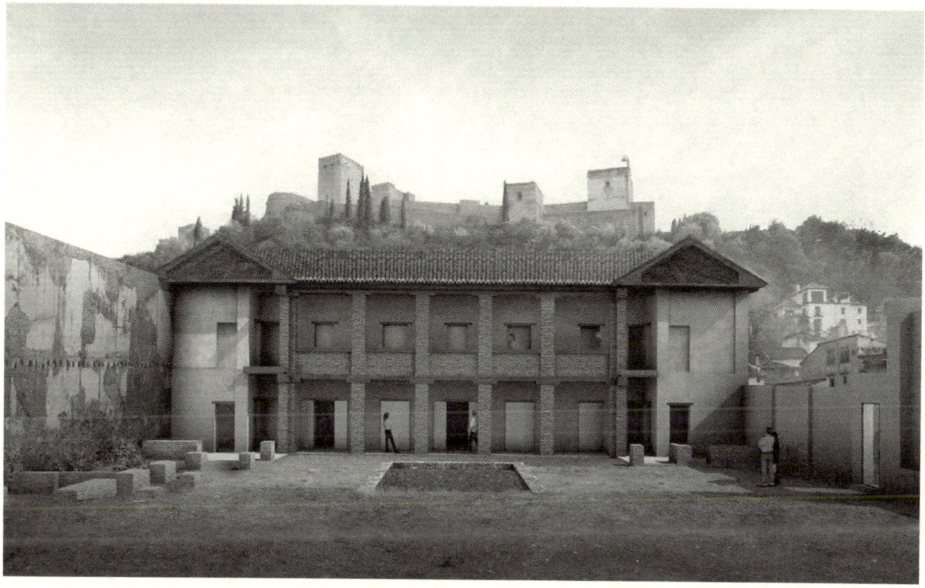

Fig. 9. Diagram of the longitudinal section of the Māristān of Granada, in contrast to the drawing by Francisco Enríquez. Image obtained from MARTIN, GARCÍA, 1984: 24.
Fig. 10. Virtual recreation of the recovered southern pavilion by Pedro Salmerón, Lucía Balboa and Antonio Jiménez. Image obtained from SALMERÓN et al. 2020: il. 18.

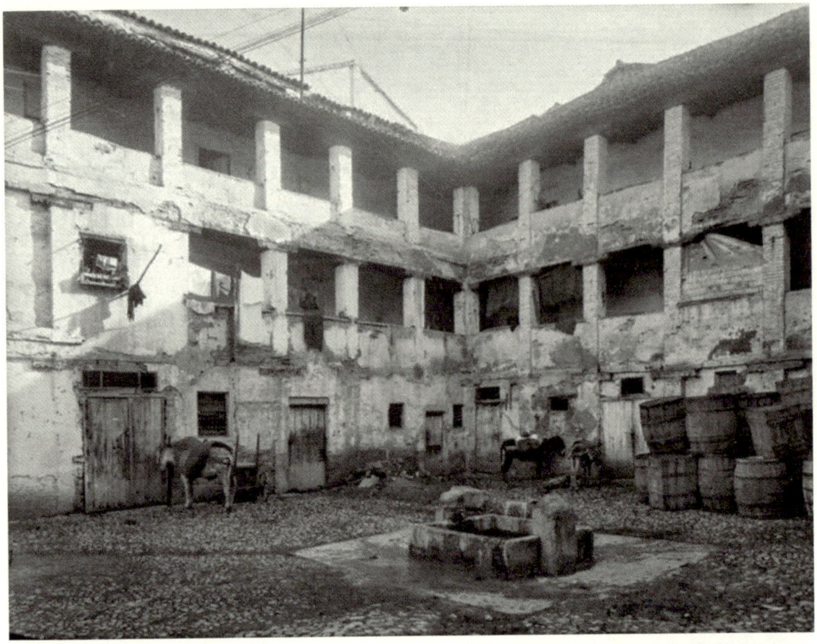

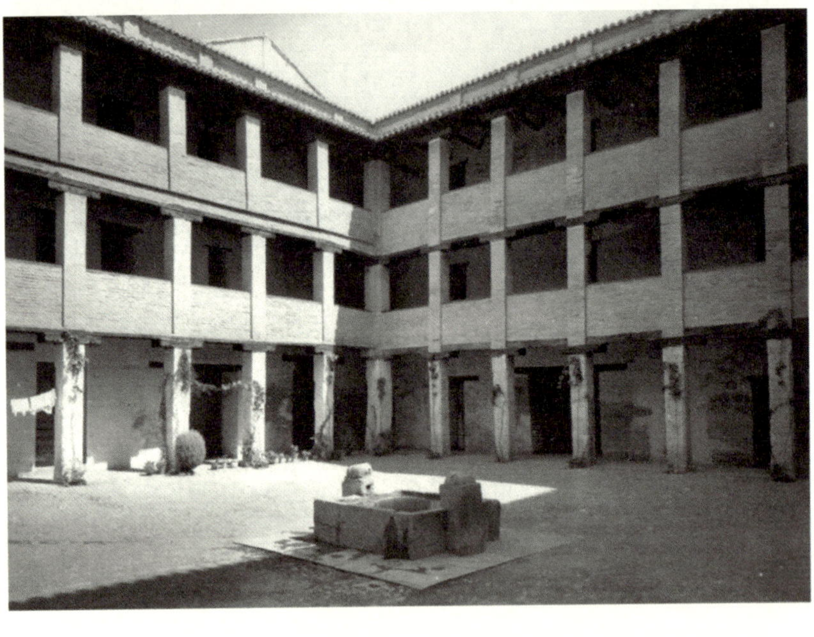

Fig. 11. Granada, Corral del Carbón before the restoration (1920-1930). Image obtained from Salmerón et al. 2020: 80.
Fig. 12. Granada, Corral del Carbón, (1930-1933?). Image obtained from Salmerón et al. 2020: 80.

# III
# *Territory and Documentary Sources*

Esther Diana

# The «Misericordia e Dolce» Hospital of Prato: A Physical and Symbolic Space (1218-2013)

The hospital between the 13th and 18th centuries was an institution with a medical and welfare mission that was framed within a context that was religious, economic, political, and, in the broadest sense, cultural. Its primary role, to manifest the *pietas* inherent in the act of care, was followed by that of the celebratory intentions of the promoter, be it public or private, secular or the representative of a religious body. The specific site in which the building or structure was placed, whether urban or extra-urban, was never an accident but always guided by its economic and social opportunities. These considerations also hold true in the history of the hospital of the Misericordia e Dolce of Prato.

## 1. *The Foundation*

Between the 13th and 14th centuries, the city of Prato, located about 20 kilometres from Florence, enjoyed a flourishing economy, based around the manufacturing of textiles (Carlesi 1904; Fantappié 1991; fig.1). This led to an important demographic increase that required an enlargement of the defensive city walls between 1192-1196, incorporating tiny settlements and scattered buildings that had arisen near the city. This is the case of a group of houses that were built between the 12th and 13th centuries at the corner of the south-west wall, near the Porta Fuja, then a nexus of an important road network. This strategic point hosted the hospital of the Misericordia (fig. 2). The institution was well placed to serve travellers on the network of pilgrimage roads that made Prato an important junction between Florence, Pistoia and Lucca, together with those who moved on the trans-Apennine Road to Bologna. Both of these roads connected at this exact spot (fig. 3).

A side road of the Via Cassia crossed the river Bisenzio at Ponte Petrino. Rather than entering Prato, it ran parallel to the river and, after passing the Castle of Pratum, seat of the Alberti family (at that time outside the city walls), headed south. It skirted the charcoal kiln near the city's southern walls, until it crossed the Roman cardo, which run from the gate of the Santa Trinità.[1] It then continued

1. Two important roads came from Pistoia: the via Romea Nonantolana, which went to the Passo della Croce Arcana, and the via Francesca della Sambuca which threaded the valleys of Ombrone, della Limentra Occidentale and del Reno (Stopani 2014: 55-76; Bologni 2007: 29-34).

towards the abbey of Santa Maria a Gricignano,[2] and ran in front of a Romanesque church devoted to Saint Barnabas. From there, it met the main route of the Via Cassia, leading to Pistoia, near the village of Petriccio and the oratory of Saint Paul, built in 1180 on the remains of the older parish church of the same name, also known as "a Stagnana".[3]

The hospital of the Misericordia was founded in 1218 by the municipality of Prato at the juncture of the two aforementioned roads with a road coming from the city center out of Porta Fuja. A canal carrying the city's water supply from the river Bisenzio, the Gora Gello, flowed along this spot. This secular hospital was immediately placed under the protection of the Virgin of Mercy (Maria Misericordiosa, hence its Italian name of Spedale di Santa Maria della Misericordia) and Saint Barnabas and commanded to be placed «*intra ecclesiam S. Barnabis*» (Bologni 1995: 21, 53, n. 37).

Saint Barnabas is usually depicted with the pilgrim's staff, the palm branch, and the gospel of Saint Matthew, and was venerated as a thaumaturge. Therefore, he was an especially appropriate figure to represent the hospital. The small Romanesque church consecrated to this saint had a single nave and a portal made of two-tone green and white marble; it was built at approximately the same time as the hospital. In 1220, the bishop destined it to serve the hospital as a religious place intended for the service of the sick and those who would find shelter there.

The place of worship provided an immediate comfort to the pilgrim, as expressed in the 'blessing hand' of the wayfarer imprinted on the lintel of the entrance portal along the road (fig.4). Anyone would have readily understood this iconography. Inside the church, a cycle of frescos was painted in the first half of the 13th century to celebrate the life of Saint Mary Magdalene (fig.5).

The cult of Mary Magdalene had been on the rise since 1050, when the Vézelay Abbey in Burgundy (along the Via Lemovicense to Santiago de Compostela) declared that it possessed a relic of the saint's body. In Prato, the cult was associated with the fight against the proliferation of leprosy (which pilgrimages encouraged) and the pressing phenomenon of the abandonment of children, the *gettatelli*, for whom the saint is considered as a protector. In fact, the Church of Saint Barnabas hosts Saint Mary Magdalene's oldest hagiographic cycle in Tuscany. Only two parts remain today: one depicting the saint receiving communion

2. There are no extant remains of the building, on whose grounds the Cicognini college was built in 1700.

3. Today, the site is known as Narnali. In the maps of the Capitani di Parte from 1585 (which were made by draftsmen and engineers belonging to the Magistratura degli Ufficiali dei Fiumi, founded in 1545 and charged with mapping the canals and roads of Tuscany). the oratory of San Paolo continued to serve as a juncture of the roads emerging from Prato, as the hub of four roads. Presumably two were directed to Pistoia. The first was that from the church of Saint Barnabas–Borgo Petriccio–Pieve di Sant'Ippolito–Agliana mentioned above, while the second ran north through Montale. The third one went toward Poggio a Caiano and joined the road to Pisa, while the fourth was the road to Bologna, which crossed the Appennines through Vaiano–Vernio–Montepiano–Castiglion dei Pepoli–Marzabotto–Sasso Marconi.

through the hands of an angel and the other consisting of fragments of a musician angel (MARCHINI 1937: 163; MANNINI 1993: 86-87).

Mary Magdalene, as well as being the patroness of the abandoned, was invoked as the protector of penitents and "precarious" women, that is, prostitutes and exploited females. It is understandable, therefore, how the hospital, driven by the itinerant flow of pilgrims and vagrants in search of redemption, also undertook the welcoming and assistance of those children who were abandoned in its vicinity.

## 2. *The Impact of the Hospital on the City and the Territory*

The increase in the intake of abandoned children had an important impact on the development of the hospital, so much so that a little more than twenty years after its foundation, in the statues of 1244, the Misericordia was already defined as a hospital «in which all the sick are received and cared for, and the orphaned and abandoned infants are nursed» (BOLOGNI, 2016: 23, CARRARA 1993:32).

This process of medicalization is present in the iconographic themes of the small church of Saint Barnabas, dating back to the second half of the 14th century. The fresco (fig.6) shows the attributes of saints who were invoked for specific diseases and conditions: Saint Steven for bladder stones; Saint Dominic as the protector of pregnant women; Saint Sebastian, the rescuer *par excellence*; Saint Nicholas, protector of unmarried women; and, finally, Saint Anthony of Padua, here invoked as a thaumaturge.

This increase in the social and medical-assistance roles of the hospital caused the progressive expansion of its fabric (fig.7). The hospital's original nucleus consisted of a two-story house behind Saint Barnabas, the ground floor of which was intended for women, while the upper floor was meant for men, for a total of twenty-three beds.[4] It had a cloister and a portico. In 1240, a *hospitale novum* was built, perhaps parallel to the church, on the opposite side of the road.

In 1310, the construction of the third and final circle of Prato's walls began, which brought the *Misericordia* within its confines, thus becoming one of the city's points of reference.

The building activity from the 14th and 15th centuries underlines, in fact, this development. In 1338, a yard was destined for a new refectory and a vast room lodge to accommodate pilgrims and the sick, which Francesco di Tieri, director of the hospital, entrusted to the master builder Arrighetto, who finished it in 1345.

The large rectangular infirmary had a row of five windows on each side, and between one bed and another, a niche had been carved out of the thick walls for the patient to keep whatever was needed during the hospital stay: this was called an *arredo* and it can be found in other hospitals, as it is the case in Siena, for

4. The first inventory dates back to 1273: Archivio di Stato di Prato (from now on ASP), Diplomatico, Spedali di Prato, 1273, doc. XI, also reported by: BOLOGNI 1995: 50.

example, at the female infirmary of Sant'Ansano in Santa Maria della Scala, dating from the late 12th century. This demonstrates the circulation of workmen who exchanged ideas, tips, and building know-how for what, in the following century, would be known as "hospital architecture".

In the same year, Bonaccorso di Cino began the painting of the wall's frescoes, which have only been preserved in parts of a *Last Judgement*. The theme is particularly significant, as it brings illness and sin together. It illustrates, within the hospital environment, the path to redemption, throughout which the sick person was to be guided in recovery of lost health. It depicts the sacred space of the hospital complex, replete with those pictorials and/or sculptural images that were thought to have the greatest impact on the patient. In this context, two polyptychs by Bernardo Daddi, one depicting a *Madonna and Child with Saints Francis, Bartholomew, Barnabas, Saint Catherine of Alexandria* (1325-1335), and one polyptych by Giovanni da Milano, depicting a *Madonna and Child with Saints Catherine of Alexandria, Bernard, Bartholomew and Barnabas* (c. 1355-1360), were commissioned for the female and male wards. This shows the emergence of a Marian cult, which underlined the Virgin's attributes as a protector of maternity and mercy. This can be linked to a process that took the hospital towards greater specialization. Pilgrims would still stay in the hospital, but they increasingly shared it with other groups: abandoned children and women and sick people afflicted by different pathologies. Logically, next to the image of Mary and the patron saint, Barnabas, the polyptychs depict other saints: Saint Catherine of Alexandria, often invoked by nurses and the mother and protector of abandoned children, Saint Bartholomew, again as a protector of children, and Saint Bernard, confessor saint *par excellence*, who was directly inspired by the Virgin and was a leading exponent of Marian devotion.[5]

This does not mean, however, that the hospital stopped catering to the needs of vagrants. However, the road network that, at the beginning of the 13th century, had had such a decisive impact on the hospital's location had by then become obsolete. With the construction of the last city walls, the roads were detoured and were then far from the hospital itself. Nonetheless, the *Books of the Sick* of the years 1401-1481 (Paolucci 1989: 113) attest to a substantial presence (more than 35-45% of patients out of a total of 2374 who registered a place of origin) of travelling patients, who mostly came from the rest of Tuscany, Italy, Northern Europe and especially Germany.

*Books of the Sick 1401-1481* = total admissions 3079
Hospitalizations with a declared place of residence: 2374 distributed as follows:
City of Prato: 508 = 21.3%
Prato County: 405 = 18.5 %
Tuscany: 659 = 27.7%

5. The hospital would function as an orphanage until 1817.

Italy: 367 = 15.4%
Germanic area: 282 = 11.8%
Other European countries: 153 = 6.4%

A stream of people who had no ties of residence or profession with Prato and its territory ended up requiring assistance while in the city. These were merchants, the itinerant poor, and other travellers, but presumably also pilgrims who were *en route* to Pistoia and Lucca, which were part of the most important pilgrimage routes of Northern Europe. These people found their way to the hospital, despite the fact that it was now far from the crossroads. In fact, the old path that rang along Saint Barnabas had now become a private space owned by the hospital, in which the *Spedalinghi* palace was built in 1468. This new building transformed the public image of the Misericordia, which ceased to be associated with the little church of Saint Barnabas and became linked to the aforementioned palace, a public and emblematic site, and the square it overlooked.

The subjugation of Prato to Florence in 1351 and, later on, the dramatic episode of its siege and sack by the pro-Medicean Spanish troops in 1512, followed by the plague of 1526, marked an all-time low point for the city. However, the *Misericordia*, after a temporary period of neglect, came to thrive more than ever before. In 1545, it merged with the other main hospital of Prato, founded in the mid-13th century by Dolce di Mazzamuti (BOLOGNI 2016: 85, DE BENEDICTIS, DIANA 2018: 23-63), the buildings of which had been severely damaged. Thc continued support of the Medici family was decisive for the success of the *Misericordia*, a protection that only increased with the establishment of the Grand Duchy of Tuscany (1569). In this context, the hospital's artistic patrimony came to represent more than simply the redemption of the sick: it was also an expression of the economic role of the *Misericordia,* but also of the founder, Dolce di Mazzamuti, and consequently became an emblematic celebration of its administrators and the institution as a whole.

## 3. *The Hospital and Its Image: The Hegemony of the Medici Family*

The 16th century was therefore a time of growth, which, from an artistic perspective, resulted in the commission of the portraits of the directors of the hospitals and the grand duke, together with paintings of the Medici's coat of arms (DE BENEDICTIS, DIANA 2018). Court painters such as Zanobi Poggini (doc. 1540-1563), Ludovico Buti (1550-1611) and Giovan Maria Butteri (1540-1606) were called in and commissioned for works where the aggregation of the two hospitals was celebrated through the effigy of their respective patrons: Saint Barnabas for the Misericordia and Saint Sylvester for the hospital founded by Dolce di Mazzamuti (fig. 8-10).

New developments were undertaken between 1558-84 and continued in the following century until the end of the eighteenth century. The year 1558 is the probable date of the enlargement of the building and the construction of the large quadrilateral cloister and loggia, consisting of six archways along the longer side and five on the shorter side. In the upper level there is a matching row of columns along three sides, with the fourth closed off by a row of windows with a large Medici coat of arms in the middle. Though we cannot be certain of the name of the architect, the simple but severe style recalls Alfonso Parigi the Elder (?-1590) of Prato, shortly thereafter employed in the building of the lateral chapels for Santa Maria delle Carceri, also in Prato. This important enlargement might have served as an update for the services intended for pilgrims, which included a dispensary and specialised rooms for certain pathologies.

As we have said, the 16th century was a period of intense artistic activity, resulting in the commission of portraits, coats of arms, and works in which the union of the two hospitals was celebrated. However, this period was also marked by the increasing interference of Florence in the hospital's internal affairs: a clear example of this is the nomination of the hospital's magistrates, which from 1584 was brought under the influence of the Florentine *magistrato del Bigallo*, who came to direct all of the welfare institutions of the State. The century also saw great donations, such as that of Pier Francesco de' Ricci, who, not by chance, was the first secretary of Cosimo I, preceptor of his son Francesco, and from 1549, rector of the *prepositura di Prato*. During his tenure as rector, he lobbied, among other projects, for a new church to be built in 1558, which would be positioned behind the great cloister and adjacent to the original chapel dedicated to Saint Barnabas. Between 1612 and 1619, the architect Ottaviano Cernieri built a new dormitory and refectory for "maidens" behind the original nucleus of the 11th century hospital.

The enlargement of the *pellegrinaio* was only undertaken at the end of the century, triggered by the 1630 outbreak of the plague and the economic and demographic crisis that followed. The building was completed between 1696 and 1703 with the construction of its south side, which included the baroque altar that displayed *La Probatica Piscina,* a canvas by Alessandro Gherardini (1655-1726).

The accession of the house of Habsburg-Lorraine to the Tuscan throne (1737) coincided with the development and growth of institutions that were increasingly oriented toward supporting the medical progress of the time. A meticulous *regolamento* (regulations) was adopted in 1776 by Marco Girolami Covoni, as desired by the Grand Duke Peter Leopold. It included modernising norms –both functional and administrative– for the hospital, which had now returned to the management of the municipality of Prato, and, therefore, was removed from the aegis of the *magistrato del Bigallo*.

To comply with the patients' pressing requests, the hospital incorporated in 1783 a new complex nearby the monastery of Saint Catherine, which was then transformed into an infirmary for infectious patients (tuberculosis, smallpox, typhoid fever, etc.) and utility rooms. During the same century, a new ward called San Giuseppe completed the southern perimeter of the square, finally burying all that was left of the Gora Gello.

The 17th and 18th centuries also saw the first efforts to dispose of ancient artwork, due to the change in fashion that led to the destruction of the medieval frescoes. Of the 60 paintings listed in the 1739 inventory, only 19 remained nine years later. This was the moment when the hospital turned from an artwork purchaser to a seller. However, donations continued to come thanks to direct bequests such as the Miniati inheritance and indirect ones such as those received from the suppressions of religious orders at the end of the eighteenth century and the subsequent suppressions imposed by Napoleon's laws. A substantial artistic heritage was then subject to theft, sales, or donations, but it still remained substantial at least until 1897, when 132 works of art were transferred to the city, to be displayed in the Municipal Gallery.

## 4. *And now?*

The Misericordia ended its healthcare activity in 2013, when the new hospital of Santo Stefano was built. Then, a debate about the destination of the institution's rich artistic and structural heritage began. What role could such an institution, so rooted in the history of Prato, play? The Region of Tuscany, together with the Documentation Centre for the History of Assistance and Healthcare, has initiated a project of musealization of the Misericordia, as part of a plan to include ancient medieval Tuscan hospitals in cultural tours. A 1960s-era wing of the building is to be demolished, liberating a very large area that, in the past, was part of the hospital's farmlands. This recovered space will form part of an 'urban park' planned by the municipality of Prato, which has been planned as a pole of attraction for the entire city and its tourists. Therefore, the complex of the Misericordia has to become an historical reference within the contemporary image of Prato.

## *Bibliography*

BICCI, Alessandro; SARTI, Claudio, 2019. *Prato: storia di un ospedale mai inaugurato*, Florence, Polistampa.

BOLOGNI, Giuseppe, 1995. *Lo Spedale della Misericordia*, Prato, Masso delle Fate.

BOLOGNI, Giuseppe, 2007. "Il percorso della via Cassia e della via Clodia in Toscana e nel territorio pratese", *Bollettino Roncioniano*, 7: 29-34.

BOLOGNI, Giuseppe, 2016. *Gli antichi Spedali della "Terra di Prato"*, Prato, Masso delle Fate.

CARLESI, Ferdinando, 1904. *Le origini della città e del comune di Prato*, Prato, Arnaldo Forni.

CARRARA, Francesca; MANNINI, Maria P., 1993. *Lo Spedale della Misericordia e Dolce di Prato*, Prato, Masso delle Fate.

DE BENEDICTIS, Cristina; DIANA, Esther, 2018. *Architettura e arte nei luoghi della salute. Gli ospedali dell'area Fiorentina,* Florence, Nardini.

DIANA, Esther (a cura di), 2015. *Il corpo e l'anima. I luoghi della e le opere della cura ospedaliera in Toscana dal XIV al XIX secolo,* Prato, Pacini.

FANTAPPIÉ, Renzo, 1991. "Nascita e sviluppo di Prato", ed. Giovanni Cherubini. *Prato, storia di una città. Ascesa e declino del centro medievale dal Mille al 1494*, Prato, Le Monnier: 79-299.

MANNINI, Maria Pia, 1993. "L'ospedale della Misericordia e Dolce. Le collezioni d'arte", Francesca Carrara, Maria Pia Mannini (ed.), *L'ospedale della Misericordia e Dolce di Prato*, Prato, Masso delle Fate: 79-130.

MARCHINI, Giuseppe, 1937. "Affreschi inediti in Prato", *Rivista d'Arte*, 19: 163-169.

MORSELLI, Piero, 1987. *Tommaso di Piero Trombetto. Aspetti della pittura pratese (1485-1530)*. Prato, Azienda Autonoma del Turismo.

PAOLUCCI, Giulio, 1989. "Gli infermi della Misericordia di Prato (1401-1491), Giovanni Pinto (ed.), *La società del bisogno*, Florence, Salimbeni: 101-129.

STOPANI, Renato, 2014. *De strata Francigena. Monachesimo e viabilità nella Toscana del Medioevo*, Florence, Centro Studi Romei.

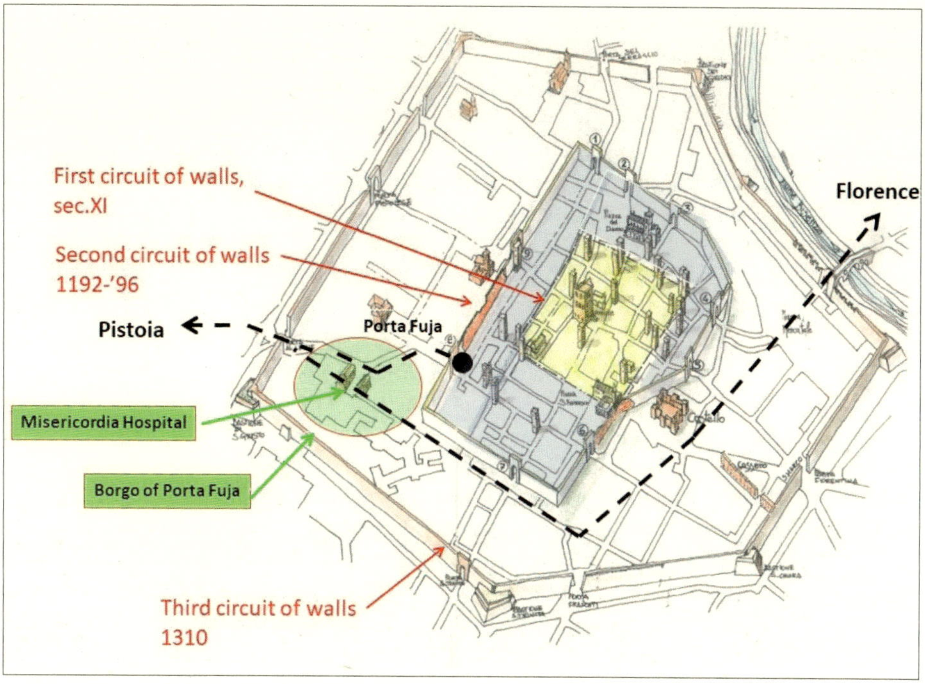


Fig. 1. Roads and urban growth: the Borgo of Porta Fuja at the intersection of the city streets and the Via Cassia, coming from Florence towards Pistoia-Lucca (12th-13th centuries). Graphic elaboration by the author.

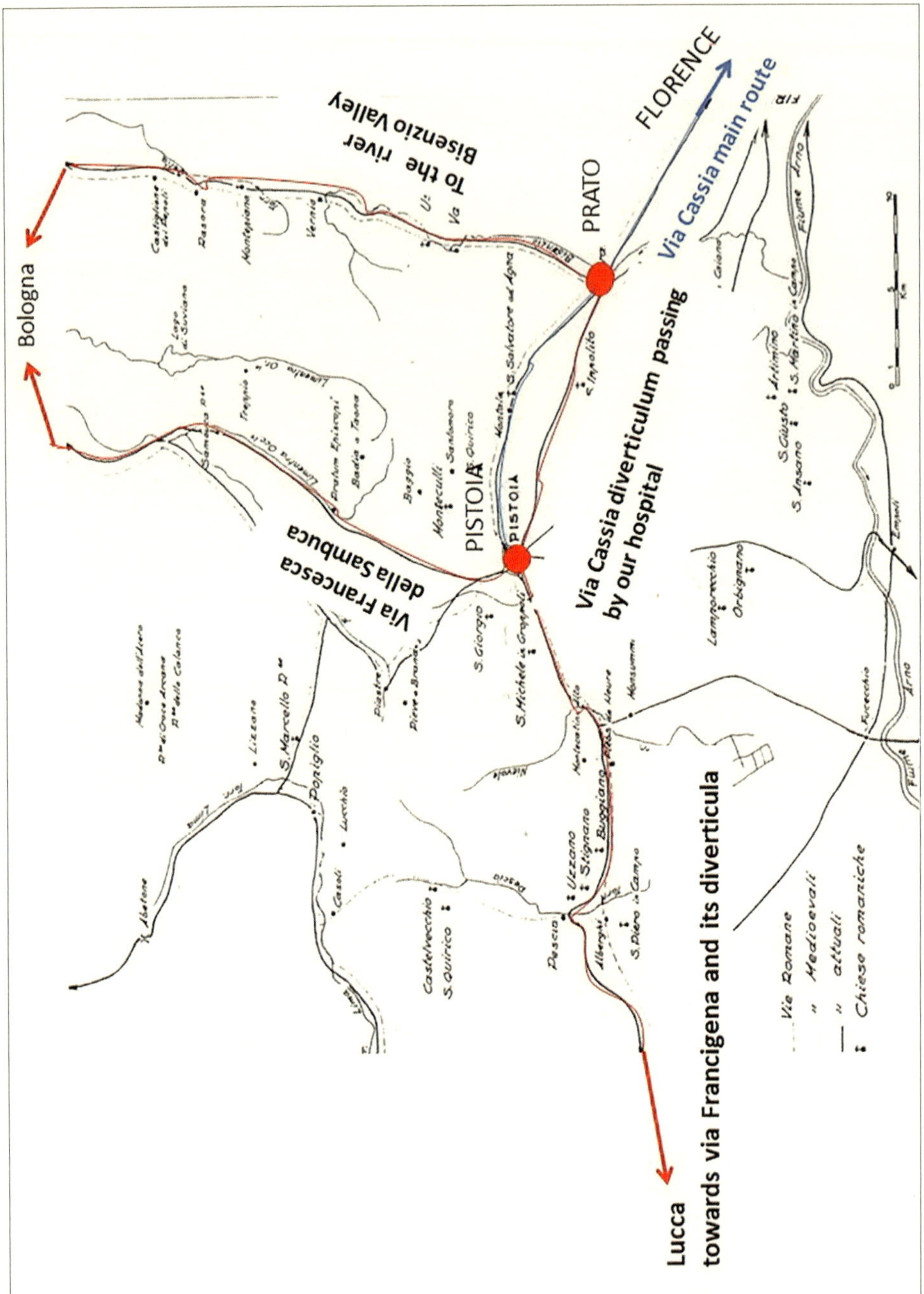


Fig. 2. The main pilgrimage routs passing by Prato in the 12th-13th centuries. Graphic elaboration by the author.

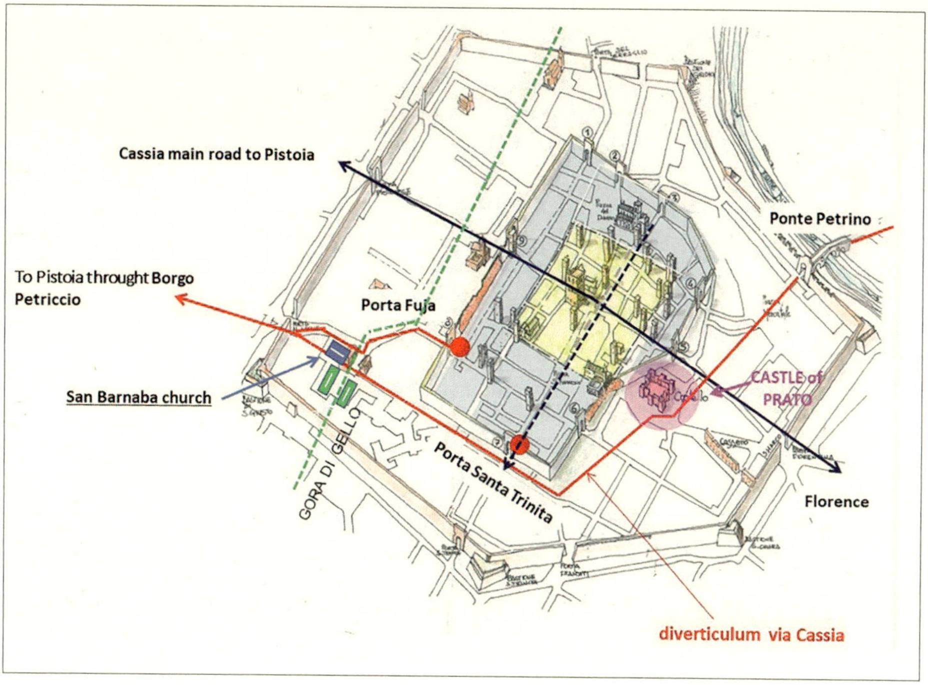


Fig. 3. 13th century: the foundation of the hospital in relation to the transit of pilgrims. Graphic elaboration by the author.

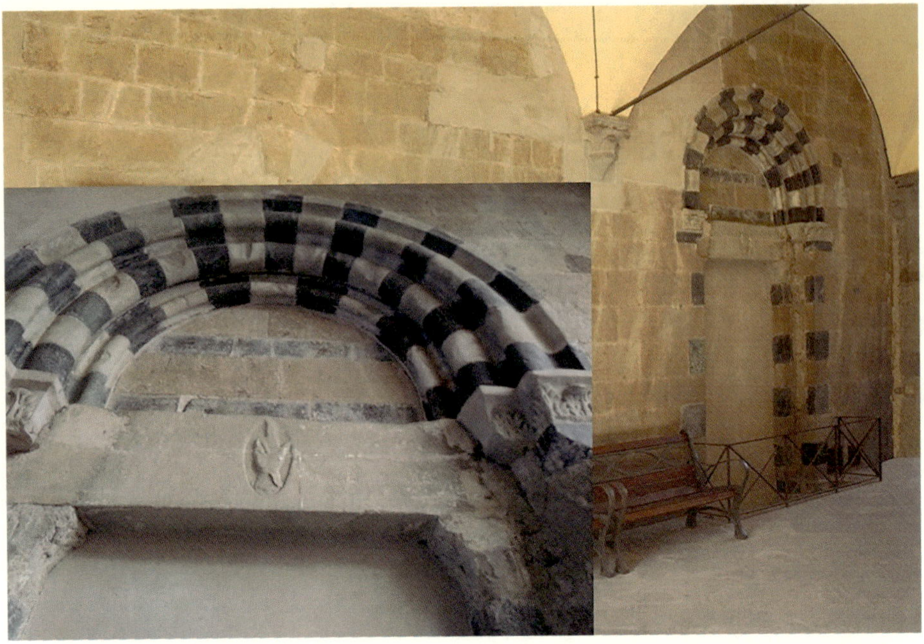

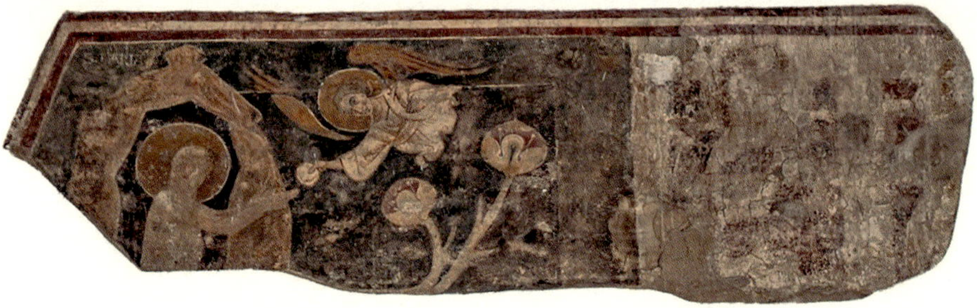

Fig. 4. Hospital as place of rescue and redemption. Church of Saint Barnabas: «blessing hand» imprinted on the lintel of the entrance portal along the road. Photograph by the author.
Fig. 5. Tuscan School: "Communion received by St Mary Magdalene through the hands of an angel", fresco, 13th century (Prato: Hospital of the Misericordia e Dolce, interior of St. Barnabas Church). Artistic representation was a path for catechesis, but was also careful to emphasize the increasing medicalization of the institution. Photograph by the author, authorized by the Hospital direction.

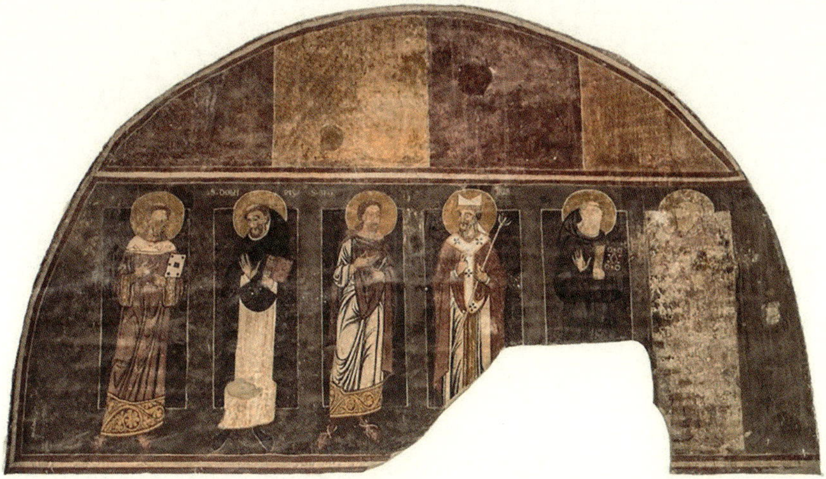
SANTO STEFANO
(for urinary calculosis )
SAN DOMENICO
(protector pregnant women)
SAN SEBASTIANO
(rescuer for excellence )
SAN NICCOLO'
(protector of unmarried women)
SANT'ANTONIO ABATE
(thaumaturge)

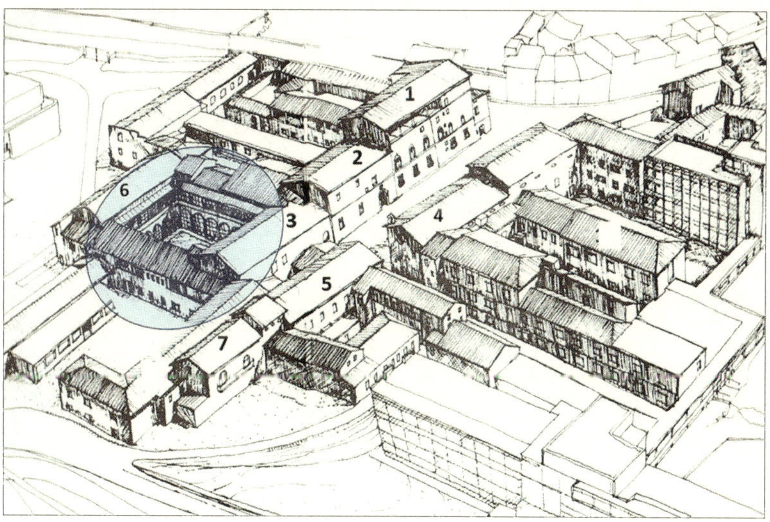


Fig. 6. Tuscan School: "Theory of the five saints", 14th century (Prato: Hospital of the Misericordia e Dolce, interior of St. Barnabas Church). Photograph by the author, authorized by the Hospital direction.

Fig. 7. Building expansions promoted by the Medici Gran Dukes. 1. Palace of Spedalinghi (1468); 2. Old church of St. Barnabas (13th century); 3. Old hospital (1218) and, behind it, the new church of St. Barnabas (1588): 4. *Pellegrinaio*, male infirmary (1345); 5. New hospital (1244); 6. Cloister and outbuildings (1558); 7. Residence for females (1612-1619). Elaboration by the author, based on a drawing by Antonio Caputo.

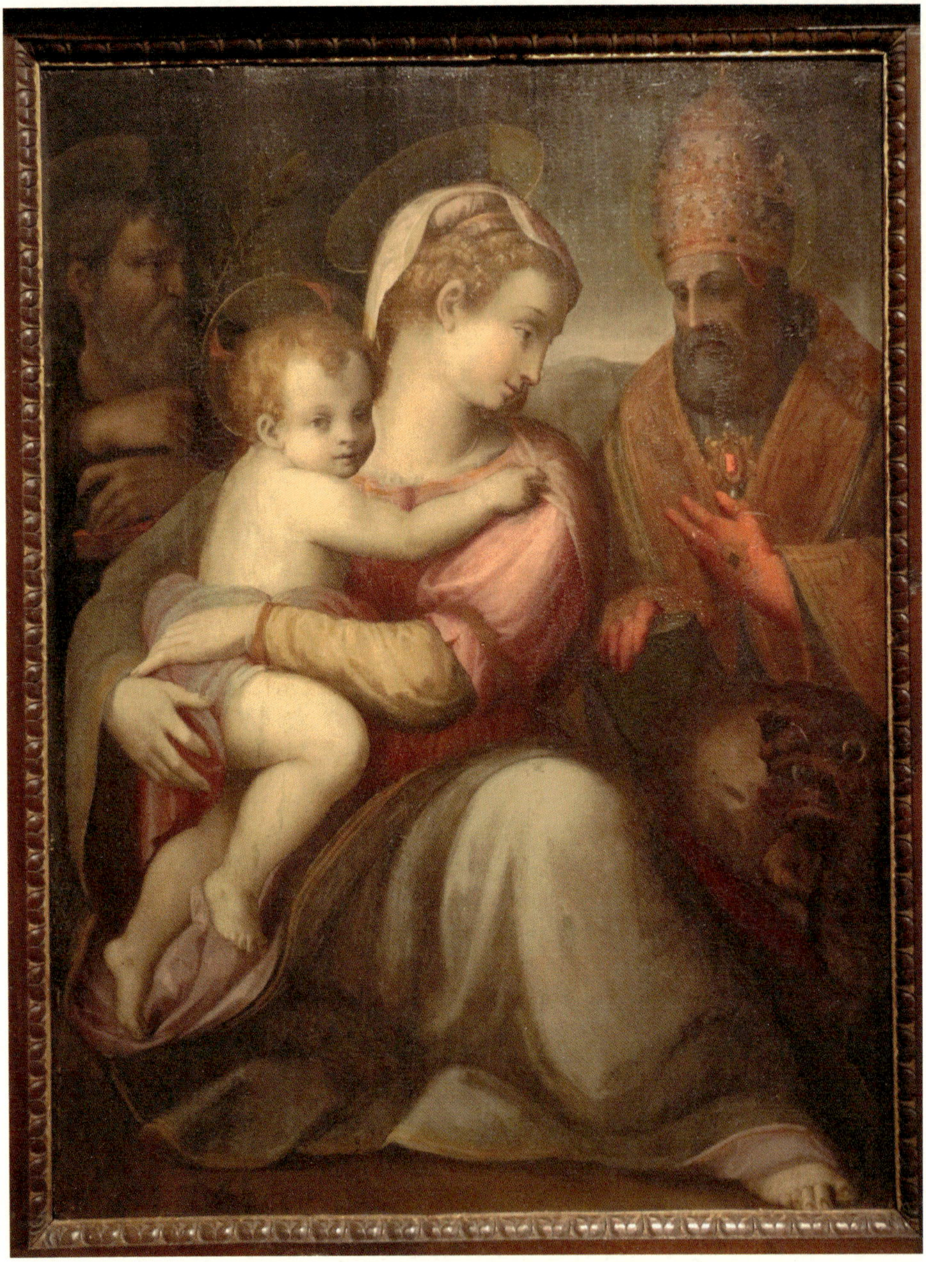

Fig. 8. Ludovico Buti: “Madonna and Child between saints Barnabas and Silvestro”, 1577 (Prato: Hospital of the Misericordia e Dolce, from 1858 to the Town Hall). The hospital’s role as a provider of healthcare and political encoding. Photo: © Wikimedia Commons.

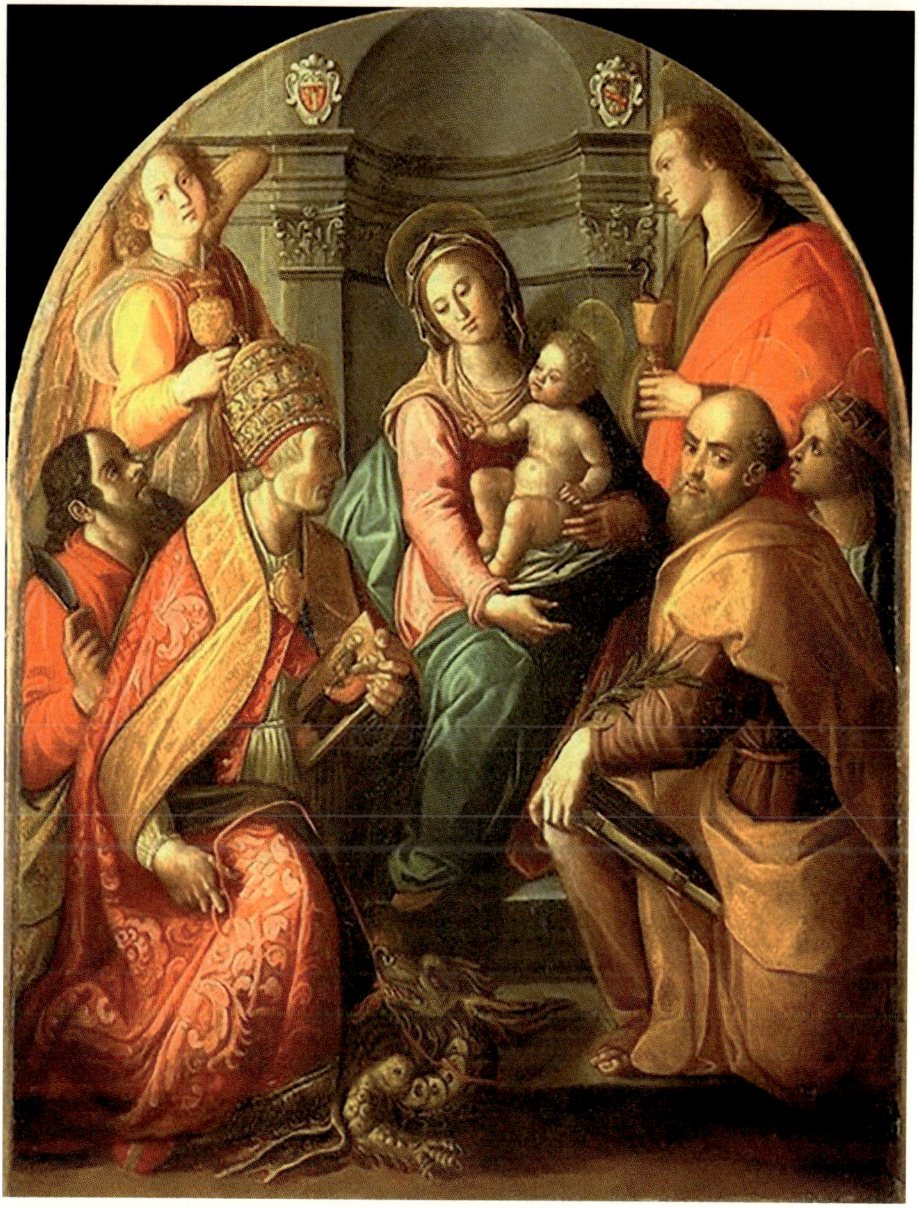

Fig. 9. Leonardo Mascagni: "Madonna with Son between saints Catherine of Alexandria, Bernard, Bartholomew, Barnabas, Silvestro, John the Evangelist and archangel Raphael", oil painting, 1618 (Prato: Hospital of the Misericordia e Dolce, from 1897 onwards at the Town Hall). Image obtained from DIANA 2015, 87.

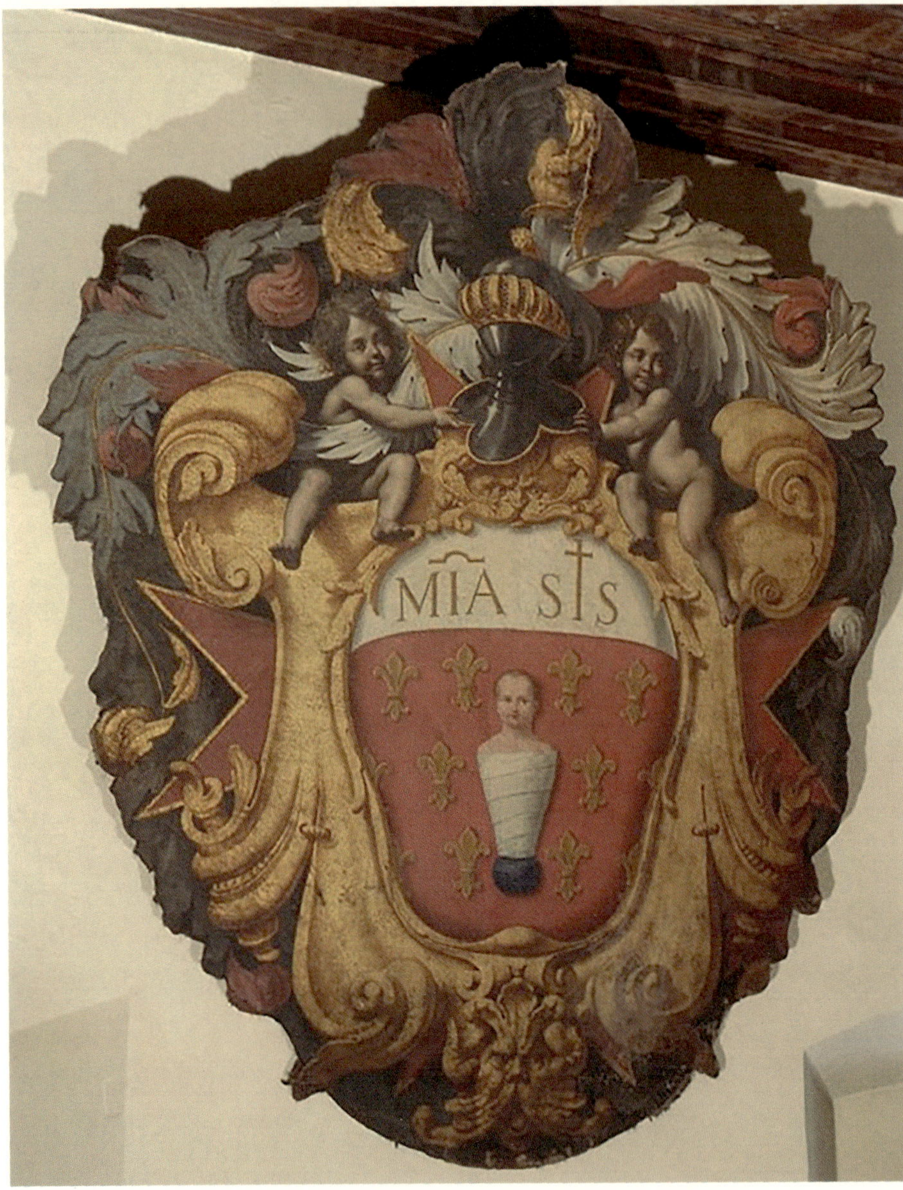


Fig. 10. Gian Pietro Naldini (attr.): "Heraldic coat of arms of the hospital", c. 1600 (Prato, Hospital of the Misericordia e Dolce, Palace Spedalinghi, Audience Hall). Photograph by the author, authorized by the Hospital direction.

Giuliana Albini

# Costruire e custodire i ponti.
# Le *domus pontis* nell'Italia settentrionale (secc. XI-XIV)

## 1. «*Sacralità dell'acqua, sacrilegio dei ponti*»: *dall'antichità alla cristianizzazione*

Prendendo l'avvio dal titolo di un classico degli studi antropologici sul tema, il volume di Anita Seppilli (1977), si possono cogliere alcune delle relazioni profonde che legano, in età medievale, la costruzione di un ponte alla tradizione di miti e rituali antichi, recepiti e mediati nella cristianità. In età antica, le fondazioni di edifici erano ritenute un sacrilegio, in quanto violavano la sacralità della terra. Nella costruzione di un ponte a ciò si aggiungeva la percezione della profanazione dell'acqua, simbolo di vita e purificazione, di rinascita e di morte. La sfida dell'uomo contro la natura portava con sé il timore di vendetta delle divinità quando oltraggiava l'acqua, il mare, i fiumi, i torrenti; percepita come un sacrilegio, ogni azione che turbava l'elemento fondamentale per la vita, l'acqua, doveva essere in qualche modo compensata da un sacrificio, anche umano. Cosa rimane di ciò nel Medioevo cristiano?

Negli sforzi condotti dalla Chiesa per sradicare i culti pagani, Gregorio di Tours comprendeva la difficoltà di opporsi ai miti che all'acqua facevano riferimento (Bartolomei 2017: 4). E molte leggende coniugano la costruzione di un ponte ad eventi soprannaturali. Come nel caso di san Colombano e del "ponte del diavolo" di Bobbio, che sarebbe stato costruito con l'aiuto appunto del diavolo, che chiedeva in cambio l'anima di chi per primo l'avesse attraversato. Il santo riuscì ad ingannare il diavolo, sacrificando la vita di un cane. Leggenda, certo, che però contiene in sé molti degli elementi presenti anche in altri racconti agiografici relativi alla costruzione dei ponti (Dinzelbacher 1900: 52). Spesso i demoni intervenivano e vite umane erano messe in gioco. Sacralità e sacrilegio richiedevano, comunque, di seppellire nelle fondamenta i cosiddetti "tesori di fondazione" o di porre edicole, cappelle, croci all'acceso ai ponti: il mondo divino pre-cristiano si trasformava, ma non si cancellava. Ai sacrifici umani e ai simboli pagani si sostituivano oggetti simbolici benedetti, spesso la croce, come si vedrà nel caso della fondazione del ponte sulla Staffora (Merlo 1987).

Il punto di attraversamento di un corso d'acqua, quali fossero le ragioni per le quali era stato prescelto e le modalità di superamento dell'ostacolo naturale (un guado, un *portus*, ossia un traghetto, un ponte), generava a sua volta una trasformazione dello spazio. Prendevano vita strutture che dovevano ottemperare a funzioni diverse, materiali e spirituali. Vi erano spesso edifici dedicati all'accoglienza dei viandanti, che necessitavano di ristoro e di ospitalità su una strada di lunga percorrenza. Altre funzioni, come l'assistenza durante l'attraversamento del corso d'acqua o il ricovero dei materiali necessari per la manutenzione o la riscossione di dazi e pedaggi, richiedevano spazi appositi. Ma oltre a ciò queste aree diventavano luoghi di religiosità, di preghiera e di carità. *Xenodochia, domus, hospitalia* insieme a chiese o cappelle caratterizzavano dunque le aree poste in prossimità degli attraversamenti dei corsi d'acqua come spazi sacri cristiani. Lo spirito di carità che per larga parte dei secoli medievali fu la spinta che sostenne la costruzione, la manutenzione dei ponti, insieme all'accoglienza ai poveri, ai viandanti, ai pellegrini. Come tali, dunque, essi erano sotto la giurisdizione ecclesiastica, anche in ragione della progressiva perdita di controllo sulle acque da parte del potere pubblico.

L'Italia padana, area sulla quale si concentra questo saggio, è caratterizzata da una notevole ricchezza di corsi d'acqua, di diversa entità. Non solo vi era la presenza del fiume Po (Greci, 2016), ma di tutti i numerosi affluenti di destra e di sinistra, e anche di numerosi corsi d'acqua minori, che creano un reticolo fitto e scomposto, che si intrecciava con una altrettanto ricca rete di strade e vie minori. La configurazione del territorio era tale da rendere necessario, a coloro che percorrevano le vie di più antica tradizione (come la Postumia) o la cosiddetta via Claudia o Romea o Francigena, l'attraversamento dello stesso fiume Po e dei suoi numerosi affluenti come necessità per continuare il loro viaggio verso l'Italia centrale, verso Roma, verso il sud dell'Italia (e di lì per la Terrasanta). Strettamente legata con l'evolversi della rete viaria (Szabò 1990; 1992a) fu la costruzione di ponti, in legno (Coppola 1996) e/o in muratura, che ne consentivano la percorribilità in corrispondenza di fiumi, torrenti, canali, che si intersecavano con il tracciato viario.

È possibile individuare tre periodi all'interno dei quali si mostrano alcune tendenze chiare:

- Secoli V-X: nella crisi del sistema stradale romano, si assiste a un deterioramento del patrimonio delle strutture in pietra (Inglese, Paris 2020) fino ad una loro quasi totale sparizione. Sono secoli nei quali il potere pubblico rinuncia, in questo come in altri ambiti, ad esercitare le proprie prerogative, cedendole via via, in varie forme, alla Chiesa.
- Secoli XI-XIII: in relazione alla ripresa generale della società europea e alla conseguente esigenza di ripristinare una rete viaria, si moltiplicano le imprese di costruzione di ponti. La nota rilevante, come si vedrà, è che tali opere furono nella quasi totalità gestite dalla Chiesa, o tramite ordini che si erano votati a questo compito, fra tutti i frati di Altopascio (Cenci 1996), o, più frequentemente, grazie ad iniziative di singoli individui o di comunità religiose

che individuarono nella costruzione e nella cura dei ponti un'opera di carità, dando vita ai cosiddetti ospedali di ponte.

- Secoli XIII-XIV: il controllo dei ponti sulle principali vie di comunicazione è oggetto di attenzione da parte dei poteri pubblici; in Italia centro-settentrionale sono i comuni ad intervenire e a determinare un nuovo sistema di gestione, che determina in molti casi la crisi degli ospedali di ponte.

## 2. *Un'età "senza ponti": la crisi dei manufatti romani*

Allo stato attuale delle indagini, si registrano nell'Italia settentrionale scarse presenze di ponti costruiti in età romana nell'Italia settentrionale, ovviamente con le dovute eccezioni, quali il ponte sul Ticino a Pavia. Alcuni ponti sono stati rintracciati nel Piemonte settentrionale, in Liguria e in Veneto, mentre era quasi assenti lungo il corso del Po e dei suoi affluenti, con l'eccezione della Romagna.[1] Più in generale, progressivo fu il deteriorarsi, in età altomedievale, dei manufatti esistenti, sino alla loro scomparsa: pur essendo strutture spesso possenti, in laterizi, soprattutto laddove si collocavano su strade di comunicazione importanti, gli stravolgimenti sia della rete viaria sia dei corsi d'acqua portarono a un pressoché totale abbandono di pur imponenti strutture, sostituite da più agili, seppur meno sicuri, mezzi di attraversamento, quali i traghetti posti in prossimità dei *portus*. Se tradizionalmente era il potere pubblico a occuparsi della manutenzione, nei secoli di crisi la capacità di controllo da parte di re e imperatori è andata via via perdendosi. Scarsi dunque i ponti, se non del tutto assenti, così come estremamente ridotti erano i luoghi di accoglienza (*xenodochia*) posti nelle vicinanze degli attraversamenti dei corsi d'acqua.[2] Un segno forte di tale stato di abbandono si può leggere nelle parole dell'imperatore Ludovico II, che concedeva alla moglie Angilberga di usare le macerie e tutte le pietre presenti sul territorio di Piacenza, e in particolare quelle del ponte sul fiume Nure, per costruire in Piacenza il monastero di S. Siro:[3] «[...] macerias omnesque petras et cymenta, quantocumque pre eundem comitatum Placentinum [...] Pontem vero Nuri ut supra ad supplementum eiusoperis proficere volumus ita ut quantum futuri monasterii strucura exigerit, libere ac potestative de quibus praediximus auferre liceat [...]».

Il potere pubblico non era dunque in grado di provvedere né alla manutenzione delle strutture viarie e dei ponti, né all'assistenza di viaggiatori e pellegrini lungo le vie di transito; sempre più frequentemente le istituzioni ecclesiastiche entrarono in possesso di diritti sulle acque e di compiti di custodia dei ponti.

1. Inglese, Paris 2020: 6, fig. 2. Così risulta sulla base della localizzazione dei ponti di età romana nella penisola condotta dagli autori.

2. Ancora in età carolingia, forse già segno di inversione di tendenza, l'imperatore Carlo il Calvo con un capitolare dell'865 chiedeva a monasteri e chiese di occuparsi della cura delle strutture di accoglienza (Albini 2016: 143).

3. *Monumenta Germaniae Historica* (da ora in poi MGH), Diplomata Karolinorum, DD, Lo II, 4, München, MCMXCIV, Corteolona, 874 ottobre 13: 198.

Significativo è il caso del monastero di San Colombano di Bobbio che aveva l'obbligo a mantenere in efficienza una parte del ponte di Pavia sul Ticino. Non si conosce l'origine di tale obbligo, che era comunque legato alla concessione della libera circolazione di propri prodotti su imbarcazioni sui fiumi Po e Ticino (Gazzini 2015: 487). Fu lo stesso imperatore Ludovico II a riconfermare tale obbligo, limitandolo però, contro evidenti pretese di altri, alle consuetudini precedenti all'860.[4]

Un esempio interessante riguarda il fiume Sesia e il cosiddetto Ponte di Notingo, dal nome del vescovo di Vercelli che ne divenne proprietario dai primi decenni del IX secolo. I resti sono stati recentemente individuati, a una decina di chilometri dalla confluenza nel Po.[5] Il manufatto era dunque posto sulla strada che collegava Pavia a Vercelli e Torino, servendo quindi da tramite viario tra Pavia, capitale del regno, Milano e le Alpi (Ferrari 2016: 90). Con diploma datato 6 marzo 882 Carlo il Grosso confermava alla chiesa vercellese *proprio iure* beni, diritti e privilegi; tra questi il ponte di Notingo: «[...] reddimus et confirmamus pontem Notingum, quem Notingus episcopus eiusdem Vercellensis ecclesie mirabiliter super eum equitando per legem recepit».[6]

La frase può essere stata interpolata nella copia trecentesca sulla quale si base l'edizione, ma è evidente testimonianza (come la conferma di Carlo il Grosso ribadisce) della dismissione da parte del potere imperiale dei diritti sul ponte. Ancor di più: come fa notare Aldo Settia (2016: 110), la vicenda si inseriva in un più ampio contesto di rinuncia da parte del potere pubblico alla costruzione e al controllo dei ponti. Nonostante i continui richiami nei capitolari, di fronte all'incapacità da parte degli ufficiali pubblici a gestire tali strutture, da Ludovico il Pio in poi si autorizzarono i privati a costruire ponti e si donarono ponti a persone o enti (spesso ecclesiastici) in grado di provvedervi.[7]

Una parabola si era compiuta (Szabò 1990), con la progressiva rinuncia da parte dei sovrani (imperatori e re) al controllo della rete viaria di tradizione romana e, con essa, dei ponti che consentivano l'attraversamento dei corsi d'acqua. La costruzione e la manutenzione dei ponti, in piena sintonia con la più generale crisi dell'ordinamento pubblico e con la diffusione dell'allodialità del potere (Tabacco 1993), passarono via via nelle mani della Chiesa, complice anche la dimensione religiosa che il ponte aveva mantenuto nel passaggio dal paganesimo al Cristianesimo. Lo sviluppo dei pellegrinaggi così come l'accento posto sulla carità come impegno dei laici finì per sostenere, come vedremo, un nuovo indirizzo di azione.

4. MGH, Diplomata Karolinorum, DD, Lo II, 4, München, MCMXCIV, Marengo, 860 ottobre 7, n. 31: 127-132.

5. Lungo circa 120 m, a 6 arcate, presumibilmente costruito nel I sec. aC (Panero, 2016: 42) i resti sono emersi nel letto del fiume tra Mantie e Motta de' Conti.

6. MGH, Diplomata regum et imperatorum, DD KIII, n. 54: 92-94, 93.

7. L'uso della locuzione *per legem* non presupporrebbe neppure un atto di concessione *ad personam* da parte del sovrano, ma un'acquisizione sulla base di una norma generale (Settia 2016: 110).

## 3. *La costruzione di ponti e di ospedali di ponte come opere di carità*

La crescita economica, che si fa sentire in modo particolarmente vivace nell'Italia centro-settentrionale dell'XI e XII secolo, portò ad un nuovo interesse per la viabilità e per la costruzione/ricostruzione di ponti (Szabò 1990; 1992b). Tale tendenza si coniugava alla vivacità della religiosità dei laici, che si manifestava, più ampiamente, in una "religiosità delle opere" che sostenne la fondazione di numerosi ospedali, in ambiente cittadino così come rurale. È un periodo nel quale muta anche la sensibilità verso la santità, che s'indirizza sempre più verso un riconoscimento delle figure attive nelle azioni concrete di carità: tra di essi anche i "santi della strada e del ponte" (Vauchez 2003).

La ripresa della costruzione di nuovi ponti in legno o in pietra, il ripristino e la manutenzione di quelli esistenti, la trasformazione dei guadi e dei traghetti con strutture stabili: sono tutte attività che trovano ampia testimonianza in tutta l'Italia centro-settentrionale e riguardano così i grandi fiumi (con l'eccezione del Po) come i fiumi, i torrenti, i corsi d'acqua (anche artificiali).

Interessanti i riferimenti alla presenza di manufatti preesistenti, caduti in disuso e progressivamente riattivati, o di ponti che furono costruiti su precedenti romani, ad esempio di una *statio* in un percorso stradale. È questo il caso del ponte sul Mella, vicino a Brescia, sulla strada che si dirigeva verso Bergamo e Milano, presso il quale era attestato un ospedale di S. Giacomo dei Romei, sorto probabilmente dove si trovava una *statio* romana. Si trattava di una comunità di *fratres* e *sorores*, che fu poi aggregata all'ospedale di S. Antonio di Vienne (Forzatti 2001: 49).

Il ponte sul Nure, che era in rovina nei secoli precedenti, acquistò nuova vita tra XII e XIII secolo grazie alla nascita di una *domus pontis*, che raccoglieva l'attenzione dei testatori nei loro legati. Il caso è interessante perché alla gestione del ponte si interessò il priore dei Cavalieri di S. Giovanni di Gerusalemme (1235), ordine che ne acquisì il controllo strappandolo alle mire del paratico dei *callegari*, che aveva contribuito alla gestione dell'opera. Che al centro degli interessi della *domus* vi fosse la gestione del ponte è chiaramente indicato al momento dell'acquisizione da parte dei cavalieri di S. Giovanni, che se ne assumeva i debiti (Albini 2002: 140):

> Quod ipse nomine dicti hospitalis solvet debita domus et pontis de Nuro et quod pro dicto hospitali et ipsum hospitale manutenebit pontem de Nuris bene apertum et refectum ad utilitatem peregrinorum et omnium aliorum hominum transeuncium et generaliter omnium hominum de Placentia et de districtu et hospitale similiter quod est ibi ad opus peregrinorum et pauperum perveniente ipsa domo et ponte in dominio et possessione dicti hospitalis.

Può essere difficile immaginare che la costruzione di un ponte possa essere considerato un'opera di carità. In realtà vi sono ragioni che ci devono portare a considerare come ciò fosse assolutamente congruente con la religiosità del tempo. Al permanere nella tradizione cristiana di una percezione della sacralità dell'acqua e dei ponti si univa un'altra eredità antica, ossia le pratiche di evergetismo tra i quali il sostegno alla costruzione di edifici pubblici, anche strade e ponti. Le concrete manifestazioni di carità cristiana si modellavano in parte sulla tradizione evergetica, che si trasformava secondo i modelli cristiani, ma pesava soprattutto nella sua dimensione civile (ALBINI 2016). A queste considerazioni si deve aggiungere la dimensione della carità cristiana come sostegno ai pellegrini e ai viandanti, a coloro che, lontani dalle loro case e dei loro affetti, cercavano aiuto e sostegni: accogliere lungo la strada coloro che necessitavano di aiuto era uno degli atti caritatevoli che avevano sostenuto la nascita di *xenodochia* e *hospitalia* lungo le vie di pellegrinaggio, anche in prossimità dei transiti dei corsi d'acqua. Alla luce di queste riflessioni forse possono apparire più chiare le ragioni che spinsero molti laici devoti a impegnarsi in un *opus pontis.*

Gli attori delle vicende sono diversi, ma in tutti i casi si possono individuare alcune costanti:

- La presenza di singoli o di piccoli gruppi di uomini e donne religiose, che dedicano i propri beni e se stessi alla costruzione o alla manutenzione di ponti, collegati spesso con la presenza di una struttura di accoglienza (*domus, hospitale*).
- Lasciti testamentari e donazioni che beneficiano queste opere al pari di monasteri, ospedali, chiese.
- L'interessamento da parte di enti ecclesiastici (pievi, monasteri, chiese cittadine), che, come accadeva per ospedali sorti al di fuori degli ordini religiosi ad opera di laici, tentavano di porre sotto il proprio controllo tali opere e i gruppi religiosi che le gestivano.

Il caso più noto è quello dell'ospedale di Altopascio, sorto negli ultimi decenni dell'XI secolo, lungo la via Francigena, vicino a Lucca, tra le paludi di Fucecchio e la valle dell'Arno. Dalla fondazione a opera di laici, cittadini di Lucca, e di canonici (SPICCIANI 2007), luogo di accoglienza per i pellegrini, la comunità ospedaliera si sviluppò, sino a divenire un ordine, con ospedali e *domus* in tutta Europa (CENCI 1996), favorita anche dall'appoggio di papi e imperatori. L'ospedale sviluppò, come noto, una finalità particolare, quello dell'impegno nella costruzione e nella custodia dei ponti e delle strade. A dimostrazione degli interessi che ruotavano intorno a tali funzioni basti ricordare che, a metà Duecento, l'ospedale di Altopascio era l'ente ecclesiastico più ricco della diocesi di Lucca (SALVESTRINI 2008: 392), con un'intensa attività economica, anche di prestito di denaro (SPICCIANI 2009). La sua rete si estendeva in tutta Europa, sostenuta anche dalla diffusione di un sistema di riscossione di elemosine legata alle concessioni di indulgenze,[8] che avevano uno scopo preciso, come emerge dalla bolla

8. Molti ospedali ottennero dai pontefici la concessione di raccogliere elemosine concedendo indulgenze (ALBINI 2016).

di Clemente IV del 1266:[9] «ad opus pauperum et infirmorum in eodem hospitali (Altipassus) degencium necnon pro constructione cuiusdam magni pontis lapidei, quem de novo super flumen Arni, ubi multi periclitari solebant, opere sumptuoso inceperunt construere».

In effetti, sono attestati questuanti che in tutta Europa (Francia, Inghilterra, Germania) raccolgono elemosine, in cambio di indulgenze, destinate al ponte di Fucecchio sull'Arno, a nome dell'ospedale di Altopascio (MEYER 2007a: 198). L'opera, iniziata nei primi decenni del XII secolo in collaborazione con altri due ospedali, di Rosaia e Campugliano, sul finire del secolo era appannaggio del solo ospedale di Altopascio, che aveva acquisito tutti i diritti sul transito di persone e merci. Il pedaggio non era richiesto ai pellegrini, ma era dovuto da mercanti e viaggiatori (MEYER 2007b): le entrate erano notevoli. Interessi economici ruotavano intorno alla gestione del ponte, mediati attraverso la gestione di enti ecclesiastici: non tanto monasteri ma piuttosto nuove realtà, come l'ordine di Altopascio, capaci di inserirsi in dinamiche non solo locali.

Fondazione di un ospedale, costruzione di un ponte: un binomio che spesso troviamo associato tra XII e XIII secolo, pur con variabili diverse da luogo a luogo alcuni elementi sono sempre presenti, ossia la religiosità di laici devoti e il rapporto, spesso conflittuale, altre volte di collaborazione, con un ente ecclesiastico. Si potrebbero richiamare molti esempi che gli studi hanno analizzato, così come molti che ancora attendono di essere indagati. Ne uscirebbe un panorama assai variegato nel quale emergono esigenze nuove e, insieme, antichissime istanze, che hanno il comune denominatore in una evoluzione del rapporto con l'acqua e con il ponte: una natura che sempre più frequentemente deve essere piegata all'esigenza degli uomini, al di là di ritualità più o meno soprannaturali, ma concretamente immerse in una religiosità delle opere che individua nell'*opus pontis* una modalità di esercizio della carità cristiana che è insieme servizio per una comunità e per le sue esigenze economiche.

Così il caso della fondazione dell'ospedale di S. Giacomo di Stura, fondato nel 1146 da un cittadino torinese, Pietro Podisio, che lo aveva donato all'abate vallombrosano di S. Benedetto di Piacenza (CASIRAGHI 1999). L'ospedale, dotato di un notevole patrimonio dallo stesso Podisio non era solo uno dei molti ospedali fondati da laici in quel periodo, perché aveva una caratteristica particolare: l'abate vallombrosano doveva istituirvi uno xenodochio a favore dei poveri e organizzare un traghetto sul fiume Stura, con imbarcazioni sempre pronte per le esigenze di viandanti e pellegrini che percorrevano "la via di Francia" (SERGI 1996). Un paesaggio in trasformazione, un territorio suburbano in espansione che gravitava intorno ad un fiume, ma che era nel contempo un'area importante per le comunicazioni (ramo della Francigena) verso la pianura padana. Ma non ci si ferma qui. All'inizio del Duecento, altri laici, appartenenti a famiglie di prestigio

9. Citazione da MEYER 2007a: 199.

torinesi,[10] sostennero il progetto di una sostituzione del traghetto con un ponte e l'istituzione di un ospedale di ponte, che avrebbe preso la titolazione di S. Maria del Ponte di Stura e acquisito autonomia di gestione, con il pieno sostegno dei ceti dirigenti cittadini. L'opera, sotto il manto della carità cristiana, rispondeva a esigenze economiche che vennero sostenute dall'intera comunità cittadina. La manutenzione del ponte, in legno, spesso distrutto, fu oggetto di conflitti con l'abate vallombrosano e diede luogo a diversi arbitrati, che si conclusero di fatto con un progressivo distacco del nuovo ente (chiesa, ospedale, ponte) di S. Maria della Stura.[11]

Meno noti, ma non per questo meno importanti, sono i casi di esperienze religiose nell'area del corso centrale del Po e dei suoi affluenti, area nella quale il transito delle acque era elemento fondamentale per consentire il proseguimento del viaggio e/o del pellegrinaggio verso Roma e Gerusalemme.

Una *domus pontis* sul fiume Trebbia è attestata nella metà del XIII secolo: della custodia del ponte (posto in località di Quartazzola) si dedicava una comunità religiosa di *fratres*, governata da Niccolò, *minister dicti pontis*. Ciò emerge con chiarezza da un atto solenne, datato 8 febbraio 1143,[12] presente nel *Registrum Magnum* di Piacenza (ed ivi registrato per volontà dei consoli) con il quale il vescovo di Piacenza giungeva ad un accordo per il controllo del ponte, concedendo l'ente, con tutti i suoi beni e diritti, all'abate di S. Salvatore, dell'ordine pugliese di S. Maria di Pulsano, monastero da poco sorto nella località di Gossolengo.[13] L'atto è interessante, dal momento che attesta sia la nascita spontanea di una comunità che si occupava della cura del ponte sia l'intervento dell'ordinario diocesano per inquadrare l'esistenza di tale gruppo in un ordine religioso. È un percorso usuale, attestato per diverse comunità "di ponte", che nel caso particolare presenta il carattere di un vero e proprio accordo, con il quale non si vuole (o non si può) estromettere il ministro della *domus*, ma si vuole nel contempo garantire la sicurezza della gestione del ponte. L'atto, infatti, insisteva ripetutamente sul fatto che al ministro, Niccolò, e dopo di lui alla comunità sarebbe continuata a competere la gestione dell'opera di ponte, salvo che non si dimostrasse in grado di mantenere in efficienza il ponte; in tal caso il vescovo poteva decidere di affidarne ad altri la cura:

> Quod ipse sanctus conventus qui ibi fuerit prenominatum pontem facere et retinere debet; set donec Nicolaus predicti pontis minister adviserit, ad ipsum pontem stare debet et facere et retinere; post autem eius decessum, prenominatus sanctus conventus similiter ipsum pontem facere et semper retinere debet et prefatam possessionem predicti pontis habere. Set, si contigerit in aliquo tempore quod prefatus sanctus

10. Sul contesto economico e sociale si veda di Torino nel periodo; v. Bordone 1997a; 1997b.

11. Le vicende qui rapidamente sintetizzate sono attentamente analizzate in Casiraghi 1999.

12. Falconi, Peveri, 1986, III, doc. 892: 600-603.

13. Fondato intorno al 1130, sarebbe entrato a far parte dell'ordine dei Cistercensi (Cariboni 2003: 90, 100). Nell'atto citato si precisa che il suddetto monastero *subiacet et obedit* al vicino monastero cistercense di S. Maria della Colomba.

conventus predictum pontem non fecerit vel non retinuerit, sicuti facere debuerit secundum sensum episcopi qui nunc erit et clericorum atque laycorum sapientum civitatis, episcopus qui tunc fuerit, cum conscilio clericorum et aliorum sapientum civitatis, ad istum pontem alias persona ordinare et collocare debet, que administracionem pontis habeant [...].[14]

Intorno al fiume Trebbia, in prossimità del suo attraversamento a poca distanza da Piacenza, presso Gossolengo, si era creata un'«area di ponte» (MERLO 1987), con l'insediamento non solo della comunità di ponte, ma anche di una nuova comunità monastica. I segni religiosi andavano crescendo: l'ospedale si dotava di una chiesa, con la presenza di un sacerdote. La presenza del monastero portava con sé nuovi interessi, economici oltre che religiosi. Aree che erano marginali diventarono oggetto di interesse da parte da parte della Chiesa cittadina e degli esponenti delle più note famiglie cittadine.[15]

Si tratta di dinamiche individuate in altre aree, come nelle vicende che riguardano il ponte sulla Staffora e l'area circostante. La costruzione del ponte sulla Staffora presso Voghera fu avviata da Giovanni Raviolo, un canonico della chiesa di S. Marciano di Tortona,[16] che intendeva «laborare in honorem Dei et Sancti Marciani et huius plebis» e a vantaggio del comune di Voghera e dei poveri (MERLO 1987: 215). Attorno all'impresa si muovevano interessi diversi: di controllo su un territorio, dal punto di vista ecclesiastico e civile, che coinvolgeva le città che vi facevano riferimento (Pavia, Voghera, Tortona) e le autorità che le governavano; economici, legati al miglioramento delle comunicazioni, ma anche all'espansione dell'agricoltura; religiosi, in quanto l'area che al ponte faceva riferimento era luogo di sperimentazione di modelli diversi di vita cristiana, con un coinvolgimento forte dei laici. Insomma, paiono coagularsi intorno al ponte scelte di vita assai diverse, che rimandano a comportamenti religiosi e sociali espressione di una volontà di rinnovamento che pervadeva la società del tempo. Con tale spirito si intraprendevano imprese ardite, come il progetto di Giovanni di costruire un ponte in pietra, a tre pile, servendosi della competenza di due esperti, Bongiovanni di Milano e Alberico di Michele. Il progetto non fu fermato neppure da una piena del torrente, che fece momentaneamente preferire un tentativo diverso, quello di Giovanni Paradiso, ministro dell'ospedale di S. Bovo, che si dedicò alla costruzione di un ponte in legno (MERLO 1987: 216). Ma il disegno originario, il ponte in pietra, sarebbe stato portato avanti nei decenni successivi, con nuovi interventi e nuovi uomini disposti a impegnarsi per la sua realizzazione:[17] e l'area circostante ne fu completamente trasformata. La presenza del ponte e della *domus* portò a una trasformazione dell'habitat, da incolto ad antropizzato. Diverse testimonianze, rese in occasione della controversia che nel 1183 oppose il vesco-

14. FALCONI, PEVERI, 1986, III, doc. 892: 601.

15. FALCONI, PEVERI, 1986, III, doc. 892: 602-603.

16. Non è chiara la sua collocazione, perché le fonti danno informazioni apparentemente contraddittorie. Si trattava comunque di un ecclesiastico.

17. Non seguiamo nel dettaglio le vicende, ricostruite con maestria in MERLO, 1987.

vo di Tortona al monastero del Senatore di Pavia per il possesso dell'ospedale e del ponte, così descrivevano l'abitato che si era venuto creando:

> Est quidam pons hedificatus in fluvio Stafole. Sunt et quedam domus iusta pontem in ierbo, ubi caput pontis positum est. Est et alia domus ultra stratam veterem, in quadam clausura que est e(m)pta a Moro, nomine pontis, postquam hedificavit pontem.[18]

Altre realtà erano presenti nel gerbido di proprietà del monastero di San Senatore: la chiesa, alla quale gli atti fanno spesso riferimento[19] e gli spazi dedicati all'accoglienza dei lebbrosi, già testimoniati prima dell'avvio dei lavori per il ponte. La *mansio pontis* si sviluppava anch'essa su terre del monastero (come ampiamente attestato dai testimoni) e si poneva come antagonista dei "malsani", tanto che il ministro ne aveva chiesto alla badessa l'allontanamento al di là del fiume, ottenendo però solo un loro spostamento oltre la *strata vetus* (Merlo 1987: 229).[20] Tutt'altro che pacifica fu l'occupazione di spazi, dal momento che la costruzione di case e recinzioni era osteggiata dagli abitanti. Pietro Sordo dedicatosi al ponte per continuare l'attività intrapresa da Giovanni aveva ottenuto dalla badessa una casa e un terreno; Pietro aveva recintato tutto con una siepe, suscitando con ciò la reazione delle persone che risiedevano lì vicino, perché ciò impediva loro di usare quelle terre come beni comuni per pascolare gli animali e per raccogliere prodotti spontanei. Dopo essere stato danneggiato nei suoi beni, Pietro fu costretto ad andarsene per intervento della stessa badessa di San Senatore.[21]

Dalle testimonianze del processo si apprendono notizie interessanti sull'area di ponte. Si trovano riferimenti a *cassine*, a una fornace, a mulini; a diritti di estrazione dell'acqua dalla Staffora e alla costruzione di una roggia: insomma a una trasformazione profonda dell'insediamento generato dalla costruzione del ponte e dalla presenza di una comunità di *fratres* ospedalieri che si occupavano di tale opera.

Molti testimoni nel processo del 1183 sottolineavano la dimensione religiosa dell'impresa, a partire dalla cerimonia di sacralizzazione del ponte. Tra gli altri, era la stessa badessa a descrivere con dovizia di particolari cosa accadde. Moro (o Mauro), colui che con la moglie, in una scelta religiosa condivisa, si era dedicato all' *opus pontis* e per anni ne era stato l'anima, attirando attorno a sé una comunità di converse e conversi, aveva richiesto alla badessa di dare solennità sacrale al lavoro compiuto. E la badessa aveva acconsentito, organizzando una liturgia

18. Le testimonianze rese al processo sono state edite e sono disponibili in Ansani, Baretta 2008. Il documento al quale si fa riferimento è *Allegationes iuris et dicta testium*, 1183 gennaio 21, Novara, doc. 111.

19. *Le carte del monastero di S. Maria del Senatore,* Instrumentum subiectionis, 1175 luglio 19, Voghera, n.79 (Ansani, Baretta 2008).

20. *Le carte del monastero di S. Maria del Senatore*, Breve iurisiurandi, 1178 aprile 29, Voghera, n. 89 (Ansani, Baretta 2008).

21. *Le carte del monastero di S. Maria del Senatore,* Instrumentum ad testes authenticandos et publicandos, 1183 febbraio 21, Novara, n.114 (Ansani, Baretta 2008).

che attestava, in pieno XII secolo, come la costruzione di un ponte fosse percepita come azione che si iscriveva in una dimensione religiosa:

> Insuper etiam sine dubitacione allegat abb(atiss)a se in inicio fundacionis ipsius pontis publice ivisse ad pontem cum suo sacerdote, convocatis hominibus et mulieribus, ca(m)panis sonantibus, deferendo crucem; et cum fuit ad pontem primum lapidem in ipso ponte posuit, missam per suum sacerdotem celebravit, pontem per eundem benedixit, aquam benedictam in ipso proiecit; missa finita, oblaciones quas ibi habuit Moro nomine pontis dedit. Iussit etiam suo sacerdoti ut ibi missam deinceps celebraret in omni die lune. Devotos et alios ibi sepultos idem sacerdos sepellivit [...].[22]

Gli elementi della sacralità sono molti: suono della campana, processione fino al ponte, con la croce, celebrazione della messa, aspersione con acqua benedetta, offerte. A conclusione di ciò i due capi del ponte furono dotati ciascuna di una croce, simboli di un luogo sacro, tale da consentire la raccolta delle elemosine a favore dell'opera; la celebrazione settimanale della messa e la sepoltura dei devoti completavano la dimensione religiosa del contesto nel quale veniva costruito il ponte.

Infine un ultimo esempio può aiutare a riannodare le fila dello stretto legame tra costruzione di un ponte e religiosità. Le notizie si evincono da una lettera pontificia di Alessandro III, in risposta ad una richiesta pervenutagli da un gruppo di ecclesiastici di Nonantola tra il 1173 e il 1179. Un uomo devoto, del quale non ci è nota l'identità, si era votato alla chiesa di S. Maria di Nonantola, con l'intento di collaborare alla sua ricostruzione, dopo la sua distruzione durante uno dei tanti episodi del conflitto tra Modena e Bologna per il controllo della zona (BONACINI 2000). Non sappiamo le ragioni per le quali egli decise di venir meno al voto fatto,[23] recandosi altrove, vicino a Parma, sul fiume Taro, dove era difficile l'attraversamento delle acque per dedicarsi a un ospedale di ponte «super fluvium Tari supra Parmam ubi solebant multi submergi cum auxilio Domini pontem construxit et multa operatus et que Deo et hominibus beneplacita de accepta videntur».

Sappiamo da altre fonti che esisteva già nel 1141 un *hospitale iuxta Taronem*, dipendente dai canonici di Parma, sotto la giurisdizione della pieve di S. Pancrazio. Attestato nel secolo successivo da diversi atti, era nel 1230 censito nelle *Rationes decimarum* come non sottoposto ad alcuna pieve, ma direttamente sottoposto al vescovo;[24] attorno al ponte, qui come altrove, sorse più di una comu-

22. *Le carte del monastero di S. Maria del Senatore*, Allegationes iuris et dicta testium, 1183 febbraio 21, Novara, n. 111. Si veda anche Instrumentum ad testes authenticandos et publicandos, 1183 febbraio 21, Novara, n. 112 (ANSANI, BARETTA 2008).

23. Traggo la citazione da AFFÒ III, LXXXII, p. 381, che a sua volta afferma di utilizzare la trascrizione riportata dal Tiraboschi, t. II, p. 257. Si veda anche KEHR, 1906, V: p. 354, che data il documento tra il 1173-1179. Il testo indica genericamente le difficoltà alle quali egli andava incontro: «Decurso autem longo temporis spatio cum non posset tentationes que superveniebant varias substinere [...]».

24. Le vicende dell'ospedale, i suoi rapporti con il pontefice, la distruzione e la ricostruzione sono descritte in: ALBINI 2002: 140-143.

nità ospedaliera e il controllo dell'ospedale di ponte fu qui come altrove oggetto di conflitti giurisdizionali.

Tornando al laico devoto che aveva lasciato la chiesa di Nonantola per dedicarsi al ponte sul Taro, la questione che era stata posta al pontefice riguardava la possibilità di sciogliere dal vincolo del voto fatto nei confronti della chiesa di S. Maria. La risposta del pontefice fu una chiara approvazione:

> Verum quoniam dubium vobis et incertum existit an de priori vero servaturum discretioni vestre presentibus litteris innotescat, quia idem P. votum non fregit in eo quod ad locum se alium transtulerit in quo Domino fructificare amplius potest et fructum reddere digniorem.[25]

Le parole del pontefice sottolineano come la nuova opera fosse più degna rispetto alla precedente e consentiva quindi l'assoluzione dal precedente voto. La costruzione di un ponte e la cura di un ospedale non solo eguagliavano il servizio per ricostruire una chiesa, ma erano considerate come maggiormente meritevoli agli occhi del pontefice.

## 4. *La crisi degli ospedali di ponte e il progressivo intervento dei comuni*

Già nel corso del XII secolo è possibile cogliere segni dell'interesse dei comuni cittadini a controllare la rete stradale e i punti di attraversamento dei corsi d'acqua (ponti e porti). La pace di Costanza (1183) sancì, in virtù delle concessioni imperiali, i diritti dei comuni ad esercitare tale potere. La via era segnata: i ponti da opere di carità si avviavano a diventare (o meglio a ritornare ad essere) opere pubbliche. E le comunità di ponte, ospedali, *domus*, *mansiones*, perdettero progressivamente le loro prerogative, pur continuando la loro esistenza.

Tale cambiamento si comprende solo se messo in relazioni alle trasformazioni in atto, sia dal punto di vista economico, sia da quello istituzionale. I comuni cittadini tendevano ad ampliare progressivamente gli spazi di intervento, acquisendo competenze in ambiti precedentemente appannaggio della Chiesa. Come per la gestione degli ospedali, sui quali si faceva sempre più pressante la volontà di controllo da parte delle autorità comunali, così avvenne anche per gli ospedali di ponte. Ciò è assolutamente comprensibile nel momento in cui controllare i ponti significava, per i comuni, garantire la sicurezza delle vie di comunicazioni (necessarie per i rapporti commerciali, e non solo) e ricevere anche, tramite pedaggi, introiti fiscali.

Concludo con un esempio, riprendendo il caso del ponte sul fiume Taro (*pons Taronis*). Qui si vede con chiarezza il progressivo intervento da parte del comune di Parma, che inizialmente agì utilizzando la presenza di quei gruppi di 'costruttori di ponte' che ancora erano in grado di garantire la manutenzione dei ponti e l'accoglienza ai viaggiatori. Le trasformazioni sarebbero avvenute in modo

25. Affò, III, LXXXII, p. 381.

graduale, così come attestato dagli statuti cittadini: «De pactis inter Commune Parma et Pontem Taronis de strata Claudia observandis. Capitulum quod potestas teneatur adtendere in perpetuum omnes promissiones et pacta et transactiones factas et facta inter Commune Parmae et Pontem Taronis de Strata Cluadia ipsi Ponti seu ministris ipsius pontis, secundum quod continetur in carta facta per manum Rolandi Gilli».[26]

Dunque era stato stipulato un atto notarile[27] tra il comune e *l'opus pontis* sul Taro, manufatto importante per la città perché garantiva il transito lungo la via Aemilia (detta anche via Claudia). Siamo alla metà del XIII secolo e il podestà cittadino dimostrava di avere poteri di controllo su enti ecclesiastici con una decisa vocazione civile, quali erano gli ospedali di ponte. Anche il vescovo aveva dovuto sottostare alle richieste del comune e farsi garante della corretta utilizzazione dei fondi raccolti per la manutenzione dei ponti loro affidati, di fronte alle evidenti difficoltà degli ospedali. Di ciò vi è ancora indicazione chiara negli statuti:

> [...] et ordinare cum eis et cogere eos ad reaedificationem ipsorum poncium de bonis dictorum poncium et domorum ipsorum, ita quod commode transiri possit per eos ad pedem et ad caballum. Et si dicti ponterii hoc nollent facere, potestas teneatur possessione ipsorum poncium obligare pignori et obligatas defendere quibulibet volentibus reaedificari ipsos pontes et reaedificari facere, quousque satisfactum fuerit de expensis factisin ipsis pontibus et utilitati ipsorum».

La spinta religiosa che aveva sostenuto la nascita di molte comunità che si erano dedicate alla costruzione e alla cura dei ponti, superando le difficoltà che fiumi e torrenti non ancora irregimentati opponevano alla viabilità (SZABÒ 1992a) e contribuendo a creare una rete di comunicazione, si era esaurita. Gli ospedali esistenti presso i ponti, quando sopravvissero, avrebbero svolto funzioni di accoglienza ai poveri e ai pellegrini, rinunciando alla loro originaria vocazione.

## *Bibliografia*

AFFÒ, Ireneo, 1792-95. *Storia della città di Parma*, Parma, 4 voll. Ristampa anastatica, Bologna, Forni, 1971-72.

ALBINI, Giuliana, 2002. "Strade e ospitalità, ponti e ospedali di ponte nell'Emilia occidentale (secc. XII-XIV)", *Carità e governo delle povertà (secoli XII-XV)*, Milano, Unicopli: 117-154.

ALBINI, Giuliana 2016. "L'economia della carità e del perdono. Questue e indulgenze nella Lombardia bassomedievale", Marina Gazzini, Antonio Olivieri (ed.), *L'ospedale, il denaro e altre ricchezze. Scritture e pratiche economiche dell'assistenza in Italia nel tardo Medioevo*, in *Reti Medievali Rivista*, 17/1: 155-188.

ALBINI, Giuliana, 2016. *Poveri e povertà nel medioevo*, Roma, Carocci.

ANSANI, Michele; BARETTA, Mirella (a cura di), 2008. *Le carte del monastero di S. Maria del Senatore = Le carte del monastero di S. Maria del Senatore di Pavia (714-1200)*, Codice Diplo-

26. RONCHINI 1856: 119.
27. Purtroppo l'atto non si è conservato o, comunque, non è ad oggi reperibile.

matico della Lombardia medievale (secoli VIII - XII), https://www.lombardiabeniculturali.it/cdlm/edizioni/pv/pavia-smariasenatore/ [link visitato settembre 2022].

Bartolomei, Alessandra, 2017. "L'acqua nell'immaginario dei monaci tra tardoantico e alto medioevo (secoli IV-IX)", Concetta Bianca, Francesco Salvestrini (a cura di), *L'acqua nemica. Fiumi, inondazioni e città storiche dall'antichità al contemporaneo, Atti del Convegno di studio a cinquant'anni dall'alluvione di Firenze (1966-2016), Firenze, 29-30 gennaio 2015*, Spoleto, Fondazione Centro Italiano di Studi sull'Alto Medioevo: 1-31.

Bonacini, Pierpaolo, 2001. "Il confine militare tra Modena e Bologna nel secolo XIII", Paola Foschi, Renzo Zagnoni (a cura di), *Il confine appenninico: percezione e realtà dall'Età antica ad oggi*, Porretta Terme-Pistoia: 71-92.

Bordone, Renato, 1997a. "Caratteri della società urbana fra XI e XII secolo", Giuseppe Sergi (a cura di), *Storia di Torino*, I, *Dalla preistoria al comune medievale*, Torino, Einaudi: 465-498.

Bordone, Renato, 1997b. "Vita economica del Duecento", Giuseppe Sergi (a cura di), *Storia di Torino*, I, *Dalla preistoria al comune medievale*, Torino, Einaudi: 751-783.

Cariboni, Guido, 2003. "Esenzione cistercense e formazione del *Privilegium commune*. Osservazioni a partire dai cenobi dell'Italia settentrionale", Nicolangelo D'Acunto (a cura di), *Papato e monachesimo "esente" nei secoli centrali del Medioevo*, Firenze, Firenze University Press: 65-107.

Casiraghi, Giampietro, 1999. "I Vallombrosani nel Piemonte occidentale: S. Giacomo di Stura e le sue dipendenze", Giordano Monzio (a cura di), *L'Ordo Vallisumbrosae tra XII e XIII secolo. Gli sviluppi istituzionali e culturali e l'espansione geografica (1101-1293), Atti del convegno II Colloquio Vallombrosano, Abbazia di Vallombrosa, 25-28 agosto 1996*, Vallombrosa, Edizioni Vallombrosa: 619-675.

Cenci, Alessandra (a cura di), 1996. *L'ospitalità in Antopascio. Storia e funzioni di un grande centro ospitaliero. Il cibo, la medicina e il controllo delle strade*, Lucca, Cassa di Risparmio di Lucca.

Cognasso, Francesco, 1958. "Ospedali di ponte", *Studi di storia ospedaliera piemontese in onore di Giovanni Donna d'Oldenico* = Annali dell'Ospedale Maria Vittoria di Torino, vol. 51: 109-115.

Coppola, Giovanni, 1996. *Ponti medievali in legno*, Roma-Bari, Laterza.

Dinzelbacher, Peter, 1990. "Il ponte come luogo sacro nella realtà e nell'immaginario", Sofia Boesch, Lucetta Scaraffia (a cura di), *Luoghi sacri e spazi della santità*, Torino, Rosenberg-Sellier: 51-60.

Falconi, Ettore; Peveri, Roberta (a cura di) 1986. *Registrum Magnum del comune di Piacenza*, Milano, Giuffré, 1986-1997, 3 voll.

Ferraris, Giovanni, 2016. "La Sesia e i confini orientali della diocesi di Vercelli", Riccardo Rao (a cura di), *I paesaggi fluviali della Sesia fra storia e archeologia. Territori, insediamenti, rappresentazioni*, Firenze, All'Insegna del Giglio: 75-94

Forzatti, Giovanna, 2001. "L'ospitalità della Chiesa. Pievi e canoniche bresciane sulle vie dei pellegrini", Gabriele Archetti (a cura di), *Lungo le strade della fede. Pellegrini e pellegrinaggio nel Bresciano, Atti della Giornata di studio, Brescia, 16 dicembre 2000*, in *Brixia Sacra. Memorie storiche della diocesi di Brescia*, s.III, VI/3-4: 33-68.

Frati, Macro, 2004. "Spazi medievali di accoglienza: ospedali urbani e rurali lungo le strade tra le Alpi e il mare", Elena Dellapiana, Pier M. Furlan, Marco Galloni (a cura di), *I luoghi delle cure in Piemonte*, Torino, Celid: 61-83

Gazzini, Marina, 2015. "*La rete ospedaliera di Bobbio fra alto e basso medioevo*", *La diocesi di Bobbio. Formazione e sviluppi di un'istituzione millenaria.* Firenze, Firenze University Press: 481-507.

Gazzini, Marina, 2021. "Ospedali di passo sull'Appennino tosco-emiliano. Prato del Vescovo e Croce Brandegliana nelle proiezioni ecclesiastiche, economiche e militari di Pistoia (secoli XI-XIV)", *Quaderni degli Studi di Storia Medioevale e di Diplomatica*, 5: 321-355.

GRECI, Roberto, 2016. “Porti fluviali e ponti in età medievale. Il Po e l'area padana”, *Hortus Artium Medievalium*, 22: 238-248.

INGLESE, Carlo; PARIS, Leonardo (a cura di), 2020. *Arte e tecnica dei ponti romani in pietra*, Roma, Sapienza University Press.

KEHR, Paulus F., 1906. *Italia pontificia sive Repertorium privilegiorum et litterarum a romanis pontificibus... concessorum, Aemilia sive privincia Ravenna*, vol. V, Berolini, Apud Weidmannos.

LE BLÉVEC, Daniel, 2000, *La part du pauvre. L'assistance dans les pays du Bas-Rhône du XIIe siècle au milieu du XVe siècle*, Roma, École Française de Rome.

SERGI, Giuseppe (a cura di), 1996. *Luoghi di strada nel Medioevo fra il Po, il mare e le Alpi occidentali*, Torino, Paravia-Scriptorium.

MERLO, Grado G., 1987. “Esperienze religiose e opere assistenziali in un'area di ponte tra XII e XIII secolo”, *Esperienze religiose e opere assistenziali nei secoli XII e XIII*, Torino: 213-234.

MESQUI, Jean, 1996. “Grands chantiers de ponts et financements charitables au Moyen Âge en France”, *Tecnología y sociedad: las grandes obras públicas en la Europa medieval*, Pamplona: 153-178.

MEYER, Andreas, 2007a. “Altopascio, Lucca e la questua organizzata nel XIII secolo”, *Ricerche dell'Istituto Storico Germanico di Roma*, 3: 195- 209.

MEYER, Andreas, 2007b. “Organisierter Bettel Und Andere Finanzgeschäfte Des Hospitals Von Altopascio Im 13. Jahrhundert (Mit Textedition)”, *Hospitäler In Mittelalter Und Früher Neuzeit [Hospitäler In Mittelalter Und Früher Neuzeit. Frankreich, Deutschland Und Italien. Eine Vergleichende Geschichte - Hôpitaux Au Moyen Âge Et Aux Temps Modernes. France, Allemagne Et Italie. Une Histoire Comparée*, herausgegeben von G. Drossbach, München: 55-105.

PACINI, Gian P., 2002. “I Crociferi e le comunità ospedaliere lungo le vie dei pellegrinaggi nel Veneto medioevale secoli XII-XIV”, Antonio Rigon (a cura di), *I percorsi della fede e l'esperienza della carità nel Veneto medievale*, Padova, Il Poligrafo: 155-172.

PANERO, Elisa, 2016, “Il territorio di *Vercellae* in età romana: studio e ricostruzione di una città d'acque”, Riccardo Rao (a cura di), *I paesaggi fluviali della Sesia fra storia e archeologia. Territori, insediamenti, rappresentazioni*, Firenze, All'Insegna del Giglio: 31-54.

RONCHINI, Amadio (a cura di), 1856. *Statuta Communis Parmae digesta anno MCCLV*, Parma, Monumenta Historica ad provincias Parmensem et Placentinam pertinentia

SALVESTRINI, Francesco, 2008. “La proprietà fondiaria dei grandi enti ecclesiastici nella Tuscia dei secoli XI-XV. Spunti di riflessione, tentativi di interpretazione”, *Rivista di Storia della Chiesa in Italia,* 2: 377-412.

SEPPILLI, Anita, 1977. *Sacralità dell'acqua e sacrilegio dei ponti,* Palermo, Sellerio.

SETTIA, Aldo A., 2016, “La Sesia, il Po e il ‘Ponte di Notingo’”, Riccardo Rao (a cura di), *I paesaggi fluviali della Sesia fra storia e archeologia. Territori, insediamenti, rappresentazioni*, Firenze, All'Insegna del Giglio: 107-124.

SPICCIANI, Amleto, 1999, “L'ospedale di Altopascio nella Lucchesia del secolo XII: donazioni, acquisti e prestiti”, *Gli spazi economici della Chiesa nell'Occidente mediterraneo (secoli XII-metà XIV), Atti del XVI Convegno Internazionale, Pistoia, 16-19 maggio 1997,* Pistoia, Centro Italiano di Studi di Storia e d'Arte: 509-528.

SZABÒ, Thomas, 1990. “Costruzioni di ponti e di strade in Italia fra il IX e il XIV secolo. La trasformazione delle strutture organizzative”, Jean-Claude Maire Vigueur, Agostino Paravicini Bagliani (a cura di), *Ars et ratio. Dalla torre di Babele al ponte di Rialto*, Palermo, Sellerio: 73-91.

SZABÒ, Thomas, 1992a. “Strade e potere pubblico nell'Italia centro-settentrionale (secoli VI-XIV)”, *Comuni e politica stradale in Toscana e in Italia nel Medioevo*, Bologna, CLUEB: 71-112.

SZABÒ, Thomas, 1992b. “Xenodochi, ospedali e locande: forme di ospitalità ecclesiastica e commerciale nell'Italia del Medioevo (secoli VII-XIV)”, *Comuni e politica stradale in Toscana e in Italia nel Medioevo*, Bologna, CLUEB: 285-319.

TABACCO, Giovanni, 1993. *Sperimentazioni del potere nell'alto medioevo*, Torino, Einaudi.

VAUCHEZ, André, 2003. "La santità dei laici nell'Occidente medievale: nascita ed evoluzione di un modello agiografico (secoli XII-XIII)", *Esperienze religiose nel Medioevo*, Roma, Viella: 15-26.

Marina Gazzini

# Quando l'ospedale è la meta del viaggio. Processioni e pellegrinaggi nella Lombardia medievale

Il nesso tra ospedali e *utentes stratis* (utenti della strada) è acclarato. Le testimonianze storiche, archeologiche, artistiche, documentarie, rivelano l'intensificarsi delle fondazioni assistenziali in quei contesti, sia urbani sia rurali, che risultavano attraversati da importanti vie di comunicazione, terrestri, fluviali e marittime.[1] Prima e dopo la nascita delle locande a pagamento, infatti, gli ospedali rappresentavano un punto di riferimento imprescindibile per chi percorreva una strada: pellegrini, mercanti, soldati, studenti, maestri, artigiani, lavoranti, artisti, ma anche banditi e fuorilegge, tutti –a modo loro– utenti delle strade e bisognosi di punti di ricetto e cura. A dispetto di una narrazione successiva, il medioevo fu un'era di grandi spostamenti: e gli ospedali entrarono a pieno titolo in questo panorama di gente in movimento (Mazzi [1997] 2016). La presenza di un'utenza forestiera e non solo locale è testimoniata in ospedali di città, di campagna, di montagna: in queste strutture troviamo traccia della presenza di stranieri sia tra le persone assistite sia tra quelle che assistevano, *fratres* e *sorores*, ruoli che, come sempre accadeva negli ospedali medievali, erano spesso interscambiabili (Taddei, Ghermani 2019).

In questa sede non è mia intenzione soffermami sul ruolo degli ospedali come tappa del viaggio, una tappa funzionale all'assistenza di viaggiatori e forestieri. Molto è già stato scritto, spesso anche enfatizzando in verità, perché molti ospedali che la storiografia ha a lungo ritenuto destinati all'assistenza dei pellegrini in realtà servivano soprattutto le popolazioni locali e assolvevano compiti di amministrazione fondiaria. È il caso dei dieci *xenodochia* altomedievali del monastero di Bobbio, sparsi su una vasta area padana, in contesti urbani come rurali, descritti dalla storiografia come esclusivamente preposti all'assistenza di pellegrini, soprattutto irlandesi, in viaggio da terre lontane verso la tomba di san Colombano; un'attenta lettura degli inventari monastici rivela invece che essi erano in primo luogo –insieme a pievi e cappelle parimenti dipendenti dal monastero– perni di gestione delle terre monastiche e luoghi di assistenza sanitaria per gli uomini che lavoravano e vivevano su queste terre (Gazzini 2015). Sempre riferendosi all'area nord italiana, ma in questo caso a strutture bassomedievali, eguale prevalenza di utenze e interessi locali si rintraccia nei servizi offerti dagli

1. Per il contesto qui trattato cf. Greci 2000.

ospedali di montagna, eretti su importanti valichi delle Alpi e degli Appennini (Gazzini, Frank 2021). Lo dimostrano fonti diverse, come inventari multilingue di suppellettili e di beni fondiari, disposizioni comunali, atti notarili, unificazioni ospedaliere, liti sulla nomina dei rettori, visite pastorali: laddove un ospedale era collegato a una forte comunità locale –ospedaliera, monastica, di villaggio o di castello– aveva molte chances di prosperare nel tempo; in caso contrario, laddove il nesso con l'ambiente locale era debole, l'ente ospedaliero era destinato a seguire il fluttuante destino delle vie di comunicazione che, anche nel caso delle direttrici più importanti, come la via Francigena, si disperdevano in ampi fasci di strade e non coincidevano con itinerari fissi. Se l'area di strada manteneva la sua ragione d'essere indipendentemente dal mutare dei poteri, delle economie, del clima, il singolo percorso era soggetto a frequenti cambiamenti, inglobando nel suo mutevole destino la sopravvivenza o la scomparsa dei luoghi e delle strutture sorte parallelamente ad esso (Sergi 1996).

Ora vorrei invece formulare qualche osservazione sul ruolo degli ospedali come meta stessa del viaggio. Le domande da cui parto sono le seguenti: vi erano persone che si mettevano in cammino proprio per raggiungere un ospedale? individui che lasciavano la propria casa perché sapevano che altrove, ad esempio nell'ospedale di una grande città, avrebbero potuto ricevere aiuti di differente natura, dal ricovero all'assistenza medica, dalle elemosine ad un'occupazione retribuita? La risposta è: ovviamente si. L'ospedale medievale distribuiva cibo, vesti, denaro, rimedi farmacologici. In ospedale si trovavano medici e soprattutto chirurghi e barbieri che curavano ferite, ossa rotte, febbri ignote. Donne in stato interessante e prive di assistenza casalinga si muovevano per partorire entro le strutture ospedaliere. Famiglie povere, o donne senza marito, lasciavano le loro dimore per andare ad abbandonare i propri figli alla ruota di un ospedale: alle volte l'addio era definitivo, altre volte si trattava di una cessione mascherata perché la madre si riproponeva come balia del suo stesso bambino, ripercorrendo quindi in senso inverso e con spirito diverso il viaggio di abbandono dell'andata (Piccinni 2020).

L'ospedale offriva inoltre lavoro (quello delle balie appena menzionato è appunto uno di questi). L'impiego di uomini e donne forestieri come personale di servizio nelle istituzioni assistenziali è abbondantemente testimoniato a Venezia, a Firenze, a Roma, città che per diversi motivi –religiosi ed economici soprattutto– furono meta di forestieri provenienti da terre più o meno lontane (Gazzini 2019). Un'occupazione presso la struttura ospedaliera veniva spesso trovata grazie al tramite di conduttori di osterie e locande dove il forestiero aveva in un primo tempo cercato alloggio. Le modalità di impiego di questo personale di servizio forestiero erano varie –in corsia ma anche nella gestione del patrimonio fondiario–[2] ed assumevano i contorni non solo del rapporto di lavoro ma anche dell'assistenza: un privato infatti difficilmente era disposto a ricorrere alle prestazioni di uno straniero appena arrivato e senza referenze. In tale forma di

2. Si vedano ad esempio i dipendenti di origine corsa al servizio come bovari, vaccari e fattori per l'ospedale di Santo Spirito in Sassia di Roma (Esposito 2014).

assistenza tuttavia non mancava un certo tornaconto da parte della struttura caritativa che in tal modo si assicurava manodopera a basso costo, risparmiando così sul capitolo di spesa del personale salariato (Sandri 1988).

Molte persone dunque viaggiavano per curarsi, per ricevere aiuti, per garantirsi assistenza, avendo come meta una struttura ospedaliera. La nostra idea della versione medievale del turismo sanitario odierno non sarebbe però completa se non includessimo accanto alla cura del corpo anche la cura dell'anima. Nei secoli di mezzo, furono infatti numerosi gli ospedali che divennero meta di processioni se non di veri e propri pellegrinaggi.

Nei centri maggiori come in quelli minori, si svolgevano periodicamente processioni che coinvolgevano gli ospedali quali tappe importanti di percorsi civici che segnavano un'ellissi sacrale tra chiese cattedrali, parrocchie, pievi, luoghi pii e ospedali. Prendendo come riferimento l'area padana da me meglio conosciuta, posso ricordare la processione del *Corpus Domini* che a Parma dal 1332 ebbe due mete fisse, la cattedrale di Santa Maria, sita nell'antica *civitas* romana, e l'ospedale dei Quattro Mestieri, sorto nel quartiere suburbano di Capodiponte: si trattava di due fuochi della religiosità civica, la chiesa cattedrale e un ospedale di patronato comunale.[3]

Esempio ancora più emblematico di come queste processioni[4] –vedendo la partecipazione dei poteri civili, delle autorità ecclesiastiche, della cittadinanza con le sue varie rappresentanze– non fossero semplici cerimoniali, ma importanti momenti di comunicazione politica, è sicuramente dato dalla celebrazione della Festa del Perdono di Milano: la solennità, istituita a Milano a partire da metà Quattrocento, ebbe come meta il nuovo Ospedale Maggiore in alternanza alla Fabbrica del Duomo, una soluzione ideata nel 1459 da Pio II per omaggiare e finanziare due simboli della *caritas* cittadina evitando competizioni fra loro. Il pontefice, per sostenere sia la costruzione della nuova cattedrale, iniziata nel 1385, sia i lavori del nuovo ospedale grande, fondato nel 1456 dal duca Francesco Sforza e da sua moglie Bianca Maria Visconti, stabilì infatti che al 25 marzo (solennità dell'Annunciazione) degli anni pari fosse concessa l'indulgenza plenaria a coloro che compissero donazioni per la costruzione del Duomo; e che al 25 marzo degli anni dispari, l'indulgenza fosse concessa a coloro che donassero all'ospedale. La celebrazione si alterna da oltre cinque secoli: fino alla seconda guerra mondiale, la bolla pontificia che aveva originato la Festa del Perdono veniva portata in processione dal Duomo all'ospedale del Filarete, nel cui cortile venivano anche esposti i ritratti di tutti i benefattori che avevano contribuito alla sua costruzione. Questa processione bicefala, alla quale partecipavano le tre principali componenti della società milanese –il duca, l'arcivescovo, i cittadini–, era una sorta di mediazione trovata dal pontefice tra le esigenze della Fabbrica del Duomo e quelle del neo istituito ospedale. L'approvazione papale del nuovo

3. Il percorso, così come la data, variavano invece di anno in anno (Gazzini 2013).

4. Si veda in questo stesso volume il contributo di Raúl Villagrasa "El loco, el niño y el hospital: la inclusión del pobre verdadero en el espacio urbano renacentista".

ente ospedaliero era stata infatti a lungo osteggiata proprio da esponenti della stessa società civile milanese che si appellarono al papa per difendere le esigenze di una costruzione, come quella del nuovo Duomo, che originò dal cuore della stessa cittadinanza, contro quelle di un edificio ospedaliero che, insieme ai lavori di ricostruzione del castello visconteo, simboleggiava il potere del duca più che quello dei cittadini (Somaini 2005; Saltamacchia 2017).

Ma vi furono anche processioni che, coinvolgendo comunità estranee alla società locale, assunsero la fisionomia di piccoli pellegrinaggi. Tipicamente, ciò accadeva quando intorno alla figura dei fondatori ospedalieri, spesso ancora in vita, si diffondeva una fama di santità. Fra i vari casi ai quali si può fare riferimento, mi soffermerò ora sull'ospedale del beato Gerardo Tintori, fondato nel 1174 a Monza, località prossima a Milano, perché fornisce un esempio molto interessante sul lungo periodo. Si tratta infatti di un ente caratterizzato da una straordinaria durata: non solo l'edificio medievale sopravvisse fino al XIX secolo, ma l'intitolazione a Gerardo, che si fece strada a poco a poco accanto a quella originaria a sant'Ambrogio per poi soppiantarla del tutto, perdura ancora oggi dal momento che il principale ospedale di Monza (e il quarto per dimensioni in tutta la Lombardia) si intitola sempre a san Gerardo (Mambretti 2011).

Le premesse per questa storia di attaccamento ininterrotto furono gettate fin dalle origini (risalenti al 1174), quando l'ente andò a collocarsi fra i principali simboli municipali. Esso sorse infatti grazie a un patto stipulato da Girardus Tinctor, converso di un *hospitale pauperum* da lui stesso fondato «*in loco et fundo Modoetie ultra flumen Lambri prope ecclesiam Sancti Ambroxi*» (nella terra di Monza, oltre il fiume Lambro e vicino alla chiesa di Sant'Ambrogio), con l'arciprete della chiesa di San Giovanni Oberto da Terzago, e due consoli del comune, Arderico Fidelis e Arnaldo Lanterius.[5] La successiva fortuna dell'ospedale, il suo ruolo di simbolo per la società locale e di faro per comunità anche lontane, dipesero dal fortunato connubio dell'ente assistenziale con il culto sorto intorno alla figura del laico fondatore, Gerardo Tintori. Come rivela il cognome (Tinctor significa tintore), egli proveniva dal ceto medio dei lavoratori e dei piccoli proprietari[6] che nella Lombardia del suo tempo si riconosceva nel gruppo sociale e politico del "popolo". Non è un caso se dalle fila del Popolo dell'Italia centro-settentrionale siano provenuti, fra XII e XIII secolo, molte figure di santi che la moderna storiografia ha definito "della carità e del lavoro", individuando nell'aiuto al prossimo bisognoso e nell'onesto esercizio della propria professione gli elementi caratteristici di un nuovo modello agiografico che incontrò un grande favore nella popolazione (Vauchez 1989).

5. L'atto, stipulato dal notaio Iunio *iudex* presso la canonica di San Giovanni, costituisce anche la prima menzione nota dell'esistenza del comune monzese. L'originale del documento –fortunatamente trascritto da A.F. Frisi (1794, II, doc. LXXII, 70-71)– è andato perduto: presso l'Archivio capitolare di San Giovanni di Monza si conserva solo una copia in pergamena del XIV secolo.

6. Il gruppo parentale dei Tinctores è attestato a Monza fin dalla metà dell'XI secolo. Per dettagli, si veda Gazzini 1993: 48, n. 17.

Monza, soffocata per tutto il medioevo (e anche oltre) dalla vicina Milano, che le impedì di raggiungere l'agognato riconoscimento a *civitas* (ovvero a centro dotato di autonomia ecclesiastica e politica),[7] affidò le sue ambizioni cittadine alla pervicace difesa di due tradizioni: la memoria della regina Teodolinda e la memoria di Gerardo Tintori.

Teodolinda incarna l'orgoglio di un centro minore che, in età gota e longobarda, venne elevato a sede regia accanto a centri di più antico riconoscimento. Ogni pietra in cui ancora oggi si inciampi a Monza viene attribuita all'evergetismo architettonico di Teodolinda e del consorte Agilulfo che portò alla ricostruzione (o molto più probabilmente al restauro) del palazzo regio del goto Teodorico, e all'edificazione dell'annessa basilica di San Giovanni (BROGIOLO 2005; GASPARRI 2002). Il radicamento del ricordo della regina longobarda, oltre che su avanzi manufatti (agli edifici vanno aggiunti stupendi oggetti di oreficeria), poggiò anche su avanzi scritti, dalle storie di Paolo Diacono alla cronaca di Giovanni Villani, senza dimenticare naturalmente la corrispondenza intrattenuta dalla stessa Teodolinda con papa Gregorio Magno che conferì alla regina un ruolo fondamentale nel processo di "cattolicizzazione" del popolo longobardo; molto fece infine la rievocazione trecentesca da parte della famiglia Visconti, desiderosa nel proprio processo di ascesa politica di collegarsi alla fama legittimante dei re longobardi (GASPARRI 2000).

A questa memoria "nobile" fece da contraltare l'affermazione della figura "popolare" di Gerardo Tintori. Espressione di una devozione sorta dal basso e coniugatasi subito con le istanze del nuovo potere comunale, Gerardo fu oggetto sin dall'epoca della sua morte, avvenuta il 6 giugno 1207,[8] di un culto popolare coronato nel 1582 dalla canonizzazione ufficiale.[9] Ma già nei secoli precedenti Gerardo era assurto al rango di patrono del borgo di Monza, insieme a san Giovanni Battista.[10] Gli statuti trecenteschi del comune di Monza menzionano infatti la celebrazione, da parte delle autorità e della popolazione, di una festa dedicata al Tintori che si svolgeva –e si svolge a tutt'oggi– il 6 giugno. Questa festa prevedeva una processione che aveva come suo capo la chiesa e l'ospedale di San Gerardo e vedeva la partecipazione della popolazione, delle autorità civili e di quelle ecclesiastiche.[11]

7. Ricordo che in Italia il concetto di *civitas* fu più forte che altrove: centri demici che in Europa avrebbero potuto venire tranquillamente chiamati città, in Italia erano indicati come *burgi, terrae, castra*, nel momento in cui non erano sede di diocesi e non erano centro del potere di un conte o di un altro pubblico rappresentante (CHITTOLINI 1996).

8. *Necrologium Modoetiense*, secolo XII e compilato fino al secolo XVI, edito da Frisi (1794, III, 122). In questa data veniva, e viene ancora oggi, celebrata una festa in onore del santo, come riporta la rubrica *De diebus festivis celebrandis* degli statuti di Monza (*Liber statutorum communis Modoetie*, Mediolani 1579, rist. anast. Milano 1993, cc. 27v-28r).

9. Il Tintori venne poi canonizzato nel 1582: *Sancti Gerardi Modoetiensis acta, Beati Caroli Cardinalis Borromei archiepiscopi Mediolanensis iussu confecta*, Mediolani 1603.

10. Per la figura di questo santo, a tutt'oggi patrono del centro brianteo insieme a san Giovanni Battista, v.: MODORATI 1918; 1925; RIVA, 1930: I, 19-79; *Gerardo Tintore* 1979.

11. *Liber statutorum communis Modoetie*, cc. 27v-28r.

La fama di Gerardo varcò presto i confini del borgo. Una fonte trecentesca, il *Chronicon modoetiense* di Bonincontro Morigia, che fornì il dossier informativo sulla vita e i miracoli di Gerardo su cui si sarebbe basato anche il processo di canonizzazione moderno (Zabbia 2012), ci riferisce di pellegrinaggi alla tomba del santo collocata nella chiesa del complesso ospedaliero. Questi pellegrinaggi erano compiuti da parte degli abitanti di paesi situati nei dintorni di Como, Milano e Varese, importanti centri posti lungo le principali direttrici stradali che si dipartivano da Monza. Secondo Bonincontro Morigia, la tradizione sarebbe stata inaugurata ad appena quaranta giorni dalla morte del santo quando uomini e donne di Olgiate Comasco, piccola località distante 20 miglia (quasi 50 km) da Monza, per guarire da un male che li aveva colpiti (una misteriosa infermità denominata dalla fonte *syncoposis*) seguirono il consiglio di un anacoreta residente nei dintorni e si recarono in pellegrinaggio collettivo a Monza per chiedere aiuto a Gerardo.[12] Ottenuto il miracolo, la popolazione riconoscente stabilì di reiterare il pellegrinaggio annualmente. La tradizione è ancora in vita.

Non sappiamo in realtà quando il rituale abbia avuto inizio perché la prima fonte che ce ne parla è proprio la cronaca trecentesca. Esso venne comunque confermato nei processi informativi alla causa di beatificazione indetti da Carlo Borromeo nel XVI secolo. Al Seicento risale invece l'identificazione dell'anonimo eremita ricordato dal Morigia nella figura del beato Manfredo da Settala, sacerdote morto nel 1217. Le scarsissime attestazioni di questo personaggio impediscono di capire se egli appartenesse all'antica e nobile famiglia milanese che diede alla città consoli e arcivescovi (Alberzoni 2018: 312-316), o se fosse semplicemente originario della località di Settala, posta a sud est di Milano: è invece certo che dalla fine del secolo XII, Manfredo fu prete di Cuasso, nella pieve di Arcisate, in diocesi di Milano, vicino al ramo sud-occidentale del lago di Lugano.[13] In entrambi i casi si tratta dunque di attestazioni più tarde rispetto ai fatti narrati che lasciano aperti vari interrogativi e in particolare quello relativo ai motivi per cui gli abitanti di un centro lontano da Monza avessero scelto quel borgo, quel santo, quell'ospedale, come meta di un cammino di guarigione fisica e spirituale. In mancanza di fonti coeve e di attestate relazioni politiche, ecclesiastiche o economiche tra i due centri lombardi, è difficile dare una risposta. I collegamenti tra Monza e il Comasco dovevano comunque essere più fitti di quel che si immagina. Allo stato attuale delle ricerche abbiamo solo qualche indicazione: alla fine del XIII secolo l'arciprete, ovvero la massima carica ecclesiastica monzese, *Advocatus de Advocatis*, noto per avere dato avvio alla ricostruzione del Duomo, veniva dalla chiesa di Como e non da quella di Milano cui Monza tradizionalmente si rivolgeva per attingere i propri alti prelati. A sua volta, la chiesa di Monza aveva qualche dipendenza in area comasca: nel XIII secolo fu difatti coinvolta in una contesa sui beni della chiesa di Santa Maria di

12. Presso la parrocchiale di San Gerardo al Corpo, anticamente intitolata a Sant'Ambrogio, dove sono conservati i suoi resti.

13. Ipotesi avanzata da Bartolomeo Zucchi (1606) e da Primo Tatti (1663), e poi ripresa nel XVIII secolo dal Frisi (1794: 99-100) che però la ritenne poco probabile.

Bizzarone, località della diocesi di Como posta a soli 8 chilometri da Olgiate Comasco (MAMBRETTI 2000). Non si esclude quindi la presenza nella canonica della cattedrale di Monza di personaggi provenienti da quelle zone ma –si avverte– si tratta di una ricerca ancora tutta da fare.

Invece, l'incertezza sull'identificazione dell'anonimo eremita trecentesco con Manfredo da Settala, unita anche all'impossibilità di attribuire a quest'ultimo un legame con la potente famiglia milanese dei da Settala, spinge a non sbilanciarsi su eventuali nessi politici ed ecclesiastici tra Milano, Monza, Olgiate mediati da questa figura. Possiamo solo incidentalmente notare che nella prima metà del Duecento, e dunque poco dopo la morte di Gerardo Tintori e di Manfredo, i rapporti tra la chiesa milanese e Monza si inasprirono proprio a causa di un da Settala, il potente arcivescovo Enrico che dapprima entrò in conflitto con il comune di Milano proprio per avere scomunicato il podestà e gli abitanti di Monza, al punto da essere costretto all'esilio, e che poi, per ottemperare a direttive papali, patrocinò le «*pauperes sorores Mediolani commorantes ordinis de Spolito*», ovvero le future Damianite o Clarisse che ottennero i beni di un altro ospedale monzese, quello di San Biagio, pertinente *nullo medio* alla chiesa romana, il quale venne soppresso con la classica accusa di un cattivo uso delle risorse dei poveri.[14]

Le vie che da Olgiate Comasco conducono a Monza sono dunque, come quelle del Signore, infinite e anche un po' tortuose. E, a proposito di strade, non dobbiamo trascurare i collegamenti viari, terrestri e fluviali, che si diramavano in Brianza, il ricco territorio di cui Monza era perno e che già all'epoca aveva dato luogo a un sistema integrato, fatto di flussi di persone, beni, energie (PRACCHI 1954; BOSISIO, VISMARA 1969-1979). L'ente ospedaliero era stato infatti eretto nella parte dell'abitato monzese rivolta verso nord, da dove partiva una direttrice di traffico di un certo rilievo che metteva in comunicazione Milano e Lecco, città posta sul ramo orientale del lago di Como, e che si congiungeva con la Como-Bergamo, aprendosi a est con i maggiori centri veneti, a nord-ovest con i valichi alpini. Lo stesso fiume Lambro che lambiva l'ospedale, e che viene ricordato in un miracolo dello stesso Gerardo,[15] nasce in territorio lariano (anche se non passa da Olgiate, ma più a est).

Il legame tra il personaggio Gerardo Tintori, vivo e morto, e l'ospedale da lui fondato fu saldo fin dalle origini. La nascita subitanea di una devozione ver-

14. Biblioteca Trivulziana di Milano, Fondo Belgioioso, cart. 221, fasc. III: bolla *Licet ex suscepte* originale (edito in: FRISI 1794: II, doc. CIX); *ibidem*, 1233 febbraio 18; 1233 febbraio 21. Sulla vicenda e su altre simili: GAZZINI 2017: 147-166.

15. Consistente nell'arresto delle acque del Lambro che straripando avevano travolto un ponte collegato con l'ospedale e minacciavano lo stesso edificio ospedaliero (MORIGIA 1728: col. 1086). L'ergersi a baluardo contro le catastrofi naturali fa parte della fenomenologia dell'evento miracoloso propria di santi, vivi o morti (VAUCHEZ 1989: 470). Tra gli altri miracoli attribuiti dalla tradizione a Gerardo alcuni si ricollegano alla sua attività assistenziale, come la moltiplicazione di grano e vino da distribuire ai poveri durante una carestia e la guarigione di numerosi malati (MORIGIA 1728: coll. 1086-88).

so il fondatore ospedaliero è attestata ad esempio dall'evolversi delle denominazioni assunte dall'ente assistenziale, indicato come «*hospitale pauperum de Sancto Ambrosio*» (dal nome della chiesa presso la quale venne eretto l'istituto) fintanto che Gerardo visse (Riva 1930: 64-66), passando quindi a «*hospitale beati quondam Girardi*» già nel 1230 (Frisi 1794: II, doc. CIII), per assumere l'intitolazione definitiva di «*hospitale Sancti Girardi*» a partire almeno dal 1247 (Frisi 1794: II, doc. cxxvi). Il nesso tra la fortuna del nuovo culto e il successo dell'ospedale è riconducibile, almeno in parte, a quei sentimenti che anche altrove spinsero gruppi o istituzioni –famiglie, confraternite, opere di carità– a premere affinché venisse riconosciuta, per ragioni di prestigio ma anche di affetto, la santità del loro fondatore o di colui che avevano scelto come protettore ufficiale (Merlo 1989: 207). Per lungo tempo l'ospedale restò l'unico sito ad attestare la venerazione per il santo. Solo alla fine del Quattrocento vennero intitolati in sua memoria una chiesa, un ponte, entrambi già esistenti ai tempi della fondazione ospedaliera, e una delle porte di Monza (Frisi 1794: 233-238; Modorati 1918: 30 e ss.).

Santo e ospedale si diedero una mano reciproca nel loro processo di affermazione e radicamento presso la società locale. Nel Quattrocento, l'ospedale assurse esplicitamente a simbolo di un centro minore in affannosa ricerca di separazione da Milano. Le vicende legate all'unificazione dell'ente all'Ospedale Maggiore ne sono testimonianza. Dopo l'approvazione papale nel 1459 della riforma ospedaliera voluta dal duca di Milano che, tra il resto, previde la centralizzazione amministrativa di tutti gli ospedali della diocesi di Milano nel nuovo ospedale grande costruito a Milano, l'ospedale di Gerardo Tintori ottenne infatti di continuare a essere governato come in passato da un capitolo di amministratori laici di estrazione locale che sarebbero stati però da quel momento scelti dai deputati dell'Ospedale Maggiore di Milano e non dal comune di Monza. Il patteggiamento parla chiaro. La comunità difese nei limiti del possibile l'autonomia della fondazione ospedaliera che rappresentava lo spirito municipale in maniera più degna di un ente comunale privo di reale peso politico e di una chiesa monopolizzata da elementi estranei alla società locale (Gazzini 1997: 179-207).

La Lombardia medievale fu teatro di altre vicende ospedaliere nelle quali si coniugarono storie di viaggi, di assistenza, di devozioni, di rivendicazioni sociali e politiche. Tra le montagne bergamasche e la pianura del fiume Po si snodò la vita di un altro santo laico di estrazione popolare, il portatore di brente Alberto. Originario di Villadogna, in valle Seriana, Alberto emigrò a Cremona dove morì nel 1279 in fama di santità: i suoi colleghi di Parma e Piacenza organizzarono processioni che a Parma portarono alla creazione di un ospedale da campo provvisorio che ospitava pellegrini ammalati speranzosi in un intervento taumaturgico del defunto Alberto. Il comune, retto al tempo dalle Arti, intuì la portata politica del fenomeno e si fece carico sia della devozione sia dell'ospedale, trovando per questo una sistemazione più degna in muratura.[16]

16. Si veda il mio lavoro in corso di stampa *La leggenda del santo Brentatore. Arti, Chiesa e Popolo nell'Italia dei comuni.*

Mentre l'ospedale di frate Alberto di Parma e la devozione per la figura del brentatore ebbero vita breve, legati com'erano a una specifica parte politica e sociale della società locale, l'ospedale di Gerardo Tintori di Monza presenta, come già scritto, una durata eccezionale nel tempo. Qualcosa sembrò cambiare a fine XIX secolo quando, nel 1890, una donazione del re d'Italia Umberto I diede avvio alla costruzione di un nuovo edificio ospedaliero che venne a lui intitolato e che sostituì l'ospedale di San Gerardo nel ruolo di principale ente assistenziale cittadino. Non possiamo dire che il generoso gesto abbia portato fortuna al sovrano italiano. Il 29 luglio 1900 re Umberto I fu assassinato dall'anarchico Gaetano Bresci proprio a Monza, dopo essere già scampato ad altri due attentati. E la sua memoria fu definitivamente cancellata quando nel 1946, dopo i risultati del referendum in cui gli italiani si espressero per la forma costituzionale da dare al loro stato, scegliendo la repubblica al posto della monarchia, l'amministrazione comunale di Monza cambiò il nome dell'ospedale cittadino, decidendo di eliminare l'intitolazione in onore di un re estraneo all'identità locale, Umberto I di Savoia, e di tornare all'antico: Gerardo Tintori, il santo di casa. Dopo qualche decennio, l'ospedale ottocentesco subì una graduale dismissione per l'edificazione di un nuovo ente che comunque avrebbe portato nel titolo il riferimento al passato: si tratta dell'Ospedale odierno di San Gerardo, che ospita anche la facoltà di medicina dell'Università di Milano-Bicocca. I cambiamenti edilizi non hanno dunque portato, se non per un brevissimo periodo, a un mutamento dell'intitolazione a San Gerardo, confermando lo strettissimo legame municipale tra la città, l'ospedale e il suo santo.

## *Bibliografia*


Alberzoni, Maria P., 2018. "Settala Enrico", *Dizionario biografico degli Italiani*, Roma, Istituto dell'Enciclopedia Italiana: 312-316.

Bosisio, Alfredo; Vismara, Giulio, 1969-1979. *Storia di Monza e della Brianza*, Milano, Il Polifilo, 6 vol.

Brogiolo, Gian P., 2005. "Capitali e residenze regie nell'Italia longobarda", *Alto medioevo mediterraneo*, Firenze, Firenze University Press: 233-250.

Chittolini, Giorgio, 1996. "Quasi-città. Borghi e terre in area lombarda nel tardo medioevo", *Città, comunità e feudi negli stati dell'Italia centro-settentrionale*, Milano, Unicopli: 85-104.

Esposito, Anna, 2014. "Le minoranze indesiderate (corsi, slavi e albanesi) e il processo di integrazione nella società romana nel corso del Quattrocento", *Cittadinanza e mestieri. Radicamento urbano e integrazione nelle città bassomedievali (secc. XIII-XVI)*, Roma, Viella: 283-297.

Frisi, Antonio F., 1794. *Memorie storiche di Monza e sua corte*, Milano.

Gasparri, Stefano, 2000. "I Longobardi tra oblio e memoria", *Studi sul Medioevo per Girolamo Arnaldi*, Roma, Viella: 237-277.

Gasparri, Stefano, 2002. "L'alto Medioevo: da Teodorico a Berengario (secoli VI-X)", *Monza. La sua storia,* Monza, Silvana: 48-73

Gazzini, Marina, 2019. "Aiutare il forestiero. L'assistenza di ospedali e confraternite nel medioevo (Italia centro-settentrionale)", Ilaria Taddei, Naima Ghermani (dir.), *Hospitalité de l'étranger au Moyen Âge et à l'époque moderne: entre charité, contrôle et utilité sociale. Italie Europe*, Roma, École Française de Rome: 407-416.

GAZZINI, Marina, 1997. "L'esempio di una 'quasi-città': gli ospedali di Monza e i loro rapporti con Milano (secoli XIII-XV)", Allen J. Grieco, Lucia Sandri (a cura di), *Ospedali e città. L'Italia del Centro-Nord, XIII-XVI secolo*, Firenze, Le Lettere: 179-207.

GAZZINI, Marina, 2017. "La maleficenza. Malversazioni e altri illeciti negli ospedali della Lombardia medievale", *Storie di frodi. Intacchi, malversazioni e furti nei monti di pietà e negli istituti caritatevoli tra medioevo ed età moderna*, Bologna, Il Mulino: 147-166.

GAZZINI, Marina, 2013. "La nascita del quartiere di Capodiponte: spazi materiali e scenari simbolici", *Andare Oltretorrente. Archeologia e storia a Parma*, Parma, Monte Università Parma: 87-98.

GAZZINI, Marina, 1993. "L'ospedale di S. Gerardo di Monza (secoli XII-XV)", *Archivio Storico Lombardo*, 119: 45-69.

GAZZINI, Marina, 2015. "La rete ospedaliera di Bobbio fra alto e basso medioevo", *La diocesi di Bobbio. Formazione e sviluppi di un'istituzione millenaria*, Firenze, Firenze University Press: 481-507, www.ebook.retimedievali.it.

GAZZINI, Marina; FRANK, Thomas (a cura di), 2021. *Ospedali e montagne. Paesaggi, funzioni, poteri in età medievale*, Milano-Torino, Pearson.

*Gerardo Tintore*, 1979. *Il santo di Monza*, Monza, Il Bulino.

GRECI, Roberto (a cura di), 2000. *Un'area di strada. L'Emilia occidentale nel Medioevo. Ricerche storiche e riflessioni metodologiche*, Bologna, Clueb.

MAMBRETTI, Renato, 2011. "Alle origini di un mito borghigiano. Gerardo Tintori e l'hospitale pauperum di Monza nei secoli XII-XIV", *Aevum*, 85: 509-525.

MAMBRETTI, Renato, 2000. "«Cum questio diu fuisset ventillata». La contesa sui beni di Santa Maria di Bizzarone agli inizi del XIII secolo", *Archivio Storico della Diocesi di Como*, 11: 127-158.

MORIGIA, Bonincontro, 1728. *Chronicon Modoetiense ab origine Modoetiae usque ad annum 1349 ubi potissimum agitur de gestis priorum vicecomitum principum*, RR.II.SS., XII, Milano: 1061-1184.

MAZZI, Maria Serena, [1997] 2016. *Oltre l'orizzonte. In viaggio nel Medioevo*, Torino, Paravia/ Scriptorium.

MERLO, Grado Giovanni 1989. "Religiosità e cultura religiosa dei laici nel secolo XII", *L'Europa dei secoli XI e XII fra novità e tradizione: sviluppi di una cultura*, Milano, Vita e Pensiero: 197-215.

MODORATI, Luigi, 1924. *Dell'ospedale di S. Gerardo e di altre istituzioni benefiche di Monza*, Monza, Istituto Artigianelli.

MODORATI, Luigi, 1918. *Memorie intorno alla chiesa e al culto di S. Gerardo di Monza*, Monza, Tip. Soc. Monzese.

MODORATI, Luigi, 1925. *Vita di S. Gerardo. Cenni storici*, Monza, Tip. Soc. Monzese.

PICCINNI, Gabriella (a cura di), 2020. *Alle origini del welfare (XIII-XVI secolo). Radici medievali e moderne della cultura europea dell'assistenza*, Roma, Viella.

PRACCHI, R. 1954. *La Brianza. Primi risultati di un'indagine geografica*, Como, Sagsa, Soc. Arti grafiche S. Abbondio.

RIVA, Giuseppe, 1930. "S. Gerardo e il suo ospedale nei documenti dei secoli XII-XIII della Congregazione di Carità di Monza", *Saggi critici e narrativi di storia monzese*, Monza, I: 19-79.

SALTAMACCHIA, MARTINA, 2007. *Milano. Un popolo e il suo Duomo. Storie di uomini che costruirono la cattedrale*, Milano, Marietti1820.

SANDRI, Lucia, 1988. "Stranieri e forestieri nella Firenze del Quattrocento attraverso i libri di ricordi e di entrata e uscita degli ospedali cittadini, *Forestieri e stranieri nelle città basso-medievali*, Firenze, Salimbeni: 149-161.

SERGI, Giuseppe, 1996. *Luoghi di strada nel Medioevo fra il Po, il mare e le Alpi occidentali*, Torino, Scriptorium.

SOMAINI, Francesco, 2005. "Alle origini dell'Ospedale Grande: il duca, il papa, la città", *La Ca' Granda. Vita ospedaliera e informazioni culturali*, 46/2: 19-34.

TADDEI, Ilaria; GHERMANI, Naïma (a cura di), 2019. *Hospitalité de l'étranger au Moyen Âge et à l'époque moderne: entre charité, contrôle et utilité sociale. Italie Europe*, in *Mélanges de l'École Française de Rome - Moyen Âge*, 131/2: 407-416, https://journals.openedition.org/mefrm/5494.

TATTI, Primo, 1663. *Degli annali sacri della città di Como*, Como, per gl'heredi di Nicolò Caprani.

VAUCHEZ, André, 1989. *La santità nel Medioevo*, Bologna, Il Mulino.

ZABBIA, Marino, 2012. "Morigia, Bonincontro", *Dizionario Biografico degli Italiani*, 76, Roma, Istituto dell'Enciclopedia Italiana: 836-837.

ZUCCHI, Bartolomeo, 1606. *Vita et miracula sancti Gerardi Tinctorii Modoetiensis*, Milano, Pontius & Piccaleus.

Frederic Aparisi Romero

# Mapping the Hospitals of the Agro-towns and Villages of Medieval Valencia*

## 1. *Introduction*

Finding medieval rural hospitals or even small-town hospitals is not easy. The written trace that these institutions have left is quite weak. This is one of the reasons behind the strong imbalance in the studies of urban and rural hospitals, the former being far more numerous. Indeed, the study of hospitals in the Middle Ages has a long historiographical tradition throughout Europe and in Valencia more specifically (Garcia Ballester 1989).[1] Traditionally, the healthcare institutions of large cities have attracted more attention, as is the case in Valencia itself, the capital city and central node of its Kingdom. In the specific case of Valencia, and beyond the Kingdom's capital, the hospitals of towns such as Castelló de la Plana (Revest 1947) and Gandia (Olaso 1988) have been studied as much as their extant written sources have allowed it. Despite this, the institution of the rural and small-town hospital has yet to be considered as a subject, except for the work of Max Satchell (2007) in the English context.

The contribution we are presenting here attempts to map the hospitals of Valencia's countryside and agro-towns, since the 13th century conquest of the Kingdom and until the beginning of the 16th century. We are working with the assumption that hospitals were not static institutions and, therefore, this network of assistance underwent changes during this time period. These hospitals, although autonomous in their institutional nature, coexisted and, therefore, they had a specific presence in common imaginaries. People knew where they were located, in what conditions their buildings were, and what kind of treatment they provided to those whom they admitted. The circulation of this kind of information among wayfarers and travellers denotes the existence of an informal network (Villagrasa 2016; Roca 2021).

* This work is part of the research project *Mercados, instituciones e integración económica en el Mediterráneo occidental (siglos XIII-XVI)*, ref. PID2021-128038NB-I00 (MCI/AEI/FEDER, UE).

1. See also Carmel Ferragud's chapter in this volume.

In this paper we use the term "agro-town" as a synonym for small town, with the added intention of stressing the rural nature of these settlements. Their role as marketplaces made them towns in their own right, but their main economic activities tied them to the rural world. Besides, technically speaking, only Valencia, Xàtiva, and later Oriola enjoyed the legal title of city. Other settlements were known as *viles* in Catalan, including important towns such as Morella, Alzira, and Morvedre and, more commonly, small towns such as Alcoi, Llíria, and Dénia, among others. Villages *–llocs* in Catalan–, corresponded to a third level in size and importance, and were applied to settlements such as La Jana, Rossell, and Russafa.

Beyond these introductory clarifications, we can proceed with the main aim of this chapter, that is, inventorying the rural hospitals of the Kingdom of Valencia in medieval times. The list of documented hospitals between 1238 and 1500 includes 78 institutions. This list is inevitably incomplete, but it allows us to sketch the broad contours of mediaeval Valencia's rural hospital network. According to their type and date of foundation, these hospitals can be grouped into three large groups. In the Kingdom's first stage, local councils were behind the creation of most hospitals, a trend that changed after 1300, when seigniorial and private foundations became commonplace. Finally, the 15th century saw a more varied landscape of foundations that depended on each case. The rural nature of these towns and villages did not prevent them from initiating processes of hospital fusion, as large cities had done on similar dates. Furthermore, their local governments constructed and promoted new municipal hospitals.

## 2. *A Century of Municipal Hospitals*

The military conquest of Valencia was followed by a process of colonization. The arrival of Christian settlers was a constant through the 13th century and the first decades of the 14th century, when new communities were created both ex novo and in previous Muslim settlements. Communities that needed buildings and spaces to develop their communal needs and issues and reinforce their collective identity. Local courts of justice, council halls, churches, and indeed, hospitals, were among the first buildings to be constructed.

These first hospitals had a triple function. For starters, they provided assistance and healing to the sick and poor. Secondly, hospitals were also places of worship, as they had a small chapel or at least an altar. And thirdly, in addition to this religious and health significance, they had marked political implications, since the building materialised the collective identity of the new settlers and, at the same time, constituted an architectonic manifestation of the main character of the dominant Christian feudal society (Rubio Vela 1984: 41-42).

Although in most cases we cannot determine the precise moment of foundation due to the scarcity of written sources, later evidence suggests that they took place during the first decades following the Christian conquest. In Alcoi, for instance, we can document how the hospital was already housing a number of sick people even before the local church was finished in 1262. In Dénia, the earliest reference to the hospital dates from 1275, but since the document refers to one of the hospital's landholdings, the institution itself had to be built and operational years before.[2] In Gandia, the hospital's location suggests that it was built during the immediate post-conquest period. An 18th century land survey does indeed confirm that the hospital was built a few years after the town's foundation (Olaso 1988: 14).

However, communal action was not the sole force behind the foundation of the medieval hospitals of Valencia in this first stage of their history. As it happened in the city of Valencia, monastic orders, and particularly Mercedarian monks, promoted the construction of hospitals. Following the express wishes of King James I, these monks founded a hospital in Dénia in 1245, just one year after the conquest of that small town (Aparisi 2018: 61). The same happened in Cullera in 1256 (Aparisi 2018: 61). It is not clear if these hospitals coexisted with the aforementioned municipal foundations, but it seems likely that their continuity was linked the presence of the Mercedarians, who left both towns after 1300. Therefore, it is possible that James I gave lands to the Mercedarians, together with the command to build hospitals in them, to give a rapid response to the needs of these communities. Both Dénia and Cullera were natural harbours where fishermen and sailors might have been in need of assistance, especially in relation with the frequent piracy-related kidnappings.

The management of these municipal hospitals was in the hands of the local authorities, represented by the administrator of the institution. In Gandia, for instance, one of the aldermen was appointed as the manager of the hospital. This administrator was in charge of everything related to the hospital except taking care of the inmates and wayfarers. That task fell on the so-called *hospitaler* and his wife. At best, they had basic health care, but not much more. Surgeons and barbers were called to inspect the patients and apply physical cures, but their presence depended on the budget of the institution and the local administration.

The importance of local authorities in the creation and management of hospitals did not mean that the Church was not very present. As it has been said, hospitals were places for healing both the body and the soul, and this spiritual care had to be provided by clergymen. Indeed, all hospitals had spaces of worship, and portable altars were frequently deployed. Besides, pastoral visits were conducted by priests, sent by their bishops, who reviewed the living conditions of the hospital's inmates (Galiana 2009; Aparisi 2018). The documents produced by these visits inform of the hospital's number of beds, its general state, or if gender separation was enforced, among other issues. Most agro-town hospitals used to have

2. In spite of not knowing the foundation date of the hospital, we do know that it was built before 1275. It is mentioned indirectly in a document that refers to a piece of land that belonged to the hospital: «*et afrontat dicta hereditas cum honore que fuit hospitalis*» (Arxiu de la Corona d'Aragó; ACA from now on), Cancelleria, reg. 20, f. 328.

between 10 and 15 beds for both genders, but hospitals in villages such as Xert or Benicàssim had between 2 and 6 beds in total (Aparisi 2018: 62-63; table 1).

## 3. *Private and Seigneurial Hospitals*

From the last quarter of the 13th century onwards, we detect a new phenomenon in the foundation of hospitals. This is the time when the post-Conquest generation entered the final stages of their lives and began to write their last wills, in which they established the foundation of new hospitals. This practice, which was commonplace in 13th century feudal Europe, emerged in force in the newly feudalised Kingdom of Valencia from the 14th century on. Therefore, through this new wave of private and personal foundations, the hospital landscape of Valencia accentuated its secular character, which had already started with its first municipal foundations. In many cases, the administration of the newly founded hospitals was given to a family member, and the Church only had authority when it came to worship. In some cases, however, the patron delegated the administration to a clergyman. For instance, a prosperous neighbour of Alzira, called Escuder, founded a hospital in 1404, named after Saint Catherine but popularly known as the hospital d'en Escuder, and gave its administration to a priest (Aparisi, Ferragud 2018: 38).

The purpose of these personal foundations was twofold. On the one hand, the testator performed an act of charity towards the poor, Christ's representatives on earth, with the aim of earning, at the time of their death, forgiveness and, in short, the salvation of the soul. On the other hand, there were less pious motivations. The foundation of a hospital could guarantee lasting fame and recognition, and the survival of the donor's name after their death. Indeed, hospitals were dedicated to a particular saint, but they were popularly known by the name of their founder. Some examples of this pattern are the hospital d'en Dahers, in Vila-Real, founded by Pere Dahera in 1275, and the hospital d'en Trujols in Castelló de la Plana, erected before 1390 (Revest 1947: 8).

The 14th century also saw a wave of what I have called "seigneurial founding", that is, new hospitals founded by manorial lords for the sake of the communities they ruled over. In all the documented cases, we have not found any evidence of other coexisting hospitals. Therefore, we can safely assume that this type of seigneurial initiative emerged when local communities had insufficient funds to erect a hospital.

Examples of this pattern can be detected as early as 1292, when Pere de Benviure and Constança d'Anglesola founded the hospital of Albalat de la Ribera, in the manor they owned and ruled (Aparisi, Ferragud 2018: 35). In 1341, another noblewoman, Margarida de Llúria, refounded the hospital of her manor of el Puig, since the already existing hospital was financially and physically derelict. She bequeathed 500 annual *sous* to the «*hospitali pauperum*» to support the building and those poor people that «*confluentibus in eodem*». Later, in a codicil of 1343, she granted an additional yearly rent of 50 *sous*, aimed at rearing the building and feeding its inmates. After her death in 1409, the manor was taken over by the city of Valencia and, consequently, the management of the hospital was left in the hands of the aldermen of the Kingdom's capital. They continued to appoint local administrators until the hospital was dissolved in 1450 (RUBIO VELA 1996-1997: 8-9).

The example of Margarida de Llúria was in no way exceptional. Other local lords became involved in the rebuilding of hospitals during periods of extreme necessity for their vassals, particularly after the war with Castile (1355-1366). This was the case of Bernat de Bonastre, lord of Ondara, a large village that suffered major damages during the war (RICHART 2001). He «rebuilt the hospital of the village of Ondara, for which he bought and later gave a piece of land, and all together (the repairs and the piece of land) cost him 1,500 *sous* and even more».[3] There is a high chance that Alfonso of Aragon, duke of Gandia and count of Dénia, was also involved in the rebuilding of rural hospitals, since his seigneurial holdings had been devastated by the Castilian troops of King Peter I. Indeed, the hospital of Gandia was rededicated in 1378 to Saint Mark, on the behest of Jaume d'Aragó, bishop of Valencia and Alfonso's brother (APARISI 2018: 64).

It is worth saying that the involvement of seigneurial powers in the economic and architectonic restoration of hospitals did not necessarily entail that such institutions became private or personal foundations. Their management was still in the hands of the local administrations, and, unlike the previously mentioned private foundations, they were popularly known by the name of the saint they were dedicated to.

## 4. *Years of Fusion*

During the 15th century, the conditions of the hospitals in the agro-towns of Valencia were diverse. While larger agro-towns, which had more than one hospital, initiated processes of hospital concentration, smaller towns had to restore their hospitals, usually with the help of their seigneurial lord or at the initiative of local authorities.

Since the very beginning of the century, the small hospitals of the capitals and larger cities of the different territories of the Crown of Aragon underwent processes of fusion or concentration that gave way to a single, larger institution. In Barcelona, this process took place in 1401, in Zaragoza in 1425, in Lleida in 1454, and in Mallorca in 1456. In the case of the city of Valencia, its hospitals did not merge into a larger institution until 1512. The main reason under these hospital fusions was the structural lack of economic resources of these welfare institutions. Hospital merging allowed, therefore, to maximise existing funds and rationalise management.

3. Arxiu del Regne de València (from now on ARV), Governació, num. 2.195, mà 7, f. 11v; quoted in Richard 2001: 54-55.

This policy of concentrating resources was also followed in agro-towns and villages, such as Castelló de la Plana (Revest 1947), Alzira, and Cocentaina. Indeed, we can document a process of hospital concentration in Concentaina at a date as early as 1401. Unfortunately, we have no specific details of the unification process, but we do know that four pre-existing hospitals -the municipal hospital, the hospital d'en Berenguer, the hospital d'en Cepillo and the hospital d'en Rojals– were merged into a new, larger hospital, placed under the administration of the local municipal authorities.

In Alzira, a failed effort to merge the town's two hospitals -one managed by the municipality and the other, the hospital d'en Escuder, under ecclesiastical control- was started in 1454. Despite this initial upset, the local aldermen used the foundation of a new private hospital in 1465 to reopen the possibility of a hospital merger, this time involving three hospitals. Before 1471, both the city council and the church reached an agreement, and these three hospitals were concentrated into one institution, supervised by both the council and the church (Aparisi, Feragud 2018: 38-39).

As the aforementioned examples show, private hospitals struggled to survive at a higher rate than municipal ones. Their problems had to do not only with financial ruin but also with their management. Despite the fact that founders could initially appoint a family member as the hospital's patron, in due time the municipal councils tended to absorb these hospitals, and the aldermen became their administrators, becoming these municipal hospitals.

The process of hospital concentration took place mostly in larger and medium agro-towns like the aforementioned, which had a clear role as marketplaces. Conversely, other agro-towns that did not have this marked commercial character displayed other trends. This was the case, for instance, of the agrotowns of Castellfabib and Ademús and the village of Arguines. These three cases were located in the inlands of the Kingdom of Valencia and were granted the privilege of founding a new hospital by the same king, John II. Despite the lack of evidence, it is highly probable that Castellfabib and Ademús had pre-existing hospitals, given their importance in the Valencian inland. In Ademús, the royal privilege was conceded after the aldermen had requested the King to «*hedificandi hospitale licentiam et facultatem concedere*».[4] This exact same formula was also used for the privilege of Castellfabib.[5] Unfortunately, beyond these purely formal words, we do not know the details of these foundations, although it is clear that they responded to a demand of the local authorities.

In the case of the 1470 hospital of Arguines, it is clear that it was in fact a refoundation of an already existing hospital. There is evidence of a hospital in the village at least until 1418, when it was ruined due to an armed robbery that killed the two people who were in charge of it (Carbonell, Díaz 2018: 164). It took fifty years to create a new hospital, in a jointly organised action of the

4. ARV, Reial Cancelleria, num. 269 f. 56.
5. ARV, Reial Cancelleria, num. 269 f. 56v.

Mercedarian order, the lord of Arguines, the representatives of the local community, and the king, Joan II. We do not know how the people who travelled from Aragon to Valencia and frequently made use of this establishment reacted to its disappearance in 1418, but there is no doubt that the absence of a hospital in the village altered the travel routes in the area. Finally, in 1470, the king's officials dictated the features, both architectonic and financial, of the new hospital.[6] It had to provide accommodation for six inmates, each with its own bed. New buildings had to be erected, particularly a kitchen, a wood deposit, and a new house with rooms to accommodate poor wayfarers. We may assume that the royal commands were followed and the hospital built, but the continuity of the centre remains unknown.

The hospital of Gandia represents centres that, despite structural economic troubles, enjoyed a remarkable continuity. It is an exceptional case, since it is the only agro-town hospital that functioned continuously from its foundation in the 13th century to the 20th century. Indeed, the town's merchants and well-off neighbours did not create their own hospitals, as their counterparts elsewhere did, for reasons that are still unknown to us. Nevertheless, this lack of competition did not mean that the hospital of Gandia was free from the economic hurdles that were so often attached to these institutions (Olaso 1988: 15-19). Perhaps the creation of the General Hospital of Valencia in 1512 relieved some of the pressure on the hospital of Gandia, since the larger institution would deal with more difficult cases and diseases. But, beyond this very specific case, the town's hospital had to cater to the needs of the poor, sick, and disabled from not only Gandia itself, but also its surrounding area.

The 15th century hospital of the small village of La Jana is also note-worthy. It is probably the only complete medieval hospital building that is still standing in the region of Valencia, although it was slightly modified when it was turned into a small chapel. It is also illustrative of the hospitals in villages and small agro-towns. These hospitals shared some features with their urban counterparts, like being mostly located at the entryways of their settlements, so their inmates' beggarly activities could be more effectively focused. Despite this, the differences with urban hospitals abound. Rural hospitals consisted of simpler buildings, with only one ward, that were, in fact, mostly undifferentiated from other local common houses. In fact, some private hospitals were located in the original houses of their founders (Revest 1947: 8-9). These hospitals had no interior separation, since they had only one room (Aparisi 2018: 59). As a result, during pastoral visits, priests demanded that, at the very least, gender separation be enforced through the use of curtains (Aparisi 2018: 61). To cater to the inmates' spiritual needs, rural hospitals had modest altars, visible even to patients who could not stand up. In the case of the hospital of La Jana, the altar was at the end of this sole main room.

6. ARV, Reial Cancelleria, f. 102v-104 (Carbonell, Díaz 2018: 175-176). The volume of *Reial Cancelleria* is not specified.

## 5. *Conclusions*

The history of hospitals cannot be explained as a straight and unequivocal line. The existence of a hospital at a given point in time did not at all imply its continuity. Conversely, the foundation of a hospital at a certain date does not imply that there could not have been other previously existing hospitals in the same community. Consequently, the network of hospitals in a territory was not something stable but changing, in constant transformation. Some centres could emerge while others disappeared, and the material conditions of a specific hospital changed in time. Therefore, from a wayfarer's perspective, one centre could provide a better welcome at a given moment, creating a constantly changing network of welfare.

Despite the importance these pilgrims and wayfarers, hospitals were created, first and foremost, to serve the needs of local communities, and especially those who lived in poverty or suffered from disabilities. Even private foundations were created in response to communal needs.

To conclude, the Valencian network of hospitals did not necessarily reflect the economic and political evolution of the Kingdom at large. During its first century, in a context of expansion, the foundation of hospitals relied on the action of local authorities first and later on prosperous neighbours who wanted to perpetuate their names and save their souls. The difficulties of the mid-14$^{th}$ century brought certain levels of disaffection, as a decrease in private and personal foundations shows. Despite this, the economic improvements and the political stability that came with the enthronement of the Trastamaras did not imply a general increase in charitable endeavours nor any significant improvement in the material conditions of hospitals. In contrast, the 15$^{th}$ century saw the generalisation of hospital concentration processes, aimed at maximising existing resources, in most agro-towns, years before the capital city's hospital merger. It is tempting to associate the Valencian hospital concentration of 1512 with the outburst of the revolt of the Germanies in 1520, as an early symptom of a worsening economic situation. But this is not necessarily so. The 16$^{th}$ century also saw the founding of hospitals in small villages such as Teulada (Ivars 2010). As three hundred years before, the foundation of a hospital became the physical manifestation of the demographic weight and, especially, the political maturity of a community.

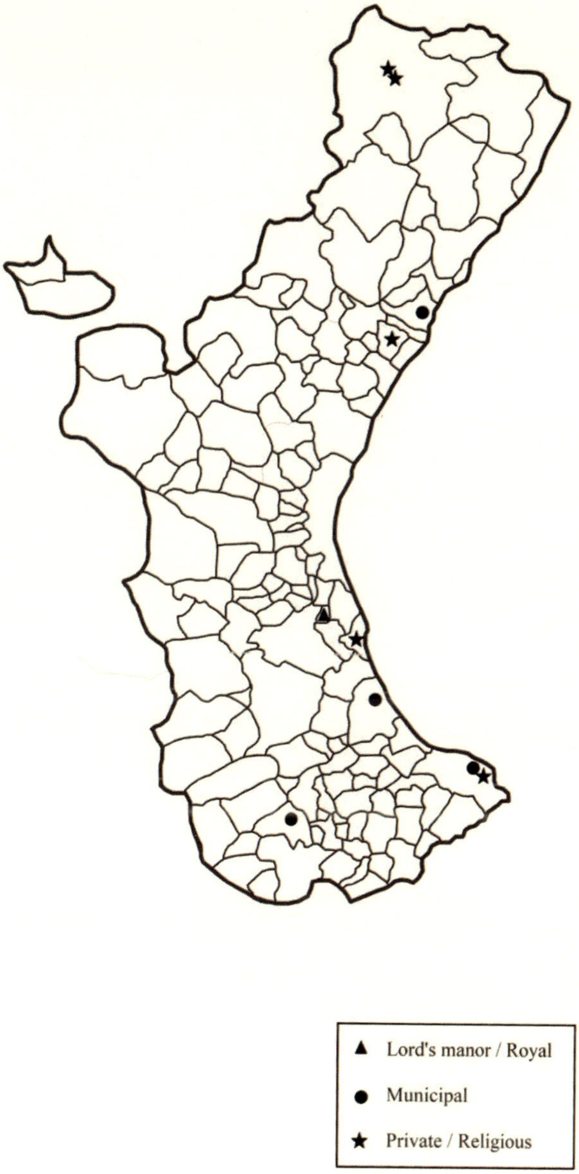


Fig. 1. The Kingdom of Valencia in the 13th century.

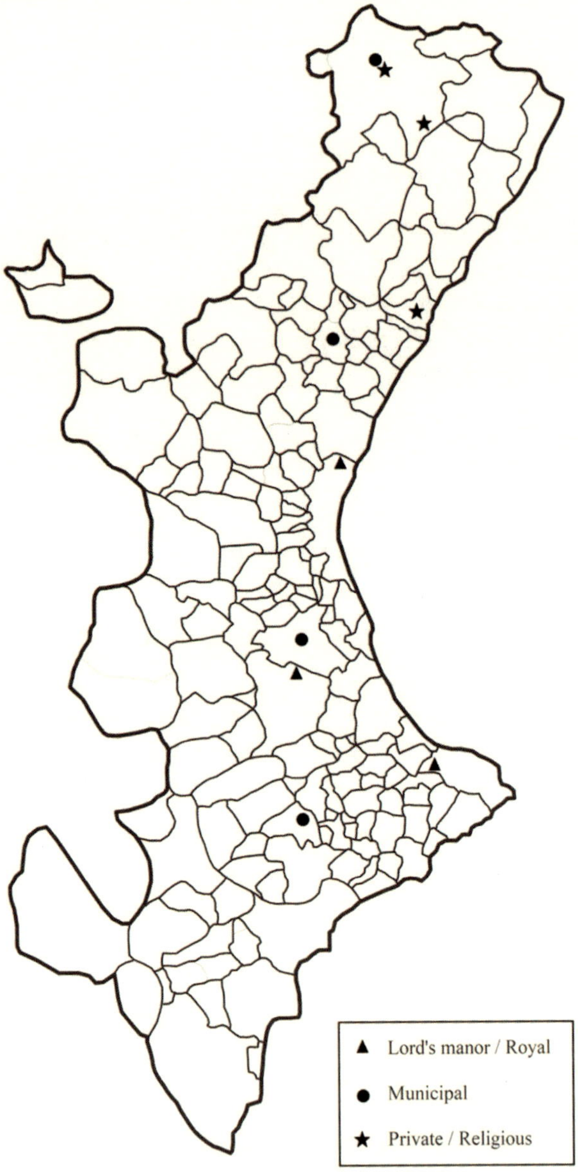


Fig. 2. The Kingdom of Valencia in the 14th century.

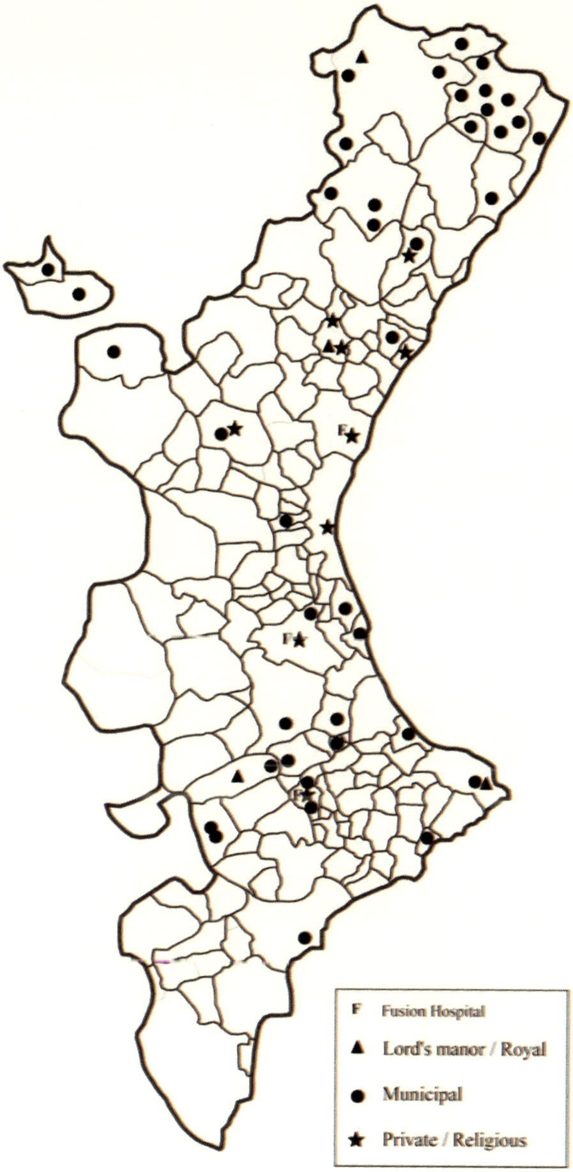


Fig. 3. The Kingdom of Valencia in the 15th century.

Table 1: List (in progress) of village and agro-town hospitals in Medieval Valencia[7]

| Name | Agro-town or village | Year of foundation<br>First reference*<br>*last reference | Founder | Women / Total beds |
|---|---|---|---|---|
| | Dénia | 1245 | Mercedarian | |
| de Sant Nicolau | Morella | 1248 | Brotherhood | |
| pobres de Crist<br>de Sant Marc (1378) | Gandia | 1254 | Municipal | |
| | Cullera | 1256 | Mercedarian | |
| de la vila | Alcoi | 1262 | Municipal | |
| d'en Dahera | Vila-real | 1275 | Private | |
| de la vila | Dénia | 1275* | Municipal | |
| de lleprosos | Morella | 1280 | Franciscans | |
| de Sant Jaume | Castelló de la Plana | 1290* | Municipal | |
| | Albalat de la Ribera | 1299* | Seigneurial | |
| d'en Segarra | Catí | 1321 | Private | |
| | Alcoi | 1322* | Municipal | |
| | Pobla Llarga | 1337 | Seigneurial | |
| hospitali pauperum | el Puig | 1341* | Seigneurial | |
| de Santa Llúcia | Alzira | 1355* | Municipal | |
| de la Santa Trinitat<br>i Sant Antoni Abat | Morella | 1365 | Brotherhood | |
| | Ondara | 1372 | Seigneurial | |
| de la vila | Sogorb | 1378* | Municipal | |
| dels Folls | Morella | 1378 | Municipal | |
| de Sant Nicolau | Cocentaina | 1383* | Brotherhood | |
| d'en Trujols | Castelló de la Plana | 1390 | Private | 11 |
| d'en Berenguer | Cocentaina | *1401 | Private | |
| d'en Cepillo | Cocentaina | *1401 | Private | |
| d'en Rojals | Cocentaina | *1401 | Private | |
| Nostra Senyora de la Misericòrdia | Cocentaina | 1401 | Fusion | |

7. Source: https://www.uv.es/fearo2/xarxahospitalsruralsVlc.html [2022, 12, 14].

| Name | Agro-town or village | Year of foundation First reference* *last reference | Founder | Women / Total beds |
|---|---|---|---|---|
| d'en Escuder o de Santa Caterina | Alzira | 1404* | Private | |
| | El Forcall | 1408 | Royal | |
| d'en Guasch | Vilafamés | 1408 | Private | |
| | Arguines | 1418 | Seigneurial | |
| de Sant Joan | Cullera | 1442* | Municipal | |
| de la vila | Oliva | 1444* | Municipal | |
| | Sueca | 1445* | Municipal | |
| de pobres de Crist | Ademús | 1446 | Municipal | |
| de pobres de Crist | Castellfabib | 1446 | Municipal | |
| | Alacant | 1448* | Municipal | |
| | Agullent | 1448* | Municipal | |
| | Alcalà | 1448* | Municipal | 4 |
| de la vila | Alpont | 1448* | Municipal | |
| de Sant Pere | Altea | 1448* | Municipal | |
| del lloc | Atzaneta del Maestrat | 1448* | Municipal | |
| | Benicarló | 1448* | Municipal | 1/5 |
| de pobres | Benifassà | 1448* | Municipal | |
| | Biar | 1448* | Municipal | |
| | Biar | 1448* | Municipal | |
| Sant Blai | Borriana | 1448 | Brotherhood | |
| | Càlig | 1448* | Municipal | |
| | Canet | 1448* | Municipal | 2 |
| | Cervera | 1448* | Municipal | |
| | Culla | 1448* | Municipal | 3 |
| | la Jana | 1448* | Municipal | 2 |
| | la Mata | 1448* | Municipal | 1 |
| d'en Bellpuig | Llíria | 1448* | Private | |
| de la vila | Llíria | 1448* | Municipal | |
| na Marzena | Morvedre | 1448* | Private | |
| de la reina | Ontinyent | 1448* | Royal | |
| de la vila | Pego | 1448* | Municipal | |

| NAME | AGRO-TOWN OR VILLAGE | YEAR OF FOUNDATION FIRST REFERENCE* *LAST REFERENCE | FOUNDER | WOMEN / TOTAL BEDS |
|---|---|---|---|---|
| | Rossell | 1448* | Municipal | |
| d'en Guiot | Russafa | 1448 | Private | |
| de la vila | Sant Mateu | 1448* | Municipal | 14 |
| de Sant Miquel | Sogorb | 1448* | Private | |
| | Traiguera | 1448* | Municipal | 1/4 |
| | Vallibona | 1448* | Municipal | |
| | Vila-real | 1448* | Municipal | |
| | Vilafamés | 1448* | Municipal | 3 |
| | Vilafranca | 1448* | Municipal | |
| de la vila | Vistabella | 1448* | Municipal | |
| | Xàbia | 1448* | Municipal | |
| | Xert | 1448* | Municipal | 2 |
| de la vila | Llutxent | 1469* | Municipal | |
| Santa Maria Merced | Arguines | 1470 | Royal | 6 |
| de la vila-Santa Llúcia | Alzira | 1471* | Fusion | |
| | Algemesí | 1475* | Municipal | |
| | Albaida | 1478* | Municipal | |
| de la vila | Pobla de Rugat | 1479* | Municipal | |
| | Castelló de la Ribera | 1489* | Municipal | |
| de la vila | Quart | 1492* | Municipal | |
| de la Trinitat | Morvedre | 1500* | Fusion | |
| de la vila | Xàbia | 1502 | Seigneurial | |

## *Bibliography*

Aparisi, Frederic, 2018. "La cultura material de los hospitales de las villas valencianas en la Baja Edad Media", *Revista de la CECEL-CSIC*, 18: 55-68.

Aparisi, Frederic; Ferragud, Carmel, 2018. "Hospitals rurals a la València baixmedieval: el cas de l'hospital de Santa Llúcia d'Alzira", Josep M. Comelles, Antoni Conejo, Josep Barceló (ed.), *Imago civitatis. Hospitales y manicomios en Occidente*, Tarragona, URV-UB: 33-55.

Carbonell, Maria J.; Díaz, Andrés, 2018. "Las instrucciones de Juan de Navarra para la reconstrucción del hospital de Arguines en 1470", María Julia Martínez et al (ed.), *Els turquets d'Algar. La redempció de captius per l'Ordre dels Mercedaris al Camp de Morvedre*, Algar de Palència, Ajuntament d'Algar de Palència: 159-176.

Galiana, José M. (a cura de), 2009. *La visita pastoral d'Otó de Montcada al Bisbat de Tortosa (1428-1429)*, Valencia, Universitat de València.

García Ballester, Luis, 1989. *La medicina a la València medieval. Medicina i societat en un país medieval mediterrani*, Valencia, Alfons el Magnànim.

Ivars, Joan, 2010. "Hospitals i cases de caritat a la Marina Alta: l'Hospital de Sant Martí, bisbe, de Teulada (s. XVI-XIX)", *Aguaits*, 29: 37-56

Olaso, Vicent, 1988. *L'hospital de Sant Marc de Gandia, una institució per a pobres malalts. Segles XIII-XX,* Gandia, CEIC Alfons el Vell.

Revest, Luis, 1947. *Hospitales y pobres en el Castellón de otros tiempos*, Castelló de la Plana, Sociedad Castellonense de Cultura.

Richart, Jaume, 2001. "Documents: Ondara i el seu castell: 1372/1407", *Aguaits*, 18: 97-103.

Roca, Guillem, 2021. *Pobresa i hospitals a la Lleida baixmedieval*, Lleida, Institut d'Estudis Ilerdencs.

Rubio Vela, Agustín, 1984. *Pobreza, enfermedad y asistencia hospitalaria en la Valencia del siglo XIV*, València, Alfons el Magnànim.

Rubio Vela, Agustín, 1996-1997. "El hospital medieval de El Puig: esbozo de su historia", *Estudis Castellonencs*, 7: 5-14.

Satchell, Max, 2007. "Towards a Landscape History of the Rural Hospital in England, 1100-1300", John Henderson, Peregrine Horden, Alessandro Pastore (ed), *The Impact of Hospitals 300-2000*, Bern, Peter Lang: 237-256.

Villagrasa, Raúl, 2016. *La red de hospitales en el Aragón medieval (ss. XII-XV)*, Zaragoza, Instituto Fernando el Católico.

Anna Maria Ester Condins

# Els inventaris de béns de l'hospital de la Santa Creu de Vic*

## 1. *Introducció*

La recerca sobre els hospitals de l'edat mitjana sovint ensopega amb una dificultat: poder descriure amb precisió els diferents espais que els conformaven i quines eren les seves funcions. Els documents conservats aporten indicis que permeten deduir-ne l'activitat que s'hi duia a terme. Malauradament, la seva estructura interna o bé s'ha perdut, o bé ha sofert nombroses modificacions i ampliacions amb el pas dels anys. El cas de l'hospital de la Santa Creu de Vic no se'n deslliura.

Aquest hospital va ser fundat el 1348 mitjançant testament atorgat per Ramon Terrades, un mercader vigatà que deixà a la ciutat 600 lliures per a la seva construcció (Junyent 1976; Prades 2000). L'edifici, que avui en dia podem contemplar formant part d'un magnífic conjunt hospitalari, també ha sofert múltiples canvis i ampliacions, que fan difícil la seva interpretació.

Tanmateix, disposem d'una font extraordinària que ens descobreix la distribució de les diferents sales i, també, la seva ubicació dins l'edifici, a més de precisar-ne els mobles, robes i eines que s'hi usaven habitualment: els inventaris de béns. Aquests inventaris, que es duien a terme periòdicament, eren una eina més de la qual disposava el Consell de la Ciutat per tal d'exercir un millor control de la gestió dels hospitalers. Es realitzaven davant de notari i en presència de testimonis i calia repetir-los sovint, ja fos quan cessava un hospitaler i n'entrava un altre, o bé per tal de registrar-ne noves donacions dels fidels. Algunes d'aquestes deixes podien ser tan bàsiques com un llit, un cobertor, o simplement, un joc de llençols.

Pel que fa al context català, la majoria d'inventaris publicats fins a la data, ja sigui de centres assistencials o d'habitatges privats, revelen una certa homo-

* Els inventaris donats a conèixer en aquest estudi formen part de la meva tesi doctoral en curs sobre l'hospital vigatà. Agraeixo a Antoni Conejo i Salvatore Marino, directors de la meva tesi doctoral, les indicacions que m'han proporcionat per l'elaboració d'aquest text. També vull adreçar el meu agraïment a Rafel Ginebra, arxiver de l'Arxiu i Biblioteca Episcopal de Vic (ABEV), pel seu suport.

geneïtat quant als mobles, roba i atuells de tota mena que s'hi documenten. Per exemple, Maria D. Santandreu (2006), a la seva tesi doctoral sobre la vila de Berga, estudià a bastament l'aixovar i la resta de béns de les cases medievals. En altres àmbits, Jordi Bolòs (2022) aconsegueix, mitjançant l'anàlisi de diversos inventaris *post mortem*, assolir una imatge aproximada de la distribució de les estances de les residències urbanes del segle XV. Per la seva banda, Flocel Sabaté (1990) ha publicat un estudi sobre els objectes de la vida quotidiana a les llars de Barcelona del tres-cents. Encara que aquestes aportacions són alienes al mon hospitalari, són d'una gran utilitat per tal de valorar què es podia trobar a l'interior d'un nosocomi de l'època, ja que, al cap i a la fi, molts dels elements eren els mateixos.

Centrant-nos en el tema que ens ocupa, són diversos els autors que han donat a conèixer inventaris d'hospitals pròpiament dits. Llur interpretació permet imaginar com es distribuïen les estances, de quin mobiliari disposaven, les robes dels llits, la seva qualitat i els colors, els estris culinaris i tot allò que hi havia al menjador o al celler. Rubio Vela (1984) ja va descriure en el seu dia les diferents estances de l'hospital d'en Clapers de València. Pel que fa a Girona, Anna Gironella (2001) publicà l'inventari de béns de l'hospital de la Seu corresponent a 1342, mentre que Jaume de Puig i Oliver (2020) donà a conèixer els dels anys 1353 i 1362. Quant a la ciutat de Lleida, Guillem Roca (2021) s'endinsa en un seguit d'inventaris de diversos dels seus hospitals urbans, tots datats el 1447. Recentment, Carmel Ferragud (2022) ha fet el propi amb un parell pertanyents a l'hospital de Sant Andreu de Mallorca de 1370 i 1451. Un cas ben curiós és el d'un inventari custodiat a l'Arxiu de la Catedral de Barcelona de l'hospital italià de Santa Maria della Scala de Siena, publicat per Antoni Conejo i Carles Vela (2021); tot i que no està datat, molt probablement es devia fer pels volts de 1400. Aquest darrer exemple revela, com també ha estat subratllat per altres autors (Piccinni 2016), que les descripcions i els inventaris d'un centre podien viatjar i anar d'un lloc a l'altre i servir de model, o no, per a establiments ubicats en geografies allunyades entre si.

A tots aquests i a molts d'altres que no esmento per no allargar-me en excés, ara hi podem afegir els inventaris de béns de l'hospital de la Santa Creu de Vic conservats a l'Arxiu de la Catedral de la capital osonenca, els quals se solien redactar amb motiu del nomenament d'un nou hospitaler.[1] Es tractava, doncs, d'una manera per controlar i detectar si, durant la gestió de la persona cessant, hom havia sostret o malmès béns pertanyents a l'hospital i, en definitiva, a la ciutat.

A la llum d'aquests documents, en aquestes ratlles en farem una descripció i una anàlisi al més acurada que ens sigui possible. A més, el fet de disposar d'inventaris de diferents anys, també ens permetrà resseguir les noves dependències que s'hi van anar afegint o construint durant els primers anys de funcionament de

1. Aquests nomenaments es poden consultar a l'Arxiu de la Catedral de Vic, concretament a l'Arxiu de la Cúria Fumada (a partir d'ara ACF), número 4489.

l'entitat.[2] Per aquesta raó n'he triat els que aporten més informació. D'una banda, històrica, ja que es para esment dels edificis més antics. I, de l'altra, social, perquè ens apropa a la vida quotidiana dels ciutadans de la Vic baixmedieval. El primer és del 1388; el segon es realitzà deu anys després; mentre que els tres restants que s'analitzaran corresponen a 1399, 1405 i 1407.[3]

Cal insistir que aquest és el primer cop en què es fa una anàlisi d'aquests instruments. Malgrat que amb anterioritat alguns autors ja s'hi havien referit, com ara Cèsar Martinell (1935) o Segimon Cunill (1931), no van entrar a valorar-ne llur contingut, "limitant-se" a emprar-los per tal justificar la data en què el centre havia començat a funcionar.

## 2. *Espais i mobiliari*

### 2.1. *Inventari de l'any 1388*

A l'inventari de l'any 1388 hi són presents Pere Estanyol, escrivà jurat, Antoni Rabes i Bernat Compte, coltellers, Joan Moles i Joan Terrers, procuradors de l'hospital, i Bonanat Vall, en representació dels consellers de la ciutat; en canvi, no hi consta cap hospitaler. Tan sols es registren els béns, pocs tot sigui dit, corresponents a una única sala de la que se'ns diu que es trobava a la planta inferior –per la qual cosa cal deduir que l'edifici constava de dos nivells–, i a la qual se l'anomena "casa maior", fet que en pressuposa una certa rellevància i grandària. Tanmateix, el document permet constatar que l'hospital ja era construït i que estava en funcionament,[4] alhora que ens informa del nombre de llits i la seva distribució.

Tal com avançava, el text s'inicia amb l'al·lusió a una «*domo maiori inferiori ipsius hospitalis res sequentes*», a l'interior de la qual hi trobem vuit llits, cinc dels quals són al costat dret i els tres restants a l'angle esquerre. Segons s'apunta, aquests comptaven amb una màrfega farcida de palla i, només un, amb un matalàs. Quasi tots disposen d'un parell de llençols d'estopa de cànem (*canapis*), dues o tres flassades blanques fetes amb llana d'Aragó i llistades de diferents colors.[5] No tots tenen coixins, i s'enumeren tres travessers i un coixí de fustani. Hi ha tres llits dels quals no es descriu cap mena de parament, tot i que es puntualitza que són «a l'antigor»; no sabem si aquest seria el motiu de no usar-los.

2. És interessant la reflexió de Josep M. Casas (1975: 215): «Els inventaris no solen ésser bons col·laboradors de la història, presos individualment, perquè d'un a un són el registre d'un moment, d'una situació. És necessària la confluència de com més millor».

3. A l'annex recullo la transcripció de l'inventari de l'any 1407, el darrer dels analitzats en aquest article.

4. ACF 4489, f. 2r «[...] venerabilium consiliariorum administratorum hospitalis vocati d'en Terrades, constructi in carrario Sancti Petri».

5. M. Dolors Santandreu (2006, 379) en relació amb els objectes quotidians documentats a la vila de Berga puntualitza que les flassades de llana d'Aragó es trobaven a cases de gent benestant.

### 2.2. *Inventari de l'any 1398*

L'inventari següent correspon a l'any 1398 i, en aquesta ocasió, detallen els béns del pis superior del que abans només en deduíem l'existència. Hi foren presents Tomàs Mateu, escrivà jurat, Joan Terrers, especier i procurador de l'hospital, Francesca, esposa de Domènec Falcó, l'hospitaler ja difunt, i Pere de Santaeulàlia i Bernat Carne manegadors.

L'autor del text ens introdueix en un nou habitacle i ho fa amb una descripció ben clara: «*Primo in capite gradarii ipsius hospicii*», és a dir, dalt les escales, per tant, el pis superior. Aquest àmbit sobirà tenia unes funcions ben diferents al de la planta inferior. La casa o sala major era un espai de grans dimensions on només hi havia llits, fet que demostra que es tractava d'una sala destinada al repòs i l'atenció dels malalts. En canvi, a dalt documentem eines i una cambra independent amb roba de dona (probablement, la de l'hospitalera). Interpreto, doncs, que devia tractar-se d'una àrea privada separada de la resta i destinada a l'ús del personal propi.

De la lectura dels objectes i estris descrits es pot conjecturar que era un espai d'emmagatzematge o de treball. Hi ha una balança de fustes, una caixa amb coberta i una altra de més petita.[6] També hi trobem altres elements, probablement penjats de la paret o bé, distribuïts en lleixes. En primer lloc, una cistella de canyes que contenia "frasques", un "gavadalot",[7] una carabassa de vi,[8] un coixí de ploma i una caixa amb tapa de flassada amb llistes vermelles. També hi ha una caixeta, una cistelleta i un morter amb el seu boix de fusta.

Quant al segon habitacle devia ser una habitació d'ús individual i en la qual hi trobem una caixa amb potes que conté, com s'ha dit, la roba de l'hospitalera i l'aixovar de llit, un "saglit" ple de palla i dos capçals de llit. També es para esment d'un banc[9] amb peus o «petyat» amb més roba de llit i també, vestits propis d'una dona. Finalment, s'esmenta una galleda o poal i un morter.

A les darreres línies consta un pagament de 2 sous, suposadament pagats a un parell de testimonis: el cirurgià Guillem Andreu[10] i el bracer Bernat Cosar.

6. Segons Flocel Sabaté (1990: 57), aquestes caixes sovint descansaven directament sobre el terra. Les més preuades serien aquelles que tenien potes.

7. Segons el Diccionari d'Alcover-Moll (a partir d'ara DCVB) es tracta d'un vas de fusta per rentar plats.

8. Segons el DCVB carabassa de vi, carabassa vinatera o vinera, o carabassa de viner o carabassa de pelegrí: és llenyosa i forma dues panxes unides per un coll estret o bé, una sola panxa i un coll llarguer. Serveix per dur vi o aigua, i també s'empra buida com a surador per banyar-se les persones que no saben nedar.

9. A les tres darreres línies d'aquest foli hi ha pèrdua de material que dificulta la lectura completa del text.

10. La presència d'un professional de la medicina exercint de testimoni fa pensar que s'hi trobava en exercici de la seva feina. Per contra, no els trobem als llibres de comptes de l'hospital cobrant el seu salari.

## 2.3. *Inventari de l'any 1399*

L'any 1399 s'inicia un nou inventari que ja presenta els espais d'una manera més ordenada, ja que es descriu tant el pis inferior com el superior, fet que ens proporciona una idea de conjunt més aproximada. En primer lloc, igual en l'inventari de 1388, es comença pel que se «atrobat en la casa maior del dit hospital on jauen los pobres ço es en l'entrada davant la porta». Hi trobem set llits, cinc de posts, una colga i un de cabirons. Sis disposen de màrfega i quatre de matalàs. Els parells de llençols –de vegades de tres teles, és a dir, de qualitat– es troben en sis dels llits que, alhora, compten amb quatre travessers o coixins llargs. Pel que fa a les flassades, habitualment en corresponen dues per llit, i es diu que eren fetes amb llana d'Aragó i llistades amb diversos colors.

Seguidament, es fa referència a una altra casa o estança destinada a les dones: «Item foren atrobats en una altra casa baxa aprés la dita casa major damunt contenguda on jaen les fembres». Així doncs, aquest retall ens permet afirmar que, almenys des de 1399, l'hospital ja disposava d'una infraestructura suficient per segregar els pobres, malalts o pelegrins per gènere. Aquesta segona casa, més baixa i situada a continuació de la *maior*, podria interpretar-se de dues maneres: bé com una sala contigua a la primera i, per tant, integrada en el mateix edifici; bé com un ambient annex i independent. Tan sols té quatre llits,[11] tres de posts i un de cabirons; tots ells amb màrfega, un amb matalàs, cadascun amb dos llençols i travessers. Les flassades, com les anteriors, també eren de llana d'Aragó i amb llistats multicolor.

Un tercer espai situat vora l'hort i anomenat "casa de les robes", s'emprava per a guardar peces tèxtils i també alguns llits en desús. Pel que fa al mobiliari, s'esmenten una taula –precisament per a plegar-hi la roba–, un llit de cabirons sense parament i diversos components de llits fets malbé, potser per reciclar-los en cas d'haver de fer alguna reparació als que estaven en bones condicions. A l'últim, també hi trobem una corriola de pou. En total, es compten vint-i-dues flassades, algunes de llana d'Aragó i dotze de borra. Totes eren blanques amb llistats molt variats: blau i vermell, negres i vermells, blaves i verdes etc. Emperò, es puntualitza que la qualitat no sempre era òptima, car n'hi ha quatre que es descriuen com a sotils o de poc valor; d'altres es diu que o bé estaven esquinçades o bé, tan sols hi quedaven alguns retalls. Així i tot, hi ha dos llençols de tres teles, a més a més de tres cobertors i un parell de vànoves.

Finalment, el text ens proporciona la descripció del celler, on hi consta una tona de quatre sesters, una altra de dos sesters, un follador de fusta i dos cercles, tot destinat a conservar i processar el vi. D'altra banda, al menjador, situat al pis superior, s'esmenten dos taüts de diferent grandària i un caixó petit sotil. I a la cuina, ubicada també a la planta noble, es registren tres olles una de coure i dues d'aram, una bacina d'aram, un morter de coure i un perol trencat.

11. Aquesta diferència a la quantitat de llits entre les dues sales (homes i dones) també és observada per Carmel Ferragud (2022: 121) a propòsit de l'hospital de Sant Andreu de Mallorca.

L'inventari el signa com a hospitalera Francesca, esposa com s'ha dit del difunt hospitaler Domènec Falcó. Cal remarcar que Francesca assumí el càrrec per contracte i de manera individual, una feina que, anteriorment, havia compartit el matrimoni. Aquest fet confirma l'acceptació de Francesca com a treballadora al mateix nivell i responsabilitats que el marit i, per tant, sense cap mena de discriminació de gènere.[12]

## 2.4. *Inventari de l'any 1407*

Amb el tombant de segle, els inventaris segueixen un ordre molt similar als que hem vist fins ara i amb continguts força superposables, raó per la qual tan sols em detindré en el darrer, corresponent a l'any 1407, any en què a més consta que s'amplia el pis superior amb una cambra addicional. En el primer habitacle, situat al costat de la cuina, s'assenten dos llits, un gran de cabirons i un altre de mides més reduïdes, de posts amb capitells i amb els seus respectius paraments. En canvi, la segona cambra consta que tenia un llit de cabirons amb el seu parament, a més d'haver-hi altres elements com un collidor de brases d'aram, una talla de pou,[13] un recipient de ferro i una carraca.

Gràcies a tots aquests inventaris, s'han pogut concretar els diferents usos de cadascuna de les estances documentades. A la taula I es mostra una relació dels diferents espais i llur funció, així com l'evolució que s'observa durant els primers anys de funcionament de l'hospital (1388-1407). D'altra banda, la taula II evidencia un augment del nombre de llits o, el que és el mateix, un increment en l'oferta d'espai per als malalts, pobres i pelegrins que truquessin a la porta del nosocomi.[14]

# 3. *Robes*

En relació a la roba descrita als inventaris, sobretot el parament dels llits, es pot afirmar tant la seva qualitat com, en alguns casos, el seu lloc d'origen. L'any 1407 consta que les flassades eren fetes de borra (41%) o llana (59%); d'aquestes últimes, almenys el 74% de les peces citades provenien d'Aragó.[15] En canvi, els llençols solien ser de cànem, i als inventaris dels anys 1405 i 1407 molts cops se n'especifica un origen borgonyó (66%) i de dues o tres teles, fet que en demostra

12. Carmel Ferragud (2022) esmenta una situació molt similar a l'hospital de Sant Andreu de Mallorca. Sibil·la, esposa de l'hospitaler, un cop mort aquest, continua gestionant el centre, essent reconeguda com administradora.

13. Segons el DCVB es tractaria d'una peça de metall on es munten les politges per pujar o moure coses feixugues.

14. Un fet destacable d'aquest inventari és la presència del mestre en arts i físic, Nicolau Perers, el qual consta com a procurador de l'hospital juntament amb Guillem de Bellver, teixidor de llana.

15. Trobem a algun assentament l'expressió «de la terra» o «nostrades» per indicar-ne l'origen local.

Taula I. Inventaris de béns de l'Hospital de Vic. Evolució del nombre de llits i diferents usos dels espais (elaboració: autora).

| Any | Nivell | Descripció d'ús | Nombre de llits |
|---|---|---|---|
| 1388 | Planta baixa | Casa major inferior | 5 |
| 1398 | Planta superior | Zona de treball | |
| | | Cambra | 1 |
| 1399 | Planta baixa | Casa major on jauen els pobres | 8 |
| | | Casa on jauen les dones | 4 |
| | | Casa de les robes | |
| | | Celler | |
| | Planta superior | Menjador | |
| | | Cuina | |
| 1405 | Planta baixa | Casa major | 11 |
| | | Casa on jauen les dones | 5 |
| | | Casa de les robes | |
| | | Celler | |
| | Planta superior | Menjador | |
| | | Cuina | |
| 1407 | Planta baixa | Casa major | 11 |
| | | Casa de les dones | 5 |
| | | Casa de les robes | |
| | | Celler | |
| | Planta Superior | Menjador | |
| | | Cuina | |
| | | Dues Cambres | 3 |

Taula II. Evolució del nombre de llits (elaboració: autora).

| | Inv. 1388-1398 | Inv. 1399 | Inv. 1405 | Inv. 1407 |
|---|---|---|---|---|
| Llits homes | 5 | 8 | 11 | 11 |
| Llits dones | | 4 | 5 | 5 |
| Cambres | 1 | | | 2 |

una bona qualitat; també hi trobem un "axaló".[16] Els travessers o coixins allargats i els matalassos eren fets de fustani; també hi trobem alguna vànova de cotonina, llençols d'estopa de cànem, estam als coixins i, en el cas de les tovalloles, lli.

A les taules III i IV hi detallo les diferents robes i procedències. Si prenem com a punt de referència els inventaris de cases urbanes lleidatanes treballats per Imma Sànchez (2016), copsem un enfilall de teles foranes originàries de França, Alemanya, Flandes i fins i tot, Egipte. Guillem Roca (2021: 218), per la seva banda, comenta un inventari de l'hospital dels preveres de la capital del Segrià, datat el 1447, en què es descriuen dus màrfegues franceses. A propòsit de l'hospital de la Seu de Girona, Anna Gironella (2001: 170) destaca robes fetes amb llana d'Aragó i de València, però no n'atesta cap de francesa.

Val a dir que la importació tèxtil d'altres àmbits geopolítics era considerat un luxe per la qualitat dels teixits i l'elevat preu del transport. De fet, gran part de la població, sobretot els pagesos, feien ús de vestimentes de confecció local o fetes a casa amb teles sense tintar (To 2016: 524). És per això que suposem que la presència d'aquests teixits de qualitat a l'hospital es deu, probablement, a les donacions fetes pels ciutadans de Vic. Aquest seria el cas del draper Bernat Vall que feu la donació d'una vànova de llana d'anyins.[17]

## 4. *Discussió*

Els cinc inventaris de l'hospital de la Santa Creu de Vic –i d'altres que afrontarem en un futur– analitzats en aquesta primera aproximació són d'un interès extraordinari. En primer lloc, perquè ens aporten informació de les primeres passes de l'hospital al segle XIV, més encara si tenim present que no disposem de cap altra font d'aquesta centúria, ja que els llibres de comptes conservats no s'inicien fins a l'any 1439. En segona instància, la descripció detallada d'objectes, robes i espais ens apropa a la realitat social i quotidiana, i a la cultura material d'aquell

16. També anomenat aixaló o xaló, chaluns, etc. Es refereix a teixits de llana fabricats a Xaló (Chalons), ciutat de França. El terme "exaló" apareix a l'inventari de l'hospital de la Seu de Girona (Puig i Oliver 2020: 205).

17. Llana d'anyell (DCVB).

Taula III. Detall de la procedència d'alguns teixits esmentats als inventaris (elaboració: autora).

| Material | Tipus | 1388 | 1399 | 1405 | 1407 |
|---|---|---|---|---|---|
| Llana d'Aragó | flassades | 7 | 30 | 34 | 26 |
| Cànem de Borgonya | llençols | | | 2 | 18 |
| Châlons | axaló | | | 1 | |

Taula IV. Robes i teixits descrits als inventaris de l'hospital de la Santa Creu de Vic (elaboració: autora).

| MATERIAL | TIPUS | 1388 | 1398 | 1399 | 1405 | 1407 |
|---|---|---|---|---|---|---|
| Borra | Flassades, matalàs | | | 19 | 24 | 24 |
| Cànem o canyamars | Llençols, vànova, matalàs, travessers | | | 5 | 28 | 6 |
| Cànem de Borgonya | Llençols | | | | 2 | 18 |
| Cotonina | Vànova | | | | | 1 |
| Estam | Coixins i cobertors | | | 2 | | 2 |
| Estopa de cànem | Llençols | 10 | | | 2 | 2 |
| Fustani | Travessers, matalassos, "cóceres" | 4 | | 18 | 16 | 20 |
| Llana | Flassades, llençols | | | | 7 | 11 |
| Llana d'Aragó | Flassades | 7 | | 29 | 34 | 26 |
| Lli | Llençols, tovalloles | | 3 | 6 | 4 | 5 |

moment. Però, allò que considero més rellevant és que ens permeten fer un seguiment de l'evolució els primers anys de vida de la institució.

En primer lloc, aquests documents palesen que l'hospital ja estava en ple funcionament l'any 1388. Sens dubte, ja devia fer temps que era operatiu, però la manca d'altres documents no permet asseverar a partir de quin any precís això fou així. Recordem que l'origen de l'hospital es remunta a la fundació testamentària del mercader Ramon Terrades (1348) i, a partir d'aquest moment, tot és silenci fins al mencionat inventari de béns de 1388.

Una altra dada interessant d'aquest primer inventari és que es fa la descripció d'un únic espai a la planta baixa. L'edifici encara devia estar en obres, i, potser per això, no ens ha de sobtar que no es digui res del que hi havia a sobre –tal vegada perquè devia estar a mig fer i sense cap funció específica– o que no es pari esment de cap cambra reservada a les dones. A priori, aquest fet podria semblar sorprenent, però altres autors, com és el cas de Frederic Aparisi (2018), han constatat també un retard en la fàbrica d'una sala per a dones en el cas de l'hospital de Gandia.

A partir del mencionat inventari de 1398, constatem l'addició de nous espais amb funcions ben diferenciades: la sala dels homes i la de les dones, sala de les robes, el celler, l'escala que puja al pis superior on hi trobem, els darrers anys, la cuina, el menjador i una o dues cambres individuals. Tanmateix, resseguint aquesta descripció, el primer pensament que ens ve al cap és si l'hospital estava conformat per un sol edifici. De ser així, posaríem en crisi la lectura tradicional que n'ha fet la historiografia, segons la qual el complex constava de dos grans àmbits separats entre si: un per a homes i un altre per dones, disposats a banda i banda d'un pati central. Amb tot, els documents són poc precisos i no ens detallen aquest punt. Tampoc no ajuda el significat polisèmic o ambigu de la paraula "casa", ja que la documentació històrica l'empra indistintament per a referir-se a una mera sala o a un immoble aïllat. En el cas que ens ocupa, si acceptem que l'accepció "casa" es refereix a una cambra, podem concloure que l'hospital comptava amb un sol edifici, almenys en el tombant del segle XIV i XV.[18]

Pel que fa al mobiliari i les robes, un fet que crida l'atenció és la seva diversitat, fet que es podria justificar perquè molts llits i robes de llit procedien de donacions privades i, per tant, havien estat d'ús personal. Des d'aquest punt de vista, doncs, els inventaris reflecteixen en certa manera la cultura material de les cases vigatanes de la tardor de l'Edat Mitjana. També sorprèn l'escassetat del mobiliari. Per exemple, tant la sala dels homes com la de les dones tan sols conten llits, fet d'altra banda, que en certifica llur ús com a dormitoris.

Un dels aspectes més sorprenents i que desconcerta d'aquests inventaris és que no es faci al·lusió a la capella, que com és sabut, es tractava d'un espai comú a tots els hospitals de l'època. Ramon Terrades havia especificat en el testament fundacional la donació de 30 lliures per la millora del paviment de la capella del convent de Santa Margarida, situada a l'altra banda del carrer i hi va fer la donació d'un pal·li de vellut vermell per l'altar. No sabem si aquesta capella, un cop restaurada, va acollir els oficis religiosos mentre no se'n disposava dins l'hospital. De fet, el 1441, tal com ja va subratllar Segimon Cunill (1931: 19), se'n va construir una dins el complex hospitalari pròpiament dit.

En definitiva, el principal valor d'aquests inventaris és que ens aporten dades per intuir com devia configurar-se a grans trets l'estructura de l'hospital, així com una relació dels objectes, robes i mobles d'ús quotidià. Però pel que fa a la qüestió de l'organització interna de l'edifici, cal reiterar l'interès de l'inventari de 1407, que permet deduir que les dues cambres del pis superior estaven destinades, probablement, a l'hospitaler i als servents de la institució. Això revelaria la intenció de separar la part "assistencial" per dir-ho així, de la de serveis comuns.[19]

18. Maria del A. Cortés (2016) fa una descripció detallada de les cases al Berguedà i assenyala la possibilitat que les cases inicialment tenien un sol bloc però que posteriorment s'hi anaven afegint noves construccions de manera que augmentava la grandària de l'edifici.

19. Aquesta distribució de llits per acollir els malalts a la planta inferior i cambres individuals pel personal també la veiem a la descripció de l'hospital de Santa Andreu de Mallorca (Ferragud 2022).

## *Annex documental*

1407 juny 13, Vic.[20]

*Inventari de béns de l'hospital d'en Ramon Terrades redactat per l'escrivà Gabriel Estanyol, en presència del notari Pere de Artigues i dels procuradors de l'hospital designats pel Consell de la ciutat: el mestre físic Nicolau de Perer i el teixidor Guillem de Bellver.*

A. Vic. ABEV, ACF4489, f. 28r-34v.

Die lune, XIII die iunii, anno a nativitate Domini Mº CCCCº septimo. | Noverint universi quod, die lune tertia decima die mensis iunii, anno a nativitate Domini millesimo quadringentesimo septimo, | presente Gabriele Stanyol, scriptore iurato sub me, Petro de Artigis, notario publico vicense, | auctoritate domini vicense episcopi. Et presentibus Iohanne Cudina, managatore, et Petro Sunyer, coltelle | rio, civibus vicensis, pro testibus ad hec vocatis, venerabilis Nicholaus de Pirario, magister in | artibus et fisicus, ac Guillemus de Bellver, textor pannorum lane, cives vicense, | procuratores constituti, ut dixerunt, per honorabiles consiliarios civitatis vicense, positi et | assignati ad regendum et administrandum hospitali Raymundi de Terradis, civitatis vicense, | volentes, ut dixerunt scire, bona sunt in dicto hospitali ipsumque hospitale et bona eiusdem recipere | cum beneficio inventarii, necnon et propter doli maculam evitandam et omnem suspicionem tollen | dam de omnibus bonis dicti hospitalis honorabili. | † Signum Crucis hic posito et impresso | presens inventarium, repertorium, seu memoriale facere procuramus. |

Et primo trobam en la casa maior del dit hospital los lits e robes sagüents: |
Primo, I lit de posts[21] ab sos capitells.[22] | Ítem, una màrfaga plena de palla. | Ítem, I matalàss amb coberta de fustani tot lista amb listes blanques e blaves ab |sotana[23] groga bo e bell | Ítem, I travesser del propedit fustani ab aquelles matexes listes. | Ítem, I cubertor de stamany vermell. | Ítem, I lit encaxat ab màrfaga plena de palla. | Ítem, I matalàs de fustani ab listes blaves manudes ab sotana de cànam blanch | de pocha valor. | Ítem, I travesser de fustani ab listes blaves e blanques. | Ítem, I parell de lansols de cànam de Bargu[n]ya[24] de tres tels. [f. 28r]

20. La transcripció s'ha fet segons les normes d'Antoni Furió i Enric Guinot (2009) per a l'edició de documents medievals: desenvolupament d'abreviatures sense indicar les lletres restituïdes; ús d'accents, apòstrof, guionet, punt volat i puntuació segons la gramàtica catalana actual; es regularitza l'ús de la *i* i *j,* de la *u* i de la *v*; ús de la *l·l* quan el terme ho requereix, i del punt volat en cas d'aglutinació de les partícules pronominals *y, u* i *us* amb la paraula anterior, si aquesta no és cap forma verbal (que·es, a·n). Es regularitza l'ús de majúscules i minúscules. S'han transcrit amb una F/f les consonants dobles Ff en noms, substantius i verbs. Als textos en llatí, les grafies *i* i *j* són transcrites sempre com *i*; les grafies c/t amb valor de c, si no es troben ben diferenciades al text; l'expressió etcètera s'ha resolt en cursiva (*et cetera*).

21. Cadascuna de les peces de fusta damunt de les quals es posa el matalàs (DCVB).

22. Capçal del llit (DCVB).

23. La tela de baix de certes peces de roba de llit com vànoves, matalassos o coixins (DCVB).

24. «Cànem de Bargunya» apareix amb diferents grafies: Bergunya, Barguya i Burgunya. Molt probablement, fa referència a Burgunya, important ducat a l'Edat Mitjana, avui dia regió del sud-est de França, d'on es citen fil, cànem, xarxes i teles de Borgonya (v. *Diccionari Gual Camarena*).

Ítem, una flassada de borra ab, a cade cap, una lista verda tota blanqua. | Ítem, una flassada de borra ab listes blaves e burelles. | Ítem, [I] lit ab cabirons ab màrfaga plena de palla. |Ítem, una cóssera[25] de fustani ab verges blaves plena de ploma. | Ítem, I travesser de fustani ab listes blaves. | Ítem, I parell de lansols de stopa de cànam de II tel·les. | Ítem, una flassada d'Aragó ab listes vermelles als caps vermelles e negres e groges. | Ítem, I parell de lansols de cànam de Bargunya de duas teles e miga. Ítem, una flassada de borra burella ab listes blaves e blanqes e burelles. | Ítem, I travasser de fustani blanch de pocha valor. | Ítem, I altro lit ab ses post e capitells. | Ítem, una màrfaga plena de palla. | Ítem, matalàs de cànam blau ab la sotana groga. | Ítem, travasser de fustani blanch ab listes blaves. | Ítem, I parell de lansols de cànam de Bergunya de dues teles e miga. | [Ítem], una flassada d'Aragó blanqa als caps ab listes negres e vermelles. | [Ítem], una flassada de borra blancha ab
[f. 28v] listes blaves e vermelles als | [caps]. |

Ítem, I altro lit ab posts e capitells. | Ítem, una màrfaga plena de palla. | Ítem, I matalàs de fustani tot listes de blau e de blanch ab sotana groga. | Ítem, I travasser de cànam tot blanc. | Ítem, I parell de lansols de cànam de duas teles e miga squinsat. | Ítem, una flassada de borro blanqua ab listes als caps verdes, blaves e vermelles. | Ítem, I lit de posts ab sos capitells. | Ítem, una màrfaga plena de palla. | Ítem, I matalàs de fustani tot barrat de blau e de blanch ab sotana groga. | Ítem, I travasser de fustani ab listes blaves e blanqes. |Ítem, I parell de lansols de cànam de Bargunya de duas teles e miga. | Ítem, una flassada tota barrada ab barres amples blaves e burelles. | Ítem, una altra flassada de Aragó blanque ab listes als caps negres e groges. | Ítem, I cubertor d'estamenya vermella ab sanyal de tasora blava. | Ítem. | Ítem, I altro lit ab posts e capitells. | Ítem, una màrfaga plena de palla. | Ítem, I matalàs tot squinsat. | Ítem, I travasser de fustani tot listat de blanch e de blau. |
[f. 29r] Ítem, I altro capsal ab listes vermelles de pocha valor.|

Ítem, una flassada per cobrir palles d'Eragó als caps ab listes negres e | groges. | Ítem, I parell de lansols de cànam de Bargunya de duas teles e miga. | Ítem, una flassada blancha d'Aragà ab listes als caps vermelles e negres. |Ítem, miga flassada de borra masclada ab una lista blancha a cada cap. | Ítem, I lit ab cabirons[26] e capitells. | Ítem, una màrfaga plena de palla. | Ítem, una cóssera de fustani blanch barrada de blau de ploma. | Ítem, un capsal d'estameny ab listes negres e vermelles. | Ítem, I parell de lansolls de Bargunya de duas tales. | Ítem, una flassada de lana blancha ab listes als caps blaves e vermelles. | Ítem, una altra flassada de lana tota listada de blanch, blau e vermell. | Ítem, I lit de posts ab sos capitells. | Ítem, una màrfaga plena de palla. | Ítem, una flassada d'Eragó ab listes vermelles a cade cap que serveix a | cobrir les palles. | Ítem, I travasser de fustani ab listes blaves. | Ítem, I parell de lansols squinsats de duas tel·les. | Ítem, una flassada de lana d'Aragó ab listes vermelles als caps. | Ítem, una flassada de borro squinsada blava ab listes vermelles
[f. 29v] e blanqes. |

Ítem, I altro lit ab posts, cabirons e capitells. | Ítem, una màrfaga plena de palla. | Ítem, una flassada de lana tota barrada de vermell e de negre per cobrir palles. | Ítem, I travasser de lana de borro blanch e vermell. | Ítem, I parell de lansols de drap de Bargunya de II teles e miga. | Ítem, una flassada blancha d'Aragó ab listes als caps negres e groges. | Ítem,

25. Vànova (DCVB).

26. Peça de fusta que sosté les llates de la teulada (*Diccionari de la llengua catalana* de l'Institut d'Estudis Catalans [DIEC2]).

una altra flassada d'Aragó de pocha valor ab listes vermelles als caps. | En l'altra casa, aderent a la propdita casa on jauen les | dones, trobam les cosas següents. | Ítem, I lit de posts ab sos capitells. | Ítem, una màrfaga plena de palla. | Ítem, I cobri pales de borra de cànam. | Ítem, I travasser tot listat de listes blaves de fustani. | Ítem, I parell de lansols de Burgunya de duas teles e miga. | Ítem, una flassada de lana burella ab listes blaves e verdes e vermelles | de pocha valor. | Ítem, una altra flassa de borra tota listada de blau, vert e groch. | Ítem, una flassada de borra tota listada de blau, blanch e vermell. | Ítem. | Ítem, I lit de cabirons. | [f. 30r]

Ítem, una màrfaga plena de palla. | Ítem, I cobri palles o flassada de borro squinsat ab listes blaves de | pocha valor. | Ítem, I travasser de canamàs blanch. | Ítem, I lansol squinsat. | Ítem, una flassada d'Aragó ab listes vermelles e groges als caps. | Ítem, una altra flassada d'Aragó ab listes negres e vermelles als caps. | Ítem, I altro lit de posts ab sos capitells. | Ítem, una màrfaga plena de palla. | Ítem, un cobri palles, o flassada d'Aragó, ab listes als caps vermelles, negres | e grogues. | Ítem, I capsal de lana de pocha valor ab listes vermelles als caps. | Ítem, una flassada de lana blancha ab listes vermelles als caps. | Ítem, I lit de posts ab sos capitells. | Ítem, una màrfaga plena de palla. | Ítem, cobri palles de lana squinsat. | Ítem, I travasser de fustani tot listat de listes blaves e blanques. | Ítem, una flassada de Aragó ab listes negres e vermelles als caps. | [Ítem], I altro lit ab posts e capitells. | [Ítem], una màrfaga plena de palla. | [f. 30v]

Ítem, I matalàs sotill de fustani barrat de blau. | Ítem, I travesser de fustani ab barres blanqes e blaves. | Ítem, una flassada de lana ab barres als caps negres, groges e vermelles. | En l'altra casa contigua a la propdita apellada le casa de les | robes trobam les cosas següent. | Primo, un matalàs de fustani tot vergat de listes o verges blanques e | blaves ab sotana groga. | Ítem, una flassada de borra ab listes als caps blanques e blaves e lo camp | burell. Ítem, una altra flassada de bora mansclada ab listes als caps | blanques e blaves. | Ítem, una altra flassada de lana de la terra ab listes tota listada de blanqes | e burelles. Ítem, una altra flassada de borra burella ab listes als caps blanques. | Ítem, una altra flassada de borra tota listada de blau, blanch e vert. | Ítem, una altra flassada de borra burella e masclada als caps ab listes | blaves e blanqes. | Ítem, una altra flassada de lana de la terra blancha ab listes negres als caps. | Ítem, una flassada de borro de blau clar ab listes als caps de blau scur. | Ítem, una altra flassada de borra tota listada de blanch, de vermell e blau e v[ert]. | Ítem, una altra flassada de lana blancha ab listes blaves als caps. | [f. 31r]

Ítem, una flassada d'Eragó blancha ab listes vermelles e negres. | Ítem, una altra flassada de borra tota listada de bares blanques, blaves e vermelles, | la qual dixe lo spitaller que despuix que ell ragia lo spital la'n havia donada | lo senyor en Pere de Santa Eulàlia, la qual flassada deia qua y havia jaquida | la muller, quondam, del dit Pere. | Ítem, I drap pintat qui solia anar sobre les cossos morts quant los soterram ab sanyal de paons. | Ítem, una flassada de borra blanqua | ab listes als caps burells. | Ítem, una vàngua ab sotana groga apadassada. | Ítem, I padàs de vànova blanqua. | Ítem, una flassada de Aragó ab listes als caps negres e vermelles. | Ítem, una flassada de lana blancha ab listes burelles als caps. | Ítem, una vànova grossa de cànam. | Ítem, una flassada de borro blanqua ab listes blaves als caps. | Ítem, un barragà listat de listes groges e vermelles. | Ítem, una flassada d'Aragó ab listes als caps vermelles negres e grogues. | Ítem, I barragà[27] listat de listes vermelles,

27. Tela de llana impermeable (DCVB).

verdes e blanques e blaves, apadassat. | Ítem, una flassada d'Aragó ab listes als caps vermelles, | negres e grogues. | Ítem, una altra flassada d'Aragó blanqua pell rase ab listes als caps vermelles | e negres. | Ítem, I barragà listat de listes vermelles, verdes e blanques e blaves, apadassat. | Ítem, una altra flassada d'Aragó blancha ab listes vermelles als caps, sotill. | Ítem, una flassada d'Ara blancha ab listes vermelles e negres als caps. | [Ítem], una
[f. 31v] flassada d'Aragó blanqua squinsada ab listes vermelles e groges | als caps. |

Ítem, una altra flassada d'Aragó blanqua sotill ab listes als caps vermelles. | Ítem, un vanovot de pocha valor. | Ítem, una altra flassada d'Aragó blanqua als caps ab listes negres e vermelles. | Ítem, una altra flassada blanqua d'Aragó sotil ab listes als caps vermelles e | negres. | Ítem, una altra flassada de lana d'Aragó ab listes negres e vermelles | als caps. | Ítem, una altra flassada de lana d'Aragó ab listes vermelles e negres als caps. | Ítem, una altra flassada d'Aragó blanqua squinsada ab listes vermelles e negres. Ítem, una altra flassada d'Aragó blancha ab listes als caps vermelles, negres, | blaves e verdes. | Ítem, una altra flassada d'Aragó blanqua ab listes vermelles, negres e groges. | Ítem, una altra flassada d'Aragó blanqua ab listes vermelles e negres als | caps. Ítem, miga flassada squinsada tota barrada de blau, vermell e blanch. | Ítem, una flassada d'Aragó squinsada ab listes vermelles e groges als caps. | Ítem, una taula o plaga[28] en que stan les dites flassades. | Ítem, I parell de lansols de brm (*sic*) de cànam de III tel·les. | Ítem, I parell de lansols squinsats tots. | Ítem, un altra parell de lansolls tots squinsats. |Ítem, una caxa gran ab peus
[f. 32r] on stan les robes sagüents ab I calaxó | e un travesser. |

Primo una vànova de belli plene de cota tota ondada ab una creu de | fill blave a cada cap de III tel·les e miga.| Ítem, una altra vánova de cotonina ondada de IIII tel·les plena de cotó. | Ítem, un parell de lansols de li de III tales e miga bons e bells. | Ítem, I altra parell de lansols de li de III teles ab senyal a cada cap de fill | blau. Ítem, unas thovalles de li scacades e al caps ab listes blaves scacades | ab una creu de fill blau cade cap. |Ítem, I coxi de ploma ab cuberta de drap de li ab randa engir[29] |e entorn ab botons als caps. | Ítem, unas thovalloles de li tota stessa. | Ítem, unas thovallas scacades ab listes als caps blaves. | Ítem, un coxí blau. | Ítem, un altre coxí blanch de pocha valor. | Ítem, I travasser barrat de blau e blanch de pocha valor. | Ítem, una altro travasser. | Ítem, I altro travesser. | Ítem, I altro travesser. | Ítem, I altro travesser tots de pocha valor. | Ítem, III o IIII saclits tots esquinsats e de pocha valor. | Ítem, un matalassot squinsat de pocha valor. | Ítem, III i IIII
[f. 32v] artificis de lits tots sgavallats. |

Entram en lo saler contiguu a la dita casa on trobam | les coses següents: |
Primo, una thona de IIII sesters. | Ítem, una altra thona de IIII sesters. | Ítem, una altra de capassitat de set botes. | Ítem, un foladoret patit sgavallat. | Ítem, un barricó patit sgavallat. | Muntan alt al cap de l'scala en lo mangador |on trobam les cose sagüents |
Primo, una thaüt de dos calaixes de tanir blat. | Ítem, una altra thaüt ab dos calaxos per tanir blat. | Ítem, una caxeta patita de pocha valor.| Entram en la cuyna del dit spital contigua a la propdita casa | on trobam les coses sagüents | Primo, I morter de coura ab sa mà bo e bell. | Ítem, una paella de aram. | Ítem, duas olas de aram la una gran e l'altra pocha. | Ítem, una
[f. 33r] conqueta d'aram trenquada. | Ítem, una ola de coura trenquada. | Ítem, I ast de ferro. |

28. Taula o armari de plega on es guarden coses plegades (DCVB).
29. Al voltant (DCVB).

Entram en la cambra contigua a la dita cuyna on trobam | les cosas sagüents: | Primo, un lit de cabirons. | Ítem, una màrfaga plena de palla. | Ítem, I travasser de fustani tot listat ab listes blanques e blaves. | Ítem, un parell de lansols de cànam de Bargunya de II teles e miga. | Ítem, una flassada de borra ab listes blaves, burelles e verdes. | Ítem, miga flassada sotil tota blava. | Ítem, I lit patit de posts ab capitells. | Ítem, una màrfaga plena de palla. | Ítem, I matalàs sotil. | Ítem, I lansol de canamas gros de duas tel·les. | Ítem, una flassada sotill d'Aragó blancha ab listes negres e vermelles als | caps. | Ítem, I flassadot de Aragó squinsat. | Entram en una cambra contigua a la propdita on trobam | les cosas sagüents | Ítem, un lit de cabirons. | Ítem, una màrfaga plena de palla. | Ítem, una matalàs de fustani tot listat ab listes blaves | e blavues. [f. 33v]

Ítem, I travasser de fustani blanch ab listes blaves. | Ítem, I parell de lansols de III tel·les de Burgunya. | Ítem, una flassada blanqua de lana nostrada ab listes vermelles a cade cap. | Ítem, una flassada de borra burella tota listada de blau. | Ítem, I parell de lansols de duas teles e miga de stopa de li. | Ítem, una flassada de llana blancha ab listes burellas e ab senyal de serra. | Ítem, un coiydor de brasquer de aram de pocha valor. | Ítem, una talla de pou. | Ítem, una bancha trognada. | Ítem, una farrada. | Ítem, una carreca. | Et haec bona et non alia invenerunt dicti procuratores in hospitali antedicto | retinentes sibi et protestantes quod si decretur *et cetera.* [f. 34r]

## *Bibliografia*


Aparisi, Federic, 2018. "La cultura material de los hospitales de las villas valencianas en la baja Edad Media", *Revista de la CECEL*, 18: 55-68.

Bolòs Masclans, Jordi; Sánchez Boira, Imma, 2022. "Entrem dins d'una casa medieval", *L'Erol*, 151: 21-27.

Casas Homs, Josep M., 1975. "Interpretació històrico-geogràfica d'un inventari medieval", *Miscel·lània Pau Vila*, Barcelona, Institut d'Estudis Catalans: 215-219.

Conejo da Pena, Antoni, 2002. *Assistència i hospitalitat a l'Edat Mitjana. L'arquitectura dels hospitals catalans: del gòtic al primer Renaixement*, Tesi Doctoral, Universitat de Barcelona.

Conejo da Pena, Antoni, 1994. *El "spital del coyl de Balaguer" de l'infant fra Pere*, L'Hospitalet de l'Infant, Ajuntament de Vandellòs i l'Hospitalet de l'Infant.

Conejo da Pena, Antoni; Vela Aulesa, Carles, 2021. "Un informe barcelonés del «venerabile hospitale Sancte Marie della Scala de Sene»: ca. 1401", Roberta Mucciarelli, Michele Pellegrini (a cura de), *Il tarlo dello storico. Studi per Gabriella Piccinni*, Arcidosso, Effigi: 567-592.

Cortés, Maria del A., 2016. *Espai domèstic i cultura material. Una aproximació històrica a les cases rurals del Berguedà*, Tesi doctoral, Universitat Autònoma de Barcelona.

Cunill, Segimon, 1931. *El Sant Crist de l'hospital de Vich*, Vic, Gazeta de Vich.

Dcvb. *Diccionari català-valencià-balear*, A. M. Alcover i F. de B. Moll, Palma de Mallorca, Moll, 1968-1969, https://dcvb.iec.cat/ [enllaç actiu el setembre 2022].

Ferragud, Carmel, 2022. *L'hospital, la dona i el capellà. Sant Andreu de Mallorca (1230-1445)*, Catarroja, Afers.

Furió, Antoni; Guinot, Enric, 2009. *Normes de presentació, edició i transcripció,* València, Publicacions de la Universitat de València.

Gironella, Anna, 2001. "La cultura de la caritat: inventari dels béns de l'Hospital de la Seu (Girona, 31 de gener 1342)", *Annals de l'Institut d'Estudis Gironins*, 42: 163-177.

Gironella, Anna, 2020. "Els antics hospitals de Girona: diferències i semblances, segle X-XV", *Annals de l'Institut d'Estudis Gironins*, 61: 49-76.

Gual Camarena, Legado. *Vocabulario de comercio medieval*, https://www.um.es/lexico-comercio-medieval/index.php/vocabulario [enllaç actiu el setembre 2022].

Junyent, Eduard, 1976. *La ciutat de Vic i la seva història*, Barcelona, Curial.

Marino, Salvatore, 2018. "Trabajo y aprendizaje en los hospitales de la Baja Edad Media. Aproximación comparativa entre Barcelona, Milán, Nápoles y Siena", *Reti Medievali Rivista,* 19/2: 171-205

Martinell, César, 1935. "Les hôpitaux", *L'architecture gothique civile en Catalogne,* Mataró, Minerva: 51-67.

Piccinni, Gabriella, 2016. "I modelli ospedalieri e la loro circolazione dall'Italia all'Europa alla fine del medioevo", Gregoria Cavero (coord.), *'Civitas Bendita'. Encrucijada de las relaciones sociales y de poder en la ciudad medieval*, León, Universidad de León: 9-26.

Prades, Isidre, 2000. Llegats testamentaris i obra material a *Hospital de la Santa Creu de Vic. Història d'una institució assistencial*, Vic, Arxiu Històric Comarcal d'Osona.

Puig i Oliver, Jaume de, 2020. "Els inventaris de l'hospital de la Seu de Girona dels anys 1353 i 1362" *Annals de l'Institut d'Estudis Gironins*, 61: 161-218.

Roca Cabau, Guillem, 2021. *Pobresa i hospitals a la Lleida baixmedieval*, Lleida, Pagès.

Rubio Vela, Agustín, 1984. *Pobreza, enfermedad y asistencia hospitalaria en la Valencia del siglo XIV*, València, Institució Alfons el Magnànim.

Sabaté, Flocel, 1990. "Els objectes de la vida quotidiana a les llars barcelonines al començament del Segle XIV", *Anuario de Estudios Medievales*, 20: 1-56.

Sánchez Boira, Imma, 2016. *Aproximació als espais i objectes de les cases urbanes de Lleida. Des del final del segle XIV fins al segle XVI: del món real a la representació de les imatges*, Tesi doctoral, Universitat de Lleida.

Santandreu Soler, Maria D., 2006. *La vila de Berga a l'edat mitjana. La familia dels Berga*, Tesi doctoral, Universitat de Barcelona.

To Figueres, Lluís. 2016. "Wedding Trousseaus and Cloth Consumption in Catalonia around 1300", *Economyc History Review*, 69/2: 522-547.

Mariangela Rapetti, Maria Beatrice Artizzu

# L'ospedale S. Antonio abate di Cagliari: dalle carte d'archivio al museo virtuale

## 1. *L'ospedale S. Antonio abate di Cagliari, una storia lunga cinque secoli*

L'8 febbraio 1338, da Valenza, Pietro il Cerimonioso concedeva a Nicola di Saluzzo, procuratore dell'abate di Saint-Antoine-et-Saint-Pierre di Lézat, Poncius de Vilamuro, di edificare, alle appendici di Castell de Caller, un ospedale «*sub invocationi Beati Anthoni*».[1] Ne dava comunicazione all'arcivescovo cagliaritano Gondisalvo, annunciando la raccolta di questue per il sostentamento dei poveri dell'ospedale. L'8 aprile successivo, Pietro scriveva al governatore generale del Regno di Sardegna, Raimondo de Ripellis, ordinandogli di concedere a frate Nicola l'acquisto di terreni o altre proprietà per la costruzione dell'ospedale (Rapetti 2017: 145-148). Frate Nicola rappresentava una comunità affiliata alla congregazione cluniacense e proclamatasi detentrice, come i canonici di S. Antonio di Vienne, delle spoglie del santo egiziano (Foscati 2013). L'assenza di ulteriori fonti sui cluniacensi di Lézat a Cagliari e la presenza in Sardegna, in quegli anni, dei canonici di Vienne, che raccoglievano questue da inviare alla casa madre (Rapetti 2017: 156), lasciano spazio a dubbi sui primi anni di gestione del nuovo ospedale.

Dobbiamo aspettare il 1365 per trovare, tra le rendite della mensa arcivescovile, la prima menzione di un ospedale di S. Antonio nell'appendice "di Lapola", ovvero il quartiere portuale cagliaritano (fig. 1-2), così chiamato dalla presenza di una *leppula* o *lapola*, una gru girevole, necessaria per il carico e lo scarico delle merci (Cadinu 2019: 66). Un documento del 1366, mutilo, ci informa di una controversia tra l'arcivescovo e la città di Cagliari sul patronato dell'ospedale. Secondo i consiglieri civici, l'ospedale S. Antonio era stato «anticamente» fondato come struttura laica, destinata ai poveri e ai malati, in alcuni locali già di proprietà di tale Iacopo Stefani, che li aveva donati alla città per questo scopo. L'arcivescovo, invece, sosteneva che l'ospedale era stato edificato in gran parte da Bernardo Galceran –forse un antoniano di Vienne?– che, da molti anni, racco-

1. Il presente lavoro è frutto di una collaborazione tra le autrici. Sono da attribuirsi a Mariangela Rapetti i paragrafi 1-2, a Maria Beatrice Artizzu i paragrafi 3-4.

glieva, sotto il segno di sant'Antonio, le offerte degli abitanti di Lapola (Rapetti 2017: 85).

Nel 1382, l'amministratore dell'ospedale era un laico, il barbiere Pere Polit (Ferragud 2005: 483). Su un documento dell'infante Giovanni, a lui destinato, leggiamo che l'ospedale era destinato a «*pobres desolats e dolents*» (Rapetti 2017: 166). Lo stesso Polit lasciò delle proprietà immobiliari all'ospedale, ubicate «in villa Lapole in vico dels Cavallers» (Rapetti 2017: 168), l'odierna via Cavour (Scano 1934: 118, 119).

I consiglieri della città e gli arcivescovi cagliaritani si contesero i diritti sull'ospedale di Lapola per alcuni secoli. Nel corso del Quattrocento, in modo discontinuo, la struttura era affidata agli ospedalieri antoniani di Vienne, che detenevano il favore regio e vescovile, ma non quello dei consiglieri della città. Negli anni 30 del Cinquecento, i consiglieri riuscirono a dimostrare la negligenza dei canonici di Vienne e li estromisero completamente dalla gestione (Rapetti 2020). Da quel momento, e per i tre secoli successivi, è possibile ricostruire la storia dell'ospedale, detto del glorioso S. Antonio o di S. Antonio abate, grazie alla conservazione di buona parte dell'archivio ospedaliero.[2]

Per circa un secolo, i consiglieri della città mantennero la gestione diretta, nominando ogni anno un clavario per il controllo delle spese e la tenuta dei registri dell'ospedale. Il clavario raccoglieva gli affitti, assegnava al maggiordomo la dotazione economica per le spese giornaliere, pagava i medici, gli infermieri, le balie (o dide) e tutto il personale che a vario titolo contribuiva alle attività ordinarie e straordinarie dell'ospedale.[3]

La gestione, però, non fu sempre ottimale, e si rese necessario intervenire in modo radicale: fu così che, nel 1636, i consiglieri della città affidarono la struttura –unico ospedale attivo a Cagliari– agli ospedalieri di S. Giovanni di Dio (Russotto 1956: 129-136). L'attività dei Fatebenefratelli fu rivolta a tutta la popolazione della città, del circondario e dei forestieri. Trovavano accoglienza al S. Antonio abate i poveri, i malati, i marinai, gli esposti, i pazzi e gli incurabili. Traccia di questi ricoveri rimane nei registri d'ingresso, ma le altre fonti d'archivio testimoniano, in generale, un quadro desolato: se, da un lato, abbiamo la certezza della presenza del personale chirurgico e medico –tra i quali i professori di medicina

2. Gli avvicendamenti amministrativi e gestionali hanno comportato la dispersione della documentazione ospedaliera in tre Istituti di conservazione: l'archivio ospedaliero propriamente detto, il cui documento più antico è del 1499, è conservato dall'Archivio di Stato di Cagliari (ASCa); buona parte della documentazione amministrativa prodotta tra Cinquecento e Settecento si conserva all'Archivio Storico Comunale di Cagliari (ASCCa); una terza parte si conserva presso la Curia generalizia dell'Ordine ospedaliero di S. Giovanni di Dio (OHSJD), che ha amministrato direttamente e successivamente gestito l'ospedale cagliaritano. A questi nuclei si aggiungono i carteggi della Regia Segreteria di Stato e di Guerra del Regno di Sardegna, conservati in ASCa e presso la Sezione Corte dell'Archivio di Stato di Torino (ASTo), relativi agli anni 1720-1848.

3. I libri del clavario sono in ASCCa, Sezione antica, voll. 347-350, cf. Tasca, Rapetti 2019: 146-150; Rapetti 2020: 134.

dello Studio generale cagliaritano– dall'altro è evidente quanto la struttura fosse povera e sovraffollata.

Nel frattempo, nel 1720, il Regno di Sardegna passava a Vittorio Amedeo II di Savoia. Dopo alcuni decenni, il suo successore Carlo Emanuele III fece avviare una serie di istruttorie e successive riforme che coinvolsero anche gli ospedali, a partire proprio da quello cagliaritano. Il S. Antonio abate, a seguito dell'ennesima lamentela contro i Fatebenefratelli presentata dai consiglieri, fu riformato e posto sotto il controllo di una apposita Congregazione sopra l'ospedale, istituita nel 1765, mentre gli ospedalieri di S. Giovanni di Dio furono mantenuti come infermieri.[4] Nel 1806, con Carta Reale del 15 settembre, Vittorio Emanuele I restituì ai Fatebenefratelli l'amministrazione diretta dell'ospedale, sostituendo la Congregazione con una Regia Delegazione (RUSSOTTO 1956: 55-57). La Congregazione venne ripristinata con Carta Reale del 19 maggio 1820, ma dal 1847, con le disposizioni del sovrano Carlo Alberto volte al «miglior governo degli Ospedali Civili del regno», furono abolite le Congregazioni e l'amministrazione economica e finanziaria dell'ospedale di S. Antonio fu posta nelle mani di un Consiglio di Carità, i cui componenti rappresentavano la nobiltà locale.[5] Rimasero immutate le funzioni. Come ha notato Russotto:

> Il passaggio dell'amministrazione e della direzione diretta dai Fatebenefratelli alla speciale Congregazione presieduta dall'arcivescovo (1765); da questa nuovamente ai Religiosi (1806) e poi ancora alla Congregazione (1820), certamente non contribuì al miglioramento economico ed assistenziale dell'ospedale (RUSSOTTO 1956: 140).

In effetti, già dalla fine del Settecento, la struttura si trovava in continua emergenza, tanto economica che di spazi, inoltre era sempre più difficile garantire la salubrità degli ambienti. Si vagliarono diverse ipotesi: adattamento della struttura, trasloco, nuova costruzione.[6] Appurata l'impossibilità di adattare l'antico ospedale alle nuove esigenze, e l'assenza di altra struttura idonea, si optò per una nuova costruzione. Si scelse un'area ai margini della città, e la progettazione fu affidata a Gaetano Cima (DEL PANTA 1983: 284-285). I lavori iniziarono nel 1844,[7] ma la costruzione andò avanti un po' a rilento, con alcuni significativi

4. ASCa, Segreteria di Stato e di Guerra del Regno di Sardegna, Serie II, vol. 82, cc. 39-46; RAPETTI 2018.

5. *Regie Patenti colle quali S. M. provvede al miglior governo degli ospedali civili del Regno, conferendone esclusivamente l'amministrazione economica e finanziera ai Consigli di Carità instituiti con Carta Reale delli 17 giugno 1837, in data 27 luglio 1847*, cfr. ASCa, Segreteria di Stato e di Guerra del Regno di Sardegna, Serie II, vol. 89, *Riforma degli Spedali Civili dell'Isola* (1847-1848); ASTo, Sez. Corte, Materie Ecclesiastiche, Luoghi pii ed Opere Pie, Opere Pie in genere n. 21, *Istituzioni di carità e di beneficenza dell'isola di Sardegna. Progetto di instruzioni onde agevolare e rendere uniforme in tutta l'isola l'eseguimento delle Regie Patenti del 7 luglio 1846* (1848); ASTo, Sez. Corte, Materie Ecclesiastiche, Luoghi pii ed Opere Pie, Opere Pie di qua dai monti n. 36, *Congregazione di carità* (1849). A livello locale, però, si mantenne l'uso del termine «Congregazione».

6. ASCa, Segreteria di Stato e di Guerra del Regno di Sardegna, Serie II, vol. 85.

7. ASCa, Ospedale S. Giovanni di Dio, s. I, b. 9, fasc. 3; s. IV, b. 177.

cambiamenti in corso d'opera.[8] Tra il 1858 e il 1859, con il nuovo ospedale civile ormai operativo, l'antico S. Antonio abate fu chiuso definitivamente.

## 2. *Architettura e carte d'archivio*

L'archivio ospedaliero *stricto sensu* si conserva solo a partire dal XVI secolo. La frammentarietà delle fonti medievali non consente di conoscere l'aspetto e le dimensioni della struttura originale. Alcuni elementi tuttora visibili, però, richiamano architetture tardo medievali, mostrando l'esigenza di una riflessione più approfondita. In assenza di fonti dirette sulle caratteristiche della prima struttura, possiamo certamente riflettere, grazie soprattutto agli studi di Maria Bonaria Urban (2000) e di Marco Cadinu (2008; 2019), sull'interazione tra l'ospedale S. Antonio e il contesto urbano tra il XIV e il XV secolo.

Il luogo scelto per l'edificazione del complesso ospedaliero non dovette essere affatto casuale. Il nuovo assetto del quartiere portuale, la *pobla nova* voluta da Alfonso il Benigno, si presentò come «una griglia di strade ortogonali» (Cadinu 2008: 162): tutta l'area era stata suddivisa in lotti, tracciati da nuove vie parallele e perpendicolari, e si era provveduto a costruire, demolire o riadattare gli edifici già presenti. L'odierna via Napoli, che corre verso il mare, rispondeva a un importante ruolo nautico, offrendo punti fissi per facilitare l'ingresso al porto. Sebbene il nome della strada –*carrer de las Moras*–, abbia dato adito a varie interpretazioni (Scano 1934: 123, 124), Cadinu, ricordando che in origine la via era detta "Demoras", associa il nome al termine catalano *demora*.[9] I punti fissi cagliaritani erano rappresentati dal campanile della cattedrale, collocata sul colle del quartiere Castello, dall'ospedale S. Antonio, e dalla chiesa di S. Lucia in Lapola. E proprio sul campanile della chiesa di S. Antonio, riedificata ai primi del Settecento (Naitza 1992: 65-67), è presente quella che sembra una traccia della struttura precedente: una statua acefala, con le mani poste sulle ginocchia, che 'guarda' verso il porto (Cadinu 2019: 72-74).[10]

L'ospedale fu costruito tra due dislivelli: a nord prospettava sull'attuale via Giuseppe Manno, anticamente *Sa Costa*, in salita verso il Portico –che ora rappresenta una sorta di confine, ma che a un certo punto fu edificato per il passaggio degli ospedalieri dal convento e ospedale alla chiesa– e si sviluppava lungo il declivio che conduce all'attuale piazza Santo Sepolcro, attraversata la quale si imbocca via Napoli (fig. 1).

8. ASCa, Ospedale S. Giovanni di Dio, s. IV, b. 178, fasc. 619.

9. «*Direcció o rumb en què està situat un objecte en relació a una embarcació, a un punt de la costa o a un altre objecte determinat*» (DCVB).

10. Marco Cadinu ha rielaborato la pianta del quartiere evidenziando, tra il campanile della cattedrale e il mare, lungo la via *Demora*, l'asse fondativo del reticolo stradale realizzato dagli aragonesi tra il 1327 e il 1331, cf. Cadinu 2019: figura 12 per la pianta e figura 13 per la statua acefala sul campanile.

Il complesso di S. Antonio dovette rivestire da subito un ruolo fondamentale per il quartiere e per i nuovi arrivati via mare, e non solo come punto fisso per un approdo sicuro. La struttura di ricovero dell'epoca precedente, affidata agli ospedalieri di Stagno e intitolata a S. Leonardo (SCHIRRU 2003: 123-125, 191-202), scompare dalle fonti a seguito dell'assedio catalano-aragonese del 1324: probabilmente fu abbandonata, lasciando l'antico quartiere portuale sprovvisto di ospedale (FADDA, RAPETTI 2020).

L'area incontrò da subito una notevole espansione edilizia, e anche la toponomastica fu fortemente influenzata (fig. 3). Dal Quattrocento, infatti, la chiesa e l'ospedale, così come il *carrer de Sant'Antoni* o *de Sant'Anthoni de Vianes*, attualmente tratto di via Manno (SCANO 1934: 122), e il *vico de Sancti Anthoni* o *descensus/abaxada hospitali Santi Antoni*, dove oggi sono le scalette S. Sepolcro (SCANO 1934: 117), compaiono menzionati in diversi atti di compravendita (URBAN 2000: 271-274). Uno di questi riguarda gli amministratori dell'ospedale, e menziona un patio[11] situato nei pressi di una fontana. Il dato è interessante perché, nel XVI secolo, uno dei maggiori problemi del quartiere portuale era rappresentato dalla penuria di acqua potabile: le poche fontane pubbliche non erano sufficienti, ed erano presenti molte cisterne, private, che raccoglievano l'acqua piovana (TASCA 2020: 43). Un altro atto di compravendita, relativo a una casa ubicata accanto all'ospedale, illustra il sistema di raccolta dell'acqua piovana attraverso un sistema di canalizzazione collegato direttamente al tetto (TASCA 1990: 140-141). La fontana pubblica più vicina all'ospedale era in quella che oggi è piazzetta Savoia, nell'Ottocento detta Piazza della Fontana Nova (SCANO 1934: 127), «perché anni addietro vi stava in mezzo una fontana o pozzo per il pubblico» (SPANO 1861: 223). L'ospedale, per ovvie ragioni, faceva un grande consumo d'acqua, per questo acquistava quella potabile (RAPETTI 2021: 101), ed era dotato di una cisterna di acqua pluviale e di un pozzo, indicato nelle piante settecentesche come «pozzo d'acqua salmastra».[12]

Le prime notizie riguardanti interventi alla struttura risalgono alla seconda metà del Cinquecento. Grazie ai libri della clavaria, per esempio, apprendiamo che nel 1568 furono messe le inferriate alle finestre[13] e fu realizzata la «*estufa por als qui tenen mal fransès*».[14] Pochi anni dopo, nel 1583, compaiono a libro paga alcuni

11. Il patio era stato donato all'ospedale, in passato, da Pere Pilita: potrebbe trattarsi di un'altra casa appartenuta al già menzionato barbiere Pere Polit?

12. ASTo, Sez. Corte, Paesi, Sardegna, Ecclesiastico, categoria XII Immunità, cartella 2, *Nuovo Progetto per l'ingrandimento dello Spedale detto di Sant'Antonio esistente nella Città presente di Cagliari, e nella Contrada detta della Costa agregata alla Marina* (*Cagliari li 6 feb 1773, Architetto Giuseppe Viana Misuratore per S.M.*). La cisterna è indicata con la lettera M nella *Pianta del Pian Terreno* (fig. 5). Nel 1830 un'altra cisterna di acqua potabile fu fatta collocare nei pressi del portico, «affinché i poveri vi potessero attingere acqua gratuitamente durante l'estate» (RUSSOTTO 1956: 113).

13. ASCCa, Sezione Antica, vol. 347/II, c. 10r.

14. ASCCa, Sezione Antica, vol. 347/II, c. 7v. La «*estufa*»: «*Cambra o lloc clos a una temperatura més o menys elevada i generalment graduable, on es posen persones o coses per a assecar-se, desinfectar-se, rebre l'acció d'un gas medicinal, etc.*» (DCVB, 1), costruita per curare i malati

*picapedrers* per la stima dei lavori da farsi nella casa di Antonio Matzutzi, destinata all'ospedale. Le azioni rendicontate sono la misurazione delle pareti e la stima di «*sostres y llenyam*».[15] Altri interventi hanno riguardato, per esempio, il cimitero: nel 1601 il clavario registrava i pagamenti effettuati per gli scavi appena eseguiti.[16] Il cimitero era accanto all'ospedale, in quella che è ora denominata piazza S. Sepolcro: la consacrazione avvenne nel 1583, come ricorda un'epigrafe ubicata nella chiesa del S. Sepolcro, prospiciente la piazza (Arru et al. 2020: 95-96).

Notizie sui primi interventi edilizi eseguiti dai Fatebenefratelli si ricavano dalle memorie di Fra Giusto Santa Maria, al secolo Diego Duque de Estrada:

> L'ospedale venne fabbricato in parte e restaurato dove si trovava in cattive condizioni; si fecero gran quantità di letti di ferro, materassi, lenzuola, federe, tende, biancheria e nuove officine. A tale scopo mi recai a Napoli, da dove portai croci, piattini d'argento per la Comunione e tutto l'occorrente per ornare gli altari (Estrada 1982: 459).

Il numero dei letti dell'ospedale si attestava intorno a 38-40. La notizia di un aumento dei letti fino a 100 dopo l'arrivo dei Fatebenefratelli è certamente un falso storico, infatti è messa in discussione dallo stesso padre Gabriele Russotto, che la riporta: «evidentemente è stato scambiato il numero dei malati presenti con quello dei letti» (Russotto 1956: 138).

Ulteriori lavori furono eseguiti negli anni 70 del Seicento, sotto il priorato di frate Nicolò Pulcasio. L'archivio dell'ospedale conserva un registro dei lavori eseguiti per la nuova infermeria, nel quale il priore annotò il dettaglio delle spese affrontate per i progettisti, i manovali, le pietre, la calce «et ogni altra cosa appartenente alla fabbrica».[17] Il nuovo dormitorio era stato disegnato da Domenico Spotorno, indicato come capomastro della cattedrale di Cagliari, pagato 25 lire;[18] la cappella dell'infermeria grande era stata affidata allo stuccatore siciliano Onofrio de Amato, che aveva ricevuto la retribuzione di 50 lire;[19] dal pittore Antonino Serqui erano stati acquistati tre grandi quadri, raffiguranti la Purissima, san Giovanni di Dio e san Nicola di Bari.[20] Questi lavori dovettero riguardare il reparto

di sifilide attraverso le fumigazioni, sarebbe divenuta, col passare del tempo, la «stufa», ovvero la stanza riservata alla segregazione dei folli (Tasca, Rapetti 2018: 137).

15. ASCCa, Sezione Antica, vol. 347/IV, c. 7r.

16. ASCCa, Sezione Antica, vol. 348/I, c. 24r.

17. ASCa, Ospedale S. Antonio abate, s. I.1, n. 1. La descrizione degli ambienti è stata rintracciata in un minutario notarile dall'archivista Nicola Settembre, e illustrata da Marcello Schirru in occasione dell'XI edizione del convegno internazionale *Abrils de l'Hospital* (Cagliari, 6-7 giugno 2022).

18. Ivi, c. 3r. Il ligure Spotorno era impegnato nel rifacimento della Cattedrale (Naitza 1992: 18).

19. Ivi, c. 3r. Sull'attività a Cagliari di Onofrio de Amato ci sono varie testimonianze, e sappiamo che nel 1677 fu incaricato di realizzare la cappella di Nostra Signora degli abbandonati nella chiesa del S. Sepolcro (Virdis 2017: 283-284).

20. Ivi, c. 23v. Del pittore Antonino Serqui è noto che ha dipinto, nel 1678, il retablo della chiesa parrocchiale di Pirri, realizzato insieme allo scultore Agostino Carta e allo scultore e doratore Saturno Lochi (Estofado de oro 2001: 258, 267, 279).

maschile. Ancora nel 1692 le donne si trovavano al piano inferiore, nell'«*hospital de bajo de les mujeres*» (KIROVA 1984: 22).

Un'epigrafe sulla facciata dell'ospedale, oggi perduta, ricordava i lavori fatti eseguire da Pulcasio:

> S. Ioannis Dei Religiosorum comoditati ac pauperum utilitati edificium hoc septem cubiculis septemque tabernis suis cum cellulis digestum R.mo P. Angelo Corrampulla Generali et R.do Fr. Nicolao Pulcasio Priore administrante curiose ac diligenter extructum anno MDCLXXIIII (SPANO 1861: 230).

Restano, invece, alcuni stemmi medievali, distribuiti su tre livelli e posizionati sopra una delle porte che affacciano sul portico. La posizione degli stemmi lascia intendere che siano stati spostati, ma non se ne conosce l'ubicazione originaria, né il momento di trasferimento. Inoltre, non sono indicati in bibliografia prima del Novecento (SCANO 1934: 117). Su un totale di dodici stemmi, ne sono stati identificati sei: quelli d'Aragona e delle Città di Cagliari e Barcellona (PLAISANT 1989: 30) e quelli delle famiglie Battle, Palou e Pujades, che hanno rivestito importanti cariche cittadine (FADDA, RAPETTI 2020: 200-202).

Nel corso dell'età moderna, soprattutto nel Settecento, il quartiere mutò il suo assetto (fig. 4). Gli interventi sul complesso S. Antonio furono molteplici ma, fatta eccezione per il rifacimento della chiesa, i lavori eseguiti furono di emergenza. Nel 1742 fu riparato il tetto, «che minacciava rovina» (KIROVA 1984: 20, 25-26). Tra il 1765 e il 1775 si intervenne a più riprese per la spezieria, il refettorio, la «stanza dei pazzi» (KIROVA 1984: 20). Nel 1777 le stanze destinate ai malati psichiatrici erano «ristrette e malsane, per prive d'aria libera, e talmente umide», che si pensò di realizzare per loro un'altra stanza, ricavata nel cortile, e terminata nel 1779.[21] Poco dopo, fu sistemato l'antico camerone delle donne per essere destinato alle cure mercuriali.[22]

Giuseppe Cossu (1739-1811), nelle sue notizie sulla città di Cagliari, pubblicate nel 1780, scriveva che l'ospedale cresceva «tutti gli anni in fabbriche» (KIROVA 1984: 21). Lo stesso può dirsi per i primi decenni dell'Ottocento, con interventi mirati a sanare situazioni di emergenza. Ancora nel 1853, il consiglio di carità dell'ospedale acquistò due nuovi cameroni, dotati di un cortiletto ciascuno, per ricoverare rispettivamente fino a tre uomini e tre donne affetti da mania (RAPETTI 2015: 295-296), ma si trattò dell'ennesima toppa su un tessuto ormai inservibile.

> Tutto questo vasto locale di proprietà dell'ospedale sarà ora venduto a particolari per edificarvi case che daranno un buon aspetto alla strada mentre attualmente quelle misere e basse celle dei Frati deturpano molto quella bella e ricca contrada di Cagliari (SPANO 1861: 230).

21. ASCa, Segreteria di Stato e di Guerra del Regno di Sardegna, Serie II, vol. 82, cc. 201-229.

22. Ivi, c. 254v.

Così scriveva Giovanni Spano poco dopo il trasporto degli ultimi malati nel nuovo ospedale civile, appena edificato. Le spese di trasferimento dei degenti furono sostenute dalla locale Congregazione grazie alla messa in vendita dall'antico complesso ospedaliero. Il fabbricato fu diviso in lotti e valutato. L'Archivio di Stato di Cagliari conserva, nel fondo Ospedale S. Antonio abate, le minute della Congregazione, la relazione e l'estimo compilati dagli ingegneri nonché il decreto del ministro Rattazzi del 30 dicembre 1859, che autorizzava la vendita a seguito di parere positivo del Consiglio di Stato.[23]

## 3. *Descrizione degli ambienti e cartografie settecentesche*

Nella primavera del 1751 il priore dei Fatebenefratelli, Paolo Murru, compilava un *Inventario del Convento di Cagliari*.[24] La descrizione sembra condurre dentro la famosa *Relatività* di Escher, certamente a causa della morfologia dell'area in cui insiste l'intero complesso architettonico. Per una corretta lettura dell'inventario e anche, come vedremo, della cartografia di Giuseppe Viana[25] del 1773 –progetto non realizzato, ma riferimento cartografico più antico– è necessario richiamare l'ubicazione dell'edificio tra due dislivelli: la salita di via Manno a nord, il declivio che conduce alla piazza S. Sepolcro a est. I dislivelli comportano una serie di piani, non immediatamente interpretabili, che vanno dai sotterranei ai due superiori. È importante fare una corretta distinzione tra il «Piano Terra» sulla via Manno e il «Piano Terreno della Corte» dell'ospedale, essendo indicato il primo nelle carte Viana al livello della strada *Sa Costa*, e il secondo a un livello inferiore, visto appunto il declivio che inizia con le scale del Portico e la discesa verso la piazza S. Sepolcro (fig. 5-6).

La descrizione di padre Murru partiva dalla chiesa, prospiciente la via Manno, dentro la quale erano presenti un battistero per gli esposti, una cantoria con l'organo, sette altari e la sacrestia. Il priore passava successivamente alle scalette che conducevano all'ingresso principale del convento, al lato del quale si trovava una campanella «per suonare alla carità dell'ospedale»; da lì passava all'ospedale

23. ASCa, Ospedale S. Antonio abate, s. I.1, n. 8.

24. ASTo, Sez. Corte, Paesi, Sardegna, Ecclesiastico, categoria 13, mazzo 1, fasc. 3, Ospedale di Cagliari, n. 6, 1751-1752. Il documento è annesso alla *Rappresentanza della Città di Cagliari la quale, stante li disordini che nascevano dalla cattiva condotta de' religiosi di S. Giovanni di Dio pregiudiziali alla direzione di quell'Ospedale di Sant'Antonio, pretendea doversi questo restituire all'amministrazione della medesima città.* L'inventario, segnato E, consta di 14 cc.

25. Giuseppe Viana (1735-1803) arrivò in Sardegna nel 1770 come misuratore ed estimatore delle Fortificazioni e Fabbriche militari. Fu subito coinvolto in due importanti progetti, riguardanti la fabbrica del nuovo seminario e il completamento della nuova facciata della cattedrale (Medde 2020). Nel 1773 Viana presentò dei progetti, rimasti lettera morta e oggi conservati in ASTo, Sez. Corte, Paesi, Sardegna, Ecclesiastico, categoria XII Immunità, cartella 2, relativi a strutture di assistenza: la conversione dell'antico seminario in ospizio di carità (Cavallari Murat 1960: 397) e due varianti alla fabbrica dell'ospedale. Queste ultime, già note (Kirova 1984; Pescarmona 1984), sono qui riesaminate grazie agli elaborati tridimensionali quotati.

degli uomini, dotato di una grande bussola all'ingresso. Nell'ospedale maschile vi erano un altare e 28 letti in ferro, un surplus di materassi (36 in tutto) e di paglhericci (42). Tramite una scala si saliva all'infermeria delle donne, costituita da otto letti in ferro, un piccolo altare, e altre due stanze: una ad uso delle infermiere, l'altra destinata alle pazze, con catene e due casse usate come letti. Venivano poi descritte la stanza del terziario e la stanza dei pazzi, questa con quattro casse a uso di letto e le catene attaccate al muro. Il priore passava a descrivere il corridoio del convento o «dei Reverendi Padri», ricco di quadri raffiguranti i frati, che si trovava al piano terra (quindi a livello di via Manno e sopraelevato rispetto alla corte), per poi descrivere la scala che conduceva al piano superiore, dove erano presenti il dormitorio, la stanza del padre commissario e altre otto stanze, indicate come occupate dal padre segretario, dal mastro, dal procuratore, da un forestiero, da frate Francesco, dallo spenditore, dal padre provinciale (composta da 3 ambienti) e da frate Giorgio.

Separato dal dormitorio dei frati era il noviziato, con «una stanza fatta a guisa di coridore» con le celle per i novizi e il loro maestro. Ai piedi della scala del noviziato era l'ambiente concesso al gremio dei sarti;[26] di fronte a questa si trovava il magazzino del grano, mentre sopra era un'altra stanza, usata talvolta per le provviste di grano, ma che in quel momento era destinata «al Sepulcro».[27] Da questo ambiente era possibile scendere in un'altra piccola stanza, occupata da vecchie cose.

Senza illustrare la via di collegamento, il priore si ritrovava all'ospedale degli uomini, per descrivere la stanza del padre Alessandro e un piccolo corridoio chiuso, adibito a guardaroba nel quale conservare i fagotti dei ricoverati e «una Pietà dorata che serve per li moribundi». Seguono poi la stanza dei padri Alberto e Giovanni Battista, e quella detta dell'ufficio priorale, che tra le tante cose, custodiva anche l'archivio dei frati, con «tutte la scritture, spectanti al Convento, libri di administrazioni ed altre diverse». La descrizione seguiva poi con un'altra camera e il professario, entrambi disabitati ma ricchi di oggetti. Sotto il professario stava la cantina, poi venivano descritti il refettorio, la cucina, due cortili (uno con cisterna, pozzo e mulino a ruota per tirare l'acqua), un giardino con piante da frutto, agrumi e rose, e infine la stalla, dalla quale si accedeva al carcere, munito

26. «Al piede della scala di detto Noviciato vi è una stanza grande spectante al gremio dei Sartori, ceduta a i medesimi per loro comodo da esso convento in occasione della nova Chiesa, in cambio d'altro sito da essi ceduta già diversi anni a profitto e comodo di convento». Tra il 6 e il 12 gennaio 1683, i Fatebenefratelli e il gremio dei sarti pattuivano il trasferimento di questi ultimi in altri locali, sempre attigui alla chiesa di S. Antonio abate, azione necessaria in vista del rifacimento della chiesa (ASCa, Ospedale S. Antonio abate, s. I.1, n. 2).

27. «Sopra quella dei sartori vi è una altra stanza grande, quale alcuna volta serve per mettervi grano. Presentemente sonovi diverse cose spectante al Sepulcro, tiene la sua serratura e chiave». Non è chiaro se si riferisse a un uso da parte della chiesa del Santo Sepolcro o, più probabilmente, della confraternita del Crocifisso e dell'Orazione o della Morte, detta del Santo Sepolcro (Rapetti 2022: 513).

di catenaccio e ceppo. Risultavano, inoltre, due magazzini affittati: uno si trovava sotto la chiesa, l'altro sotto l'ospedale.

L'ubicazione di questi ambienti è comprensibile se si collaziona l'inventario con le cartografie delle due varianti volte all'ingrandimento e modifiche dell'ospedale S. Antonio abate firmate da Viana il 6 e 15 febbraio 1773,[28] sulle quali ci si è basati per la ricostruzione tridimensionale del convento e ospedale di S. Antonio abate. Il primo progetto comprende le planimetrie dei piani terra, primo e secondo, e tre sezioni, mentre il secondo comprende la planimetria del primo piano, che funge da base per gli altri due, i cui ambienti sono descritti in una legenda. Nei disegni è possibile riconoscere la planimetria dell'ospedale esistente, perché vengono utilizzati colori diversi per le parti esistenti e per quelle da realizzare o da modificare.[29]

Al piano terra erano presenti una spezieria, che comunicava direttamente con l'ospedale e con un ingresso pubblico che dava sul portico, diversi locali di servizio, disposti intorno a un cortile quadrato, per il quale era previsto anche un passo carraio, la «porta rustica». Gli ambienti indicati nella carta del «piano Terreno» sono: granaio, cucina, con «tombarello per somministrare vettovaglie alla infermeria», «stalla per conservare Bovi e vitelli, con magazzeno per riporre Paglia e Orzo», macelleria, «bugadiera con suo camerino», magazzino per la legna, «paneteria e Pastino», «magazeno a Paglia per i pagliarici», cisterna d'acqua pluviale, magazzino del carbone, cantina. L'ingresso principale era lo stesso indicato nell'inventario del 1751, ossia dopo la rampa delle scale nel Portico. Al piano superiore, come dal documento del 1751, si trovavano l'ospedale degli uomini, l'infermeria e alcuni ambienti del convento, al secondo piano il convento e il noviziato.[30]

Nel secondo progetto del Viana,[31] vicino alla «porta rustica», sono i nuovi «luoghi comuni» (segnati con la lettera Z) che indicano i bagni, ma risultano esistenti altri bagni (con la lettera T) in diversi punti nei «poggioli servienti per li convalescenti» (a loro volta indicati con la lettera V). Altro elemento importante da segnalare è il Tombarello «per alzare e abbassare le vettovaglie dalla cucina alle infermerie». Forse il nome dell'adiacente via Tagliolas o *Tallolas*, ovvero carrucole (Scano 1934: 120), indicava come dalla parte dell'attuale piazza S. Sepolcro e via Dettori fosse necessario, a causa del forte pendio, avere delle carrucole per le merci.

Dalle carte Viana si riconoscono la scuola di Medicina, ubicata al secondo piano, e il teatro anatomico, al primo, «qual si può demolire col terreno per

28. ASTo, Sez. Corte, Paesi, Sardegna, Ecclesiastico, categoria XII Immunità, cartella 2.

29. ASTo, Sez. Corte, Paesi, Sardegna, Ecclesiastico, categoria XII Immunità, cartella 2.

30. ASTo, Sez. Corte, Paesi, Sardegna, Ecclesiastico, categoria XII Immunità, cartella 2, *Pianta del Pian Terreno - Pianta del Secondo Piano* (fig. 5).

31. Ivi, *Altro progetto per il Ristauramento, ed ingrandimento dello Spedale di Sant'Antonio eretto nella presente Città nella Contrada detta della Costa alla Marina, lasciando interinalmente l'abitazione dei M. RR.PP. qual col tempo può servire per alloggio del'impiegati per detto Spedale mediante una Scaletta a farsi.*

ingrandire il Cortile». Si può supporre che il teatro anatomico occupasse due piani, compreso il piano sulla Corte, ma né questo né la scuola di Medicina sono menzionati nel 1751. Potrebbero essere successivi alla fondazione della scuola di Chirurgia all'interno dell'Ateneo cagliaritano (1759) o alla rifondazione dello stesso Ateneo (1764), ma non si esclude che nel periodo precedente esistessero dei locali dell'ospedale adibiti alle dissezioni, essendo l'Università di Cagliari attiva dal 1626 (TRUCAS, QUARTU, RIVA 2020: 72-86).

Nelle antiche mappe catastali, realizzate nella seconda metà dell'Ottocento, l'area dell'antico ospedale è identificata come isolato K-2365.[32] Data l'estensione e l'importanza dell'edificio e dei suoi annessi, le citazioni sono numerosissime nei documenti di fine Settecento e di inizio Ottocento. Grazie agli studi compiuti da Guido Massacci,[33] che ha rintracciato due atti notarili datati 23 settembre 1796 e 22 novembre 1797, è noto che davanti alla casa Dugoni (2415), sulla strada della Costa, vi era la «spezieria dello Spedale», quindi all'estremità ovest, verso la Porta Stampace.[34] I locali indicati dal Viana potrebbero essere di progetto e non realizzati, oppure utilizzati come ufficio dello speziale nei piani sotterranei rispetto al livello della via Sa Costa, mentre la spezieria indicata dagli atti notarili del 1796-1797 dovrebbe essere ubicata dove si trovava la Farmacia S. Antonio, ancora esistente sino a pochi anni fa.[35]

Sempre dal lato della Costa, al piano terra, erano presenti diverse botteghe date in affitto. Il 26 settembre 1806 venne redatto l'inventario dei «beni mobili, semoventi e stabili appartenenti allo Spedale della Marina sotto l'invocazione di Sant'Antonio Abate, e loro consegna al procuratore generale dei Padri Spedalieri della città», come da ordini del re del 15 settembre 1806.[36] Fra i beni denunciati

32. ASCa, Ufficio tecnico erariale, n. 105, accessibile online su http://www.archiviostatocagliari.it/archivio2/visualiz_sel_skede.php?COD=6370&M=S&q3=%20Marina [2022/07/07].

33. Importante per l'analisi dell'area dell'ospedale di S. Antonio è una ricerca condotta da Guido Massacci, pubblicata su https://storiadicase.jimdofree.com/ [2022/06/22], che presenta attraverso mappe e documenti il quartiere della Marina tra il XVIII e il XIX secolo.

34. La Porta Stampace era il varco dal quale si imboccava Sa Costa, e separava i quartieri Marina e Stampace. Il 30 agosto 1809 una bottega (e stanze annesse), sita davanti alla casa Dugoni (2415) e confinante da entrambi i lati con altre botteghe degli ospedalieri, fu concessa in enfiteusi vitalizia al negoziante Filippo Martini per 90 lire annue. Con altro atto del notaio Martini del 30 dicembre 1810, una bottega con una stanza posteriore ed un mezzanello furono concessi in enfiteusi al negoziante milanese Marco Cima e a sua moglie Giuseppa Marchisoli; la bottega era fino ad allora utilizzata dal convento, confinava con altre botteghe dell'ospedale di cui una utilizzata dal sarto Pietro Nuxis, cfr. https://storiadicase.jimdofree.com/isolati-gruppo-1-2194-2387/isolato-k-2365-2387/ [2022/06/22].

35. Di questa spezieria esiste in OHSJD un bellissimo inventario del 1815: «porta di strada con vetrate e scuri al di dentro, e ben muniti di serratura [...] vi sono 110 vasi di Maiolica, tra grandi, mezzani e piccoli, ognuno con il suo coperchio; bottiglie di cristallo e vetro, in tutte 100 [...]» (RUSSOTTO 1956: 141).

36. https://storiadicase.jimdofree.com/isolati-gruppo-1-2194-2387/isolato-k-2365-2387/ [2022/06/22].

nel 1807 dagli ospedalieri figurano nove botteghe.[37] Sempre grazie alle ricerche di Massacci, si hanno notizie sui locatari delle botteghe:

> con atto notarile del 16 luglio 1811 Domenico Rossi, Mastro del Battaglione dei Cacciatori di Savoia, prese «in locazione per 9 anni dal 15 settembre 1811 fino al 1820 tutta la bottega e piano superiore che la comunità (del Regio Ospedale) possiede nella strada della Costa, per lire 100 annue; è la casa detta del numero 4 (nel tratto che va) dal Portico del convento sino alla spezieria, che confina da una parte alla casa e bottega concessa a Marco Cima (cioccolatiere), d'altra parte a bottega del Cappellaro Michele Bonino, alle spalle il convento, e dirimpetto la casa detta di Perpignano (2413) ora di San Michele, strada in mezzo».[38]

Domenico Rossi fu sfrattato il 31 ottobre 1827, dovendo i frati eseguire alcuni lavori urgenti all'ospedale.

I coniugi Marco Cima e Giuseppa Marchisoli, concessionari di un'enfiteusi vitalizia relativa a «una bottega col suo mezzanello», nel marzo 1812 rinunciarono all'accordo e restituirono i locali all'ospedale. Infine, a metà Ottocento, tale Rosa Demelas, moglie di Efisio Frau, risultava proprietaria di una parte dell'unità 2365, dove aveva una bottega.[39]

Per quanto concerne il teatro anatomico è possibile dedurre l'ubicazione nel lato ovest della corte dai documenti compresi in un fascicolo relativo a una lite civile fra i negozianti Giuseppe Chessa e Giovanni Battista Franco,[40] iniziata nel 1803.

Dai documenti si apprende che il Chessa stava eseguendo degli importanti lavori nella sua casa della Costa, numero catastale 2386: egli ammise di aver distrutto, per ingrandire la sua casa, uno "splendido giardinetto pieno di alberi da frutto e fiori", di sua proprietà; oltre ad aver già "oscurato" alcune finestre del primo piano della casa Franco, unità 2378 sulla strada Tagliolas, con l'innalzamento della nuova costruzione avrebbe tolto luce anche ad alcune finestre più alte della stessa casa; costrinse quindi l'Ospedale a intervenire nella lite in quanto le fondamenta della «fabbrica del Chessa distavano dall'ospedale solo 13 palmi [cosicché la nuova costruzione], avrebbe privato di luce anche la camera anatomica dove sogliono fare operazioni di parti sottilissime, e priverebbe di ventilazione un

37. ASCa, Segreteria di Stato e di Guerra del Regno di Sardegna, Serie II, vol. 83, cc. 13-18, in https://storiadicase.jimdofree.com/isolati-gruppo-1-2194-2387/isolato-k-2365-2387/ [2022/06/22].

38. https://storiadicase.jimdofree.com/isolati-gruppo-1-2194-2387/isolato-k-2365-2387/ [2022/06/22].

39. *Ibidem*. Per le specifiche delle particelle catastali indicate si rimanda alla mappa catastale e alla rielaborazione di Massacci in https://storiadicase.jimdofree.com/le-strade-e-le-mappe/mappe-catastali-rielaborate/mappa-nord-ovest/ e https://storiadicase.jimdofree.com/le-strade-e-le-mappe/mappe-catastali-originali/mappa-3-isolati-i-k-i1-l1-v1-x1-y1-z1-a2-b2/ [2022/06/22].

40. Giovanni Battista Franco (1769-1830), marmorario originario di Lanzo d'Intelvi (Como). Tra le sue opere a Cagliari: l'altare maggiore in preziosi marmi policromi nella chiesa di S. Efisio in Stampace e l'altare in cui risiede il simulacro del Santo; l'altare maggiore dell'Oratorio delle Anime Purganti (Piazza S. Giacomo); l'altare marmoreo nella cappella del Crocifisso della Cattedrale di Cagliari (Pasolini 2011).

ambiente inquinato dalle esalazioni putride dei cadaveri, e la camera d'infermeria delle donne».[41]

Le ricerche di Massacci danno ragione di credere che la costruzione del Chessa rimase bloccata per diversi anni: un atto notarile del 1808 dimostra che il Chessa vendette la sua casa (2386) e «diversi materiali "non ancora messi in opera"» e che «sul suo cortile si affacciavano due stanze dell'Ospedale, "una per le donne ammalate, l'altra per l'anatomia"».[42] Una carta del 26 settembre 1822, tra le ultime relative alla lite, cita l'intervento del negoziante Giovanni Calb (Kalb), proprietario della casa dell'ormai defunto Giuseppe Chessa, che intendeva chiudere la questione con il Franco. Franco morì nel 1830, a metà Ottocento la casa risultava appartenere a suo figlio Giovanni, negoziante, nato nel 1794.[43]

L'unità catastale 2386, invece, stimata 5.577 lire, fu venduta il 13 novembre 1784 dai fratelli Marramaldo Toufani a quel Giuseppe Chessa che già la abitava. La casa confinava da un lato con la casa Arthemalle (2385), e dall'altro con una casa di Eligio Allemand (2387), mentre aveva davanti la casa Scarpinati del Capitolo Cagliaritano (2417). Secondo Massacci, si può ipotizzare «che all'inizio del secolo XVIII ci fosse un terreno ancora non edificato, magari un giardino», al posto dei lotti 2385 e 2386.[44] L'ipotesi è plausibile: nelle cartografie del XVI secolo, come quella famosa di Cagliari di Sigismondo Arquer,[45] è ben visibile come il complesso di S. Antonio, segnato con la lettera F, fosse isolato rispetto alla strada del Tempio di S. Leonardo (G) e quella di Barcellona (D) che si conclude con la Piazza di *Gliapola* e la *Palizada* del Porto.

Quanto agli ambienti destinati all'assistenza, nei progetti Viana erano segnati come cameroni, maschile e femminile, dotati di altare (come da descrizione del 1751), mentre ai pazzi e ai malati di sifilide erano destinati ambienti più piccoli e separati, confinanti con il portico.[46] I due progetti, tra le varie modifiche, prevedevano una nuova ala, perpendicolare alla corsia degli uomini, e un nuovo ospedale per le donne al piano superiore. In corrispondenza dello «Spedale degli Uomini» si trova l'unità catastale 2366, confinante con le attuali scalette di S. Sepolcro. Un donativo dell'Arciconfraternita del Sepolcro, proprietaria dell'attigua casa (2367), dimostra che questa era confinante con una proprietà dell'ospedale, e ulteriore conferma arriva dall'Ufficio tecnico erariale: ancora dopo il 1859, l'unità 2366 apparteneva all'Ospedale Civile.[47]

41. https://storiadicase.jimdofree.com/isolati-gruppo-1-2194-2387/isolato-k-2365-2387/ [2022/06/22].

42. *Ibidem*.

43. *Ibidem*.

44. *Ibidem*.

45. https://www.unica.it/unica/it/multimedia_foto_s1.page?contentId=GAL175539 [2022/06/22].

46. ASTo, Sez. Corte, Paesi, Sardegna, Ecclesiastico, categoria XII Immunità, cartella 2, *Nuovo Progetto* (figg. 5-6).

47. https://storiadicase.jimdofree.com/isolati-gruppo-1-2194-2387/isolato-k-2365-2387/ [2022/06/22].

Nel progetto Viana del 6 febbraio 1773 la ruota degli esposti e la stanza del didoto[48] venivano indicate come esistenti accanto all'ingresso principale, mentre nella variante del 15 febbraio una nuova ruota e la stanza del didoto furono disegnate accanto all'ingresso della chiesa (da convertirsi in oratorio dell'ospedale), e non più nel portico.[49]

Le modifiche più evidenti attualmente, rispetto alla situazione dei secoli XVIII e XIX, sono legate alla cessata attività ospedaliera a seguito della costruzione del nuovo ospedale. Gli edifici sulla via Manno vennero venduti a privati, con la costruzione di palazzi che hanno sostituito la fila di botteghe un tempo affittate a piccoli commercianti. Nel Progetto per la divisione e vendita, l'ex ospedale S. Antonio è diviso in 3 porzioni (indicate coi colori blu, verde, rosso): sono evidenti i due palazzi attuali prospicenti la via Manno, le porzioni verde e rossa formano il palazzo al numero civico 68, mentre la porzione blu corrisponde al palazzo con il numero civico 60, che incorpora l'ingresso al portico.[50]

La parte meridionale che prospetta sulla corte fu adibita prima a caserma e poi, fino al 1992, a scuola pubblica.[51] Attualmente la struttura, riaperta al pubblico dopo la ristrutturazione nel 2009, ospita l'Hostel Marina e il portico, che ha visto nel 2017 la ricollocazione della statua marmorea di S. Antonio abate nella sua nicchia, è ritornato a pullulare di vita.[52]

## 4. *Il Progetto Hostel*

Il Liceo Artistico Musicale Foiso Fois di Cagliari ha attivato, dall'anno scolastico 2016-2017, un progetto di *Alternanza scuola-lavoro* dedicato allo studio e valorizzazione del complesso monumentale S. Antonio abate.[53] L'*Alternanza*

48. Da *didot*, «derivat de *dida* amb el sufix augmentatiu i masculinitzador *-ot*» (DCVB), ospedaliere incaricato degli esposti. Il nome della carica rimase immutato in età sabauda. Sull'infanzia abbandonata a Cagliari cfr. Durzu 2011.

49. L'abbandono degli esposti nella ruota del S. Antonio è documentato dal 1576 (ASCCa, Sezione Antica, vol. 347/III, cc. 20r-37v) e il pagamento delle dide dal 1549 (ASCCa, Sezione Antica, vol. 281, c. 118v), ma questo è l'unico documento che localizzi con certezza la ruota.

50. ASCCa, Fondo Cartografico, serie G, edifici pubblici, G 21 I-III, *Tipo del fabbricato detto l'antico spedale civile sito in via La Costa quartiere Marina Rilevato ed estimato per provvedersi alla sua vendita dividendolo in tre porzioni come si vede indicato in linee rosse*, disponibile su https://mediateca.comune.cagliari.it/serieg.html [2022/06/22].

51. L'Istituto Tecnico Commerciale Pietro Martini ha occupato la sede fino agli anni 30 del Novecento. Nel secondo dopoguerra gli spazi sono stati occupati dal Liceo Ginnasio Giovanni Siotto Pintor, trasferito nel 1968 in viale Trento. Successivamente, l'edificio ha ospitato la Scuola Media Giovanni Spano e, infine, l'Istituto professionale Domenico Alberto Azuni (Artizzu 2000).

52. La statua è realizzata in marmo pregiato e poco usato nella scultura sarda. Potrebbe essere ascritta al XV secolo, e le sue caratteristiche la collocano come immagine devozionale (Pillittu 2015). Fu donata dalla signora A. Carossino e posta nella nicchia dal Gruppo archeologico sardo nel 1946. Non è ancora noto quando e come la signora Carossino, forse Angela (Cagliari, 1883-1964), sia entrata in possesso della statua.

53. Hanno lavorato al progetto gli studenti dell'indirizzo di Design (3I, 4I, 5I nel triennio

*scuola lavoro* (ASL) è una modalità didattica innovativa, consistente in un periodo di formazione teorica in classe e un periodo di esperienza pratica sul campo in cui si decide di svolgere l'attività, introdotta nella scuola secondaria di secondo livello con la Legge 107/2015, ridenominata «percorso per le competenze trasversali e per l'orientamento» (PCTO) a decorrere dall'anno scolastico 2018-2019 (DM 774 del 4 settembre 2019). I progetti ASL/PCTO, obbligatori per le classi dell'ultimo triennio, sono strutturati in maniera tale da avvicinare gli studenti al mondo del lavoro, consentendo loro di acquisire un'esperienza utile per le professioni future attraverso il consolidamento delle conoscenze, la scoperta e/o lo sviluppo delle attitudini personali.

Il progetto dedicato al complesso monumentale, denominato "Progetto Hostel" in ragione dell'attuale destinazione d'uso, è stato concepito come un veicolo attraverso cui gli studenti potessero acquisire competenze disciplinari in campo ambientale, territoriale, urbanistico, architettonico, design, artistico, storico-letterario, musicale, grafico, digitale e multimediale, nonché competenze trasversali di tipo organizzativo, sociale, etico-civile. Il coinvolgimento attivo degli studenti li ha visti partecipi in termini di progettazione degli spazi, esposizioni, laboratori, comunicazione, ecc., fermo restando l'aspetto didattico-pedagogico dell'iniziativa (ARTIZZU 2020; 2021). Nell'ambito dell'ASL, il complesso architettonico è stato l'epicentro di una serie di laboratori creativi e progettuali delle discipline di indirizzo del Liceo Foiso Fois (in particolare Architettura, Design, Discipline pittoriche), con il coinvolgimento di diversi soggetti, la condivisione e l'interazione. I risultati di questo lavoro sono fruibili in loco nonché attraverso il portale https://progettohostel.jimdo.com/, i cui assi portanti sono le sezioni *Monumento*, *Museo Virtuale* e *ASL*.[54]

*Monumento.* La sezione presenta quattro capitoli dedicati, rispettivamente, alla storia dell'antico ospedale, all'ordine canonicale ospedaliero di S. Antonio di Vienne, alla festa di sant'Antonio abate e ai locali ubicati sotto la chiesa di S. Antonio, un tempo appartenuti al convento. Sono inoltre presenti i collegamenti alle altre sezioni, come gli *Eventi*, tra i quali è messa in risalto la XXI edizione di *Monumenti aperti*,[55] alla quale aderì anche il Progetto Hostel.[56]

2016-2019), le classi 4A, 5A di Architettura e Ambiente nel biennio 2016-2018, la classe 3A nel 2019. Importante anche la partecipazione di due ex studentesse, Marta Deias e Greca Nathascia Meloni, che hanno coadiuvato i lavori del museo virtuale e realizzato il sito.

54. Il portale offre, inoltre, le seguenti pagine: Eventi, Concorsi, Notizie, Contatti, Partnership (Eccellenze e Associazioni).

55. https://progettohostel.jimdo.com/home/eventi/monumenti-aperti-2017/ [2022/06/22]. La manifestazione prevede l'apertura gratuita dei monumenti. Nata grazie all'associazione culturale Imago Mundi, costituita nel 1993 da un gruppo di studenti universitari cagliaritani interessati a diffondere la cultura e le tradizioni storiche nell'ambiente cittadino, è giunta alla XXVI edizione, coinvolgendo ormai quasi tutta la Sardegna, nonché diverse località della penisola, cfr. https://monumentiaperti.com/it/ [2022/06/22].

56. https://progettohostel.jimdo.com/home/eventi/monumenti-aperti-2017/ [2022/06/22]. Il progetto è stato poi presentato per La Settimana delle Culture Digitali del 2018 (https://progetto-

I contenuti delle pagine sono stati realizzati interamente dagli studenti, che hanno attinto dalla bibliografia scientifica, dalle informazioni presenti sui portali web di taglio divulgativo, e dal ricco patrimonio fotografico, audiovisivo e iconografico raccolto, nel tempo, da diversi soggetti –pubblici e privati– a vario titolo coinvolti nelle attività che si sono svolte all'interno dei locali del complesso monumentale.[57] Tali materiali di studio completano i testi composti dagli studenti e sono offerti al visitatore del portale e, attraverso i QRcode presenti sui pannelli espositivi posti all'ingresso dell'Ostello, anche agli ospiti e ai visitatori della struttura.

*Museo Virtuale.* Nel 2023, dopo l'esperienza della pandemia da Covid-19, per parlare di 'museo virtuale' o 'visita virtuale' non sono necessari lunghi preamboli. Eppure, appena sei anni fa, era necessario definire il museo virtuale come «entità digitale che condivide alcune caratteristiche del museo tradizionale e ha lo scopo di completare, migliorare e aumentare l'esperienza attraverso forme di personalizzazione, interazione ed arricchimento dei contenuti».[58] Lo scopo del lavoro svolto dagli studenti all'interno di questo ambito del Progetto Hostel è stato quello di rendere accessibile il complesso monumentale, raccogliendo ed elaborando informazioni e materiali per poterli presentare al grande pubblico con una nuova veste, più immediata, facilmente raggiungibile e soprattutto comprensibile: le informazioni, offerte con un taglio divulgativo, sono fruibili sia nel sito, ovvero il luogo fisico della mostra, sia online, attraverso l'uso di smartphone, tablet e PC. Attualmente, dal portale e grazie all'applicativo *Thinglink*, si può effettuare una visita virtuale e prendere visione dei pannelli espositivi ubicati all'ingresso dell'Hostel Marina. È possibile, inoltre, sfogliare le gallerie fotografiche relative ai diversi eventi espositivi realizzati nella struttura. A causa dell'obsolescenza tecnologica, non è più possibile accedere ai contenuti in realtà aumentata realizzati con Aurasma-*Hp Reveal*, ma il lavoro digitale rimane comunque archiviato per essere utilizzato con altri sistemi, dato che la tecnologica è in continua evoluzione e il digitale permette di essere rielaborato.

*ASL.* La sezione relativa al progetto di *Alternanza scuola-lavoro* entra nel vivo delle attività svolte dagli studenti del Liceo Foiso Fois all'interno della struttura che oggi ospita l'ostello. La ricerca bibliografica e d'archivio è stata completata dalle attività di indirizzo del Liceo, che comprendono, per esempio, il Design, con il restyling dell'ostello. I lavori di progettazione sono durati un anno, dopodiché si è dato vita ai laboratori in loco. Il portale offre sia le schede di presentazione e le schede tecniche, immagini e video di ciascun progetto di restyling, che il diario dei laboratori, arricchito dalla galleria fotografica con le camere prima, durante e dopo l'attività.[59]

hostel.jimdo.com/home/eventi/scud-2018-1/) e del 2019 (https://progettohostel.jimdo.com/home/eventi/scud-2019/) [2022/06/22].

57. https://progettohostel.jimdo.com/progetto-asl-1/monumento/ [2022/06/22].

58. https://progettohostel.jimdo.com/progetto-asl-1/museo-virtuale/ [2022/06/22].

59. https://progettohostel.jimdo.com/progetto-asl-1/progetti-restyling/laboratorio-camere/ [2022/06/22].

Le classi di Design e Architettura e Ambiente, negli anni scolastici dal 2016 al 2019, hanno elaborato i progetti tridimensionali con il programma *SketchUp* e le successive elaborazioni di rendering di immagini e video con *Light Up* e *kerkythea*. Sempre all'interno del file *SketchUp* sono state elaborate le 'scene' per la formazione del video, fruibile anche nell'applicazione *Kubity*. Tale applicazione permette, inoltre, di vedere gli ambienti con il visore 3D e in Realtà Aumentata. Tutte queste applicazioni sono open source, scaricabili gratuitamente.

Allo stato attuale sono stati ripresi i lavori da alcuni studenti della classe 5A di Architettura e Ambiente,[60] che si sono cimentati nella ricostruzione in 3D virtuale, render e video render degli ambienti della Corte. La cartografia di base è quella relativa ai progetti settecenteschi del Viana, ma sono state analizzate anche le descrizioni del 1751 già citate.

In questa nuova fase del lavoro si evidenzia l'importanza del digitale nell'evoluzione delle elaborazioni, perché sono stati utilizzati i file .skp dei lavori eseguiti dagli studenti negli anni precedenti, ma con la possibilità di incrementare le elaborazioni digitali grazie all'evoluzione tecnologica, con l'ausilio di un laboratorio professionalizzante presente nella sede centrale del Liceo, la possibilità di avere PC performanti per l'uso di *SketchUp PRO 2022* e il programma di renderizzazione *Twinmotion*. Tali elaborazioni permettono anche un'esperienza immersiva con l'ausilio del visore 3D e con sistemi più performanti come *Oculus* o *HTC Vive*.

Sono state realizzate immagini e video render del corridoio dei Reverendi Padri e degli ambienti di servizio dell'ospedale ubicati nella Corte al piano terreno (fig. 8-10). Con la pianta del secondo progetto[61] si è elaborata la ricostruzione grafica delle murature «in gialo da demolirsi» per evidenziare l'antica struttura,[62] ma si ritiene necessario ampliare lo studio con il supporto della cartografia ottocentesca realizzata in occasione della messa in vendita ai privati.[63] I rilievi e le misure sono quelle tratte dalla cartografia attuale e antica, sarebbe auspicabile un lavoro di rilevo più complesso e la possibilità di esplorare gli ambienti sotterranei e limitrofi per attuare una ricostruzione scientificamente più realistica, ma è necessario avere il supporto dell'Università e la sinergia di differenti figure professionali.

60. Gli studenti, coadiuvati da M. Beatrice Artizzu, sono: Samuele Lupinu, Alessia Manni, Filippo Marceddu e Gianluca Menga. Hanno presentato il lavoro in occasione del convegno XI *Abrils de l'Hospital*, il 6 Giugno 2022.

61. ASTo, Sez. Corte, Paesi, Sardegna, Ecclesiastico, categoria XII Immunità, cartella 2, *Altro progetto*.

62. Fig. 7. In occasione dell'XI edizione degli *Abrils de l'Hospital*, è stato inaugurato presso l'attuale Hostel Marina un pannello esplicativo che riporta la cartografia antica analizzata e le elaborazioni digitali. È possibile prendere visione del materiale all'url: https://www.profbix.it/progettohostel-cagliari-antico-spedale-sant-antonio/ [2022/06/22].

63. ASCCa, Fondo Cartografico, serie G, edifici pubblici, cfr. https://mediateca.comune.cagliari.it/serieg.html [2022/06/22].

Il Progetto Hostel vuole offrire un modello alternativo: agendo sin dalla scuola secondaria[64] si vuole offrire una visione del patrimonio culturale e artistico come sistema di nuove professioni correlate alle tecnologie digitali (Artizzu 2021), allineandosi agli obiettivi culturali e formativi finalizzati ad avvicinare i giovani al patrimonio culturale, educandoli alla tutela attraverso un percorso virtuoso di conoscenza e valorizzazione, sviluppando in loro sia una cultura del digitale per la conservazione e valorizzazione del patrimonio culturale, sia la consapevolezza che la cultura digitale contemporanea produce anch'essa patrimonio culturale, trasmettendo loro il valore che il patrimonio ha per le comunità del presente e del futuro (Artizzu 2020; 2021).

## *Bibliografia*


Arru, M. Grazia; Masala, Franco; Mura, Lucia, Nonne, Claudio, 2020. "Inquadramento storico-topografico dell'area", Rosanna Martorelli, Donatella Mureddu (a cura di), *Archeologia urbana a Cagliari. Scavi nella chiesa di Sant'Eulalia alla Marina. Il quartiere dalle origini ai giorni nostri:* status quaestionis *all'inizio della ricerca*, Perugia, Morlacchi: 45-159.

Artizzu, M. Beatrice, 2000. "Adotta un Monumento. Complesso monumentale S. Antonio, Marina, Cagliari", Maria Antonietta Calledda, Pino Calledda (a cura di), *Io vivo in Sardegna e ne faccio parte. Dall'accoglienza al viaggio*, Cagliari, CUEC: 49-55.

Artizzu, M. Beatrice, 2020. "Didattica con la Realtà Aumentata al Liceo Artistico Musicale 'Foiso Fois' di Cagliari", *Progetto IDEA: Innovazione Didattica E Apprendimento*, a cura del Programma di Educational Techonology - ISOC CRS4: 33-38, https://www.logus.it/progetto-idea-innovazione-didattica-e-apprendimento/.

Artizzu, M. Beatrice, 2021. "Didattica Digitale al Liceo Artistico Musicale Foiso Fois di Cagliari. Architettura e Ambiente: 3D Realtà Virtuale e Realtà Aumentata", *Culture Digitali*, 1: 44-48, https://www.diculther.it/rivista/culture-digitali-n-1/.

Cadinu, Marco, 2008. "Il nuovo quartiere aragonese sul porto nel primo Trecento a Cagliari", *La città europea del Trecento. Trasformazioni, monumenti, ampliamenti urbani*, Bologna, Kappa: 162-172.

Cadinu, Marco, 2019. "Strutture portuali, architetture e forme urbane medievali tra XI e XIV secolo. Lo spazio tirrenico toscano, la Sardegna, le isole", *RODIS. Journal of Medieval and Post-medieval Archaeology*, 2: 57-88, https://doi.org/10.33115/a/26046679/2_3

Cavallari Murat, Augusto, 1960. "G. V., architetto sabaudo in Sardegna", *Atti e rassegna tecnica della Società Ingegneri e Architetti in Torino*, n.s., XIV: 395-415.

DCVB. *Diccionari català-valencià-balear*, Antoni Maria Alcover i Francesc de Borja, Palma de Mallorca, Moll, 1968-1969, https://dcvb.iec.cat/.

Del Panta, Antonella, 1983. *Un architetto e la sua città. L'opera di Gaetano Cima (1805-1878) nelle carte dell'Archivio comunale di Cagliari*, Cagliari, Edizioni della Torre.

Durzu, Annalisa, 2011. *Orfani e trovatelli nella Sardegna moderna*, Milano, FrancoAngeli.

Estofado de oro, 2001. *Estofado de oro. La statuaria lignea nella Sardegna spagnola*, Cagliari, Janus/Ministero per i beni e le Attività Culturali.

Estrada, Diego Duque de, 1982. *Comentarios del desengañado de sì mismo. vida del mismo autor*, Madrid, Castalia.


64. Conferenza *Tutti A Iscol@*, https://progettohostel.jimdo.com/home/notizie/conferenza-idea-ar/ [2022/06/22].

Fadda, Bianca; Rapetti, Mariangela, 2020. "Le strutture di assistenza ospedaliera", Rosanna Martorelli, Donatella Mureddu (a cura di), *Archeologia urbana a Cagliari. Scavi nella chiesa di Sant'Eulalia alla Marina. Il quartiere dalle origini ai giorni nostri:* status quaestionis *all'inizio della ricerca*, Perugia, Morlacchi: 195-205.

Ferragud, Carmel, 2005. *Medicina i promoció social a la baixa edat mitjana (Corona d'Aragò, 1350-1410)*, Madrid, CSIC.

Foscati, Alessandra, 2013. "I tre corpi del santo. Le leggende di traslazione delle spoglie di sant'Antonio abate in Occidente", *Hagiographica*, 20: 144-181.

Kirova, Tatiana K., 1984. "I Fatebenefratelli e l'ospedale di S. Antonio Abate in Cagliari", a cura di Tatiana K. Kirova. *Arte e Cultura del '600 e del '700 in Sardegna*, Napoli, Edizioni Scientifiche Italiane.

Medde, Silvia, 2020. "Viana, Giuseppe", *Dizionario Biografico degli Italiani*, Roma, Istituto della Enciclopedia Italiana: *ad vocem*.

Naitza, Salvatore, 1992. *Architettura dal tardo '600 al Classicismo purista*, Nuoro, Ilisso.

Pasolini, Alessandra, 2011. "Marmorari Intelvesi in Sardegna: le botteghe di Spazzi e Franco dal 1740 al 1830", *Artisti dei Laghi – Rivista online*, 1: 908-935.

Pescarmona, Daniele, 1984. "Nuovi contributi alla conoscenza dell'attività degli ingegneri militari piemontesi in Sardegna nel secolo XVIII", *Bollettino d'Arte*, s. 6, 69/28: 71-90.

Pillittu, Aldo, 2015. "Una nuova scultura marmorea tardomedievale: il Sant'Antonio abate del complesso antoniano di Cagliari", Rosanna Martorelli (a cura di), *Itinerando. Senza confini dalla preistoria ad oggi. Studi in ricordo di Roberto Coroneo*, Perugia, Morlacchi: 1055-1068.

Plaisant, Maria Luisa, 1989. "Lo sviluppo del quartiere dell'insediamento medioevale al secolo XVIII", *Cagliari. Quartieri storici. Marina*, Silvana Editoriale: 27-30.

Rapetti, Mariangela, 2017. *L'espansione degli Ospedalieri di Sant'Antonio di Vienne nel Mediterraneo Occidentale fra XIII e XVI secolo. Archivi e documenti*, Perugia, Morlacchi.

Rapetti, Mariangela, 2018. "La riforma delle Opere pie nel regno di Sardegna e suoi riflessi nella produzione documentaria degli ospedali", *Studi e Ricerche*, 11: 43-63.

Rapetti, Mariangela, 2020. "Gli ospedali civici in Sardegna (secoli XIV-XVI)", *Alle origini del welfare. Radici medievali e moderne della cultura europea dell'assistenza*, Roma, Viella: 125-145.

Rapetti, Mariangela, 2021. "Le forniture alimentari dell'ospedale di Cagliari dai registri del clavario e del maggiordomo (1535-1635)", Mariangela Rapetti, Andrea Pergola (a cura di), *Ospedali e assistenza nei territori della Corona d'Aragona. Fonti archivistiche, archeologiche e artistiche*, Perugia, Morlacchi: 93-103.

Rapetti, Mariangela, 2022. "Medieval and Early Modern Confraternities in Sardinia", David D'Andrea, Salvatore Marino (a cura di), *Confraternities in Southern Italy: Art, Politics, and Religion (1100-1800)*, Toronto, Centre for Renaissance and Reformation and Studies & Victoria University in the University of Toronto: 507-556.

Russotto, Gabriele, 1956. *I Fatebenefratelli in Sardegna*, Roma, Ordine ospedaliero di S. Giovanni di Dio.

Scano, Dionigi, 1934. *Forma Kalaris*, Cagliari, Società editrice Italiana.

Schirru, Valeria, 2003. "Le pergamene relative alla Sardegna nel Diplomatico San Lorenzo alla Rivolta dell'Archivio di Stato di Pisa", *Archivio Storico Sardo*, 43: 61-339.

Spano, Giovanni, 1861. *Guida della città e dintorni di Cagliari*, Cagliari, Tipografia A. Timon.

Tasca, Cecilia, 1990. "La situazione idrica di Cagliari nei secoli XV-XVIII: epigrafi e documenti", *La Sardegna nel Mondo Mediterraneo. Atti del 3. Convegno Internazionale di studi geografico-storici (Sassari-Porto Cervo-Bono, 10-14 aprile 1985)*, Sassari, Gallizzi: 117-151.

Tasca, Cecilia, 2020. "Le fonti documentarie dal 1990 al 2015: venticinque anni di scavi archivistici", Rosanna Martorelli, Donatella Mureddu (a cura di), *Archeologia urbana a Cagliari. Scavi nella chiesa di Sant'Eulalia alla Marina. Il quartiere dalle origini ai giorni nostri:* status quaestionis *all'inizio della ricerca*, Perugia, Morlacchi: 35-44.

TASCA, Cecilia; RAPETTI, Mariangela, 2018. "La stanza dei pazzi. Folli ed emarginati nell'hospital del Glorios Sant Antoni di Cagliari tra Medioevo ed Età Moderna", Josep M. Comelles, Antoni Conejo, Josep Barceló-Prats (a cura di), *Imago Civitatis. Hospitales y manicomios en Occidente*, Tarragona, URV & UB: 129-145.

TASCA, Cecilia; RAPETTI, Mariangela, 2019. "Archivi ospedalieri e fonti assistenziali nella Sardegna medievale e moderna", *RiMe. Rivista dell'Istituto di Storia dell'Europa Mediterranea*, 4 n.s./I: 131-154.

TRUCAS, Marcello, QUARTU, Marina e RIVA, Alessandro, 2020. *Anatomia Clavis et Clavus Medicinae. Storia dell'Anatomia nell'Università di Cagliari*, Cagliari, UNICApress

URBAN, Maria Bonaria, 2000. *Cagliari fra Tre e Quattrocento*, Cagliari, Istituto sui rapporti italo-iberici.

VIRDIS, Francesco, 2017. *Documenti sull'architettura religiosa in Sardegna, Cagliari, 1 (1569-1721)*, Lanusei, L'Ogliastra.

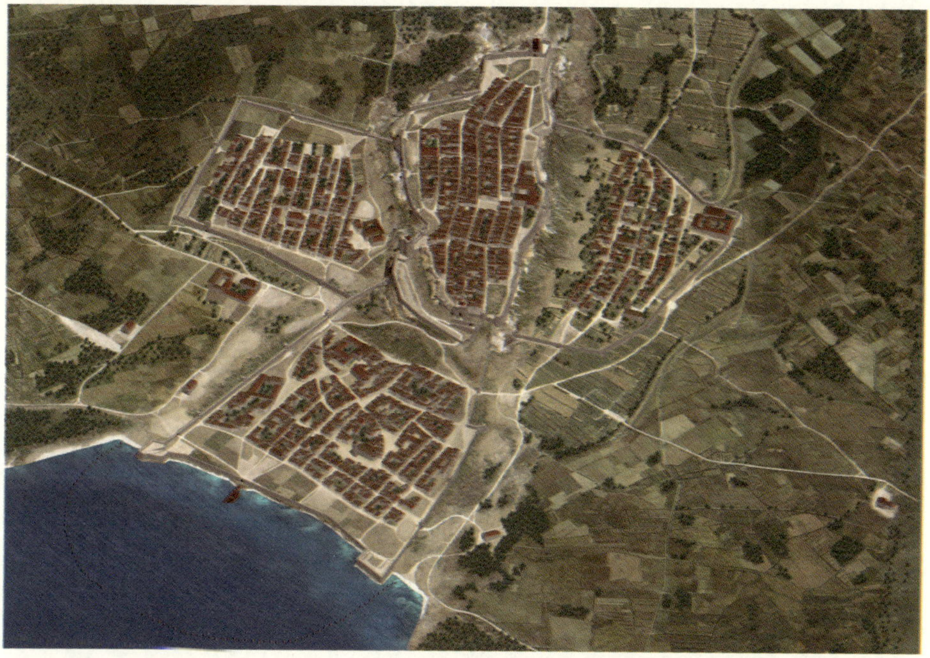

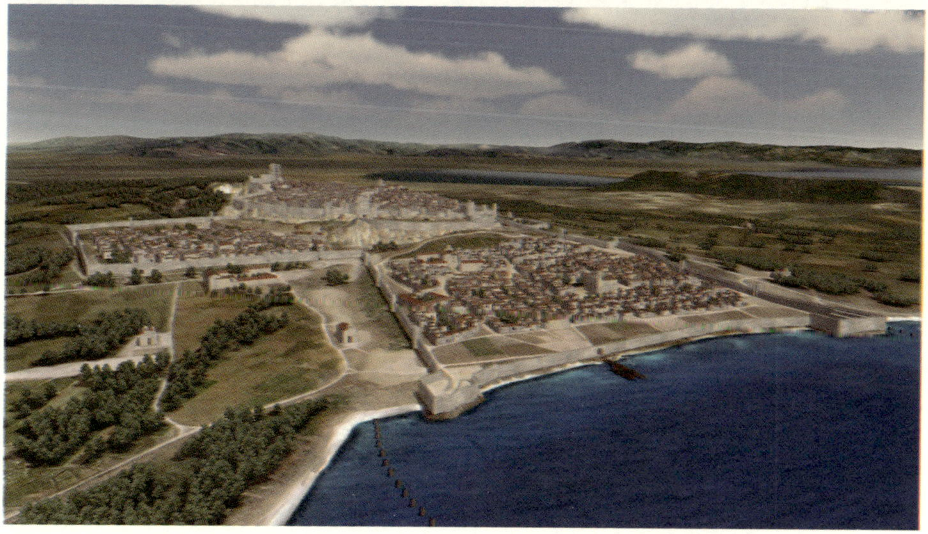

Fig. 1. Cagliari Storica 3D. XV secolo. SjmTech, architetto: M. Beatrice Artizzu. https://www.sjmtech.net/portfolio/cagliari_storica/. Planivolumetrico 3D con i 4 quartieri storici: Castello, Stampace alla sinistra, Villanova a destra, Marina, quartiere portuale, in basso.
Fig. 2. Cagliari Storica 3D. XV secolo. SjmTech, architetto M. Beatrice Artizzu. https://www.sjmtech.net/portfolio/cagliari_storica/. Vista dal Mare 3D, in primo piano il quartiere Marina e il porto.

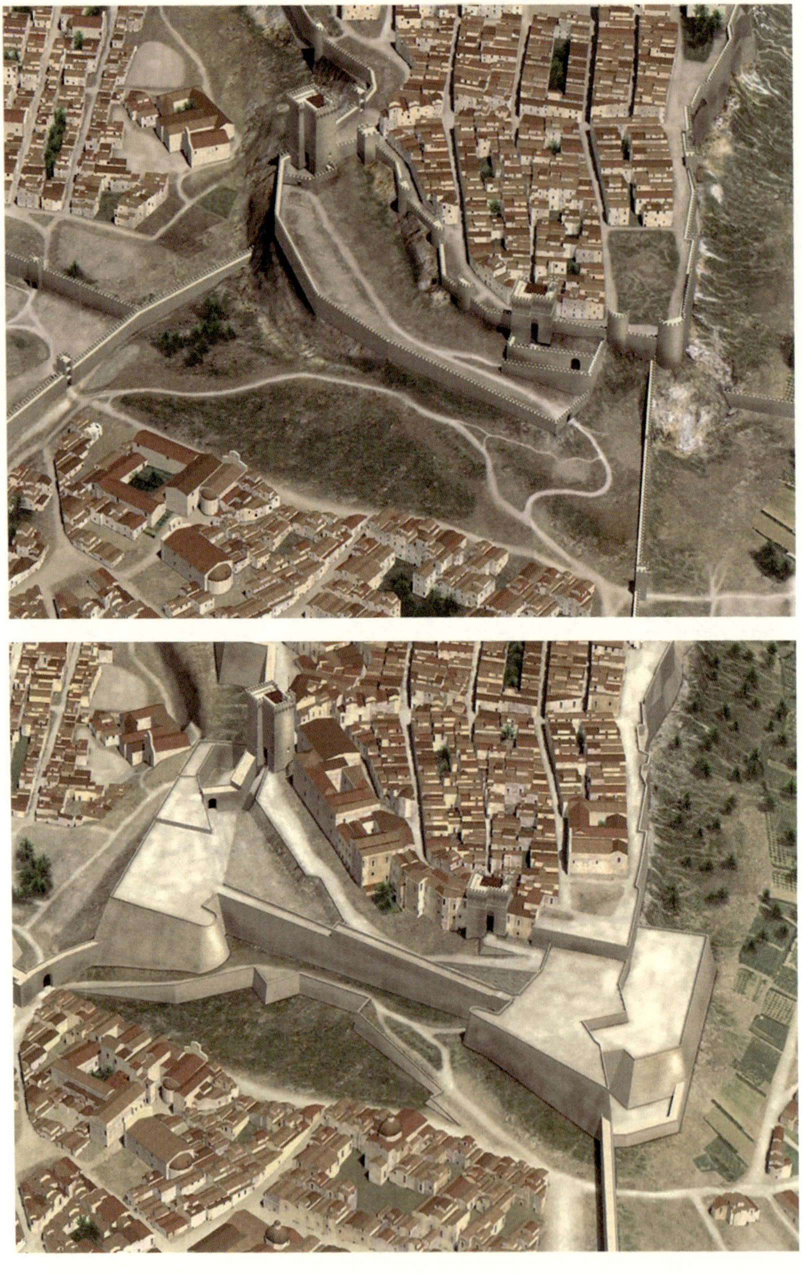

Fig. 3a-b. Cagliari Storica 3D. XV-XVII secolo. SjmTech, architetto M. Beatrice Artizzu. https://www.sjmtech.net/portfolio/cagliari_storica/. Particolari lungo la linea della strada "Sa Costa" con chiesa e ospedale di S. Antonio evidenti in basso a sinistra.

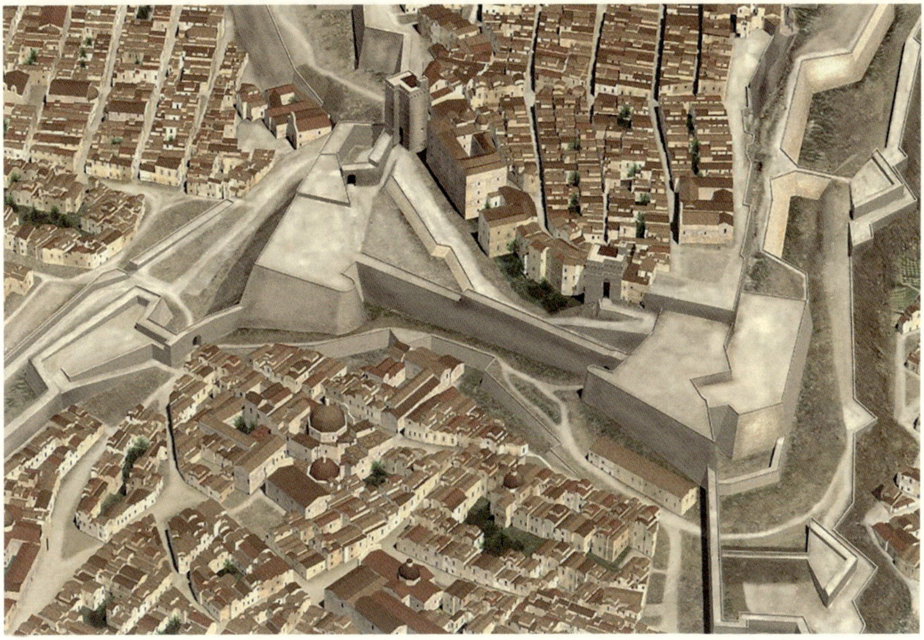

Fig. 4. Cagliari Storica 3D. XVIII secolo. SjmTech, architetto M. Beatrice Artizzu. https://www.sjmtech.net/portfolio/cagliari_storica/. Particolare lungo la linea della strada "Sa Costa" e i Bastioni, l'ospedale e la nuova chiesa di S. Antonio sono evidenti nella parte centrale, in corrispondenza delle cupole vicine delle chiese di S. Antonio e di S. Sepolcro.

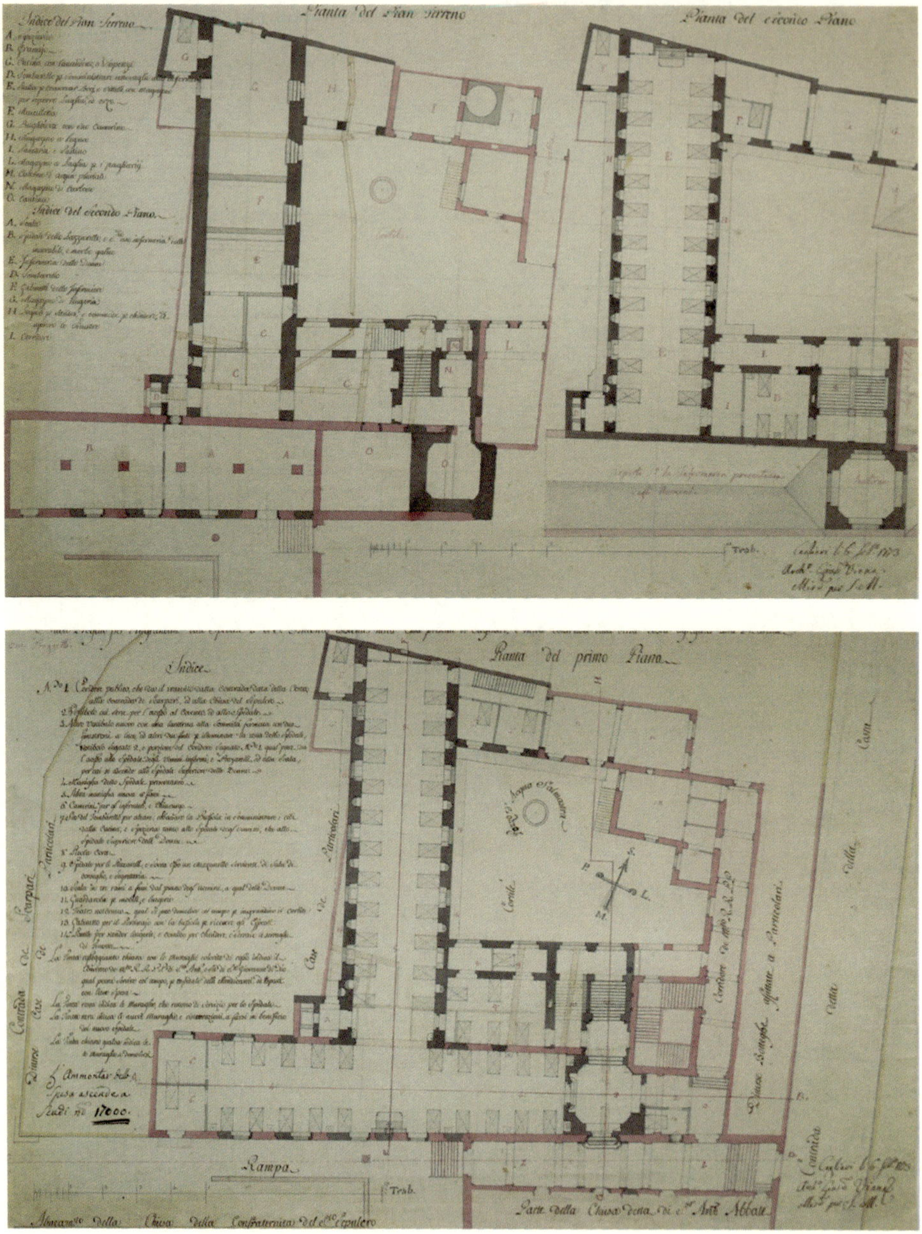


Fig. 5a-b. "Nuovo Progetto per l'ingrandimento dello Spedale detto di Sant'Antonio esistente nella Città presente di Cagliari, e nella Contrada detta della Costa agregata alla Marina (6 Febbraio 1773)" (ASTo, Sez. Corte, Paesi, Sardegna, Ecclesiastico, categoria XII Immunità, cartella 2). In alto *Pianta del Pian terreno - Pianta del Secondo piano.* In basso *Pianta del Pian Primo.*

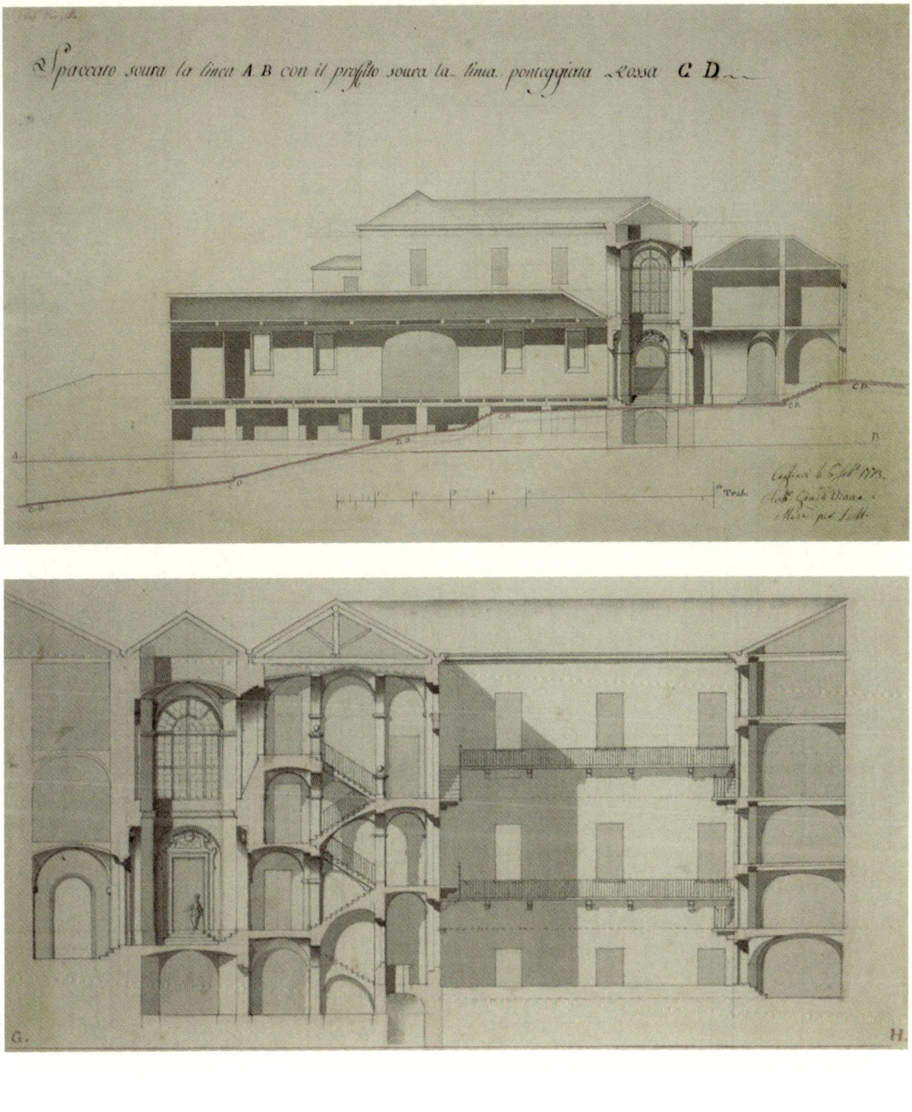


Fig. 6a-b. Spaccato sovra la linea A. B. con il profilo sovra la linea ponteggiata Rossa C. D." In basso "Spaccato G. H" (ASTo, Sez. Corte, Paesi, Sardegna, Ecclesiastico, categoria XII Immunità, cartella 2).

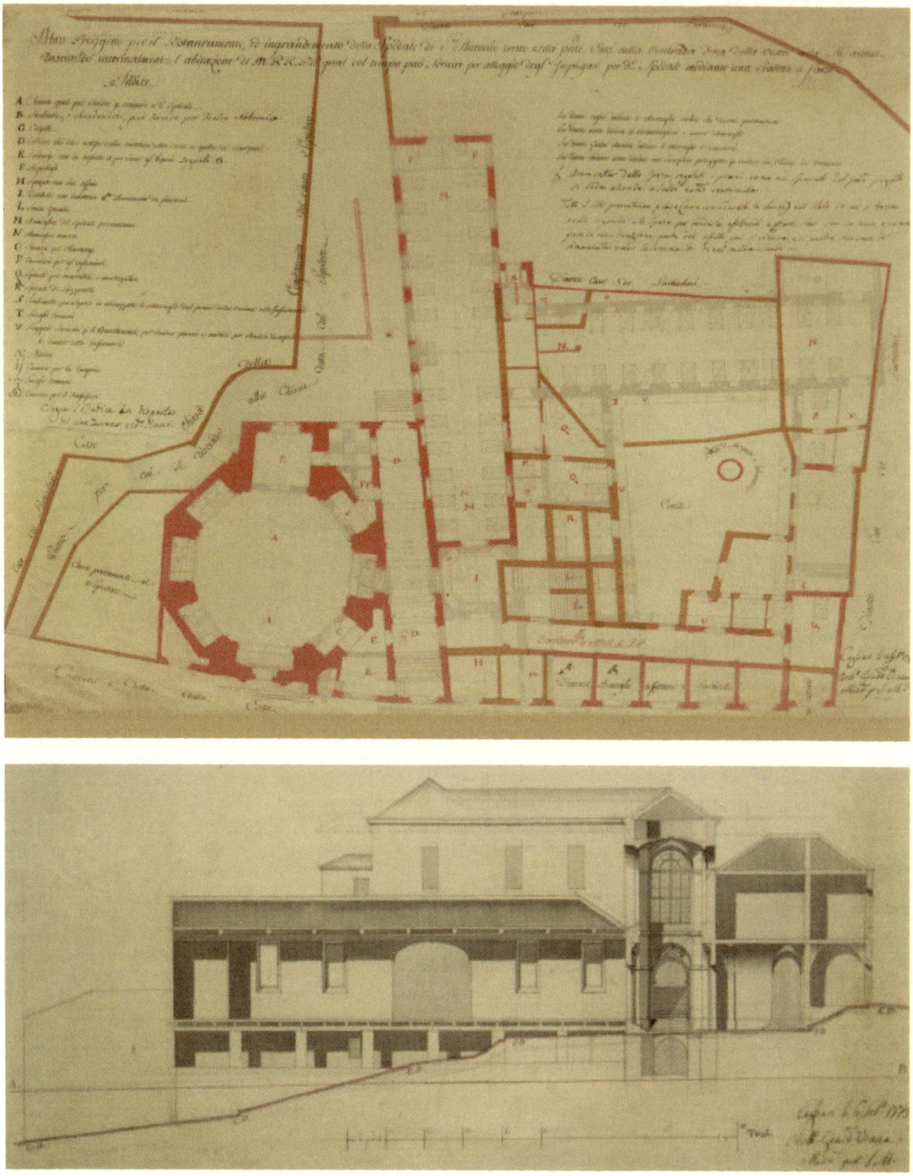

Fig. 7a-b. "Altro progetto per il Ristauramento, ed ingrandimento dello Spedale di Sant'Antonio eretto nella presente Città nella Contrada detta della Costa alla Marina, lasciando interinalmente l'abitazione dei M. RR.PP. qual col tempo può servire per alloggio del'impiegati per detto Spedale mediante una Scaletta a farsi (15 febbraio 1773)" (ASTo, Sez. Corte, Paesi, Sardegna, Ecclesiastico, categoria XII Immunità, cartella 2). La cartografia del Viana è stata rielaborata per evidenziare le «strutture esistenti», indicate in rosso, e quelle «da demolirsi», indicate in giallo, ossia lo stato di fatto precedente ai progetti, indicati in grigio, di cui sono stati realizzati solo interventi parziali.

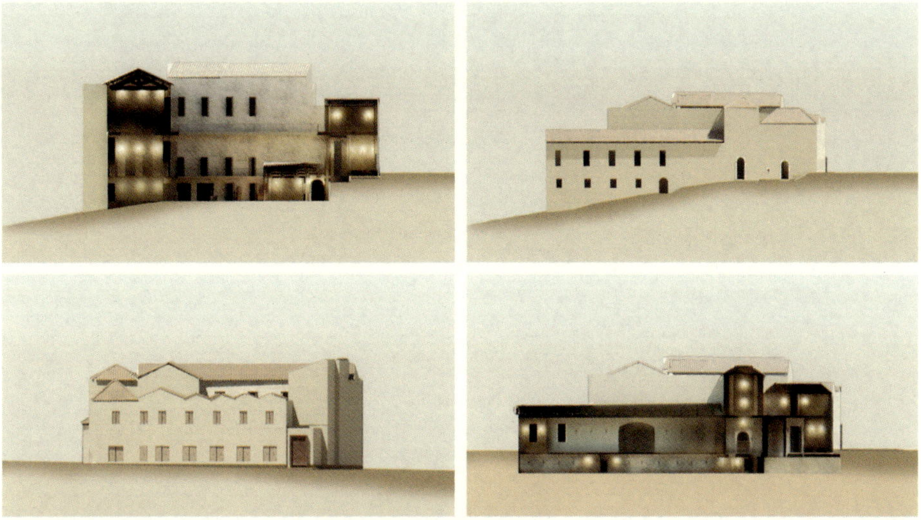

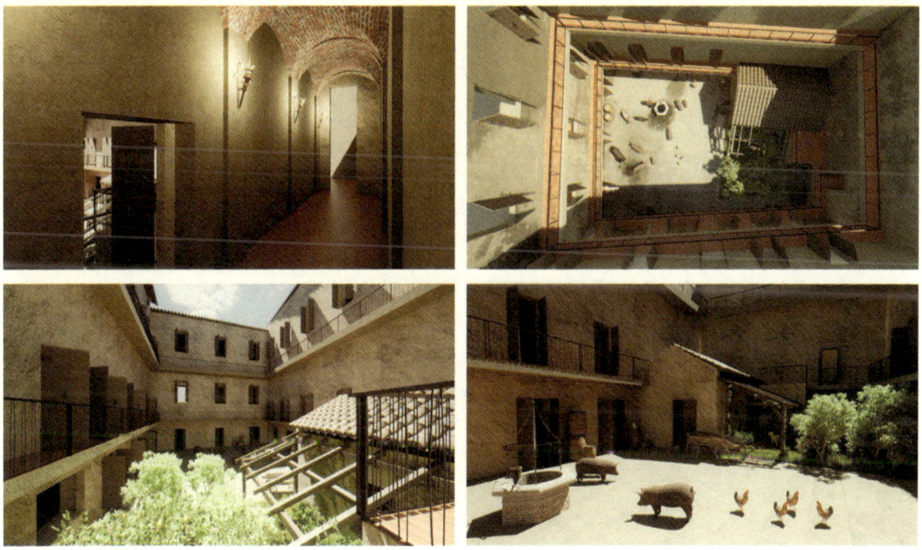

Fig. 8a-d. Elaborazioni 3D e ricostruzioni 3D quotate. In alto a sinistra, *Sezione sulla corte interna*; a destra, *Prospetto lungo il Portico*; a sinistra in basso, *Prospetto sulla via "Sa Costa"*; *Sezione lungo la «Maniga dell'Ospedale» e il blocco scale.* Elaborazione: studenti del Liceo Artistico Musicale Foiso Fois sotto la direzione di M. Beatrice Artizzu.

Fig. 9a-d. Elaborazioni 3D e ricostruzioni 3D quotate. Da sinistra in alto, «corridoio dei Reverendi Padri», con le finestre che affacciano sulla corte interna; vista dall'alto della corte interna; vista prospettica verso il corridoio dei Reverendi Padri; vista prospettica lato opposto. Elaborazione: studenti del Liceo Artistico Musicale Foiso Fois sotto la direzione di M. Beatrice Artizzu.

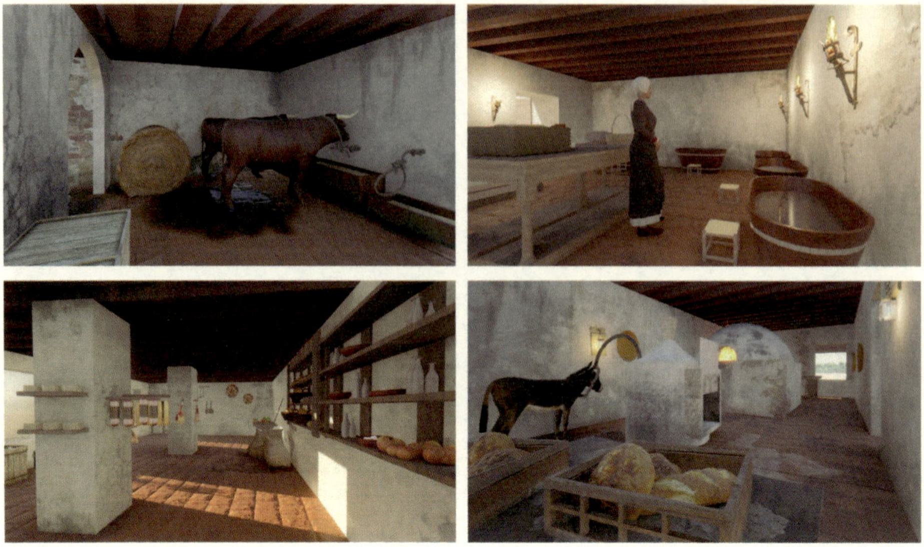

Fig. 10a-d. Elaborazioni 3D e ricostruzioni 3D quotate. Ambienti interni sulla corte: in alto a sinistra, *Stalla*, *Bugadiera* (lavanderia), *Granaio* (magazzino derrate), *Forno e Pastino* (con mola e forno sardo). Elaborazione: studenti del Liceo Artistico Musicale Foiso Fois sotto la direzione di M. Beatrice Artizzu.

# IV
## *Hospitals and Medicine*

Guillem Roca Cabau

# The Influence of Medicine and Sanitary Policies on the Structure of Lleida's Hospital Network

## 1. *Medicine and Salubrity in Lleida*

The city of Lleida was home to the first *Studium Generale* in the Crown of Aragon's peninsular territories. In 1300, King James II signed the *Studium*'s founding privilege after receiving papal authorisation in 1297. Some years before, the king had initiated transactions with the noblemen of the city of Lleida to prevent –in the monarch's own words– his subjects from having to beg for science in foreign cities (González, Busqueta 2000). The initial programmes of study included the arts, both laws –civil and canonical–, natural philosophy and medicine.

The first man to hold the chair of medicine was the physician Guillem de Béziers, trained in Montpellier and a possible disciple of Arnau de Vilanova. The need to plan a still-incipient programme of study allowed Guillem to request royal permission to ask the Jews of the Crown for the books of Arab medicine they possessed. It was essential to endow the *Studium* with a good library; to do so, they would have to expand the number of texts and correct the Latin copies, probably brought from Montpellier, which were part of this incipient library. This task required of a group of scholars with medical knowledge, who were headed by the aforementioned professor (Busqueta 2003).

It bears noting that Lleida was home to a significant number of medical professionals, a corps of experts established in the 13th century and chronicled by James I in the *Llibre dels feits.* During the conquest of Valencia, King Zayyan marvelled at the great army James had gathered around the city. It was not without reason, according to the experience of King James I: «no vim anc neguna saó host tan bé bastada con aquella, de les coses que eren mester per ajuda d'home, sí que els malaltes trobaven consell d'apoticaris con si fossen en Barcelona o en

* This paper forms part of the research project of the Spanish Ministry for Science and Innovation: *Mas allá de la Peste Negra. Epidemias y crisis de mortalidad en el nordeste peninsular, siglos XI-XVI: reconstrucción de ciclos, medición de efectos y análisis de respuestas* (PID2020-117839GB-I00, IP: Pere Benito Monclús). I would like to thank the kind help provided by the Municipal Archeology Service of Lleida in the elaboration of the maps and regarding the information about the archeological excavation of the hospital of the Holy Spirit.

Lleida»[1] (LES QUATRE 2007: 331 §270). The same monarch confirmed the presence of apothecaries from Lleida in the army: «trobava hom tota cosa que hom volgués, a vendre a comprar, així con faria hom en una ciutat, sí que ipoticaris hi havia de Montpesller e de Lleida qui hi venien espècies, així con faria hom en una gran vila, també a malauts con a sans».[2] (LES QUATRE 2007: 328 § 265).

Guillem de Béziers succeeded in his task of creating a good library. In the second half of the 14th century, the library of Lleida's *Studium* was well-supplied with works on natural philosophy and medicine. There were copies of texts by Aristotle, the *Aphorisms* of Hippocrates, various works by Galen, the *Liber ad Almansorem* of Rhazes, Avicenna's *Canon*, Abulcasis's *On Surgery and Instruments*, works by Arnau de Vilanova, and Henry de Mondeville's famous manuscript on surgery, among others (BUSQUETA 2019: 164).

Despite the interests of Lleida's oligarchy, the founder of the library only remained in the city for a few years, as the royal family's repeated demands for his services and certain problems with his salary resulted in the closure of the Faculty of Medicine between 1305 and 1310/1316. The following years were somewhat unstable. Finally, these problems were overcome with the hiring of new professors, such as Pere Gavet, trained in Paris, and the creation of a second chair. By the mid-14th century, medical instruction had become an established field, as demonstrated by the hiring of prestigious professors like the Englishman Walter de Wrobruge and Jaume d'Agramunt (GARCÍA-BALLESTER, ARRIZABALAGA 1998: 22-23).

The presence of the *Studium* and a well-nurtured faculty influenced the cleaning of the streets and an improvement in the city's salubrity. Alfonso the Kind, in a 1328 document in which he defined the limits of the university's borough, stressed the need to keep it clean, as filth made studying more difficult and the neighbourhood was supposed to be «continue munda et sine femeriis seu sterquiliniis et cadaveribus ac aliis immundicis» (GONZÁLEZ, BUSQUETA 2000: 79-84). In the same document, he ordered the drying of the reservoirs –except for the reservoir of the *Suda*, which was the main source of water for the city's clerical neighbourhood– and the canals flowing through the middle of the university district for clearly sanitary purposes. It was not an unreasonable request: Alfonso the Wise, in *Las Partidas*, observed that any city where a *studium* was to be established should be characterised «de buen ayre et de fermosas salidas» so that professors and students could «golgar et rescibir placer a la tarde quando se levantaren cansados del Estudio» (GORT 2016: 64).[3]

1. English translation: «never had we seen as well-supplied a host as that one, with the things necessary to help man, where the ill found the council of apothecaries as if they were in Barcelona or Lleida».

2. English translation: «you could find anything you wanted, to sell or buy, just as a man would do in a city. There were apothecaries from Montpellier or from Lleida who sold spices there, just like they would in a great city, for both the ill and healthy».

3. English translation: «by good air and lovely open spaces/ relax and receive pleasure in the afternoon when, tired, they left the *Studium*».

Jaume d'Agramunt –one of the *Studium*'s professors– wrote a treatise to protect his fellow citizens from the arrival of the Black Death, inspired by the news of a then-still-distant terrible illness which was devastating French regions. He penned its final lines on St Mark's Eve, that is, the 24th of April of the year 1348, weeks before the plague reached the city (MALTAS 2019: 536-538). In the text, he urged municipal authorities to clean the streets of filth, and documents produced in later plague cycles evidence that certain Galenic measures were implemented by the city council (ROCA 2018: 15-39).

> Encara hi ha una altra manera de preservació molt bona e molt profitosa, ço és toldre e esquivar totes aquelles coses que poden fer pestilència ho epidímia [...] E a açò se deven esforçar los seynnos e lurs officials, l'offici dels quals és guardar utilitat e profit comunal al qual deu ésser postposat tot altre bé e proffit particular.[4]

Agramunt was no isolated case, but rather represented another link in the chain. Before the 14th century, during the reign of King James I, the planning of the urban space was influenced by Galenism. The monarch himself ordered Lleida's slaughterhouse to be moved to the outskirts because «tota civitas valet minus propter immunditiam et foetorem qua inde exit» and this –concluded the king– was a danger to the people (ROCA 2017: 437).

Prior to 1348, physicians –following the theories of Hippocrates and Galen– pointed to urban waste as a source of air corruption. Air was the first of the six non-naturals, described by Galen and systematised by later authors, whose improper management could lead to the appearance of diseases (GARCÍA-BALLESTER 1993: 105-115). The six non-natural things were air and environment, the proper use of food and drink, sleep and wakefulness, the alternation between motion and rest, the treatment of the evacuation and retention of humours and the passions of the mind (emotions). Arnau de Vilanova, in his *Speculum Medicine,* considered that excrements and dead animals corrupted the air as they warmed up and fermented. Similarly, other physicians, like Maimonides, pointed to the odours emanating from sewers, latrines, ditches into which cooking waste was poured and pits where people and animals were buried as possible sources of pestilence (GIL SOSTRES 1996: 116-118; CONTRERAS 2011: 127).

There was also another kind of moral filth, capable of reaching the physical plane and corrupting the air. It was the dirtiness which marked some social groups, such as Jews, prostitutes, pimps, card sharps, false paupers, sodomites and blasphemers. When Eiximenis referred to the sin of sodomy, he said that «porta ab si corrupció de natura humana e és tan leig que no·s deu nomenar. Car diuen los sancts que corromp l'ayre»[5] (EIXIMENIS, 1981: 339, ch. 229). The

4. AGRAMUNT 1971: 87. English translation: «There is yet another very good and very profitable means of preservation, which is to remove and avoid all things which could cause pestilence or epidemics [...] And the lords and their officials –whose vocation is to safeguard the common utility and profit, which must prevail over any other private good or profit– must be compelled to do so».

5. English translation: «It is a corruption of human nature and is so ugly it should not be named. Because the saints say it corrupts the air».

council of Lleida referred to prostitutes in the same vein, saying they infected the streets and their inhabitants.[6] We can find similar examples; in many towns, Jews, prostitutes and pimps were forbidden from touching food in the market with their hands, and were required to point at the products they desired with a rod instead (RIERA 1988: 295-311).

As we have seen, Galenism was not limited to university academic circles: various concepts went beyond the classrooms of the *Studium* and took hold in medieval society at large. The translation of certain works and the writing of texts in vernacular languages testify to this fact. One example was the translation of the handbook of Teodorico Borgognoni into Catalan by the physician Guillem Corretger (c. 1305-1306), a surgery student in Montpellier, to make it accessible to surgeons unversed in Latin. We find another example in the treatise of Jaume d'Agramunt itself, written in vernacular «a profit del poble e no a instrucció de metges»[7] (GARCÍA-BALLESTER 2001: 181-182; AGRAMUNT 1971: 48). Similarly, the use of Galenic argot in the discourses of influential preachers such as Francesc Eiximenis and Vicent Ferrer, who used it as a resource for explaining complex theological ideas, testifies to the ease with which these concepts were used and understood. The perception of the priest as a doctor of the soul and the existence of a connection between sin and illness facilitated the extrapolation of medical ideas (FERRAGUD 2014: 27-45; VIERA, PIQUÉ, CAMAÑO 2010: 179-209).

The existence of mortality crises caused by epidemics before 1348 (MALTAS 2019), the confirmation that hygienic measures were applied before the Black Death (GELTNER 2020; RAWCLIFFE 2013; ROCA 2022) and the fact that the epidemic was not perceived as a new type of mortality until the end of the 14th century (ARRIZABALAGA 1994: 243) are factors which have reduced the importance placed on the Black Plague in the implementation of new public hygiene measures, and have led to an interpretation of the event as merely consolidating these pre-existing measures. Prior to 1348, the authorities acted according to the principals of Galenism, even in non-urban contexts, in the same moment in which medical professionals were gaining social prestige and participating in some institutions, such as courts (GELTNER, WEEDA 2021; FERRAGUD 2014).

In the midst of this context in which Galenism was a tool known and used outside of medical settings, it is logical to think that the concept of the six non-naturals was also applied to hospitals. In this sense, Jacques de Vitry (1160/70-1240), in his *Sermo ad hospitalerios et custodes infirmorum*, denounced that hospital patients slept in dirty, foetid beds and that many ended up dying of «*foetore et aeris corruptione*» (ROCA 2017: 39). We are referring to actions designed to improve the passions of the mind (emotions), rest, diet and correcting the air through the cleaning of spaces and laundry (HORDEN 2007; BELLI, GRASSI, SORDINI 2010; HENDERSON 2001).

6. Arxiu Municipal de Lleida (Lleida Municipal Archive; from now on AML), Fons Municipal, Llibre d'Actes del Consell General, reg. 412, f. 60r (08/05/1436).

7. English translation: «for the benefit of the people and not for the instruction of doctors».

But what about the hospitals' location? Did their founders follow medical criteria when choosing the site where their institution would be built? In the following pages, we aim to illuminate the connection between sanitary policies and hospitals in the context of the city of Lleida. Eiximenis (c. 1327-1409) demonstrated this relationship in a very clear way, indicating the detrimental effect that hospitals and other sites –associated with filth and moral corruption– could cause to the air:

> Hespitals, lochs de lebrosos, bordells, e taffureries e escorriments de clavegueres deuen estar a la part contrària d'aquell vent qui més se usa en la ciutat, per tal que lo vent aquell no tir les infeccions del dit loch, ans les ne luny e no les hi lex acostar.[8]

## 2. *Lleida's Hospital Network (12th-15th Centuries)*

### 2.1. *The Beginnings (12th-13th Centuries)*

Our tour through Lleida's hospitals can only begin, in the absence of documentary data, with the Christian conquest in 1149. From then on, a complex system of charitable initiatives developed in the city, the hospitals being a key part of it. Lleida became an urban centre in full growth, overflowing with settlers and with a serious lack of essential facilities for serving the needs of the newly arrived population. The settlement charter issued by Ramon Berenguer IV attracted people interested in investing capital in the new possibilities offered by a recently conquered area (LLADONOSA 1972: I, 394-395). Obviously, it did not work out for everyone: some were forced to pawn their lands and ended up falling into poverty (SABATÉ 2003: 302).

The urban aristocracy and religious orders built a series of centres for taking in both hapless settlers and the pilgrims who were also beginning to arrive. With the Muslim threat eliminated, the route of Lleida arose as one of the main ways to get to Santiago de Compostela, because it linked Barcelona with Zaragoza via the plain (BENITO 2007: 119-123).

The vast majority of hospitals founded between 1149 and 1300 were built on the outskirts of the city and near the main routes of entry. Among the founders, we find figures closely associated with the local and royal power. Such is the case of Nicolau and his wife Salerna, the founders of a hospital «ad servicium Dei et pauperum Christi» in Cappont which they handed over to the bishop of Lleida in 1156. Cappont was the neighbourhood built across the river, right by the Segre, through which the road from Barcelona entered the city. In the document of donation, the bishop authorised an oratory to be built for the workers and paupers housed at the site, the construction of a bell tower with two bells for sum-

8. EIXIMENIS 1983: 190. English translation: «Hospitals, places of lepers, brothels and card houses and sewer runoffs should be downwind from the wind which blows most often in the city, so that this wind does not carry infections from those places, but rather takes them away and does not allow them to approach»

moning for the divine offices and a cemetery (TARRAGÓ 1976: 185-187). These spaces were essential for the correct spiritual practice and good management of the centre, both for healing the sick and for properly handling the remains of the deceased. Augustine of Hippo considered God the best doctor, capable of healing the soul and any illness. Therefore, the presence of holy images, altars and relics, visible from bed, permitted a constant connection between God and the patient (CONEJO 2017: 101-102; HENDERSON 2001: 191-192). Moreover, the presence of religious elements was also linked to the proper management of the passions of the soul, improving the emotional state of the patients and facilitating their recovery (HORDEN 2007; fig. 1).

Between the years 1160 and 1163, a swelling of the river swept away the hospital and part of the neighbourhood. After the disaster, a new structure was built nearby, in a more sheltered but not isolated spot. Nicolau and Salerna took advantage of the new construction to join the centre as lay brother and sister (*donats*). They offered themselves to the hospital to live in a kind of monastic community without taking vows, an option used by different individuals, often of advanced age, who wanted to end their days in a pious way (BRODMAN 1998: 57-59). In Lleida there are more examples: in 1285, at the hospital of Saint Martin there was a hospitaller and two *donades*, Dolça Coguça and Arsenda. Five years later they were joined by a male *donat*, Pere Tibola (ROCA 2019: 86-87). Logically, these workers were responsible for organisational and care tasks, in which women played a major role, employing knowledge learned empirically and through oral transmission (FERRAGUD 2022: 85-93).

Hospitals were often run by married couples; a phenomenon also portrayed in medieval literature. In Ramon Llull's *Blanquerna*, Evast and Aloma sell their house to build a hospital, in a very convenient place in the city, where they hoped to retire and attend to the poor and the ill (LLULL 2009: 129 §10).

Other illustrious figures who built hospitals in the years after the conquest were Pere Moliner, Pere Sanç and Ramon Pere de Sanaüja, all three linked to the highest circles of power. Pere Moliner was a knight who participated in the city's conquest and received various properties and estates from Count Ramon Berenguer IV. Around 1162, he built a hospital in the neighbourhood of Cappont, which he later ceded to the Trinitarians. In 1203, the Roman Curia confirmed the Trinitarian possessions in the territory of Lleida, mentioning the facility: «apud Hilerdam hospitale quod dicitur Petri Molinarii» (ROCA 2020: 89). Later, in 1174, he built another facility which was already in operation by 1179. It was located on a piece of Templar land «*extra muros civitatis Ilerde*», near the road to Zaragoza and was supplied with water carried by the Alcarràs canal –«de muro civitatis usque ad viam que vadit ad zequiam et de carrera maiore usque ad zequiam» (MIRET I SANS 1910: 139).

Pere Sanç was a notary and close collaborator of King James I from the monarch's youth until 1247, the year of his death in Lleida. Like the others, Pere founded a hospital in Cappont and, upon his death, his daughter Bernarda took over as administrator. She later ceded the site's management to Trinitarian monks (ROCA 2021: 89-91).

The Order of the Holy Spirit arrived in Lleida in 1208, when Ramon Pere de Sanaüja and his family donated a hostel in the neighbourhood of the Magdalene, near the Noguerola river, to the mother house of the Holy Spirit of Montpellier. Ramon Pere was also an influential figure: the counts of Urgell, Ermengol and Elvira, signed the donation as witnesses.[9] The Order of the Holy Spirit was organised in a bicephalous way: from 1204 onwards, the house of Rome, Santa Maria in Sassia, administered the communities of Italy, Sicily, Hungary and England, while the house of Montpellier led the convents of France, the Iberian Peninsula, Scandinavia and Germany (BRODMAN 2011: 167). At the time the donation was made, Lleida still relied on the Andalusian-era walls and, therefore, the hospital was located outside the walls, as has been shown by excavations carried out in 2004. Later on, it was protected by expansion of the walls executed between 1366 and 1367 during the War of the Two Peters (1356-1369). The so-called hospital of Sant Esperit (Holy Spirit) was identified thanks to the appearance of different structural elements pertaining to the chapel and an ossuary with multiple burials in a rather poor condition (PAYÀ 2007; RIUDOR 2014; fig. 2).

The existence of a cemetery was a shared trait with the church of Saint Thomas, also found outside the city walls, some three hundred metres from the gates of Saint Martin and just beside the road which led to Huesca. According to a document from 1168, it also possessed a «*cimiterio pauperum*».[10] It could be nothing other than the hospital of Saint Thomas, associated with the eponymous church as were the hospitals of Saint Martin and Magdalene. The latter two were located inside the walls, but near the city gates (ROCA 2020: 85-89).

Regarding the location of Lleida's hospitals in this first phase, although we have not described them all, we can conclude that their distribution clearly obeyed certain criteria and was no random fact. There was an interest in locating these centres right by the city gates, preferably on the outside, and connecting them with routes of transportation. At the same time, many were found near water-collection areas and were associated with places of worship. At some –although it was a general phenomenon– we have managed to document a staff of workers dedicated to care and management. Undoubtedly, it all boils down to the hospitals' purpose: the housing and care of outsiders separated from the networks of neighbourly help.

## 2.2. *Beginnings of the Transformations, Second Half of the 14th Century*

Lleida's economy, characterised by major growth during the first half of the 13th century, slowly began to falter. In addition to the economic crisis, the demographic crises which defined the 14th century, especially the arrival of the Black Death and its successive later outbreaks, led to a demographic downslide and the

9. Arxiu Capitular de Lleida (Lleida Chapter Archive; from now on ACL), P7-M3-P5-C05, f. 119v-123r.

10. ACL, *Llibre Vert,* LC_0022, f. 17-20.

depopulation of the neighbourhoods outside the city walls (Busqueta 2003: 258, 261). The second half of the 14th century was a period of instability. In 1379, the chief magistrate, Guillem Berenguer d'Olzinelles, complained that «molts mals se fan en la ciutat e ell terme e los malfeytós no son perseguits».[11] In this context, the pauper was perceived as a threat, a criminal or, even worse, the bearer of terrible diseases, because the nature of poverty was markedly itinerant and foreign (Mollat 1998: 177-192, 228-233). To handle the arrival of strangers, the city reorganised its hospital network.

On the one hand, there were the hospitals which moved inside the walls, possibly due to the insecurity which reigned during the night in peripheral areas, and, on the other, there were those which moved to less-central places, near the city gates. Lleida had grown significantly during the first century after the conquest, and some hospitals had become too imbricated into the urban space.

The hospital of Saint Thomas was moved inside the walls between the years 1383 and 1392, as can be extracted from two criminal processes which occurred nearby. This is confirmed by the later appearance of the toponym "old hospital of Saint Thomas", in reference to the previous location outside the walls and near the Franciscan convent (Roca 2020: 99-100, 140).

Meanwhile, the hospital of Pere Moliner, which in the 12th century was placed outside the city walls, saw itself swallowed by the city until it stood close to the urban centre. Between 1373 and 1395, the hospital was relocated west, close to the eastern wall, not far from the hospital of Saint Anthony, built outside the walls in the first half of the 13th century.

The outlying area where both hospitals were built was called Barrinou (new district) and was not included within the walled enclosure until the walls' expansion in 1366. Yet, this latest expansion still left the hospital of Saint Anthony outside the city walls. It wasn't until the end of the 15th century, in conjunction with the reparations carried out to fix the damage from the Catalan Civil War (1462-1472), when the walls were expanded to embrace the entire city (Lladonosa 2007: 156-161). We cannot place the exact site of the hospital of Pere Moliner, but a document from 1447 reveals that it faced the slaughterhouse yard, outside the walls, and, therefore, it seems it moved outside the walled enclosure, although still quite close to the so-called gates of Gardeny.[12]

Along with the various relocations, there were two new foundations: the hospitals of Guillem Vidal and Pere Serra. Both founders were wealthy members of the local bourgeoisie and shared some family ties, as Pere was Guillem's son-in-law.

Guillem Vidal wrote his testament in 1372, leaving a good part of his properties to his grandson Bernat Coll. Guillem was only survived by two daughters

11. English translation: «many ill deeds are committed in the city and vicinity and the malefactors are not prosecuted» AML, Fons Municipal, Llibre d'Actes del Consell General, 1379, reg. 403, f. 19r.

12. ACL, reg. P7-M3-P5-C05, f. 145r.

and he made his grandson adopt his name and emblem in order to become his main heir and inherit, apart from numerous possessions, the hospital he aimed to build in the square known as Plaça de la Cadena. Guillem died in 1378 and Bernat followed his wishes. He appears among the witnesses of a criminal proceeding in 1381 as «Bernat del Coyll àlies Guillem Vidal, mercader de Leyda»[13]. At that time, the facility was not yet in operation; the establishment of the new hospital was postponed until after 1384 (Roca 2020: 103). The reason for the delay was the site chosen in the will: Plaça de la Cadena, a narrow area in the upper part of the city. In a document dated in Zaragoza on 19 July 1381, the Royal Chancellery authorised the hospital's move upon the joint request of the city government and bishop. The document specifies that it was a difficult spot to access for the crippled and the sick and was too far from the main routes of transportation, from the places where these institutions had usually been built and from water collection points, «maxime necessaria est pauperibus et infirmis».[14] The fact it was a joint request from the city council and the bishop is significant, because both institutions would, in turn, become the promoters of the future construction of the general hospital of Saint Mary. Finally, the chosen place was the busy neighbourhood of Cappont, and the hospital would, from then on, be known as the hospital of Bernat Coll or Sant Marçal, totally erasing the grandfather's memory.

Pere Serra, instead of leaving money to his family's hospital, founded, through his testament of 1395, a hospital on the street of La Coltelleria Vella. Could the decision have perhaps been provoked by a family rivalry? Guillem Vidal left most of his properties to the other side of the family, headed by Bernat, Pere's nephew. Serra's hospital was located right by the Porta Ferrissa, an old gateway in the wall which once surrounded the Andalusian medina. La Coltelleria was the name given to the main road, parallel to the river, which divided the city from east to west. It did not lie far from the square of Sant Joan, which Queen Mary, in 1442, said was the most beautiful place in the city, both for its inhabitants and also for the pilgrims coming and going from Rome to Santiago.[15] It stood, therefore, in a central spot, frequently trafficked by outsiders and relatively close to the river. The neighbourhood of the Magdalene spread eastward. It was the city's industrial sector, but it had been losing dynamism and population since the 14th century (Bolòs 2008: 179-183). The hospital was beside a chapel, which Pere Serra had built years before, dedicated to the archangel Saint Michael and Saint James and which communicated directly with the facility. In his testament, Pere established the obligations of the hospitallers, a married couple who were responsible for taking in and treating the ill and also for cleaning the clothes and linens once a week and doing the laundry once a year.

13. AML, *Llibre de Crims*, reg. 789, ff. 114r-119r. Document transcribed by Roser Gort (2016, 156-160).

14. Arxiu de la Corona d'Aragó (Archive of the Crown of Aragon; from now on ACA), Cancelleria, reg. 819, ff. 120 r-v (29/07/1391). Document found thanks to the reference provided by Carmel Ferragud (2014, 311, n. 16).

15. AML, Fons Municipal, *Llibre Vert de la ciutat de Leyda*, 1691, reg. 1370, f. 426-428.

The tasks of washing clothes and furniture could not be separated from the medical aspect, in that they contributed to reducing four odours and preventing the corruption of the air. Sibil·la, a hospitaller at the hospital of Saint Andrew in Mallorca during the third quarter of the 14th century, was tasked with washing the patients themselves and their beds, allegedly without feeling disgusted by them and their filth (FERRAGUD 2022: 88-91). Another similar measure was ventilation. Some of Lleida's hospitals had galleries –like the hospital of the Magdalene– or porches –like the hospital of Saint Martin– and were located in squares to facilitate both ventilation as well as the users' arrival and recreation (ROCA 2020: 86-87, 104-105).

As we have seen, the hospital network had to adapt to the changes caused by the difficulties of the new times. Nonetheless, a good part of the earlier preferences endured when it came to their location, that is, being close to places of worship, water and main roads. One change from the earlier model was the need of some hospitals to get closer to the walls and, even, to move inside, possibly due to the insecurity which had come to dominate exterior spaces, especially at night (fig. 3)

### 2.3. *The Creation of the General Hospital (15th Century)*

If something doesn't work, it gets modified, and if it still doesn't work, it gets replaced. This maxim was followed by the city's authorities to definitively modify the hospital network. The improvements made in the second half of the 14th century proved insufficient to fix a system tensioned by the crises which occurred in the first decades of the 15th century. The testimonies given by the hospitals' neighbours, such as the notary Pere Teixidor, are representative of the system's failure: «ell, testis, ho a vist e veu que per les dites mortalitats e sterelitats de temps les propietats son diminuïdes, en tant que casi són en total en destrucció en gran part axí que los censos que solian haver cesan e han cesat».[16]

In 1435, the city council and cathedral chapter met in search of a solution to the hospitals' precarious situation.[17] As the aforementioned Teixidor had said, their revenues had languished from the harshness of the plagues, but also from the continual embezzlement by some hospitallers. This was why many paupers roamed freely through the city without being served. The intention of Lleida's nobility was to merge the hospitals into one new facility, a solution that had seen success in other places. It was a new healthcare paradigm, initiated in the Crown of Aragon by the Hospital of the Holy Cross of Barcelona in 1401, and based on the construction of large buildings designed to both beautify the city and instigate new practices to improve the health and safety of its inhabitants (CONEJO 2017:

16. English translation: «He, a witness, has seen and sees that because of the aforementioned mortalities and sterilities, the properties have been diminished for some time, to the extent that nearly all have been largely destroyed, meaning the taxes which use to be paid are ceasing to be paid or have already ceased to be paid» (ACL, P7-M3-P5-CO5, f. 13v).

17. AML, Llibre d'Actes del Consell General, 1434-1435, reg. 411, f. 56v (24/05/1435).

99-100). However, the meeting came to nothing and a year later all the city's hospitallers were obliged to take in all the paupers who came to their doors.[18]

It was not until 1445 when the bishop García Aznárez de Añón returned to the project. In 1447, with the papal permission granted the previous year, the unification project was resumed. First, a thorough report was written to determine the status of the revenues, the behaviour of the hospitallers and the assets belonging to each institution. The intention was to demonstrate not only the necessity of a general hospital but also the possibility of building it using the languished properties of the existing institutions. The authorities came up against the frontal rejection of the hospitallers and administrators who viewed the initiative with mistrust. It was not for nothing, as the building of a general hospital would put many of their privileges in danger: most of them lived off the hospitals, spending the revenues –already scant on their own– on personal matters. Finally, the bishop's perseverance made it possible to overcome the different obstacles, and the new hospital became a partial reality in 1448 (Roca 2020: 106-115).

General hospitals were relevant buildings whose placement and design were heavily influenced by Galenism. The hospital of the Holy Cross in Barcelona was built in the neighbourhood of "el Raval", far from the urban centre and taking advantage of the structures of the former hospital d'en Colom. The hospital of Our Lady of Grace in Saragossa was established in a few houses bought by King Alfonso the Magnanimous to serve this need outside the city walls, beyond the gate called «puerta Cinegia». Similarly, construction on the general hospital of Mallorca began around 1460 in Puig d'en Sitjar, a sparsely populated area in the northeast part of the city (Conejo 2014: 441; Falcón 1980: 192-193; Cassanyes 2018). Salubrity was a primary concern when choosing the location for all these centres.

Lleida followed Barcelona's lead, not because the capital city's hospital system was in crisis –a fact that has been questioned– (Bridgewater 2020: 188-203) but because its authorities decided to expand an old, pre-existing hospital instead of building a new one *ex novo*. The authorities naturally modelled their endeavours on earlier successes, as occurred in Valencia in 1482, where the local authorities followed the example of the hospitals of the Holy Cross of Barcelona and Our Lady of Grace of Saragossa. Later, in 1453, Queen Mary granted the hospital's workers the same rights of protection, safeguarding, liberties, immunities, exemptions, graces and privileges enjoyed by the workers of the aforementioned Holy Cross hospital, a sign that Lleida's facility modelled itself on Barcelona's (Gallent 2014; Conejo 2002: 63-65). Out of all the hospital centres, Bernat Coll's in Cappont was selected to house the new institution. It was no coincidence, as the space met all the requirements and was the city's most modern institution. While Serra's hospital was built at its founder's house in Coltelleria, Bernat Coll's was located in a newly constructed building. Even so, additional construction work was needed to expand the building, and stone and wood was diligently accumulated along the riverbed for this purpose.

18. AML, Llibre d'Actes del Consell General, 1436-1437, reg. 413, f. 15r (20/07/1436).

The facility was run by a canon and a citizen chosen by the chapter and the city council respectively, and a hospitaller was placed in charge of daily operations, such as keeping the hospital clean, doing laundry and taking care of the poor and sick (BERTRAN 1991: 34-35). Once again, cleanliness and care were inseparable, both essential to transform the site into a space of health, far from the prejudicial stench's hospitals were known for.

Despite these efforts, the aforementioned location was not definitive. The floods which constantly threatened the neighbourhood and the proliferation of taverns and brothels generated doubts at least as far back as 1450 (BERTRAN 1991: 39). Finally, a swelling of the river in 1452 swept away a large part of the material accumulated for construction and ended up convincing anyone still hesitant to move the site. A year later, a commission studied the possibility of building the hospital inside the walled precinct, near one of the city's main sewers, which went through Plaça del Pes del Rei and reached the Alcarràs canal and, finally, the river. After this site was properly analysed and with royal authorisation, the preparation works began in 1453.

Despite the precarious state of the hospitals' revenues, local authorities opted for a significantly more expensive option than expanding the old hospital d'en Coll: the building of a new seat for the hospital. On 13th April 1454, with a solemn procession presided over by the members of the city's most influential families, the first stone of the new hospital was laid. In spite of the initial euphoria, financial problems were a constant event, even more so with the crisis generated by the Catalan Civil War (1462-1472), especially serious in Lleida. Thus, the building was not completed until 1519, although in 1457 the first paupers began to arrive (LLADONOSA 2007: 174-175).

The architecture of the new institutions kept their users' necessities in mind; until then, the vast majority of hospitals had been located in repurposed private homes. Unlike other hospitals of the period, the general hospital of Lleida was designed, for unknown reasons, in imitation of a noble mansion. Nonetheless, it was a large square building arranged around a central courtyard –a place of solace for the patients– and well ventilated thanks to the presence of broad windows facing the riverbank (CONEJO 2017: 131-137).

Its construction put an end to the medieval hospital network defined by the great multiplicity of centres. As the 15th century came to a close, the only hospitals still providing service, apart from the general hospital, were Saint Anthony and the Holy Spirit. Both hospitals, apparently in a precarious condition, are mentioned in a document from 1483, issued by the city's general council (LLADONOSA 1974: 455; fig. 4).

## 3. *Conclusions*

In the extremely well-known fresco of the hospital of Santa Maria della Scala in Siena, Domenico di Bartolo's *Cura e governo degli infermi* (1440-1441), daily life at the hospital is put on display: the ill, wounded and moribund solicitously treated and surgeons, physicians and priests rushing back and forth. Presiding over the main scene, at medium height, there is a large, wide-open window which allows air to enter and illuminates the hospital's daily activity. There is no doubt that hospital interiors were spaces devoted to medicine, understood, as was typical in the period, in a broad sense. At the so-called hospital of Sant Marçal in Montblanc, the founder established, through his will in 1339, the construction of a hall with six beds to a side arranged in a way that let the patients contemplate, without leaving their beds, an altar with a shrine. A century before, in 1256, canon Pere Vilar from Barcelona ordered the building of a hospital, without forgetting the need to add a chapel to it (CONEJO 2017: 102, 104). They were indisputable elements of spiritual care and, along with the large windows, part of the six non-naturals.

The location of the hospitals must be analysed through the same lens. They were spots picked to favour proper ventilation and quick access to water to wash clothes and linens and free them from the most repulsive filth by throwing them into the current.

Jaume Roig, in his *Espill*, describes the journey the protagonist must make to reach the hospital d'en Clapers, founded in 1311 in a spot outside the city walls on the road called Sant Julià: «tirí camí, fora'l portal, vers l'espital, d'en Clapés dit»[19] (RUBIO VELA 1983: 377). Similarly, in 1378, King Peter the Ceremonious ordered the moving of the hospital of Saint James in Valencia to prevent infections; he indicated that it should be located «in introitu dicte civitatis» (RODRIGO 1927: 4). The case of Lleida does not seem unique: locating hospitals outside the walled enclosure, or inside the walls but near the city gates, was a typical decision influenced both by the purpose of the institution –to take in, principally, outsiders to the city– and by the prevailing medical ideas. The progressive medicalisation of the urban world and the confirmation of decisions made by different power spheres in consideration of the six non-natural things –the foundation of preventive medicine– lead us to understand the hospitals' locations as deliberate decisions (BARCELÓ-PRATS, BUENO 2021: 113-120).

In the case of Lleida, this paper's aim has been to highlight, beyond the particular location of each hospital, the shared aspects in their location as a whole. Early on, just after the city's conquest, the first hospitals were established on the road network following an orderly structure, without overlapping and covering all the city gates. There was a practical intentionality in their placement, which was no random event. In 1228, the *Consuetudines Ilerdenses* noted the importance of this superstructure, recalling that «hospitalia civitatis et domus leprosorum sunt in gubernatione et regimine consulum et universitatis nostre» (BUSQUETA 1997: 103).

It should be clarified that when we talk about a network or superstructure, we are not referring to a fixed organisation capable of managing all the hospitals, but

19. English translation: «follow the road, outside the gate, to the hospital, Clapés in name».

rather we define an interest exercised by the municipality and the cathedral chapter –occasionally together– to include all the hospitals into a working network through intermittent actions, and not with long-lasting effects strategies.

The hospital network experienced only minor changes, at least until the 15th century, and kept providing services in its principal hotspots: the gates of the walls and the roads into the city. The citizens viewed the hospitals as gears of the same machine, which could be melted in order to grease it, if doing so improved the service: «si de tots fos fet hun spital que seria mellor regit que ara no són tots e haurian allí mellor recapte los pobres que hui no han».[20]

The radical change came with the concept of the general hospital of Saint Mary in 1447, a joint initiative of the city council and the chapter. Thus, the medieval hospitals of Lleida ceased to be watchful sentries, stationed at the gates, to become a single entity of considerable size.

## *Bibliography*

Agramunt, Jaume, 1971. *Regiment de preservació de pestilencia de Jacme d'Agramont (s. XIV)*, ed. Joan Veny. Tarragona, Diputación Provincial.

Arrizabalaga, Jon, 1994. "Facing the Black Death: Perceptions and Reactions of University Medical Practitioners", *Practical Medicine from Salerno to the Black Death,* Cambridge, Cambridge University Press: 237-288.

Barceló-Prats, Josep; Bueno, Eduardo, 2021. "Epidemias, medicalización y evolución hospitalaria: bases para una historia de las culturas de la salud y de la enfermedad", *Anais de História de Além-mar,* 22: 107-135.

Belli, Maddalena; Grassi, Francesca; Sordini, Beatrice 2010. *La cucina di un ospedale del trecento, gli spazi, gli oggetti, il cibo nel Santa Maria della Scala di Siena*, Pisa, Pacini, 2010.

Benito, Pere, 2007. "Els primers pelegrins catalans a Sant Jaume de Compostel·la (segles XI-XII): identitat, perfil social i procedència geogràfica", *El Camí de Sant Jaume i Catalunya (Actes del Congrés Internacional, Barcelona-Cervera, 16-18 octubre 2003)*, Barcelona, Abadia de Montserrat: 111-123.

Bertran, Prim, 1991. "Sobre els inicis d'una institució benèfica baixmedieval: l'Hospital de Santa Maria de la ciutat de Lleida (1435-1519)", *Universitas Tarraconensis,* 10: 33-53.

Bolòs, Jordi, 2008. *Dins les muralles de la ciutat. Carrers i oficis a la Lleida dels segles XIV i XV,* Lleida, Pagès.

Bridgewater, Pol, 2020. *"Car vosaltres havets a veure sobre hospitals": El Consell de Cent i la construcció de la primera política hospitalària a la Barcelona baixmedieval,* PhD thesis, Universitat de Barcelona.

Brodman, James, W., 1998. *Charity and Welfare. Hospitals and the Poor in Medieval Catalonia,* Philadelphia, University of Pennsylvania Press.

Brodman, James W., 2011. "Crisis in Charity: Centrifugal and Centripetal Influences upon Medieval Caritative Orders", *Imago Temporis Medium Aevum,* 5: 163-173.

Busqueta, Joan J. (ed.), 1997. *Els costums de Lleida,* Lleida, Ajuntament de Lleida.

Busqueta, Joan J., 2003. *Història de Leida*, vol. 3, *Baixa edat mitjana*, Lleida, Pagès.

Busqueta, Joan J., 2019. "Sobre l'Estudi General de Lleida a l'edat mitjana: algunes qüestions",

20. "If out of all the hospitals they made just one, it would be better managed than any of them are now and the poor would receive better refuge than they do today." ACL, P7-M3-P5-CO5, f. 24v.

*Millars,* 46/1: 145-165.

CASSANYES, Albert, 2018. "Los primeros cincuenta años del Hospital General de Mallorca: desde la fundación hasta la promulgación de la Ordenaciones (1456-1514)", *En la España Medieval,* 41: 133-153.

CONEJO DA PENA, Antoni, 2002. *L'antic hospital de Santa Maria. Seu de l'Institut d'Estudis Ilerdencs,* Lleida, Institut d'Estudis Ilerdencs.

CONEJO DA PENA, Antoni, 2014. "'Lum, noblesa, ornament, laor, glòria e amplitud': los hospitales y la renovada imagen de la ciudad bajomedieval", Teresa Huguet, Pere Verdés, Jon Arrizabalga, Manuel Sánchez (ed.), *Ciudad y hospital en el occidente europeo: 1300-1700,* Lleida, Milenio: 415-445.

CONEJO DA PENA, Antoni, 2017. "'En la present ciutat hun devot e solempne spital'. Un estudi a quatre bandes sobre l'esplendor artística i arquitectònica dels hospitals baix medievals", ed. Flocel Sabaté. *L'assistència a l'edat mitjana*, Lleida, Pagès: 99-138.

CONTRERAS, Antoni, 2011. "Contaminación por cinabrio en ciutat de Mallorca (1347)", *Bolletí de la Societat Arqueològica Lul·liana,* 865: 125-136.

FALCÓN, Maria Isabel, 1980. "Sanidad y beneficencia en Zaragoza en el siglo XV", *Aragón en la Edad Media,* 3: 183-226.

EIXIMENIS, Francesc, 1981. *Lo llibre de les dones,* ed. Frank Naccarato, Barcelona, Curial.

EIXIMENIS, Francesc, 1983. *Lo Crestià,* ed. Albert Hauf, Barcelona, Edicions 62.

FERRAGUD, Carmel, 2014. "La introducción de los practicantes de la medicina en los hospitales del reino de Valencia durante la baja edad media", Teresa Huguet, Pere Verdés, Jon Arrizabalga, Manuel Sánchez (ed.), *Ciudad y hospital en el occidente europeo, 1300-1700,* Lleida, Milenio: 305-324.

FERRAGUD, Carmel, 2014. "Medicina i religió a la Baixa Edat Mitjana: rerefons mèdic de les pràctiques penitencials en els sermons de sant Vicent Ferrer", *Scripta,* 3: 27-45.

FERRAGUD, Carmel, 2014. "Expert Examination of Wounds in the Criminal Court Justice in Cocentania (Kingdom of Valencia) during the Late Middle Ages", Wendy Turner, Sara Butler (ed.), *Medicine and the Law in the Middle Ages,* Leiden, Brill: 109-132.

FERRAGUD, Carmel, 2022. *L'hospital, la dona i el capellà. Sant Andreu de Mallorca (1230-1445),* Catarroja, Afers.

GALLENT, Mercedes, 2014. "Los hospitales de la Santa Creu de Barcelona y Nuestra Señora de Gracia de Zaragoza, dos modelos asistenciales para el Hospital General de Valencia", *Aragón en la Edad Media*, 25: 41-60.

GARCÍA-BALLESTER, Luís, 1993. "On the Origins of the Six Non-Natural Things in Galen", Jutta Kollesch, Diethard Nickel (ed.), *Galen und das hellenistische Erbe*, Stuttgart, Franz Steiner Verlag: 105-115.

GARCÍA-BALLESTER, Luís, 2001. *La búsqueda de la salud. Sanadores y enfermos en la España medieval,* Barcelona, Península.

GARCÍA-BALLESTER, Luís; ARRIZABALAGA, Jon, 1998. "El *Regiment* de Jacme d'Agramont y el *Estudi* de medicina de Lleida", Luis García-Ballester, Joan Veny, Jon Arrizabalaga (ed.), *Regiment de preservació de pestilencia (Lleida 1348)*, Barcelona, Enciclopedia Catalana: 13-31.

GELTNER, Guy, 2020. "The Path to Pistoia: Urban Hygiene before the Black Death", *Past and Present,* 246: 3-33.

GELTNER, Guy; WEEDA, Claire, 2021. "Underground and Over the Sea: More Community Prophylactics in Europe, 1100-1600", *Journal of the History of Medicine and Allied Sciences,* 76/2: 123-146.

GIL SOSTRES, Pedro, 1996. "Estudi introductori", Luis García-Ballester, Michael R. McVaugh (ed.), *Arnaldi de Vilanova Opera Medica Omnia*, vol. X.1, *Regimen Sanitatis ad Regem Aragonum*, Barcelona, CSIC: 116-118.

GONZÁLEZ, Elena; BUSQUETA, Joan J. (ed.), 2000. *L'Estudi General de Lleida: ciutat i universitat en els documents de l'Arxiu Municipal de Lleida*, Lleida, Ajuntament de Lleida.

Gort, Roser, 2016. *L'Estudi General de Lleida al segle XIV,* Lleida, Universitat de Lleida.

Henderson, John, 2001. "Healing the Body and Saving the Soul: Hospitals in Renaissance Florence", *Renaissance Studies*, 15: 188-216.

Horden, Peregrine, 2007. "A Non-Natural Environment: Medicine without Doctors and the Medieval European Hospital", Barbara S. Bowers (ed.), *The Medieval Hospital and Medical Practice*, Aldershot, Ashgate: 133-145.

Les quatre, 2007. *Les quatre grans cròniques*. vol. I. *Llibre dels feits del rei En Jaume,* Ferran Soldevila (ed.), Barcelona, Institut d'Estudis Catalans.

Lladonosa, Josep, 1972. *Història de Lleida*, Tàrrega, F. Camps Calmet.

Lladonosa, Josep, 1974. *Noticia histórica sobre el desarrollo de la medicina en Lérida,* Lleida, Colegio Oficial de Médicos de Lérida.

Lladonosa, Josep, 2007. *Els carrers i places de Lleida a través de la història,* Lleida, Universitat de Lleida-Ajuntament de Lleida.

Llull, Ramon, 2009. *Romanç d'Evast e Blanquerna,* ed. Albert Soler & Joan Santanach, Palma, Patronat Ramon Llull.

Maltas, Joan, 2019. *Caresties, fams i crisis de mortalitat a Catalunya: 1283-1351. Anàlisi d'indicadors i reconstrucció dels cicles econòmics i demogràfics*, PhD thesis, Universitat de Lleida.

Miret i Sans, Joaquim, 1910. *Les cases de templers y hospitalers. Aplech de noves y documents històrics,* Barcelona, Casa Provincial de Caritat.

Mollat, Michel, 1998. *Pobres, humildes y miserables en la Edad Media,* México, Fondo de Cultura Económica.

Payà, Xavier, 2007. *Memòria INT-178. Obres Eix - Cardenal Remolins 2004,* Lleida, Secció d'Arqueologia de l'Ajuntament de Lleida [unpublished].

Rawcliffe, Carole, 2013. *Urban Bodies. Communal Health in Late Medieval English Towns and Cities*, Woodbridge, Boydell Press.

Riera, Jaume, 1988. "La conflictivitat de l'alimentació dels jueus medievals, segles XII-XV", *Alimentació i societat a la Catalunya medieval,* Barcelona, CSIC: 295-311.

Riudor, Noemí, 2014. "Les obres de les muralles i els fossats de Lleida en el context de la guerra dels Peres (1366-1367)", *Shikar,* 1: 38-46

Roca, Guillem, 2017. *Salubritat i salut pública a la Lleida baix medieval: la gestió dels espais públics, la pobresa i els hospitals,* PhD thesis, Universitat de Lleida.

Roca, Guillem, 2018. "Medidas municipales contra la peste en la Lleida del siglo XIV e inicios del XV", *Dynamis,* 31/1: 15-39.

Roca, Guillem, 2018. "La unión de los hospitales ilerdenses: el expediente de 1447", *Revista de la CECEL,* 18: 31-54.

Roca, Guillem, 2021. "El llinatge del notari Pere Sanç, gestors i administradors d'hospitals al segle XIII", *Nokaria,* 1: 87-97.

Roca, Guillem, 2022. "Salubritat i medicina a la Tàrrega del segle XIV", *Quaderns d'Urtx,* 1: 16-59.

Rodrigo, José, 1927. "Hospitales de Valencia en el siglo XV. Su administración, régimen interior y condiciones higiénicas", *Revista de Archivos, Bibliotecas y Museos*, 90: 1-49.

Rubio Vela, Agustín, 1983. "Un hospital medieval según su fundador: el testamento de Bernat dez Clapers (Valencia, 1311)", *Dynamis*, 3: 373-387.

Sabaté, Flocel, 2003. *Història de Lleida*, vol. 2, *Alta edat mitjana*, Lleida, Pagès.

Tarragó, Josep, 1976. "Segunda miscelánea sobre historia de la medicina en Lérida (siglos XII al XVIII)", *Actas del Colegio de Médicos de Lérida,* Lleida, Colegio de Médicos de Lérida: 135-178.

Viera, David J.; Piqué, Jordi; Camaño, Ramon, 2010. "Malaltia i salut en l'obra de Francesc Eiximenis", *Caplletra,* 48: 179-209.

Villagrasa, Raúl, 2016. "Entre quatre rius. Hospitals al baix Cinca i el baix Segre a la baixa edat mitjana", *Tres estudis històrics sobre el Baix Cinca i el Baix Segre. Beques Amanda Llebot,* Fraga, Institut d'Estudis del Baix Cinca: 11-61.

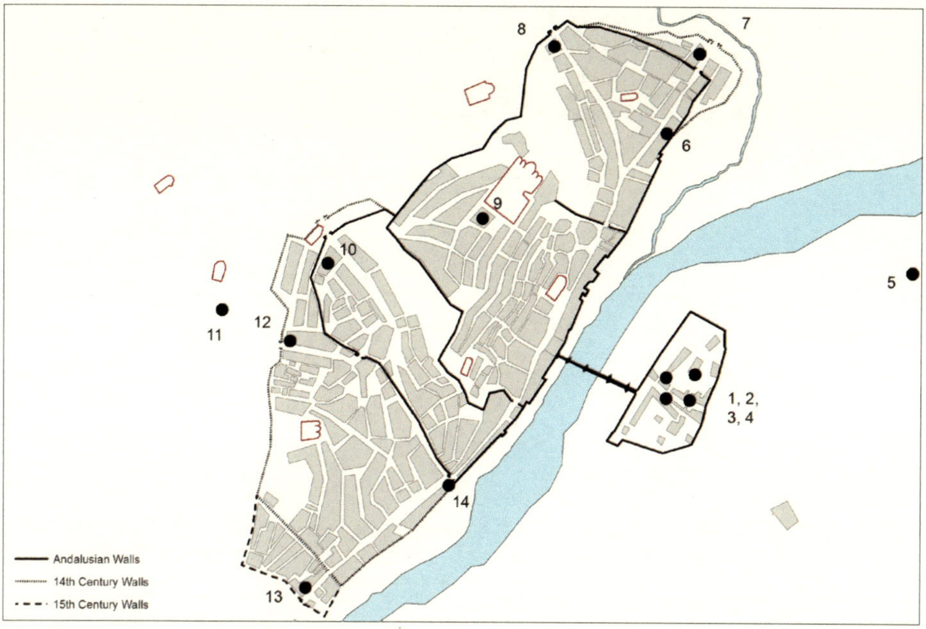


Fig. 1. Hospitals in Lleida during the 13th century. 1. Hospital of Nicolau and Salerna (1); 2. Hospital of Pere Moliner (1); 3. Hospital of Pere Sanç; 4. Hospital for Poor Priests (2); 5. Hospital of Nicolau and Salerna (2); 6. Hospital of Guillem de Fillac; 7. Hospital of the Holy Spirit; 8. Hospital of Saint Mary Magdalene; 9. Hospital of Poor Priests (1); 10. Hospital of Saint Martin; 11. Hospital of Saint Thomas; 12. Hospital of Guerau Caçola; 13. Hospital of Saint Anthony; 14. Hospital of Pere Moliner (2). Plan made by the author.

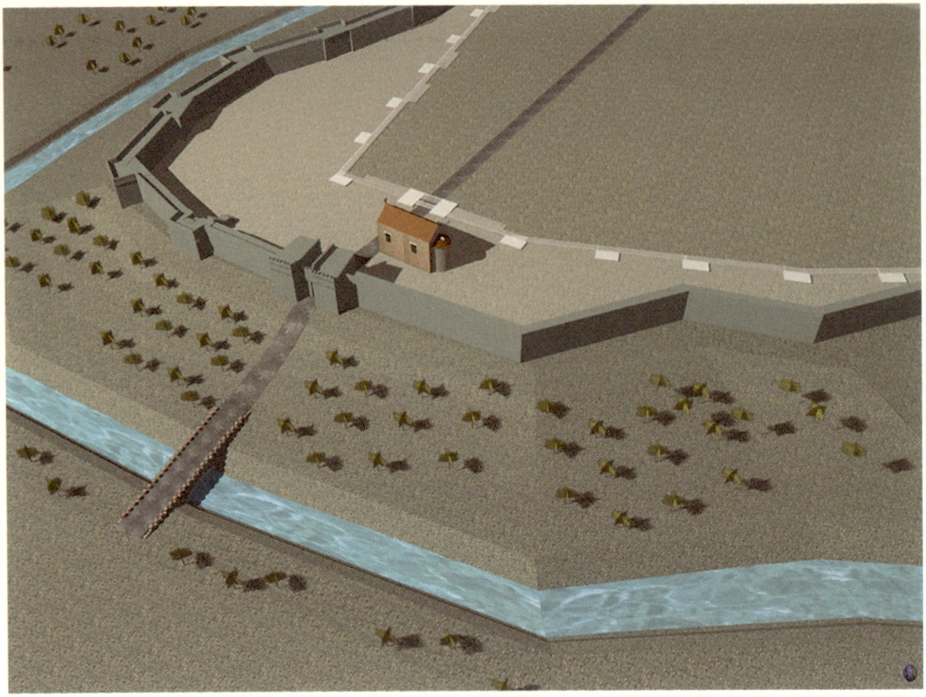

Fig. 2. Reconstruction of the location of the Hospital of the Holy Spirit, between the Andalusian wall and the 14th century wall. Image: Arxiu Arqueològic de Lleida.

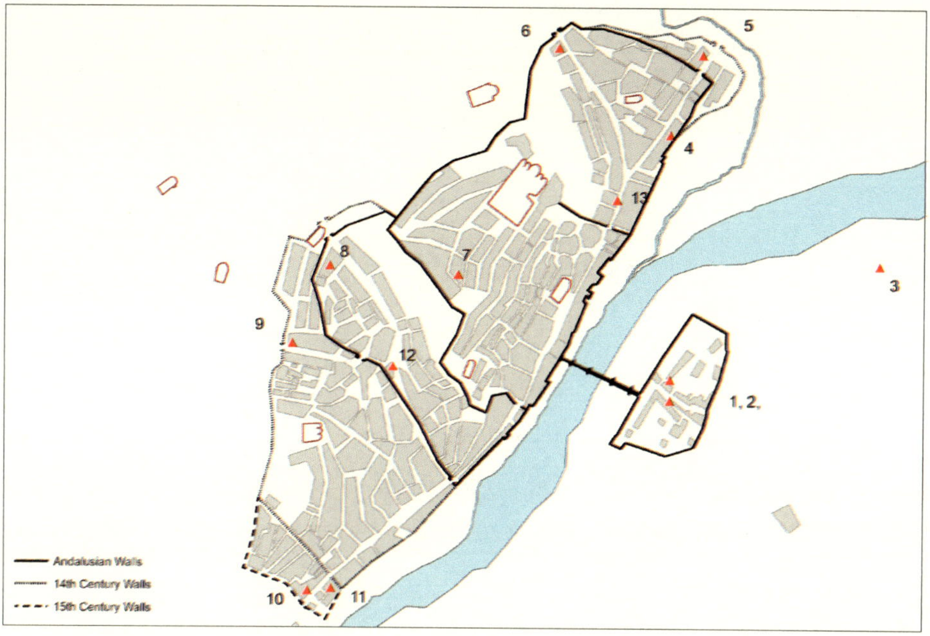


Fig. 3. Hospitals in Lleida during the 14th century. 1. Hospital of Bernat Coll; 2. Trinitarian monastery; 3. Hospital of Saint Lazarus Llàtzer; 4. Hospital of Guillem de Fillac; 5. Hospital of the Holy Spirit; 6. Hospital of Saint Mary Magdalene; 7. Hospital for Poor Priests; 8. Hospital of Saint Martin; 9. Hospital of Saint Thomas; 10. Hospital of Saint Anthony; 11. Hospital of Pere Moliner; 12. Hospital of Guillem Vidal (not built); 13. Hospital of Pere Serra. Plan made by the author.

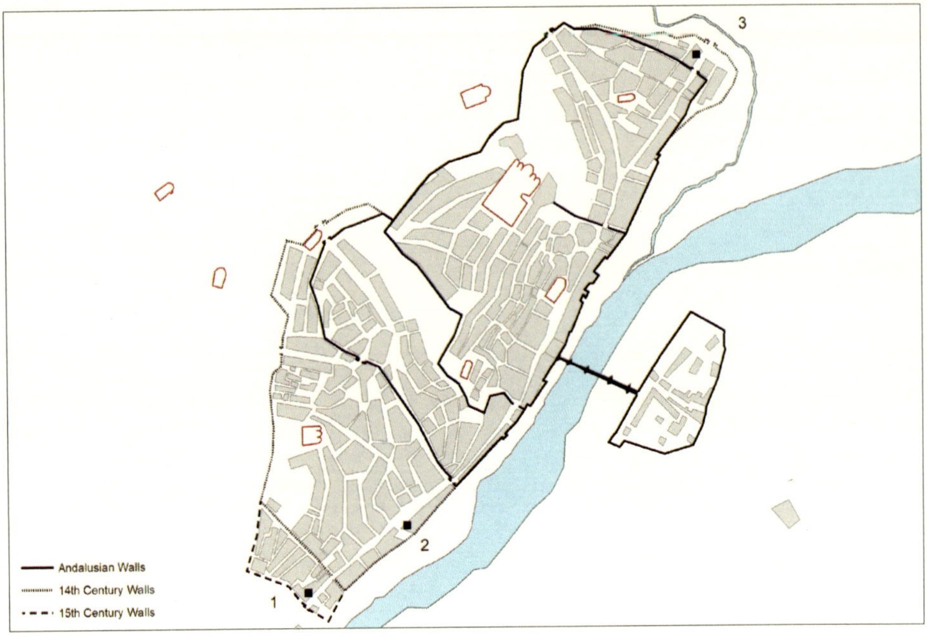


Fig. 4. Hospitals in Lleida during 15th century. 1. Hospital of Saint Anthony; 2. General Hospital of Saint Mary; 3. Hospital of the Holy Spirit. Plan made by the author.

Joana Balsa de Pinho

# Lisbon's House for the Plague Patients: A Historical, Architectural and Urban Study*

## 1. *Preliminary Considerations*

Up until the late 18th century, the terms "plague" and "pestilence" were used to define different forms of infectious diseases, such as malaria, typhus, smallpox, tuberculosis, and –most notably– bubonic plague. Epidemic outbreaks were highly contagious and spread very quickly, having huge demographic, social, and economic impacts. To respond to such crises, public health protocols promoted different measures for the prevention, control, and mitigation of such diseases that affected the population on a large scale. Preventative action involved containment measures and procedures that aimed to protect the country from external contagion, while mitigation measures aimed to minimise the effects of the epidemic in already affected areas. In other words, protocols for the prevention and containment of disease simultaneously required the royal imposition of countrywide measures, as well as the localised action of municipal authorities, a dedicated administrative structure, and suitable infrastructures for the isolation and treatment of the sick. All these measures were initially of a provisional and tentative nature.

Taking Lisbon as a case study, this paper focuses on one of the containment measures used in this context in the 15th and 16th centuries, namely the institution of plague hospitals. This phenomenon is contextualised through the systematic analysis of historical documentation that is mainly drawn from the *Provimento da saúde* (health provision) document collection, held at the *Arquivo Municipal de Lisboa* (Lisbon Municipal Archive), which provides considerable documentary evidence. However, such document collection has considerable chronological gaps, which, in some cases, are as long as a decade. In other municipal and royal documentation held at the City and Royal Chancelleries, the subject of the constitution of a plague hospital in Lisbon is absent. However, some considerations can be drawn from the available, albeit limited, documentary evidence. By the

* This chapter is written in the scope of the project *Hospitalis - Hospital architecture in Portugal at the dawn of Modernity: Identification, characterization and contextualization* (PTDC/ART-HIS/30808/2017), funded by FCT – Fundação para a Ciência e a Tecnologia, I.P.

end of the 15th century, the institution of a plague hospital in Lisbon was a central concern for both the council and the King, reflecting a paradigm shift in the way plague outbreaks had been understood and dealt with thus far. Plague hospitals became a central strategy for combating epidemics.

During this period, welfare reform also intensified, notably with the creation of a general hospital in Lisbon. Although, initially, the care of plague patients was not undertaken by a single hospital, no purpose-built structures existed for such a function, and a need for a dedicated space for plague patients became increasingly pressing. The most relevant project –although it may have remained unrealised– was proposed by King Manuel I as part of the urban renewal plan he had devised for Lisbon. The project was eventually realised by King João III, albeit in a different way, but still in the context of the promulgation of the new Health Regimen that involved the institutionalisation of the *Casa da Saúde* (House of Health), an administrative structure dedicated to the management of epidemics through prevention, control, and mitigation measures.

## 2. *A Conceptual Turn*

For a comprehensive assessment of plague responses, it is first necessary to consider the evolution in the understanding of the disease's epidemiology in order to perceive how its management changed and how this was, in turn, reflected in the establishment of regulations and structures to contain and treat it.

During the second half of the 14th century, different measures were taken to mitigate the plague. Although attempts at mitigation occurred all over Europe, Italy was the first country in which health measures were implemented in a more systematic way. Such measures included detecting the plague and its place of origin; establishing quarantine and the isolation of people and goods, and monitoring and isolating patients' contacts; closing the borders and affected areas in the city; prohibiting movement; implementing crowd control actions; arranging the burial of the dead; promoting the fumigation of patients' houses and the burning or disinfection of their clothes; enabling visits by doctors and priests; organising the transport of patients to plague hospitals or lazarettos; and ensuring the management of these institutions (Carmichael 1983; Henderson 2019; Slack 1988).

In Portugal, too, some of these measures began to be implemented. The oldest surviving evidence of this dates back to a document from Prince Dom Duarte from the beginning of the 15th century, which defines a set of measures to be applied by the city council following the arrival on the Portuguese coast of ships carrying plague patients. The document stated that, when approaching the port, the captain should report the presence of any sick or deceased people on board. Moreover, in case of suspicion of plague, the ship should be prevented from docking and should leave the Tagus estuary.[1]

1. Arquivo Municipal de Lisboa (AML), *Livro dos Pregos*, f. 258v.

From the 15th century onwards, as it became apparent that such provisional measures had become ineffective, they were codified in a structured health policy that took on a more permanent character.

This change is closely related to the emergence of a new understanding of the plague. Until the mid-15th century, medical theory on the plague stated that miasma, –the corruption of the air– was responsible for plague outbreaks, an argument that appeared in most medical treatises of the time.[2] However, governments expressed a different belief, which was reflected in the regulations they issued. Among rulers and authorities, the theory of human contagion began to gain traction. Observations of past manifestations of epidemics contributed to such a view, most notably, the fact that the plague was mainly an urban phenomenon that affected the more disadvantaged areas of cities, that it could be confined to houses, families, streets and social groups, and that more recent outbreaks were less deadly than those of the previous century. It is in such a context of paradigm change that authorities began to implement a set of laws and practices with the aim of preventing and controlling outbreaks through the establishment of dedicated administrative bodies,[3] as well as plague hospitals and lazarettos that aimed to treat and isolate the sick in order to prevent contagion (SLACK 1988), thereby providing an effective strategy for combating epidemics.[4]

## 3. *The Lisbon Plague Hospital: A Temporary, Emergency Structure*

As a port city, Lisbon was particularly vulnerable to epidemics, as it was the destination of people and goods coming from all over the world. Thus, from the end of the 14th century on, measures began to be taken to prevent epidemic outbreaks. In the context of the aforementioned healthcare measures for the prevention and mitigation of disease and of the paradigm shift in the understanding of plague transmission, attempts were made to institute a plague hospital.

Historian Jane Stevens-Crawshaw (2015: 9) identifies three categories of structures intended to fight the plague: temporary requisitioned buildings or wooden constructions that would be burned after the outbreak was over; permanent buildings that would be used only during times of epidemic; and permanent buildings that would continue to be used after the outbreak was over. The last of these structures were easier to administer, because they had permanently available staff, but they were also more costly. Urban public health systems could opt for

2. According to Ann G. Carmichael, all the treatises of this time collected by Karl Sudhoff present the miasma theory in opposition to the contagion theory as the origin of the plague (CARMICHAEL 1983: 513).

3. In Portugal, the *Provedor* (Provider) and the *Provedoria da Saúde* (Health Administration).

4. The article by Guilllem Roca, titled "The Influence of Medicine and Sanitary Policies on the Structure of Lleida's Hospital Network" and published in this same volume, is focused on urban policies to face epidemic outbreaks in the Catalan city of Lleida.

one or a combination of these solutions. In the case of Lisbon, plague hospitals first emerged as temporary structures in existing spaces that were adapted for the purpose. They were assembled and disassembled according to need, thus representing a form of emergency architecture.

As mentioned above, the first known measures to prevent and combat epidemics date back to the reign of King João I. Additional measures were developed by later monarchs. As I said, my goal is to analyse the establishment and management of plague hospitals, the function of which was to receive the sick and provide them with care and a suitable space for quarantine, as well as to disinfect their goods. In this sense, plague hospitals could be understood as early welfare institutions, emerging in the context of a broader increase in charitable initiatives towards the disadvantaged that were being promoted at the dawn of modernity (STEVENS-CRAWSHAW 2016).

Likewise, plague hospitals provided a barrier against the spread of the disease across the city, thus constituting one of its main public health structures. As spaces for isolation, they enabled the control of contagion and therefore prevented the transmissibility of the disease.

Plague hospitals appeared all over Europe during the 15th and 16th centuries, the oldest permanent example of which is the *lazzaretto vecchio* in Venice, founded in 1423. In some cases, these hospitals were temporary wooden structures intended to last for the duration of the epidemic outbreak; sometimes they occupied existing buildings. For this reason, documentary and material evidence is scarce (STEVENS-CRAWSHAW 2015: 21-24). Extant evidence suggests that King João II was the first monarch to elaborate on the need for a plague hospital in Lisbon. By the 1480s, such an institution had become a reality as the result of a greater awareness of its importance in controlling plague transmission.

In 1485, a farm in Lisbon was converted into a centre for plague patients that could host up to eight people and was furnished with equipment and staff to attend to the sick. Like most hospitals of the period, the space had a small capacity. Given these circumstances, the King ordered that the council set up another farm for the same purpose, because the existing one had already reached its full capacity. The establishment of a second institution for plague patients was motivated by a desire to keep plague patients isolated, reinforcing the theory that contagion was effectively circulating through human contact. The new farm, owned by Isabel de São Paio, was given to João Lopes and Afonso Lopes, and –just like the first farm– it was provided with beds and staff.[5]

The following year, despite the city's and the kingdom's decreasing contagion rate, the King ordered that: «the hospital where those who were sick of this disease were treated should be rebuilt immediately», indicating the precarious conditions of plague hospital as emergency constructions, temporarily built to

5. AML, Provimento da Saúde, *Livro 1.º do provimento da saúde*, f. 5-5v.

respond to health crises. The monarch also requested that this be done quickly, for if any person fell ill, «they should be taken to the said hospital to be treated».[6]

The council also took the initiative to establish a new house for plague patients, a project that rode the wave of the emerging enthusiasm for such structures and benefited from the financial help of the King. In 1493, they decided to build a house for those suffering from the plague next to the leprosy hospital of San Lázaro. In a letter about the project that the King sent to the city council, he explained that it was: «Very good and very convenient, and we consider it very well done, and we command that it should soon be realised. As for the task that was assigned to Diogo Brandão and Álvaro Pires, it seems good to us, and we believe that they are the ones who will be able to do it well».[7]

The King also appointed Afonso Leitão as the project's treasurer and immediately granted a sum for the required expenditure. The project would not involve the construction of a new building, but rather the adaptation of an existing site for the specific purpose of treating and isolating people affected by the plague. These spaces would have in-house doctors who provided patients with targeted medical care, a measure that reflects a broader turn toward the medicalization of healthcare that was taking place at the beginning of the century across Europe. This document also demanded the institution of control groups in each parish that were required to identify the sick and inform them about how they should act, enforcing penalties for those who did not comply with the given instructions.[8]

Another document from the same year confirms that, in July 1493, several houses for plague patients were available in the city, possibly because their individual capacity was limited and outbreaks were frequent. In the document, the King asked council officers to stop sick people from entering the city and that «those who come to be treated should go to the house of Sant'Antão, which is what we have ordered».[9]

Considering the risk of disease transmission through the exchange of goods, the King proposed a quarantine of goods initiative in September 1492 to prevent plague outbreaks in the city. To this end, he ordered the construction of a porch and a cross –simple but effective structures– on the outskirts of the city to expose potentially infected goods to the sun. The monarch considered that «this would be a very good thing and that we would be pleased to make a porch on top of some bunkers a little beyond Santa Maria de Belém and a large stone cross beyond Fernão Lourenço's mills so that the ships that come from dangerous places will not pass the mark of the cross and could store their goods and collect them in the porch that could be made in these bunkers».[10] This initiative aligns with Stevens-Crawshaw's argument that some of the first permanent urban structures

6. AML, Provimento da Saúde, *Livro 1.º do provimento da saúde*, f. 7-7v.

7. AML, Provimento da Saúde, *Livro 1.º do provimento da saúde*, f. 16-17v. All the quotes taken from original documents have been translated by the author from Portuguese to English.

8. AML, Provimento da Saúde, *Livro 1.º do provimento da saúde*, f. 16-17v.

9. AML, Provimento da Saúde, *Livro 1.º do provimento da saúde*, f. 8-8v.

10. AML, Provimento da Saúde, *Livro 1.º do provimento da saúde*, f. 11-11v.

for plague control were open spaces intended for the disinfection of merchandise and other goods (STEVENS-CRAWSHAW 2015: 4).

It should be noted that King João II was also the monarch responsible for the establishment of Portugal's first modern hospital, the All Saints Royal Hospital,[11] through the grant of the *Ex debito sobllicitudinis* papal bull, promulgated on 13 August 1479, which authorised the king «to build a large hospital in the city of Lisbon, with the capacity to unite and incorporate into the same building the other hospitals and centres for assistance» that already existing in the city (PAIVA 2002, 2: 51, doc. 22).[12] The merging of small hospitals into a larger structure constituted a pivotal action in the healthcare reform that would be extended to the entire kingdom by means of the *Iniunctum nobis* papal bull, dated 21 February 1486, which enabled the king to «unite the diverse hospitals for the poor and abandoned children of each city or eminent settlement in his kingdoms and dominions to the major hospital of each locality» (PAIVA 2002, 2: 54, doc. 24).[13] It is no coincidence that the monarch who promoted one of the most important initiatives in healthcare reform is the same one who, on several occasions, encouraged the institution of plague hospitals. The promotion of both of these welfare initiatives is inextricably linked to this figure, who was so sensitive to healthcare reformation.

During the reign of King Manuel I, which began in 1495, the need to address the subject of plague hospitals returned and received more consistent attention. However, for a period of around ten years during his reign, the subject does not appear in any documentation. Only in a royal document dated February 1506 is mention of plague hospitals made, in a statement that «no further obligation should be enforced on the sick to be taken to the ordered house»,[14] that is, only those who consented to be treated in plague hospitals should be taken there, and those who did not consent could be treated at home without incurring any penalties. As the plague continued to spread, the capacity of structures destined for plague patients proved to be insufficient. However, there was a concern that dedicated spaces should be «supplied and well provided as has been done hitherto», reflecting a concern for the establishment of spaces where the sick could be «provided for and well cured» that had already been expressed by the previous monarch.[15]

Years later, in 1510, King Manuel I, concerned about the situation in Lisbon, declared that «some things should be done about the plague that roams in this city».[16] To this end, he suggested that one or two more houses be built to care for plague patients. As stated in another document, the establishment of these houses

11. On the history, evolution and features of the Royal All Saints Hospital see: ALBERTO, DA SILVA, TEIXEIRA 2020.

12. Arquivo Nacional da Torre do Tombo (ANTT), mç. 12 of papal bulls, no. 8.

13. This process of merging small hospitals into new institutions occurred since the 15th century in different European geographies.

14. AML, Provimento da Saúde, *Livro 1o do provimento da saúde*, f. 33-33v.

15. AML, Provimento da Saúde, *Livro 1o do provimento da saúde*, f. 33-33v.

16. AML, Provimento da Saúde, *Livro 1.º do provimento da saúde*, f. 40-40v.

would be made at the expense of the «fee ordered for the correction of the walls» of the city.[17] The houses were to be located close to each other, so as to be served by only one physician or surgeon. The document further stated that «according to what has been seen in several parts by experience [...] so that it was not at all left to the benefit of nature».[18] It should be noted that, once again, the concern that the treatment of plague should be accompanied by a doctor's advice is evident, as is evidence that King Manuel I sought to implement measures that had been tested elsewhere. This is not an isolated case: in 1506, the King had ordered the enforcement of plague control measures similar to those implemented in Genoa in Lisbon, namely the temporary evacuation of the city, the isolation of the inhabitants who lived in its surroundings, and the installation of guards at the access gates.[19]

Less than two months later, on 4 September 1510, the monarch wrote to the City Council stating that «we believe, as we have written to you, that it would be a very profitable thing for the health of this city to have an orderly house for the cure of those suffering from pestilence and, from the messages that were sent to us regarding this, we are determined to order its construction».[20] However, because plague outbreaks were «rapidly increasing» and «due to the winter's misfortune that will enter the city from now on», the king gave up on the idea of building such houses for plague infestations.[21]

However, a later document dated 1519 and sent by King Manuel I to the council stated that work was underway for the construction of the house for plague patients. However, the council officials informed the King that «there was no longer any need for it» because the sick were not being taken there. Such a decision allowed the council to save the amount of money originally earmarked for the construction of the structure.[22]

## 4. *King Manuel I and the House for Plague Patients "Made to Last"*

In 1520, the decision to build a specialised structure to serve as a plague hospital was finally made. This would no longer be a provisional construction, but would be designed from the ground up for the specific function of admitting and treating plague patients. The project was of a remarkable scale, marking a definitive break with the typical architecture of medieval institutions, and can be better understood in the context of King Manuel I's urban renewal project for the capital. It is likely that the King looked at what was being done in Italy when he approved the project for the construction of a permanent plague hospital.

17. AML, Provimento da Saúde, *Livro 1.º do provimento da saúde*, f. 40-40v.
18. AML, Provimento da Saúde, *Livro 1.º do provimento da saúde*, f. 39-39v.
19. AML, Provimento da Saúde, *Livro 1.º do provimento da saúde*, f. 34-35v.
20. AML, Provimento da Saúde, *Livro 1.º do provimento da saúde*, f. 40-40v.
21. AML, Provimento da Saúde, *Livro 1.º do provimento da saúde*, f. 40-40v.
22. AML, Provimento da Saúde, *Livro 1.º do provimento da saúde*, f. 58-58v.

Other initiatives preceded this grandiose project. In April of the same year, when the King noticed that the plague was mainly affecting poor people and that the coexistence between the healthy and the sick was harmful, he ordered the construction of «a house in the outskirts of the city where those who fell ill could be kept, as was done in the past».[23] Following his predecessor's footsteps, the King demanded that the house should provide the sick with «all the necessary provisions», such as tables, supplies, a surgeon, and «all the other things that they need».[24]

In May and June of the same year, the King returned to the matter, authorising the house chaplain to make the wills of the sick and approve their validity.[25] This decision highlights additional levels of concern for patients: on the one hand, there was a concern for the patients' spiritual comfort, represented by the presence of a chaplain who celebrated mass and administered the sacraments. This was an important component of healing practices common to most hospitals at the time, which combined medical and spiritual care. On the other hand, the presence of the chaplain ensured the conditions for the salvation of the patients' souls as sanctioned by testamentary clauses (Vilar, Silva 1992).

In June of the same year, the King validated the council's expenses for the house of the sick, stating that it seemed to him «of so much service to our Lord and to the city that it should not be neglected».[26] However, the King also requested monthly reports from the council regarding such expenses.

In July 1520, a new project was launched by the monarch, who invited the city council to consider «how necessary and useful it would be in this city to have a permanent house where the sick could be admitted and cured», as many sick people were dying at the time owing to the absence of suitable infrastructure where they could be treated.[27] This new structure would no longer be provisional, nor would it be installed in an adapted building –as had been the case for previous houses for the sick–; rather, it would be a permanent structure built from scratch and displaying all the characteristics of a purpose-built construction, including a strategic choice of location, careful architectural design, and a financing plan that would cover the overall project from its construction to the allocation of equipment. Contrary to previous provisional fabrics, architectural form would take precedence over other issues, such as size and the quantity of sites. Thus, the structure was to be located in D. Jerónimo de Sá's vegetable garden, near the Alcântara bridge. This site had a number of advantages: it was accessible by both sea and land; it had an abundant water supply and space available for burials, and enjoyed «all the other things that are convenient for similar works».[28] For the construction and furnishing of the hospital, the King donated one million *reais*

23. AML, Provimento da Saúde, *Livro 1.º do provimento da saúde*, f. 61-61v.
24. AML, Provimento da Saúde, *Livro 1.º do provimento da saúde*, f. 61-61v.
25. AML, Provimento da Saúde, *Livro 1.º do provimento da saúde*, f. 62-62v and 63-63v.
26. AML, Provimento da Saúde, *Livro 1o do provimento da saúde*, f. 64-64v.
27. AML, Provimento da Saúde, *Livro 1o do provimento da saúde*, f. 65-66v.
28. AML, Provimento da Saúde, *Livro 1o do provimento da saúde*, f. 65-66v.

(reals) and demanded the same amount from the city council. He also warned the council that, in order to cover the five *contos* required for the hospital's construction, equipment, and staff, it would be necessary to further tax the inhabitants of the city and the surrounding areas. King Manuel I also stipulated that the council should hold meetings with the governor, noblemen, and citizens with whom the King corresponded on the matter, to define how the aforementioned tax should be levied and to appoint a clerk, a receiver and a proctor.

According to the same document, the construction would have been of significant size and would have included 160 beds, workshops, and other necessary accommodation, «as you will see from the painting of everything so that it can soon be given to the lowest bidder».[29] Unfortunately, the painting depicting the building's layout no longer exists. Two aspects of this project should be highlighted: on the one hand, this project should be understood in relation to a set of urban renovations carried out by King Manuel I, who sought to transform the capital of the kingdom into the capital of an empire (CARITA 2014: 13). These renovation projects aimed to rearrange and renew the urban space by adding civic and institutional structures, as well as religious and military buildings. On the other hand, the construction of purpose-built hospitals with specific architectural features was part of a broader healthcare reform that had been taking place in Europe since the early 15th century (BIANCHI, SŁOŃ, MAREK 2006).

Like other measures implemented by King Manuel I, the project may have been inspired by Italian plague infrastructure, in particular that seen in Milan.[30] As Stevens-Crawshaw (2015: 71) states «the general characteristics of *lazzaretti* buildings can be identified in the plan of the *lazzaretto* in Milan». However, thanks to surviving documentary evidence, such as doctors' writings, as well as descriptions and drawings of old buildings, we are able to elucidate some features of this project. The structure would have been spacious and located outside the city walls but near the port, where water would be abundant. The building would have included a chapel located at the centre of the building so that mass celebrations could be seen from different locations within the building; it had a courtyard possibly delimited by arches where goods could also be disinfected, a dedicated cemetery for the fulfilment of burial duties that also helped with the containment of the disease; accommodation for the person in charge of the space, medical staff and servants; a kitchen; and warehouses to store the goods of those undergoing treatment or quarantine. The whole building would have been surrounded by walls and would have had a quadrangular or rectangular plan. The hospital would have been constituted by a porticoed structure so that patients would have access to sunlight, and there would be separate wards for men and women. Individual and family rooms were added later on. These features were shared by most purpose-built plague hospitals in various European cities, and problably by the Lisbon project (STEVENS-CRAWSHAW 2015: 42, 51, 61-77).

29. AML, Provimento da Saúde, *Livro 1o do provimento da saúde*, f. 65-66v.
30. On the Lazareto of Milan, see Patetta, 1986: 25-42.

In spite of such careful planning, construction works were never carried out: neither material nor documentary evidence of the building's construction exist. Meanwhile, pre-existing houses for plague patients continued to function since, on 26 July 1520, the King approved monthly expenses for their maintenance, requesting that they be covered with funds obtained from the councils' rents.[31] However, the project was still considered by the municipality, given that in October 1520, as a merciful act toward the city, the King waived the aforementioned tax that he wished to levy on citizens for the construction.[32]

Until 1526, when a major new project arised, references to the existence of a house for plague patients continued to appear in scattered notes. In 1523, King Manuel I's successor, King João III, confirmed the house chaplain's authority to make wills[33] and also reinforced the obligation for those who contracted the plague in the city to be transported to dedicated houses, emphasising that «for the cure of the sick who go there, there is a good supply of medicines and of surgeons and physicians, and all other necessary things that ensure their treatment and survival»; he later added, following the council's advice, that not only «slaves and soldiers and the labourers were taken to the house».[34] He reiterated his concern that the house «be well provided with everything necessary as we have ordered and as we believe it will be in your good care».[35]

The following year, on 18 October 1524, the city council awarded Mestre Vasco, a surgeon who worked at the All-Saints Hospital, two *moios* (about 814 litres) of wheat and one of barley «for the work he [...] did in treating the plague patients in the house». The same award had previously been assigned to Mestre Gonçalo «when he was in charge of patients' treatment in the said house».[36] Aside from rewarding Vasco's work, such an initiative demonstrates the relationship that existed between different hospital institutions in the city.

## 5. *King João III's Health Regimen and the Institution of the Casa da Saúde*

Another fundamental step towards the establishment of spaces for the admission, treatment, and containment of plague patients in the city was defined by the *Regimento da saúde* (health regimen), dated 1526 and attributed to King João III.[37] This health regimen was based on notes made by Pedro Vaz during a visit to Italian cities that had been affected by the plague. The regimen involved the construction of the Lisbon plague hospital, as well as the implementation of

31. AML, Provimento da Saúde, *Livro 1.º do provimento da saúde*, f. 67-67v.
32. AML, Provimento da Saúde, *Livro 1.º do provimento da saúde*, f. 68-68v.
33. AML, Provimento da Saúde, *Livro 1.º do provimento da saúde*, f. 40-40v.
34. AML, Provimento da Saúde, *Livro 1.º do provimento da saúde*, f. 87-88v.
35. AML, Provimento da Saúde, *Livro 1.º do provimento da saúde*, f. 90-91v.
36. AML, Provimento da Saúde, *Livro 1.º do provimento da saúde*, f. 99-99v.
37. AML, Provimento da Saúde, *Livro de regimentos e posturas da Casa da Saúde*, f. 31-41v.

an administrative structure that would be responsible for the prevention, control, and mitigation of epidemics.

Pero Vaz's notes, as well as the King's writings on the subject, provide descriptions of the house for the sick and for convalescents, the latter being the place at which those recovering from illness would be kept for forty days until their symptoms were no longer evident. The house for the sick, for which more detailed documentary evidence survives, functioned as a traditional hospital and was equipped with beds, medical supplies, an apothecary, physicians, bleeders, and servants. This house could have two possible locations: the palace of *Estaus* or the houses of the King and Mestre Filipe in Santos. According to health regulations, the criteria for choosing where to erect the building had to take into account access to water, the geographical location of the building (which had to be in close proximity to the city while avoiding overcrowded areas), easy access to a burial site, and the simultaneous ability to limit and provide controlled access to the building. As previously mentioned, some of these principles had already informed the choice to locate King Manuel I's project in Alcântara. However, the two projects differed in size: while the latter had over one hundred and fifty beds, King João III's project was more modest, providing only twenty beds.

The King assigned to Pero Vaz the task of consulting with the city council to determine the most suitable location for the house and later informing the King of the decision in order to proceed with the installation. The chosen location was Santos' palace, as evidenced in a 1541 record of a payment to master architect João de Castilho[38] to carry out works, namely «the construction an infirmary for plague patients», in the aforementioned house.[39]

Such observations reveal that the initiatives of both King Manuel I and King João III to build a plague hospital were a symbolic investment –and not solely because they were sponsored by the monarchs themselves–. In Alcântara, the size of the building reinforced its architectural and artistic value, and João de Castilho's involvement in the project of Santo's palace had a similar purpose of promoting the building's aesthetic qualities. Such an artistic investment also served to guarantee the good reputation of the buildings' patrons, as noted by Gabriela Piccinni (2017) in her study of urban general hospitals. According to Piccinni, from the 15th century, governing bodies became aware that public assistance was a fundamental need and, therefore, a task of the *res publica* that was closely related to notions of common good and good government. This awareness, which promoted a redefinition of healthcare establishments, allows the origin of the welfare state to be located at the dawn of the early modern period.

Following King João III's project, other monarchs led other initiatives that had repercussions on healthcare structures in the city of Lisbon. Although outbreak prevention and control practices did not undergo substantial changes, their impact on urban life and planning is significant. The most important initiative

38. See the most recent contribution to the life and work of João de Castilho: SILVA 2021.
39. ANTT, Chancelaria de D. João III, Livro 34, f. 2-2v.

was carried out by Cardinal-King Henrique, who ordered the construction of a lazaretto in 1565 in Almada. In a document relating to this project, the King reported: «I have been informed that some people from the Kingdoms of England and other regions, who are prevented from evil deeds that our Lord wishes to keep us from, come to this city with their goods and without them», [40] thus «they must not introduce them into the city, but must place them in detention in a location where they can rest as long as necessary».[41] The monarch concludes his letter by stating that, at the border of the village of Almada referred to as *Trafaria*, a suitably sized house should be built on a portion of land belonging to Gaspar da Rua that should be evaluated for acquisition for that purpose.

## 6. *Final Remarks*

Purpose-built spaces for the admission and treatment of plague patients were an important strategy in the fight against epidemics. This phenomenon was not unique to Portugal, but was visible across Europe. In the city of Lisbon, these emergency structures originated as impromptu and temporary solutions that were built in response to health crises and were influenced by the emerging theories and practices on the treatment of contagious diseases. Such buildings were small in size, as were most of the hospital institutions of the dawn of the early modern period.

Despite such material constraints, these institutions were provided with care staff, which included health professionals and chaplains for the assistance of the sick. It was a recurring concern for several monarchs that such houses be adequately equipped to fulfill their function. Moreover, documentation shows that kings actively proposed suggestions to the council for the remodelling and construction of such houses. The monarch was more involved than the council itself.

In this context, King Manuel I's project stands out as a clearly modern institution, distinct from previous medieval institutions both in its grandeur and in its design from scratch to fulfil the function of a plague hospital. One cannot separate this measure from the urban reforms that took place during King Manuel I's reign, nor from his health concerns.

By way of conclusion, this paper has also demonstrated that the healthcare infrastructure emerging at the dawn of modernity within urban contexts is deeply related to concepts of the common good, communal welfare, and good government, while it also testifies to the proactivity of rulers in combating problems affecting their citizens and social inequalities, as well as representing an opportunity to exercise Christian charity.

40. AML, Provimento da Saúde, *Livro 1.º do provimento da saúde*, f. 155-155v.
41. AML, Provimento da Saúde, *Livro 1.º do provimento da saúde*, f. 155-155v.

## *Bibliography*

Alberto, Edite; Da Silva, Rodrigo B.; Teixeira, André (ed.), 2020. *O Hospital Real de Todos-os-Santos: Lisboa e a saúde*, Lisboa, Câmara Municipal de Lisboa.

Bianchi, Francesco; Słoń, Marek, 2006. "Le riforme ospedaliere del Quattrocento in Italia e nell'Europa centrale", *Ricerche di Storia Sociale e Religiosa*, 35/69: 7-45.

Carita, Hélder, 2014. "Da 'Ribeira' ao Terreiro do Paço: génese e formação de um modelo urbano", Miguel F. Faria (ed.), *Do Terreiro do Paço à Praça do Comércio: história de um espaço urbano*, Lisboa, Universidade Autónoma e Imprensa Nacional-Casa da Moeda: 13-35.

Carmichael, Ann G., 1983. "Plague legislation in the Italian Renaissance", *Bulletin of the History of Medicine,* 57/4: 508-525.

Da Silva, Ricardo J. Nunes, 2021. *O paradigma da arquitetura em Portugal na Idade Moderna: entre o tardo-gótico e o renascimento*, Lisboa, Associação Portuguesa de Historiadores da Arte.

Henderson, John, 2019. *Florence Under Siege: Surviving Plague in an Early Modern City*, Yale, Yale University Press.

Paiva, José Pedro, 2002. *Portugaliae monumenta misericordiarum*, Lisboa, União das Misericórdias Portuguesas, vol. 2.

Patetta, Luciano, 1986. "Nuove Ipotesi sul Lazzaretto Quattrocentesco di Milano", *Bollettino d'Arte*, n.º 35-36, 25-42.

Piccinni, Gabriella, 2017. "I grandi ospedali urbani dell'Italia medievale: all'origine del 'welfare'", F. Sabaté (ed.), *L'assistència a l'etad mitjana*, Leida, Pagès: 139-151.

Slack, Paul, 1988. "Responses to Plague in Early Modern Europe: The Implications of Public Health", *Social Research*, 55/3: 433-453.

Stevens-Crawshaw, Jane L., 2016. *Plague Hospitals: Public Health for the City in Early Modern Venice*, New York, Routledge.

Vilar, Hermínia; Silva, Maria João, 1992. "Morrer e testar na Idade Média: alguns aspectos da testamentaria dos séculos XIV e XV", *Lusitania Sacra*, 2/4: 39-60.

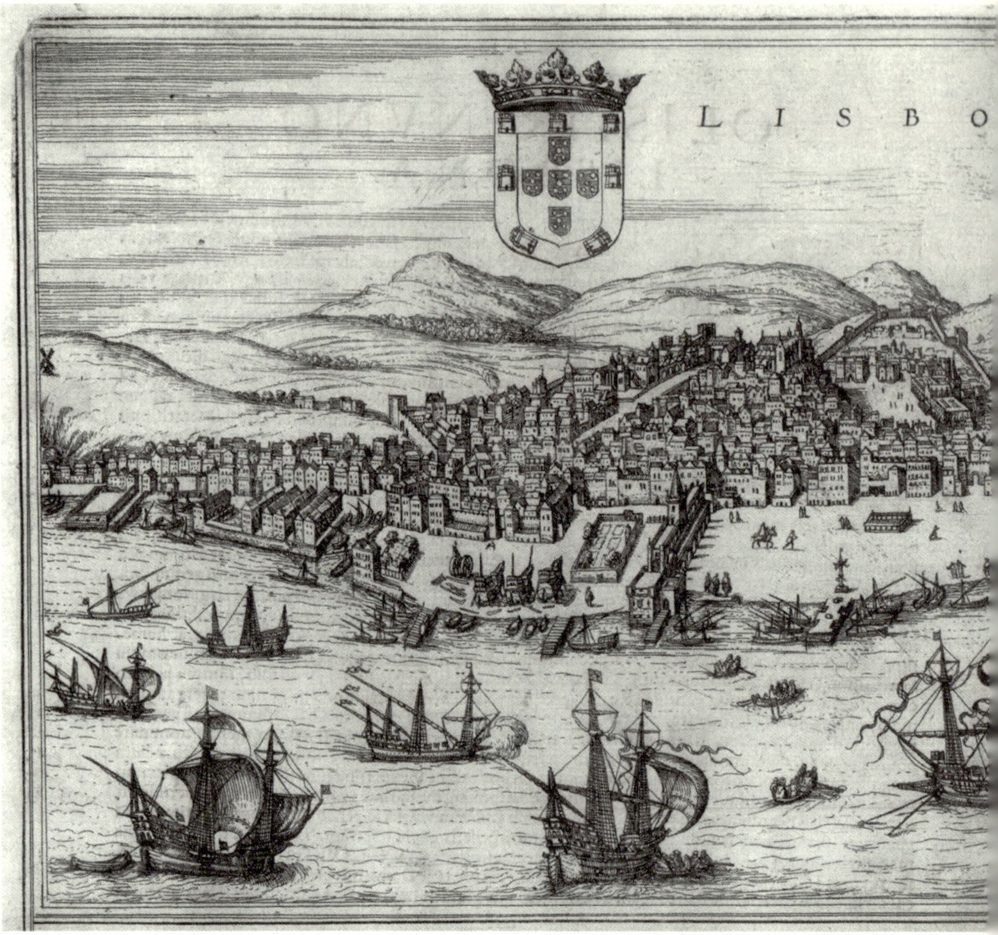


Fig. 1. Georg Braun and Frans Hogenberg: *Olisipo, sive ut persetustae lapidum inscriptiones habent, Ulysipo, vulgo Lisbona Florentissimum* [...]. Coloniae: Apud Auctores, 1572 (Biblioteca Nacional Digital, cc-798-v). Image obtained from https://purl.pt/22211/1/index.html#/1/html.

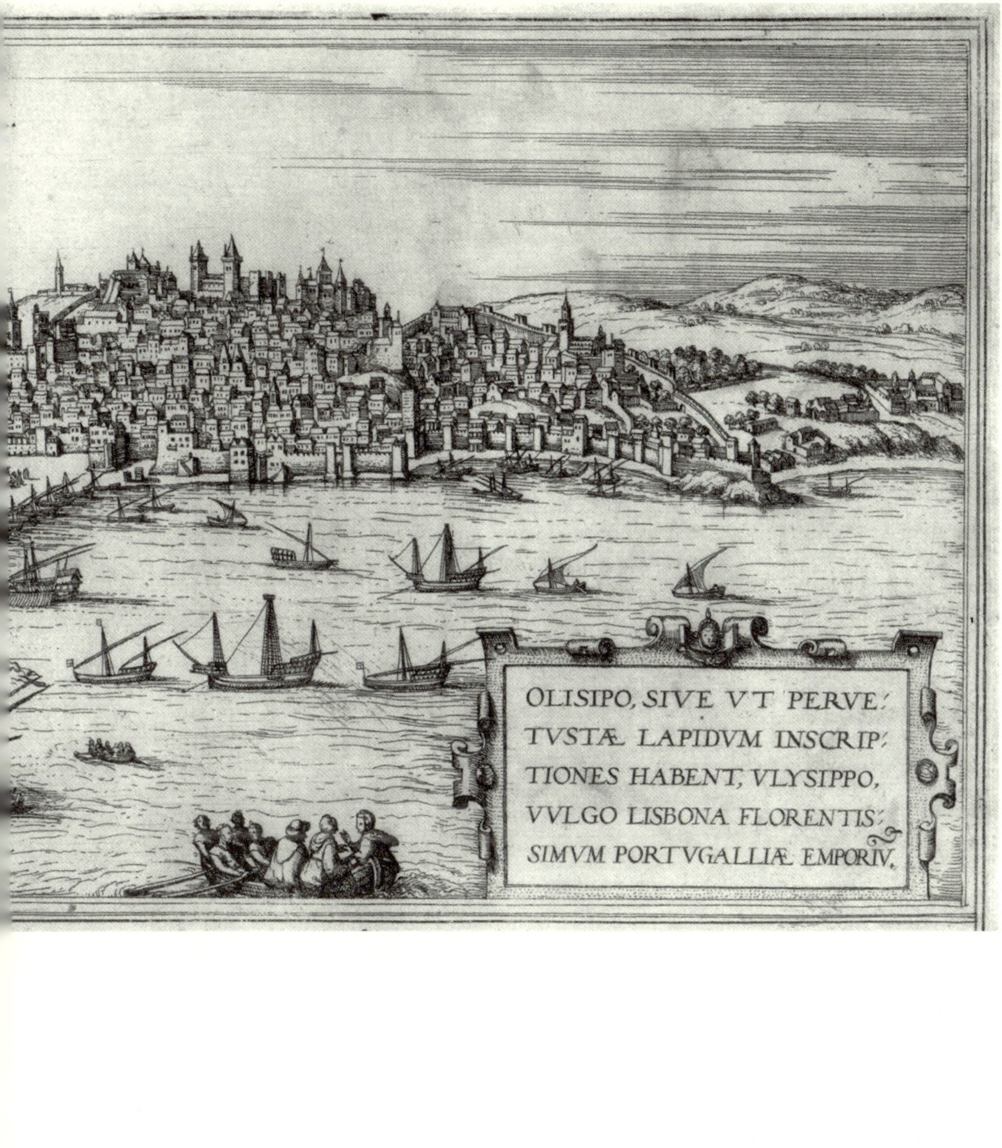
OLISIPO, SIVE VT PERVE:
TVSTÆ LAPIDVM INSCRIP:
TIONES HABENT, VLYSIPPO,
VVLGO LISBONA FLORENTIS:
SIMVM PORTVGALLIÆ EMPORIV.

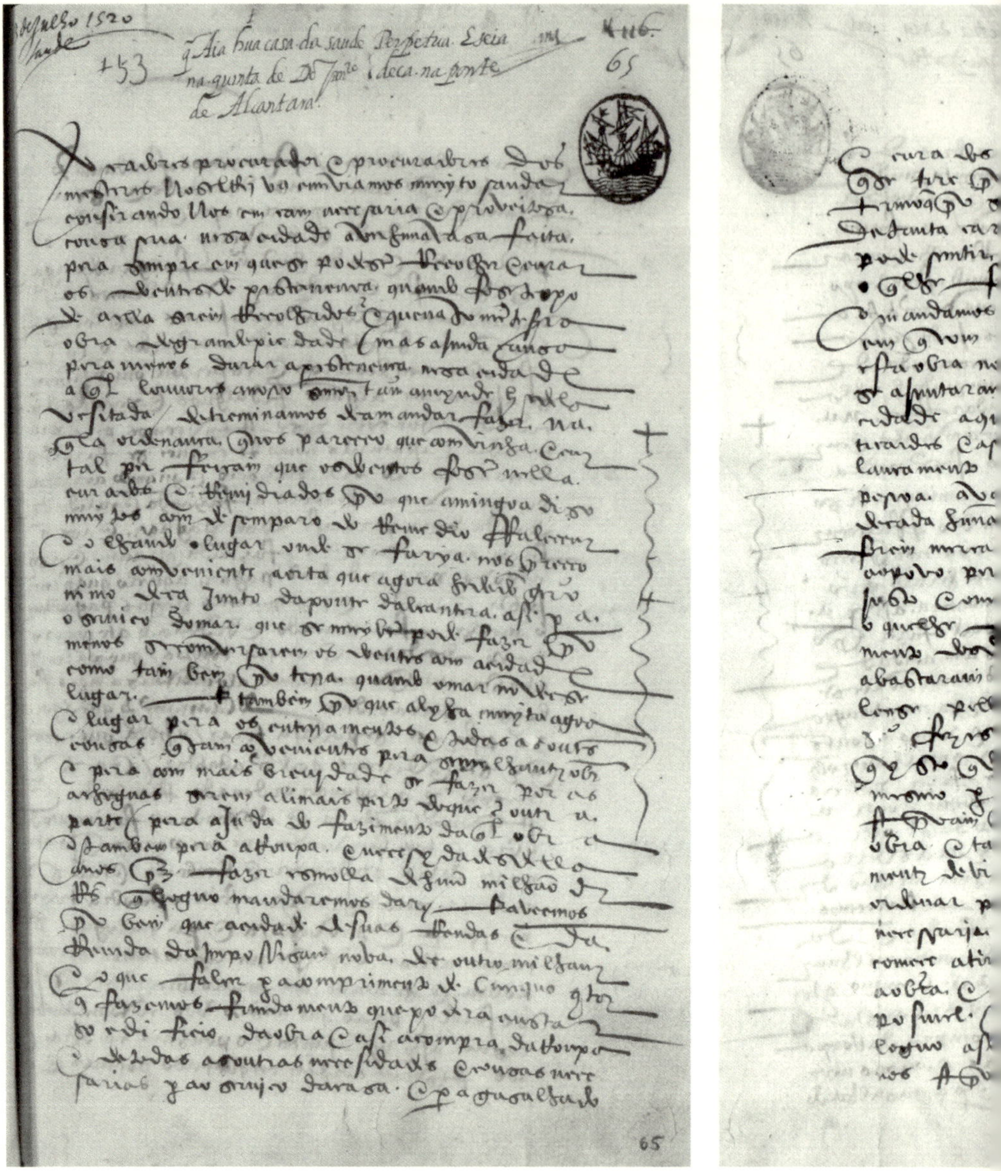

Figg. 2a-2c. AML, Provimento da Saúde, *Livro 1o do provimento da saúde*, f. 65-66v. Image obtained from https://arquivomunicipal3.cm-lisboa.pt.

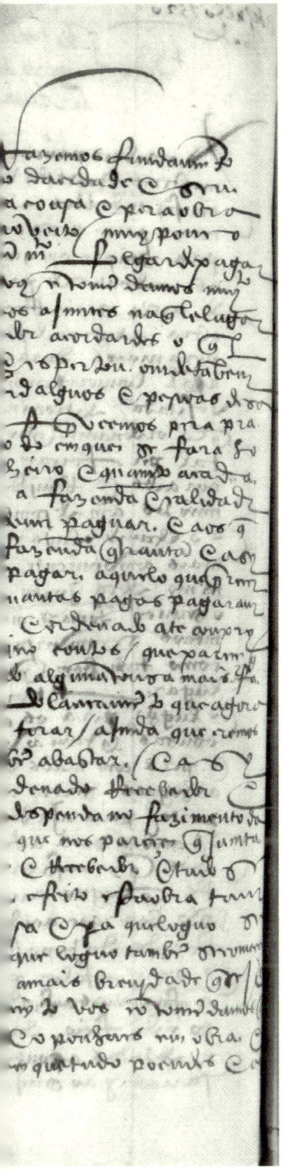

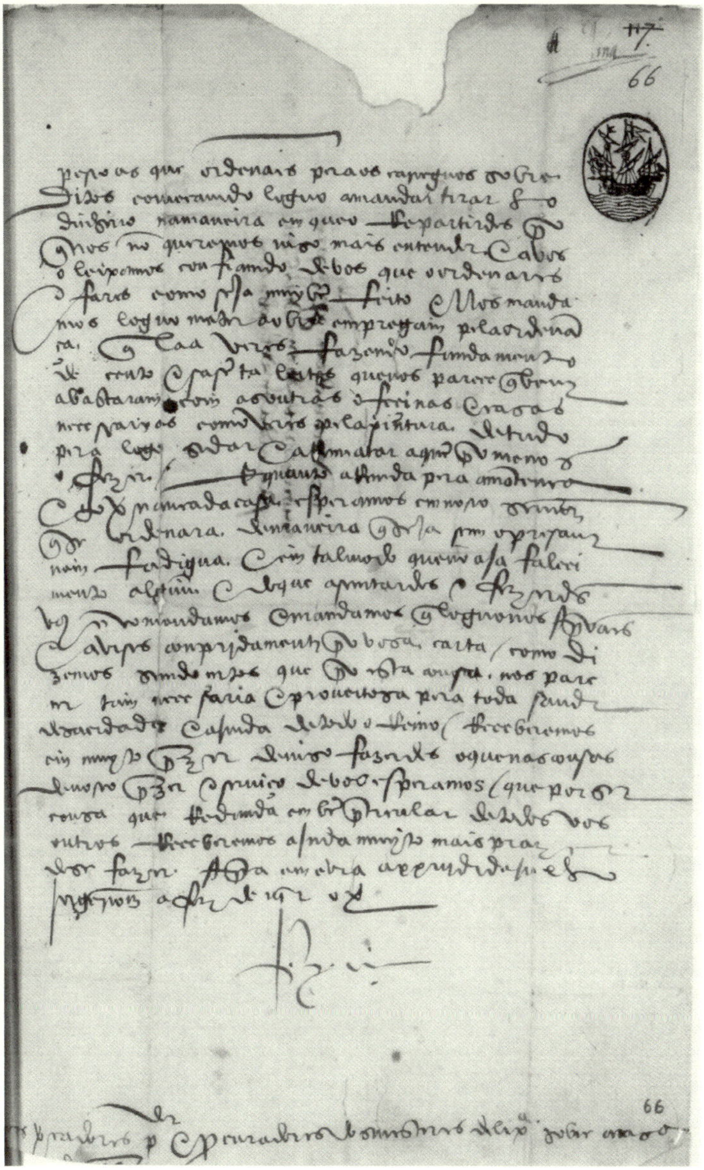

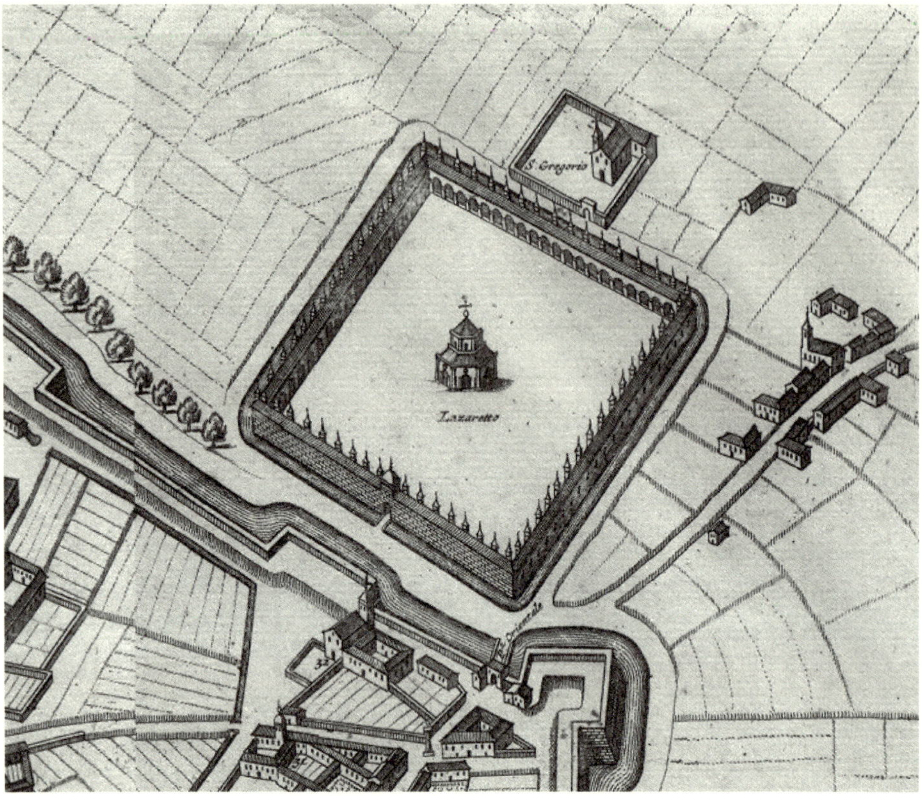


Fig. 3. *Carta di Milano*, detail of the *Lazzaretto* of Milan (1704). Image: © Wikimedia Commons.

Marialuz López-Terrada, Carmel Ferragud

# The Hospitals of the City of Valencia during the Middle Ages and the Renaissance: Academic Knowledge and Ideological Instrumentalisation*

## 1. *Introduction*

Mediaeval hospitals were linked from their origin to the Christian concept of *caritas*, and they were therefore founded and controlled by the Church until the beginning of the late Middle Ages. However, during the 13th and 14th centuries, and under the impetus of the mendicant orders, especially the Franciscans, who were to develop a central role in late mediaeval urban life and whose renewed spirituality promoted the Aristotelian idea of the common good, urban hospitals founded and run by lay people came to occupy a key position in the care of the poor. Indeed, Franciscans and Dominicans were also fervent defenders of the role of medicine in the struggle against poverty and in favour of the salvation of the soul (Arrizabalaga 2014).

The motivations that led urban elites to build hospitals in this period were much more than religious and spiritual. Civic, familiar, personal, political, intellectual, cultural, and material impulses were behind hospital foundations (Scott 2015). In many cases, hospitals served the interests of their founders, who wanted to demonstrate their power and leave a legacy, as much as the beneficiaries and recipients of charitable work. As Bernard de Mandeville declared in 1714: «Pride and vanity have built more hospitals than all the virtues together» (Conejo 2018: 74). These impulses resulted in the construction of architecturally splendorous buildings filled with a profusion of artwork. Hospitals were also tools of political persuasion, playing a crucial role in the primacy of urban oligarchs and the consolidation of civic administrations. Municipal hospitals were, in this regard, privileged spaces. They had emerged either through direct foundation by city councils or because these same municipal governments had eventually become their patrons, as a result of a development of municipal responsibilities that in-

* This study forms part of the following research projects funded by the Ministry of Science and Innovation: *Vernacularidades en la ciencia medieval y renacentista: textos, creadores, profesionales* (PID2021-123419NB-I00; Carmel Ferragud) and *Desde los márgenes. Cultura, experiencia y subjetividad en la Modernidad: género, política y saberes (siglos XVII-XIX)* (PGC2018-097445-A-C22; Marialuz López Terrada).

cluded hygiene and public health. When they worked properly and provided their services, these hospitals became public displays of civic pride. Conversely, a poorly run hospital could signify incompetence, waste, and the impossibility of caring for the needy. This identification developed, most notably, with the advent of hospital mergers and the building of general hospitals during the late Middle Ages.

The diversity of these institutions was extraordinary, and studies have shown that they need to be analysed both in a wider scope and from a microhistorical perspective, as little worlds endowed with rules, their own staff, instruments of management, and documentation. Moreover, hospitals have continued to adapt to social and economic changes and to ideas about health and disease (Rosen 1985). Indeed, in the former Crown of Aragon, hospitals founded in the Middle Ages are still in operation.

The city of Valencia is an ideal setting in which to address the phenomenon of mediaeval and early modern hospitals. The surviving archival sources are a true luxury for historians. As a result, we now count on a substantial body of research. Some publications have already summarised the current state of knowledge (Gallent Marco 2012; Hinojosa 2012). However, our approach to this historiographical tradition aims to go further. We will try to demonstrate how, all too often in recent times, different actors have succumbed to the temptation of using a laudatory, prideful tone in relation to hospitals, with the intent of justifying certain attitudes and political interests.[1] It is quite possible that the hospital-centric model that dominates healthcare nowadays has had something to do with this renewed intention to link the prestige of a city to that of its hospitals. No one can fail to notice the imposing appearance of La Fe Hospital, which greets travellers and citizens on one of the main roads into Valencia. It is now a new sign of local pride. However, we must emphasise the marked teleological nature of this view, based on projecting present categories, such as the central importance of hospitals in the provision of healthcare, back onto the past. It is important to realise that in the period being studied, hospitals did not occupy a central place in local healthcare landscapes, since most health-related resources available to the population were located within the household and the immediate community. Hospitals attended to the poorest strata of society and to people, such as travellers, who had no family and/or community networks to look after them.

Since the Francoist period, and practically up to the present day, certain sectors of the Valencian political classes have sought to instrumentalise the past by turning it into a form of collective memory. This has given rise to a certain craze for commemoration, which has served as a pretext for exhibitions, publications, and investments of public money. In short, they have elevated the role of certain

1. For the studies on hospitals in the city of Valencia that we cite and that were published before 2007, we refer the reader to Marialuz López Terrada and Tayra Lanuza (2007), where all sorts of studies known up to then are collected. In the bibliography at the end of this chapter, we only include works published after the date mentioned.

institutions, which have still kept a physical heritage in the form of buildings, archaeological remains, and important collections of documents, to allow for a particular view of the present based on a wilful reading of the past. Although resorting to the concept of "topolatry", coined by Traverso (2006: 12), might be excessive in this case, it is obvious that the aggrandisement of these places has served to construct a glorious past of political, religious, and scientific grandeur that connects with an idyllic present. Self-serving readings, a lack of perspective, and excessive academic ambition in works in this eulogistic and celebratory vein have led to the reiteration of unfounded clichés, distortions, historiographical errors, and a myriad of overall excesses.

In this study, we aim, in short, to take a critical look at different contributions to the historiography of hospitals in the city of Valencia between the foundation of the kingdom in 1238 and the end of the 16th century. Although this is an arbitrary cut, motivated by reasons of space, it is a sufficient span to show some of the problems that we would like to raise. We also aim to identify some research gaps and future lines of work. This is particularly important, given that the number of monographs and conferences on hospitals in the West has grown significantly in recent years and currently displays remarkable vigour (Abreu, Sheard 2013; Henderson, Horden, Pastore 2007; Huguet-Termes et al. 2014).

## 2. *The Medieval Hospitals Before the Unification of 1512*

The small hospitals founded in the city of Valencia during the 13th, 14th, and 15th centuries have received less attention than the Hospital dels Innocents, founded in 1409, and especially the Hospital General (HGV), dating from 1512. Indeed, we can say that apart from the seminal article by Rodrigo Pertegás (1927) on these small mediaeval hospitals, particularly during the course of the 15th century,[2] a masterly and still essential study, it was not until the 1960s that a group of professional historians intensively researched archival sources to trace their history. Father Robert Burns is responsible for some of the key works on various hospitals founded by the monarchy or military orders during the 13th century (Santa Maria de Roncesvalls and Sant Joan de Jerusalem, both very humble institutions, and especially Sant Vicent), which vanished during the same century. As early as the 1980s, Agustín Rubio Vela, Mercedes Gallent and Mateu Rodrigo Lizondo, in various works, addressed the study of some of the city's hospitals that were in operation up to the founding of the HGV, specifically those of Santa Maria or En Clapers (1311), Santa Llúcia or de la Reina (founded at the end of the 13th century or the beginning of the 14th) and the Hospital de Beguins (founded in 1334). For the latter, we must add the doctoral thesis of Iborra Pina (2003),

2. On the importance of Rodrigo Pertegás for the historiography of Valencian medicine, see: Ferragud, López Terrada 2017.

where the surviving documents can be found transcribed in sequence; this history requires a new approach.

It must be said that the book that most clearly marked the collective study of all the 13th and 14th century hospitals was probably that of Rubio Vela (1984), despite its particular focus on the Hospital d'En Clapers. The documentary appendices of this book show the wealth of Valencian sources for the study of late mediaeval hospitals. In addition, Rubio Vela was a pioneer in the use of literary sources for studying hospitals (Rubio Vela 1983), recently taken up again and expanded, by Ferragud (2022). Similarly, Gallent Marco's PhD thesis and subsequent publications became the benchmark for the 15th century. These studies focused on specific hospitals, working mainly from archive sources and with sufficient data to trace the development of these institutions, such as the Hospital d'En Clapers and the Hospital de la Reina, which soon came under municipal control. These two hospitals were undoubtedly the most important and bore the main burden of managing poverty from their foundation to their absorption into the HGV. They have subsequently been worked on from the point of view of medicalisation (Ferragud 2014). Recently, an article published by Andrea Martí Serrano (2021) has provided a new interpretative perspective by addressing the feeding of the foundlings in these hospitals and their wet nurses during the 15th century.

There were still other small late-mediaeval hospitals about which very little information has survived compared to those previously mentioned: Sant Guillem, En Guiot, En Sorell, En Bou, En Conill, Sant Antoni, and Pobres Sacerdots, for which it has been almost impossible to trace clear institutional histories. Some were short-lived and soon disappeared, or their activity was much more discreet. Others lasted much longer, although they have been less studied. The hospitals of En Bou and En Conill were amalgamated with the Hospital General on 3 August 1847, when the Hospital de Pobres Estudiants, founded by a confraternity of the same name linked to the University in 1540, was also incorporated.[3] The Hospital de Pobres Sacerdots still exists today as a residence for clergy, but in the early modern period it functioned as a hospital for sick members of religious orders. It is not clear whether it was merely a refuge for old and infirm priests and friars or whether they were given some kind of regular medical care. It contains, for example, the cell where an ill Luis Beltrán lived before he died, and where he was visited by Luis Collado, his personal doctor.

A special case is that of the leper house of Sant Llàtzer (St Lazarus), one of the hospitals that has received the most attention recently, although it had hardly been studied up until 1990, when García Verdeguer presented an undergraduate dissertation supervised by Gallent Marco. García Verdeguer's work was the first that can be considered to fall within modern historiographical parameters. Years later, and through the study of judicial proceedings, it was possible to establish

3. Arxiu General i Fotogràfic de la Diputació de València (AGFDV), "Fondo Hospital General". http://archivo.dival.es/es/fondo-documental/fondo-hospital-general.

an overview of the institution, the nature of its tenants, and their function within the leprosarium (GALLENT 2009). Rubio Vela (2014), in turn, has demonstrated the hospital's material poverty through the study of an inventory of 1427. However, these studies do not reflect the vast body of historical research devoted in recent years to the world of leprosy in the West. The most specific approach to the phenomenon of leprosy in late-mediaeval Valencia –set within the context of the Crown of Aragon and the Western world in general– has been that of Ferragud (2018b), based on published studies, archival documentation, and the sermons of St. Vincent Ferrer. In this regard, it is worth noting that in 1512 it was clearly and categorically decided that the hospital of Sant Llàtzer, though institutionally and economically merged into the HGV, should maintain its facilities and that its patients should remain there because of the contagiousness of the disease. Thanks to a 1584 inventory of the HGV's properties,[4] which was upgraded during the 17th century, it is possible to observe the changes that this hospital underwent.

## 3. *Hospital dels Innocents, Wrongly Thought to Be the First Psychiatric Hospital in the World*

The Hospital dels Innocents, founded in Valencia in 1409, has spawned a vast literature, generally characterised by hyperbolic judgements that have more to do with unbridled patriotic passion and presentist vindication than with the rigour that should be expected from professional historians. As a result, there has been a series of misunderstandings, beginning with the institution's actual name.

In fact, the earliest documents on its foundation and the first century of its existence refer to it by various names, as we can see in Gallent's collection of documents (2016). The oldest surviving reference to the name by which the institution would eventually be known (1410) calls it the hospital dels Folls, a Catalan term clearly highlighted in the Latin document, that was not used again. Instead, a papal bull of the same year and all other foundational documents refer to it by other names: *Sanctorum Innocentium* or simply *Innocentium* or *Ignoscents*; *casa dels Ignoscents* and *Beate Marie Ignoscentium* (1424), *Sancta Maria dels Ignoscents* (1427); *Sanctorum Innocentium* (1455). Despite the Marian and saintly invocation, the term that is constantly repeated is *Ignoscents*, probably because of the nature of those housed there and the tendency to simplify the names of hospitals at the time for convenience. And, despite those who insist on the archaic form of *Ignoscents, folls et orats*, it should now be transcribed as Innocents, according to modern philological rules.[5] This archaic denomination, used on many occasions, does not appear in old documents, as far as we have been able to find.

4. AGFDV, HG.III.9 Inventaris, 1584.

5. On other aspects of mental health care in medieval and early modern hospitals see Raúl Villagrasa-Elías' contribution *El loco, el niño y el hospital: la inclusión del pobre verdadero en el espacio urbano renacentista,* in this same volume.

Another misunderstanding concerns the name of the founder, the Mercedarian friar Joan Gilabert. Mateu Rodrigo made it clear in a scholarly article (2002: 41-42) that the second surname Jofre or Jofré should be rejected, as it was an entirely unfounded seventeenth-century addition, introduced by the Mercedarian author Francesc Boïl, one of his hagiographers, with the aim of linking him to a prominent family of the Valencian elite, a common practice in this type of eulogistic work. Therefore, this name Jofre (which for many has now become his first surname) should on no account be maintained, yet it is still commonly used by authors writing on the subject.

The foundation of this hospital and, in particular, the role of its founder, have attracted an inordinate amount of interest due to the ideological baggage they have carried. Thus, the initial eulogistic approach on the part of the Mercedarian friars was picked up at the height of the Francoist dictatorship by psychiatrists and scholars who supported the regime, leading to an interpretation of the Hospital dels Innocents that has come to be called "Jofrism". This interpretation, lucidly described by Polo Griñán as an ideological whole objectifiable in itself (1996: 317; 1997), identified the Catholic Church as the promoter, through Christian charity and the sublime protection of the Virgin, of a landmark in world medicine that had been the pride of Imperial Spain and an example to other countries. Key figures in this respect were the doctors Francisco Marco Merenciano, Francisco Domingo Simó, and José Calatayud Baya, who published countless works, articles in journals of psychiatry and history of medicine, and publications of a markedly local character. It is also worth mentioning that Joan Gilabert was the subject of two doctoral theses at the Complutense University of Madrid (in 1947 and 1951). All this generated an ideology that has been taken up and disseminated by many other authors up to the present day.

This way of thinking emerged at a time when Spanish and Valencian psychiatric institutions were in a deplorable state. A campaign was needed to show internationally that Spanish psychiatry had had a vigorous tradition from time immemorial. The works produced from the 1940s to the 1960s must be understood in a context in which the National Catholicism that prevailed during the Francoist period could arrogate to itself a milestone of continental magnitude. Spain, according to this line of thought, had been a pioneer of psychiatric care through the pious and masterly intervention of a friar.

The first of the pivots on which Jofrism turns is precisely that of the founder of the institution. The exaltation of this character was first reflected in art produced in the context of incipient psychiatry. In 1883, a statue of Fray Gilabert was inaugurated during the closing session of a conference entitled *Primer Certamen Frenopático Español* (First Spanish Phrenopathic Competition) in Barcelona. The young doctor Víctor Azcarreta y Colau (1884) read the biography of the Mercedarian friar at that event, as recorded by him in the proceedings of the conference. Only a few years later, the famous Valencian sculptor José Aixa Íñigo was commissioned to create a sculpture of Gilabert for the gardens of the Hospital General of Valencia. The following year, while in Italy on a scholarship granted by the Provincial Council of Valencia, the painter Joaquín Sorolla committed to painting the canvas *El padre Jofré defendiendo a un loco* (Father Jofré Protecting a Madman), an iconic image of the foundation myth. The painting was a requirement linked to the granting of the scholarship. We believe that these two commissions cannot be separated from the desire to reclaim a figure who had been glorified first in Barcelona, in the emerging context of the so-called Renaixença, a romantic movement that sought to reinvigorate Catalan culture.

Most of the literature on Gilabert is indebted to the Mercedarians; it steers a course between hagiography and the founding story, repeated and mythologised to the point of exhaustion but reaching its climax around the middle of the 20th century. The story goes as follows: after some time in North Africa working to ransom captives, Fray Gilabert returned to Valencia, where he decided to found an institution to cater for the insane and foundlings, after seeing a presumably mentally ill man being mistreated in the street. Gilabert took the man to his monastery to tend his wounds and then immediately preached a Lenten sermon in which he raised the need for a foundation for "mad people" and "maniacs." His contact with Muslim *maristans*, where the mentally ill were looked after, could have been his source of inspiration.[6] For this purpose, he had to persuade the authorities through the intervention of a character called Llorenç Salom. However, apart from the sermon preached by Gilabert and this intervention in favour of the hospital's foundation, we have no further record linking the friar and Salom to the enterprise. So much so that some authors have gone so far as to question the reliability of this story and even that of the original source (Rodrigo Pertegás 1922: 12-13; Peset 1961; Simbor 1992: 214). Nevertheless, Mateu Rodrigo (2002: 44) has insisted on the plausibility of the founding story, and the historian who has done the most and the best work on this hospital did not call these facts into question (Tropé 1994).

We must also address the obstinance with which this hospital has been considered the first psychiatric institution in the world, the first asylum to accommodate exclusively the mentally ill, and an institution where the inmates were treated in an exemplary manner.[7] In reality, this institution took in many other people who were not suffering from mental disorders but from other types of disabilities (such as blindness or paralysis), and beginning in 1493, at the request of its administrators, the hospital began to accept beggars and people who were not suffering from mental disorders (Tropé 1994: 276-77). There has even been talk of the hospital applying occupational therapy for the first time in history. Modern

6. On the *maristan* of Muslim Granada see Pere Marquès' contribution *The Architecture of the Māristān of Granada. Models, Memory, and History of a Building in Recovery*, in this same volume.

7. The Royal Academy of History's Spanish Biographical Dictionary has also perpetuated this same account since the publication in 2014 of the entry on Father Gilabert by Joaquín Millán Rubio, also a Mercedarian. Its popularisation has reached absurd extremes, such as considering Father Gilabert one of the great scientists and inventors silenced by the black legend created against the Spanish Empire (Cervera 2020).

studies disagree on this topic. Although Tropé (1994: 271-85) and Polo Griñán consider that attaching therapeutical valour to the labour of the mentally ill would be an anachronism, López Piñero (2009: 138-40) insisted that this was one of the distinctive features of this hospital, in which it surpassed that of Zaragoza. Indeed, Tropé was emphatic in stating that Father Gilabert did not intend to found an institution that specialised in the medical care of the insane, understood as sick people, but rather a place of refuge, that is, of hospitality (Tropé 1994: 31). The fact that they received medical care, as she herself shows and as was common practice in thousands of institutions all over Europe, is another matter all together. All this shows the need to dispel doubts about what has been a commonplace feature in a certain kind of historiography, which has maintained that mental illness was associated with witchcraft or demonic possession. This could not be further from the truth: European institutions that catered to the insane understood them as sick, and treated them, even if they did so poorly, with remedies, medicines, and prescriptions that were thought to be appropriate to Galenic theory.

Finally, the Jofrist narrative harped on the use of this hospital in order to turn it into an example of the glories contributed by Valencia to Spain and the world: the "universal unity of destiny", an essentialist, eulogistic discourse that connects with Claudio Sánchez Albornoz and the debate with Américo Castro on the Hispanic character and its splendours and miseries. The Spanish spirit, essentially Catholic, rose once again to universal heights through its magnificent contribution to medical science.

Not surprisingly, the celebration of events with a strong international impact, such as the celebration of the first centenary of the Washington mental hospital (1955) or the World Psychiatry Congress in Madrid (1966), was used to propagate the Jofrist paradigm far and wide (Simbor 1992: 93; Polo Griñán 1996: 320). It is also interesting to note that while professional historians of medicine have in general been fairly restrained in their assessment of the Hospital dels Innocents, a few Spanish and international psychiatrists frequently echoed the Jofrist paradigm in the 1960s and 1970s, and the occasional surprising study in the same vein can still be found today (Polo Griñán 1996: 315). However, more critical and moderate voices on the subject have recently become more prominent, emphasising the limited usefulness of disputes about priority and the need to pay more attention to the historical contexts that gave rise to the hospital, when psychiatry was not a discipline, mental illness was not regarded in the way it is now, and hospitals were very different institutions from the current ones (Pérez et al. 2012).

The foundation's sixth centennial deserves special attention for the volume of publications and exhibitions it produced. The year 2009 was declared the Year of Solidarity (*600 Anys de Solidaritat*) by the Valencian regional government, which paid homage to Joan Gilabert (Father Jofré, of course). During that year, all political rhetoric was charged: «Valencia was the world pioneer in opening a hospital dedicated to the mentally ill in June 1410. Father Jofré was the driving force behind the project» (the article published in the Valencian newspaper

*Levante EMV* on 24 February 2009 subscribed to all the claims typical of the Jofrism of the Francoist past). «The Generalitat [the Valencian regional government] wishes to lay claim to a historical constant that has characterised the Valencians, because they have always been pioneers in matters of social justice and solidarity with the weakest and neediest». In view of certain excesses on part of the Valencian government that later came to light, such statements could not be more ironic. But it was openly declared that the Hospital dels Innocents had been the model to be followed in the Crown of Aragon, Castile, and other countries. After all, it was once again a display of pride to be exhibited internationally in Valencia, a city and region that seemed to have no limits in organising events with an international impact.

José M. López Piñero, who died a year later, was tasked with publishing a book about the hospital, which was sponsored by the City Council (2009). In it, he constantly attacked the chauvinism that gave rise to those countless distortions. Severe, forceful, and determined to set things right, López Piñero sought to locate the institution within its medical context, and to this end, he introduced some details about its medical practise and its practitioners at the time of its founding. His intention was to demonstrate that the foundation arose from a process inherent in the development of medicine at the time, when the insane came to be considered within the rational logic of disease. However, the book is ultimately somewhat confusing in introducing many facts, authors, and quotations that do not quite make sense. Some of its statements, such as the considerations on the therapeutic role of work and the enormous influence of the hospital on other centres, could well be disputed. The engagement of the sick in work directed by the hospital, even in its management, was also a reality in other hospitals.

## 4. *The Hospital General and its Commemorations: A Missed Opportunity*

The construction of the HGV must be contextualised within the profound processes of transformation that mediaeval hospitals underwent over the course of the 15th and early 16th centuries throughout Western Europe.[8] The general trend consisted of the disappearance of small and no longer viable mediaeval institutions and the creation of large hospitals, where a much more diversified type of care, defined as "general", was provided. This development occurred over many years and was explained by a wide range of causes and factors, including changes in mentality towards poverty, demographic growth, increasing public health problems, and the incorporation of hospital care into the ideological and political thinking of the urban oligarchs who governed municipalities. The birth of these changes also coincided with a period of transformation in medical ideas, marked by major changes in

8. On the processes of hospital fusion and the emergence of general hospitals see Josep Barceló's contribution *The Birth of the General Hospital: Background and Development of a New Physical and Symbolic Space of Care in the Late Medieval City,* in this same volume.

relation to therapeutic practice, the emergence of new diseases, such as the French pox, and the reduced incidence of others, such as leprosy. Finally, we must bear in mind that the public authorities' intention behind these amalgamations was to both consolidate the economy of the mediaeval hospital institutions and improve their capacity (Henderson 2006; López Terrada 1999). According to Mollat (1978), once it had been accepted that healthcare was a social problem and the urban administration took responsibility for it, the amalgamation of a city's hospitals should be seen as the logical conclusion of the rationalisation of care, seeking better management of resources, a greater return on investments, and above all, more effective care (Rosen 1985; Henderson 2006; Villagrasa 2016).

Then again, the religious and moral climate of the Reformation and Counter-Reformation, between the late 16th and early 17th centuries, saw the development of a large number of new charitable initiatives aimed at different categories of the needy, a phenomenon that Pullan (1994 and 2005) has characterised as «the new "redemptive charity"». Despite the fact that laypeople were the primary architects of this two-hundred-year-old new network of welfare institutions, including unified hospitals, these initiatives have been overly attributed to religious motivations. Urban oligarchies have been portrayed as little more than executors of the will of the Counter-Reformation Church, with their behaviour being inspired by religious orders and the voice of the confessor. However, as with the foundation of the HGV, the link between welfare and privilege was a feature of charity in an *Ancien Régime* society: hospitals were associated with a social group's prestige and image (Cavallo 1989). But in a society like that of 16th century Valencia, all welfare initiatives were informed by both the will to create new spaces for the care and cure of the sick poor, since urban authorities counted public health among their responsibilities, and Christian charity, given the weight of religion in many aspects of contemporaneous life. It should not be forgotten that most of the mediaeval Valencian hospitals were of religious origin. After all, urban authorities understood the provision of care for the poor as their own responsibility and therefore intervened in the functioning of hospitals, through the control of their administration and resources, and took repressive measures against beggars (Garbellotti 2006: 118).

In the Crown of Aragon, the transformation of the mediaeval hospital network began, as in most Italian territories, much earlier than in other European territories such as Castile, thanks, in large part, to the political and economic power and dynamism of the urban oligarchies of the major cities and to the close commercial and intellectual relations between these two Mediterranean areas (Grell et al. 1999; Arrizabalaga 1999; Cavallo 1989). Moreover, it shows that the phenomenon reached small urban centres as well as big cities and both the urban and the rural sphere. And also, that the strategies of amalgamation were varied and that some places took other earlier ones as an example to create their general hospitals (Villagrasa 2016).

The doctoral thesis of Marialuz López Terrada (1986) on the HGV's first century of history was, without doubt, a turning point in the study of the institution. The surviving archival documents, absolutely exceptional for their continuity, offered the possibility of an analysis from a perspective rooted in "total history," that examined the hospital, which would take over the powers and functions of the city's aforementioned late-medieval hospitals, as a whole. The thesis has never been published in full, although some of its topics, especially those related to the hospital's patients and medical care, have been reworked as articles and book chapters (LÓPEZ TERRADA 1989; 1992; 1998; 1999; 2002; 2014). Many authors have been indebted to its legacy, though they have not always duly acknowledged it. Subsequently, other theses have addressed the hospital in the 17th and 18th centuries (VILAR 1996; CÍSCAR 1992).

Following up from that seminal investigation, many other studies have worked on HGV, such as the art history thesis and publications of Mercedes Gómez Ferrer (1995; 1998) on its architecture: according to Gómez Ferrer, the physical form of the hospital adapted to changing contexts and circumstances, and the architectural models of hospitals imitated each other. This was the case with the cruciform hospital, an important topic in the history of hospital architecture (LEISTIKOW 1967; THOMPSON, GOLDIN 1975; JETTER 1960, 1980).

The twenty-first century has seen the production of a continuous stream of works, very often characterised by offering a summary of what has already been said by others on the HGV rather than original contributions. The first of these as published in 2002 under the enigmatic title *De hospitium, folls i malalts: L'Hospital General de València*, a photographic catalogue that appeared on the occasion of the exhibition held in the Galeria del Tossal, which was connected with the archaeological excavations carried out in 1997-98 in the area of the hospital, during the construction of the *Museu Valencià de la Il·lustració i la Modernitat* (MuVIM: Valencian Museum of the Enlightenment and Modernity). The 158 photographs were accompanied by eleven articles: five offered a description and interpretation of the items discovered in those excavations, and the other six were summaries of works that were already known, with one or two that contributed things that had not yet been said. These excavations were repeated in 2012-2013, not without problems connected with political strategies unrelated to archaeological interest. These later works did not give rise to any publication.

The public presentation of this volume by the then councillor Miquel Domínguez displayed some of the clichés that have already seen: «An institution of deep significance to Valencians»; «one of the first cities to secularise healthcare»; «on the Hospital de Folls, one of the first psychiatric hospitals in Europe [...] in which the confraternity has its origins». The laudatory tone recalls that which was used during Francisco Camps' government, with Esteban González Pons as *conseller* (regional minister), when the Monastery of Santa Maria de Valldigna was turned into an emblem of Valencianness, a kind of Monastery of Montserrat with which Valencian autonomist patriotism could identify (FERRAGUD 2007).[9] One way of creating unity and cohesion in a group is through

9. The Benedictine monastery of Santa Maria de Montserrat has become one of the national emblems of Catalonia, at least since the late 19th century.

powerful symbols. Valencian politicians understood this and sought them among those that had been most conspicuous in the past but were still visible and present. Moreover, they could be used as a basis for intervention, since the attachment of Valencians to these places seemed indisputable, something that is perhaps not so obvious.

Unfortunately, the collaboration between archaeologists, architects, and historians has not been ideally fruitful, as it has resulted in an approach that has not taken into account the works published by experts on the history of hospitals. Other publications, of an institutional and non-academic nature, soon followed, marked by the approaching 5th centenary of the founding of the HGV in 2012. The previous years, and at least until 2007, had seen the proliferation of private foundations in Valencia, when the financial devastation caused by the collapse of Lehman Brothers and its subsequent shock waves were not yet foreseeable. In this context, major anniversaries were a good opportunity for self-promotion. One of such foundations was the Fundació Hospital Reial i General, which was created for the purpose of recovering and disseminating the hospital's heritage in its broadest sense. In that context, Marialuz López Terrada and Tayra Lanuza (2007), two historians of medicine and science attached to the López Piñero Institute for the History of Medicine and Science, were entrusted with preparing a compilation of the historiography of the HGV. The promoters of the Foundation announced that this would be the first of many works devoted to the study of the institution, from its earliest days to the present. We certainly cannot say that those expectations were fulfilled. The authors produced a meticulous work that collected everything written up till then on the city's hospital institutions, including all the mediaeval ones, most of which were amalgamated into the general hospital in 1512. The project turned out to be a fiasco, due to the Foundation's unfortunate interference in the text; the academic standards necessary for this type of work were not observed, the layout and publishing were amateurish, and the copies published were not distributed. The haste to obtain political returns took precedence over bringing projects of this kind to a successful conclusion. Indeed, this book was the only result of a whole wider plan that included great events, exhibitions, and publications drawn up by the Foundation in 2007 to celebrate the institution's five hundred years of existence, although an attempt was made by the then directors of the HGV to reactivate the process in 2010-11.

Soon afterwards, the Valencian medical community, and more specifically doctors who were or had been associated with the HGV, became involved in this commemorative trend. In this regard, the most notable contribution was the publication of a book by two surgeons, members of the Royal Academy of Medicine of the Valencian Community (Narbona Arnau, Tormo Alfonso 2008), which was merely a summary of previous works, whose content and documentation they used indiscriminately and without the slightest rigour. This book is a perfect example of what happens when authors with no historical training tackle a subject as complex as the historical study of hospitals. As we have already pointed out, it is an element common to many of the works published on the Valencian hospitals of all periods, produced by doctors with no training in history of any kind.

Naturally, 2012 was also marked by a new series of publications, coinciding with the anniversary of the hospital's foundation. The most notable for their size and for the financial investment involved were the two large volumes coordinated by José Hinojosa Montalvo. They were actually summaries of works already published by their authors. They did not constitute any original contribution, except for the extraordinary number of photographs, though these were placed in the book seemingly without rhyme or reason. Of course, the public presentations of these books were co-opted by politicians, who harped once again on the usual clichés.

Also coinciding with the 2012 anniversary, the archivist Francisco J. Sanchis Moreno published two notable works. The first was a facsimile of the parchment containing the arbitration award that led to the foundation of the HGV, preserved in the Arxiu General i Fotogràfic of the Diputació de València (General and Photographic Archive of the Provincial Council of Valencia) and bearing the number 3343. This was a collector's item in a luxury case, of which only a few hundred were produced. It was accompanied by a transcription and translation of the document. The second publication was a voluminous book, accompanied by a CD-ROM, about the HGV's archive, which analyses the whole collection of documents preserved right from its foundation up to 1868, also including documentary evidence of the holdings that originally came from the Hospital dels Innocents, and of all the people who in some way oversaw its development and stewardship, especially its archivists. Lists of *clavaris* (wardens), presidents, and directors up to 1900 were also provided, as were literary extracts containing information on the hospital throughout its history. This book is a long-winded and exhaustive approach to all kinds of written remnants that may allude to or have been in contact with the HGV (including various inscriptions). The author explains how and why these documents were generated, who wrote and organised them, and what they were used for.

In 2016, Mercedes Gallent Marco's book *Orígenes del sistema sanitario valenciano: documentos fundacionales del Hospital General de Valencia* was published. The author had already addressed the process of amalgamation of the mediaeval Valencian hospitals into the HGV, as well as the influences exerted by other general hospitals, in various studies, starting with her doctoral thesis (1980, 1982, 2002, 2012, 2014). On this occasion, Gallent offered a transcription of sixty documents related to the foundation of the HGV (some of them from previous hospitals and connected with the Cofradía de los Desamparados Inocentes [Confraternity of the Forsaken Innocents], linked to the hospital of the same name, which had nothing to do with the process), between 1409 and 1589, plus a final document from 1848. The author thereby intended to show that the foundation was a long process, lasting almost a century, and that the Hospital dels Innocents played a dominant role in it. We will not dispute the relevance of this contribution, although the documents lack a careful transcription in accordance with current editing criteria in Catalan philology, especially considering that most of them had already been published several times. What is more significant, as seen in the book's title, is that it suggests that the hospital-centric system of the present day gradually evolved from the mediaeval and early modern world. However, the process of social medicalisation was much more complex and extended in time; indeed, it must be dated between the last quarter of the 13th century and the beginning of the 14th, and it extended far beyond the world of hospitals (FERRAGUD 2018a, 2019).

It is also worth reflecting on the fact that during this period of heightened political interest in the subject, let alone in the following decade, there were no doctoral theses devoted to the study of the HGV in the modern period. The only three exceptions are Emma Jávega Charco's research on the hospital's foundlings, initiated with an undergraduate dissertation (2000) and continued in a doctoral thesis (2006 2010), María Teresa Pérez Villalba's thesis (2017) on French migrations to Valencia during the 16th century,[10] and the more recent work of Alfredo García Femenía (2020) on graphic culture and literacy through the study of the receipts deposited in four hospitals during the 15th and early 16th centuries (En Clapers, la Reina, Innocents and the HGV). This same author has used the HGV's sources to explore the management of the feeding of children in the hospital (GARCÍA FEMENÍA 2019). Although all three authors use sources from the hospital's archive, these are not studies of the hospital as such. In short, we can say that the political interest in the institution did not come with a parallel academic focus. All the more considering that there are still many aspects to be studied, such as the hospital's patients, who were the institution's true central figures and the reason for its existence.

The academic studies generated by the HGV has probably reached only a small audience. We should therefore highlight various works that have brought the subject closer to the general public (LÓPEZ TERRADA, FERRAGUD 2016), as well as summaries of an academic nature, such as those published in the journal *El médico* and in the history of the University of Valencia directed by Mariano Peset (LÓPEZ TERRADA 1994;1999).

## 5. *New Challenges for Future Studies*

As we have seen throughout this chapter, the hospitals of the city of Valencia up to the beginning of the 17th century have been the subject of many different historiographical approaches. However, the exceptionally rich sources available, abundant and in some cases unexplored, and the fact that many of these studies do not incorporate new historiographical make it necessary to reconsider the subject.

Despite the numerous publications (often of a commemorative nature, born as the result of institutional anniversaries), an up-to-date cataloguing and digitisa-

10. It is worth mentioning that the hospital's books had already been used as a demographic source to study migration (BENÍTEZ SÁNCHEZ-BLANCO, SALVADOR ESTEBAN 1998; BENÍTEZ SÁNCHEZ-BLANCO 2003).

tion of important documentary sources with relevant information is still needed. The Municipal Archive and that of the Diputación (Provincial Council), among others, have not yet made electronic and digital resources available to researchers. This may be one of the reasons, combined perhaps with historiographical trends, that explain why no doctoral theses have been produced in the last twenty years on some of the many issues that have yet to be studied. In contrast, the Santa Creu Hospital in Barcelona has recently been the subject of several articles, undergraduate and master's dissertations and three doctoral theses.

In this regard, we believe that the circumstances surrounding the formation of the HGV must be thoroughly reconsidered from new historiographical perspectives (Henderson 2006; Abreu, Sheard 2013; Henderson, Horden, Pastore 2007; Huguet Termes et al 2014; Horden 2020; Villanueva, Conejo, Villagrasa 2018; Comelles, Conejo, Barceló-Prats 2018). We therefore need to study why the hospital merging of Valencia occurred at a much later date than in other cities of the Crown of Aragon, without assuming traditional prejudices and uncritical eulogies, particularly those regarding the aforementioned Hospital dels Innocents. The hospital's founding has to be relocated within the new historiography of mediaeval and Renaissance hospitals, studying these institutions without falling for the teleological idea of a hospital history aimed at the triumph of modern biomedicine.

To do so, the history of the HGV should be reconsidered from a perspective that takes into account the role of the urban oligarchy and the local authorities in its governance, both economically and as a tool to manage poverty and disease (López Terrada 1999; Henderson 2006; Horden 2020). The hospital became a civic institution with a vital role in preserving urban healthcare. In replacing the small and fragmented mediaeval hospitals, the new hospital enjoyed sufficient resources to cope with both the increase in the number of poor people and the emergence of new diseases such as the French pox. We are speaking, in short, of inserting the Renaissance HGV into the history of changing attitudes towards poverty, especially on the part of the urban authorities. Luis Vives and his *De subventione pauperum*, though written in a context very far from that of Valencia, is an example of these new theories on poverty, since rather than suggesting new forms of regulation, his text prefigures a trend of the new charity policies that were to be developed by many European cities over the course of the 16th and 17th centuries. These measures, despite the author's "Valencianness", have not been analysed in relation to his home city, and can be summed up in the basic principle that the urban authorities considered it their task to provide care for poor people who needed it, and therefore cities "monitored" the work carried out in hospitals, controlled the administration of charitable resources, and took repressive measures against beggars (Garbellotti 2006: 118; López Terrada 1999). In a society like 16th century Valencia every kind of welfare strategy aimed at the poor was driven and influenced both by a need for "social control" and Christian charity. We must not forget the religious origin of most of the mediaeval hospitals of Valencia.

It is important to bear in mind that, with very few exceptions, studies on Valencian hospitals have not incorporated the new historiography that has emerged since the 1970s (Horden 1988): that is to say, a comparative, sociological, and contextual approach in a broad sense, in opposition to individualised studies of single institutions at one particular point in time. In other words, it is necessary to study hospitals within their social, cultural, religious, and medical frameworks, acknowledging from a teleological standpoint that a hospital is much more than its doctors and the medicine practised in it (Granshaw, Porter 1989). In this sense, if the Hospital del Innocents had been studied within the context of what mental illness and its care were in late-mediaeval society, and specifically in the Kingdom of Valencia, the tradition that we have exposed would have taken a very different turn. This type of study requires a longue durée approach that has never been applied in the Valencian context, but is nevertheless necessary in order to address the evolution of the city's mediaeval hospitals, up to their late disappearance and the emergence of the HGV. In the traditional history of medicine, this latter hospital has been mistakenly viewed as the beginning of the medicalization and subsequent modernization of a form of care that continues to the present day, rather than as a continuation of mediaeval hospital practices, ignoring the relationship between hospital governors and the urban administration, and similarly ignoring the role of political institutions (Garbellotti 2006: 119). We must therefore reject the notion of a radical break with the past, despite the important innovations that characterised the Renaissance hospital and, in a way, made it different from its mediaeval predecessors.

In a similar vein, several studies have been centred on the leitmotif of "medicalisation", despite that regarding the historical hospital as an exclusively medical institution is to project our own categories onto a world that thought of itself differently. However, a few studies do include a multidisciplinary perspective, in accordance with the most recent social history of medicine, to try to reach the broadest possible view of the hospital in society: "Medicine and doctors certainly appear, but as only one facet of changing varieties of therapy rather than as the defining moment in the arrival of modernity" (Henderson, Horden, Pastore 2007: 37). We therefore think that, within the history of medicine, the role of the hospital as a promoter of health needs to be researched in a much broader context than just that of doctors, to include subjects and practices that were central to the mediaeval and Renaissance world view, such as "healing the soul." Although the topic of medical treatment in the context of the hospital is indeed important, its religious component is no less so. The dedication of hospitals to the sick poor was always justified in terms of Christian charity, and all those who worked in the hospital were instructed to care for the sick "for the health of their souls." This idea must be taken into account in order to avoid an anachronistic image of the institution as essentially medical and with a purpose of healing exclusively through medicine. In line with contemporary architectural principles on the relationship between beauty and function, both the functionality and design of hospital buildings responded to reasons that were partly medical, such as high rooms to allow ventilation through the windows, and partly religious, such as providing a view of the altar from the patients' beds and enabling them to participate in mass. These principles were reflected in their façades as well as devotional images commissioned from important painters and sculptors, emphasising their dual medical and religious roles (Henderson 2006: 91).

However, there are other central issues that have been neglected by Valencian medical historiography. According to new trends, we must go beyond doctors and functions, as well as the role of the staff who cared for the sick on a daily basis, or the spaces devoted to healing, and give the patient a central role (Berco 2016; Kahlow 2020). Because –and this is perhaps one of the most striking deficiencies, given the large amount of source material available to analyse it– there are no studies centred around the patients of these institutions, apart from some aspects partially examined in some of the published monographs. So, a study of the patients of Valencian hospitals is required, emphasising the fact that practitioners and patients shared the same "Galenic" view of medicine, based on humoral theory. Therefore, as Henderson (2006: xxix–xxx) says: «In this sense the hospital itself can be seen as a "non-natural environment" in which all the various personnel made important contributions to help return the patient to health by administering physical and spiritual medicine, providing the right diet and also adjusting the temperature and air supply of his or her physical surroundings». These institutions should not be viewed as a place to die, but rather as a therapeutic option among others, depending on the patient's financial means, such as seeing a doctor, surgeon, healer, or traditional practitioner. One of the main attractions of the new Renaissance hospitals for the poor was that patients could obtain medical-pharmacological treatments there, such as mercury ointments for *morbo gallico*, to which they had no access outside of the institution. In other words, these hospitals should be seen as one more alternative in Valencian medical pluralism.

## *Bibliography*[11]

Abreu, Laurinda; Sheard, Sally, 2013. *Hospital Life: Theory and Practice from the Medieval to the Modern*, Oxford, Peter Lang.

Arrizabalaga Valbuena, Jon, 1999. "Poor Relief in Counter-Reformation Castile: An Overview", ed. Olle P. Grell et al. *Health Care and Poor Relief in Counter-Reformation Europe*, London, Routledge: 151-176.

Berco, Cristian, 2016. *From Body to Community: Venereal Disease and Society in Baroque Spain*, Toronto, University of Toronto Press.

Cavallo, Sandra, 1989. "Charity, Power and Patronage in Eighteenth-Century Italian Hospitals: The Case of Turin", Lindsay Granshaw, Roy Porter (ed.), *The Hospital in History*, London, Routledge: 93-122.

11. For the studies on hospitals in the city of Valencia that we cite and that were published before 2007, we refer the reader to: López Terrada, Lanuza 2007; here all sorts of studies known up to then are collected. In the bibliography we only include works published after the date mentioned and other general studies on hospitals.

CERVERA, César, 2020. "32 científicos e inventores españoles que cambiaron el mundo y fueron borrados por la Leyenda Negra", *ABC Historia*, 22/10/2020.

COMELLES, Josep M.; CONEJO DA PENA, Antoni; BARCELÓ-PRATS, Josep (ed.), 2018. *Imago civitatis. Hospitales y manicomios en Occidente*, Tarragona, URV-UB.

CONEJO DA PENA, Antoni, 2018. "'El orgullo y la vanidad han construido más hospitales que todas las virtudes juntas'. Patronazgo artístico y patrimonio hospitalario en la Corona de Aragón (siglos XIV-XV)", *Revista de la CECEL*, 18: 69-112.

FERRAGUD, Carmel, 2007. "La interpretació de la història: el cas del monestir de Santa Maria de Valldigna", Xosé M. Souto (ed.), *Itinerarios educativos y actividades escolares*, València, L'Ullal Edicions-Federació d'ensenyament de CCOO-PV: 31-44.

FERRAGUD, Carmel, 2014. "La introducción de los practicantes de la medicina en los hospitales del reino de Valencia durante la Baja Edad Media", Teresa Huguet-Termes et al. (ed.), *Ciudad y hospital en el Occidente europeo (1300-1700)*, Lleida, Milenio: 305-324.

FERRAGUD, Carmel, 2018a. "Los espacios de la práctica médica en la Valencia bajomedieval", Concepción Villanueva, Antoni Conejo, Raúl Villagrasa-Elías (ed.), *Redes hospitalarias. Historia, economía y sociología de la sanidad*, Zaragoza, Institución Fernando el Católico: 31-52.

FERRAGUD, Carmel, 2018b. "El predicador i la lepra. Malaltia i moral en els sermons de sant Vicent Ferrer", *Afers*, 33/90-91: 325-352.

FERRAGUD, Carmel, 2019. *Una ciutat medieval en cerca de la salut (Xàtiva, 1250-1500)*, Catarroja-Xàtiva, Afers & Ajuntament de Xàtiva.

FERRAGUD, Carmel, 2022. *L'hospital, la dona i el capellà. Sant Andreu de Mallorca (1230-1445)*, Catarroja et al., Afers.

FERRAGUD, Carmel; Marialuz LÓPEZ TERRADA, 2017. "El culte al document. L'historiador valencià Josep Rodrigo Pertegàs (1854-1930)", *Afers*, 32/86: 119-145.

GALLENT MARCO, Mercedes, 2009. "Control municipal y vida cotidiana en el hospital de Sant Llàtzer de Valencia", María I. Valdivieso, Pascual Martínez (ed.), *Castilla y el mundo feudal. Homenaje al profesor Julio Valdeón*, Valladolid, Junta de Castilla y León & Universidad de Valladolid: III, 447-461.

GALLENT MARCO, Mercedes, 2010-2011. "En el interior de los hospitales. Personas, espacios, enseres", *Saitabi*, 60-61: 81-104.

GALLENT MARCO, Mercedes, 2012. "La asistencia sanitaria a los marginados en la Edad Media", *Clio & Crimen*, 9: 135-164.

GALLENT MARCO, Mercedes, 2014. "Los hospitales de la Santa Creu de Barcelona y Nuestra Señora de Gracia de Zaragoza, dos modelos asistenciales para el Hospital General de Valencia", *Aragón en la Edad Media*, 25: 41-60.

GALLENT MARCO, Mercedes, 2015. *Orígenes del sistema sanitario valenciano: documentos fundacionales del Hospital General de Valencia*, València, Institució Alfons el Magnànim.

GARBELLOTTI, Marina, 2007. "Assets of the Poor, Assets of the City: The Management of Hospital Resources in Verona between the Sixteenth and Eighteenth Centuries", John Henderson et al. (ed.), *The Impact of Hospitals: 300-2000*, Oxford, Peter Lang: 117-34.

GARCÍA FEMENÍA, Alfredo, 2019. "La casa del portugués: una casa de dides al servei de l'Hospital General de València (1512-1522)", *Afers*, 45/92: 129-47.

GARCÍA FEMENÍA, Alfredo, 2020. *Pràctiques d'escriptura de la família Roig: alfabetització i educació gràfica en el llindar de la modernitat (València, 1450-1518)*, PhD thesis, Universitat de València.

GRANSHAW, Lindsay; PORTER, Roy (ed.), 1989. *The Hospital in History*, London, Routledge.

GRELL, Olle Peter; CUNNINGHAM, Andrew; ARRIZABALAGA VALBUENA, Jon (ed.), 1999. *Health Care and Poor Relief in Counter-Reformation Europe*, London, Routledge.

HENDERSON, John, 2006. *The Renaissance Hospital: Healing the Body and Healing the Soul*, New Haven, Yale University Press.

HENDERSON, John; HORDEN, Peregrine; PASTORE, Alessandro (ed.), 2007. *The Impact of Hospitals 300-2000*, Oxford, Peter Lang.

Hinojosa Montalvo, José (ed.), 2012. *Hospital General de Valencia 1512-2012*, València, Fundació Hospital Reial i General.

Horden, Peregrine, 1988. "A Discipline of Relevance: The Historiography of the Later Medieval Hospital", *Social History of Medicine*, 1/3: 359-374.

Horden Peregrine, 2020. *Cultures of Healing: Medieval and After*, London, Routledge.

Huguet-Termes, Teresa; Verdés i Pijuan, Pere; Arrizabalaga Valbuena, Jon; Sánchez Martínez, Manuel (ed.), 2014. *Ciudad y hospital en el Occidente europeo (1300-1700)*, Lleida, Milenio.

Javéga Charco, Emma, 2006 *Expósitos en la Valencia de la primera mitad del siglo XVI*, PhD thesis, Universitat de València.

Javéga Charco, Emma, 2010. *Expósitos en la Valencia de la primera mitad del siglo XVI*, València, Institució Alfons el Magnànim.

Jetter, Dieter, 1960. "Hospitalgebäude in Spanien", *Sudhoffs Archiv für Geschichte der Medizin und der Naturwissenschaften*, 44/3: 239-258.

Jetter, Dieter, 1980. *Geschichte des Hospitals, Band 4: Spanien von den Anfängen bis um 1500*, Wiesbaden, Franz Steiner.

Kahlow, Simone, 2020. *Archäologie des Hospitals: "Pauperes et infirmi" in Fürsorgeinstitutionen nördlich der Alpen vom 12. bis zum 19. Jahrhundert*, Berlin, Peter Lang.

Leistikow, Dankwart, 1967. *Edificios hospitalarios en Europa durante diez siglos. Historia de la arquitectura hospitalaria*, Ingelheim am Rhein, C. H. Boehringer Sohn.

López Piñero, José María, 2009. *El Hospital de "Ignoscents, Folls e Orats" (1409-1512) y la medicina valenciana durante el siglo XV*, València, Ajuntament de València.

López Piñero, José María; Soriano Sánchez, Rafaela, 2009. *VI Centenario de la Fundación del Hospital de Ignoscents, folls e orats*, València, Ajuntament de València.

López Terrada, Marialuz, 2014. "Las finanzas de una institución asistencial: la gestión económica del Hospital General de Valencia durante el siglo XVI", ed. Teresa Huguet-Termes et al. *Ciudad y hospital en el Occidente europeo (1300-1700)*, Lleida, Milenio: 263-283.

López Terrada, Marialuz; Ferragud, Carmel, 2016. "L'hospital General de València en els seus primers temps", *La Veu del País Valencià*, 01/12/2016.

López Terrada, Marialuz; Lanuza Navarro, Tayra, 2007. *Los estudios históricos sobre el Hospital General de Valencia*, València, Fundació Hospital Reial i General.

Martí Serrano, Andrea, 2021. "El treball de les dides als hospitals valencians del segle XV", *Saitabi*, 71: 105-123.

Mollat, Michel, 1978. *Les Pauvres au Moyen Âge*, Paris, Hachette.

Narbona Arnau, Benjamín; Tormo Alfonso, Vicente, 2008. *Historia del Santo Hospital General de Valencia (1512-1990)*, Valencia, Real Academia de Medicina de la Comunidad Valenciana.

Pérez, Jesús; Baldessarini, Ross J.; Undurraga, Juan; Sánchez Moreno, José, 2012. "Origins of Psychiatric Hospitalization in Medieval Spain", *Psychiatric Quarterly*, 83: 419-430.

Pérez Villalba, María T., 2017. *Franceses en Valencia durante el siglo XVI*, PhD thesis, Universitat de València.

Pullan, Brian, 1994. *Poverty and Charity: Europe, Italy, Venice, 1400-1700*, Aldershot, Variorum.

Pullan, Brian, 2005. "Catholics, Protestants, and the Poor in Early Modern Europe", *The Journal of Interdisciplinary History*, 35/3: 441-56.

Rosen, George, 1985. "El hospital: Sociología histórica de una institución comunitaria", *De la policía médica a la medicina social. Ensayos sobre la historia de la atención a la salud*, Madrid, Siglo XXI: 316-350.

Rubio Vela, Agustín, 1983. "Autobiografia i ficció en l'*Espill* de Jaume Roig. A propòsit de l'episodi en l'hospital", *L'Espill*, 17-18: 127-149.

Rubio Vela, Agustín, 2014. "El hospital de Sant Llàtzer como morada. Edificio, mobiliario y recinto de la leprosería de Valencia en el siglo XV", Teresa Huguet-Termes et al. (ed.), *Ciudad y hospital en el Occidente europeo (1300-1700)*, Lleida, Milenio: 347-364.

SANCHIS MORENO, Francisco José, 2012. *El Hospital General de Valencia y su archivo (1512-1868): 350 años de información y documentos*, Valencia, Institució Alfons el Magnànim.

SCOTT, Anne M., 2015, "Experiences of charity. Complex Motivation in the Charitables endeavour, c. 1000-c.1650", Anne M. Scott (ed.), *Experiences of Charity, 1250-1650*, Ashgate, Farnham: 1-14.

THOMPSON, John D.; GOLDIN, Grace, 1975. *The Hospital: A Social and Architectural History*, New Haven, Yale University Press.

TRAVERSO, Enzo, 2006. *Els usos del passat. Història, memòria, política*, Valencia, Universitat de València.

VERDEGUER GARCÍA, Carmen, 1990. *Una meselleria en Valencia del cuatrocientos: El Hospital de "Sent Llátzer"*, undergraduate dissertation, Universitat de València.

VILLAGRASA ELÍAS, Raúl, 2016, "Política hospitalaria en los concejos aragoneses del cuatrocientos", Paulino Iradiel, Germán Navarro, David Igual, Concepción Villanueva (ed.), *Identidades urbanas. Corona de Aragón-Italia. Redes económicas, estructuras institucionales, funciones políticas (siglos XIV-XV)*, Zaragoza, Universidad de Zaragoza: 163-176.

VILLANUEVA MORTE, Concepción; CONEJO DA PENA, Antoni; VILLAGRASA-ELÍAS, Raúl (ed.), 2018. *Redes hospitalarias: historia, economía y sociología de la sanidad*, Zaragoza, Institución Fernando el Católico.

John Henderson

# Hospitals and Plague in Renaissance Florence

## 1. *Introduction*

The hospitals of many urban centres in Italy experienced a gradual revolution during the later Middle Ages. Existing institutions and new foundations became increasingly medicalised, with the employment of a permanent staff of physicians, together with surgeons, apothecaries and a large nursing staff. This process of "medicalisation" was part of a more general specialisation in charitable initiatives in this period, characterised by a gradual move away from simply helping the Poor of Christ to concentrate on specific categories of the poor, among whom were sick adults, abandoned children, widows and girls in need of a dowry.[1]

Another aspect of specialisation was the growing realisation of the need to create separate institutions to care for those with the new epidemic diseases of plague and the French Disease or syphilis. Although there was an existing tradition in many Italian cities for the isolation of lepers, the leprosaria almost always remained on a relatively small scale. The arrival of the plague in 1347-1348 created new social and health problems for the late medieval city on a scale far greater than those caused by any previous natural disaster, with the possible exception of famine. It was the poor who suffered most during these disasters and there was a growing association in the minds of the ruling classes between poverty and disease. This led to greater intolerance towards the poor, exacerbated at the end of the fifteenth century by the arrival of the French Disease, which led to a new class of sick beggars, who crowded the streets and created, according to contemporaries, a threat to public health through their infected breath (Arrizabalaga, Henderson, French 1997; Tognotti 2018).

Although the plague posed an unprecedented threat, measures to deal with this epidemic evolved only gradually in Italian cities in the late Middle Ages. Just as it took many decades for states to develop adequate methods to quarantine entire regions or city districts, so it took time to develop adequate methods to isolate plague victims, as when they established special quarantine centres known

1. For a discussion of this development in relation to Florence see: Henderson, 1994; Albini 2016.

as *lazaretti* (fig. 1). In fact, this process varied considerably from city to city, depending partly on existing provisions for the sick poor and partly on the political will and strength of local regimes to implement strong policies. In all cases, the authorities relied quite naturally both on medical theory about the nature of the disease and on established sanitary measures. The latter included preventive measures, such as cleaning the streets and banning the slaughter of animals in city centres to avoid the creation of corrupt air (Geltner 2018).

This article will examine the role of hospitals in coping with plague in Florence, one of the largest cities in late medieval Europe, during the 180 years after 1348 in relation to measures taken by other Italian cities against plague. During this period, plague returned roughly every ten to fifteen years, but with different levels of mortality, with particularly high rates between 1360 and 1400, but with less severity for much of the fifteenth century, but followed by two periods of particularly heavy mortality in the 1490s and the 1520s, returning for the final time in 1630-1631 (Herlihy, Klapisch-Zuber 1985; Carmichael 1986; Henderson 2019).

Florence has long been associated with plague in the popular imagination, in particular with the Black Death through the famous description of the impact of the plague on society in Giovanni Boccaccio's lively Introduction to *The Decameron*. Written in 1356, he recalls the strategies adopted by the commune during the epidemic, even if the purpose of this passage was to emphasise that they were ineffective:[2]

> And in that pestilence no wisdom or measures were of any use, such as the cleaning of the streets of refuse by officials specially designated for that purpose, and the prohibition of any sick person from entering the city, and also by the advice of physicians for the preservation of health.

Boccaccio summarised a whole series of measures here. First, he speaks of «officials specifically designated for that purpose». In common with other cities in northern and central Italy, the governments appointed a magistracy to oversee the measures necessary to deal with the emergency. Indeed, when it became evident that the plague would remain a constant feature, cities appointed these public health officials whenever the plague threatened and invested them with increasing powers. Over the next two centuries, these magistracies were established on a more permanent basis. In Florence in 1448, when the plague threatened, a magistracy was appointed with the role of «preserving the health of the people and preventing [the spread of] contagion».[3] In Italy, health boards in the fifteenth and sixteenth centuries came to coordinate the general control of measures against the plague within the city, ensuring the enforcement of the complex system of

2. Giovanni Boccaccio, *Decameron*, ed. Vittore Branca (Florence, 1969); see also Henderson 1992: 136-150; Wray 2004: 301-322.

3. Archivio di Stato di Firenze (cited as ASF), Provvisioni Registri (cited as Provv. Reg.), 139, f. 125r; Corsini 1911: 32.

identifying plague victims, quarantining them and isolating those who had come into contact with the sick. In time, health passes were also introduced for goods coming from infected places and cordons sanitaire were established, borders with plague-infected neighbouring states were closed and trade with the rest of the peninsula was stopped.

City-states only gradually established policies of isolating plague victims in separate plague hospitals or *lazaretti* (STEVENS-CRAWSHAW 2012). The process that saw the birth of the *lazaretto*, however, cannot be isolated from other institutions caring for the sick poor, above all existing medical hospitals. Indeed, the important role of hospitals in the late medieval city-state's struggle against the plague has rarely been adequately recognised; most historians have focused on the emergence of the *lazaretto*. But, as we shall see in the case of Florence, hospitals were the models and often worked together with *lazaretti* to cope with the impact of the plague on a city's population.

## 2. *Florence, Hospitals, Lazaretti and Plague*

The example of Renaissance Florence is particularly interesting because it helps us combat the triumphalist view of progress that saw the inevitable development of the same public health measures throughout the Italian peninsula. What is striking about the Florentine example is that for much of the Renaissance, the city authorities seemed content to make use of the facilities provided by hospitals within the city, rather than investing in the construction of a separate *lazaretto* or even converting existing large ecclesiastical buildings.

In this period, the city had a well-developed system of hospital provision with over thirty-five institutions, ranging from the four large hospitals for the acutely ill and the famous Innocenti for foundlings to numerous smaller hostels for the poor, pilgrims and travellers. The largest, Santa Maria Nuova, alone treated over 5,500 patients a year by 1500 (HENDERSON 2006).

In Florence, measures for the isolation of plague patients evolved only gradually and for much of the fifteenth century it was the hospitals that bore the brunt of the human cost of the struggle against epidemic disease. Hospitals, and in particular Santa Maria Nuova, was used as the main place to house and to treat plague victims. In addition, their nursing staff helped the city's sick, as during the epidemic of 1448, when they distributed chicken soup to the poor in their homes (fig. 2).[4]

Already by 1448, there was some recognition that Santa Maria Nuova was not an ideal place to care for plague victims. While the idea of building a separate hospital for the infected was mooted, at the time this was not discussed in detail until the reappearance of plague in 1464.

4. ASF, Provv. Reg. 139, f. 125r; CORSINI 1911: 32.

The Priors of the city now acknowledged that because there was no place to house plague patients, those who were sick with other infirmities became ill with plague and thus many died who would not otherwise have done so.[5]

The hospital of Santa Maria Nuova was at the centre of plans to build a *lazaretto*. In 1464 the hospital director, or *spedalingo*, and five citizens were elected as workers to organise the construction of a house outside the city walls which was to be equipped with twenty beds, half for men and half for women, and all other things relevant to its operation. The staff was to include a priest, a physician, a barber, an apothecary and nurses. The day-to-day management of the *lazaretto* was to be undertaken by the hospital staff under the personal supervision of the *spedalingo*, and the entire operation was to be financed by the hospital through its holdings in the communal funded debt of the *Monte Comune*.[6]

Santa Maria Nuova's close involvement with the administration and financing of the measures against the plague also had a downside; it was ordained that while the new building was under construction, the hospital should continue to receive and treat those sick with plague. It was realised that it was not an ideal solution to treat plague victims in the centre of the city, given what was seen as their potential to infect their co-inhabitants, so the government sought to find one or more places outside Florence where they could be taken. However, this was not put in place for another half-century.

The plague continued to reappear almost every decade in the second half of the fifteenth century and Santa Maria Nuova remained central to the government's plans to deal with threats to public health. Funds were provided to Santa Maria Nuova for the construction of a new *lazaretto*, and by 1479 some progress had been made on its construction outside the city walls, to the east, in an area known as *il prato*, where criminals were traditionally executed.

Cash remained a problem not only to meet the needs of the building programme, but also to pay for the measures to cope with the plague that raged in Florence at the time, because, as the Priors admitted, «there is no provision other than that which is made for the Spedale di Sancta Maria Nuova».[7] The extent of this service can be seen in a letter written by the *spedalingo* Bonino d'Antonio di Maso Bonini to Lorenzo de' Medici in which he outlined the expenses incurred by the hospital for both internal and external patients. Part of their expenses was incurred by the distribution of bread and wine to the case *de morbati*, which probably supported about 1,500 people, and also medicines to the sick. They also complained that they had spent 500 florins on medicines and another 2300 lira on chickens to make chicken broth, and other large sums on sheets for the sick and shrouds for the dead.[8]

5. ASF, Provv. Reg. 139, f. 125r; Corsini 1911: 32.
6. ASF, Provv. Reg, 157, f. 58r: Corsini 1911: 34-35.
7. ASF, Provv. Reg. 170, f 32r, 09/06/1479.
8. ASF, Medici Avanti il Principato, xxxvii, 594, 30/07/1479.

Santa Maria Nuova was not the only Florentine hospital to be involved in the measures taken during the epidemics of the second half of the fifteenth century. Thus, a petition of 1468 from the Spedale di S. Matteo records its indebtedness, because, as was explained, during the epidemic it had been designated as a place to receive and to treat all those patients from Santa Maria Nuova who were ill from conditions other than the plague (fig. 3). The *spedalingo* complained that during the epidemic they had had to treat over 100 sick people, which meant spending over 2,000 gold florins on bills to the apothecary and suppliers of chicken and meat.[9] The same problem happened at another city hospital, Santa Maria della Scala, which was also designed as a *lazaretto*, despite the fact that it was inside the city. According to tradition, more than 20,000 corpses were buried there during the epidemic (PASSERINI 1853: 337).

This long and tortuous history of the establishment of the *lazaretto* is interesting because it emphasises the dependence of the measures taken by governments during periods of epidemic disease on the existing health structure, and especially on hospitals. This point is important both because of the implications this policy had for the hospitals themselves, and because how the Florentine experience contrasts with that of some cities in northern Italy, particularly Venice and Milan, which founded much more substantial permanent *lazaretti* during the fifteenth century (CARMICHAEL 1983: 208-225).

In 1490 when the Florentine plague hospital of San Bastiano was opened, it had only 26 beds, compared with the first *lazaretto* in Venice, the *Vecchio*, which sixty years earlier, in 1429, already had 120 beds. Then in 1471 a completely separate *lazaretto*, the *Nuovo*, was built to quarantine those who had come into close contact with the sick and those who had recovered from treatment in the *Vecchio* (fig. 4-5; STEVENS-CRAWSHAW 2012: 3-4, 19-21). It could be argued that Venice was fortunate in one respect since its location on the Lagoon gave it the possibility of creating *lazaretti* on islands, which became quarantine centres for goods and merchants during non-plague years. However, its geographical position also made it more vulnerable, for as an entrepôt benefitting from commerce between the Middle and Far East and Europe it also potentially became a focus for the arrival of plague from the East.

Perhaps the best example of a specially designed new *lazaretto* was that of Milan, which was begun around 1468 (fig. 6). It consisted of a vast square courtyard measuring about 368 x 370 metres, enclosing a single-storey structure of 280 small rooms, each measuring 8 square metre, and contained a fireplace, bed and toilet. Each room had a window which overlooked a chapel at the centre of the courtyard, which was open on all sides so that the sick could see the celebration of the Host (CIPOLLA 1978: 281-282, Table A-1; BELTRAMI 1882). However, even this was insufficient to meet the demands of really severe epidemics, such as those of the mid-1570s and 1629-1630.

9. ASF, Provv. Reg. 158, ff 212r-v, 15/02/1468; PASSERINI 1853: 156-157. On the hospital of San Matteo see: DIANA 1999.

This contrast between the size and capacity of the *lazaretti* of Venice and Milan with that of Florence cannot be put down to a great discrepancy between the populations of these three cities by the late fifteenth century for while Milan and Venice stood at about 100,000 and 110,000 respectively, Florence had already grown to about 70,000. Evidently, the Florentine public health system was inadequate in the 1490s when the city was assailed by an exceptionally severe combination of epidemic diseases of fever and plague and severe food shortages. By 1497, the city was so inundated with the poor, particularly peasants and others from further afield, that according to the contemporary, Jacopo Nardi, all the hospitals of the city were so full, their capacity provided insufficient to receive them. The authorities now made a distinction between the local poor and the peasants and foreigners whom they sent out of the city (Nardi 1842: I, 115).

Distinctions between types of poor was undoubtedly strengthened by the growing consensus of the vital need to separate those sick with the plague from those with other diseases, given that the majority of the sick were from the lower levels of society. However, in June 1497 this orderly distinction was broken when plague broke out among the patients of Santa Maria Nuova. It was only during the next significant outbreak of plague in Florence, during the 1520s, that more adequate provisions were made for plague victims. In 1522-1523 a series of isolation facilities were created. However, the *lazaretto* of San Bastiano was seen as inadequate to meet demand and four convents and monasteries north and south of the river Arno were requisitioned. Significantly, only one of these religious institutions was actually outside the city walls, despite contemporary belief in the necessity to site isolation facilities away from the general population. When plague broke out with greater severity in 1526-1527, their capacity was insufficient and the city government established a temporary village outside the city, consisting of a series of wooden and thatched huts strung along the walls and covering a distance of about 4 kilometres.[10]

## 3. *Conclusion*

This article has shown that the policies of Florentine governments towards plague in the Renaissance period were based largely on existing health facilities, and especially the city's hospitals, for which Florence was well known at the time. What is perhaps surprising, given contemporary medical theory linking disease to corrupt air, and thus the fear that the sick poor would infect the rest of the population, is the lack of urgency felt by governments to establish isolation facilities for plague victims outside the city walls, as had been recognised as early as 1464, if not before. However, one also has to take into consideration other factors which would have impacted on decision-making. In the first place, as we have seen, mortality from plague was relatively low in Florence between the epidemi-

10. On plague in the 1520s see: Henderson 1989: 165-186.

cs of 1400 and the mid-1490s, suggesting that existing charitable structures, and especially hospitals, may have been seen as sufficient to deal with the challenges of epidemic disease. Then the last quarter of the fifteenth century saw the emergence of new pressures on charitable resources with growing levels of population in the city and a fall in standards of living. The last decade was particularly challenging, given the combination of plague and war, with the invasion of the French army, and the emergence of the new epidemic of the French Disease. It was this period which in particular saw attitudes towards the poor beginning to change with the emergence of a more intolerant attitude, as echoed in the comments of the famous historian and political theorist Niccolò Machiavelli in his recollection of the plague in Florence in 1527:[11]

> The clean and beautiful districts, which used to be full of rich and noble citizens, are now stinking and brutish, filled with the poor, so that one hardly dares to walk there because of their threatening behaviour and fearful cries.

These comments also underline that it was the poor who were seen as suffering most from plague, suggesting that the charitable and isolation facilities were no longer worked properly due to the pressures from the epidemic. The poor were now seen as to be feared, as they threatened their social betters. Then, as suggested by Machiavelli's reference to stinking streets, another factor which began to emerge increasingly in the sixteenth century under the influence of the revival of neo-Hippocratic ideas, was the growing association between poverty, disease and the physical environment. This was reflected in the greater attention which came to be paid to the living conditions of the poor, as well as to structures and spaces within hospitals and *lazaretti*, as the corrupt air generated by the sick was seen as generating epidemic disease.

## *Bibliography*

ALBINI, Giuliana, 1982. *Guerra, fame, peste. Crisi di mortalità e sistema sanitario nella Lombardia tardomedievale*, Bologna, Capelli.

ALBINI, Giuliana, 2016. *Poveri e povertà nel Medioevo*, Rome, Caroccio editore.

ARRIZABALAGA, Jon; HENDERSON, John; FRENCH, Roger, 1997. *The Great Pox. The French Disease in Renaissance Europe*, London-New Haven, Yale University Press.

BELTRAMI, Luca, 1882. "Il lazzaretto di Milano", *Archivio Storico Lombardo*, 9: 403-441.

CARMICHAEL, Ann G. 1983 "Plague Legislation in the Italian Renaissance", *Bulletin of the History of Medicine*, 57: 208-225.

CARMICHAEL, Ann G. 1986. *Plague and the Poor in Renaissance Florence*, Cambridge, Cambridge University Press.

CIPOLLA, Carlo M., 1976. *Public Health and the Medical Profession in the Renaissance*. New York & London: Cambridge University Press.

11. Niccolò Macchiavelli, "Descrizione della peste di Firenze dell'anno 1527", in *Opere di Niccolò Macchiavelli cittadino e segretario fiorentino* (Florence, 1813), V: 36.

CIPOLLA, Carlo M. 1978. *Before the Industrial Revolution. European Society and Economy, 1000-1700*, London, Methuen.

CORSINI, Andrea, 1911. *La Morìa del 1464 in Toscana e l'istituzione dei primi Lazzaretti in Firenze ed in Pisa*, Florence, Claudiana.

DIANA, Esther, 1999. *San Matteo e San Giovanni di Dio, due ospedali nella storia fiorentina. Struttura nosocomiale, patrimonio fondiario e assistenza nella Firenze dei secoli XV-XVIII*, Firenze, Le Lettere.

GELTNER, Guy, 2018. *Roads to Health: Infrastructure and Urban Wellbeing in Later Medieval Italy*, Philadelphia, University of Pennsylvania Press.

HENDERSON, John, 1989. "Plague in Renaissance Florence: Medical Theory and Government Response", Neithard Bulst, Robert Delort (ed.), *Maladies et société (XIIe-XVIIIe siècles)*, Paris, CNRS: 165-186.

HENDERSON, John, 1992. "The Black Death in Florence: Medical and Communal Responses", Steven Bassett (ed.), *Death in Towns: Urban Responses to the Dying and the Dead, 100-1600*, Leicester, Leicester University Press: 136-150.

HENDERSON, John, 1994. *Piety and Charity in Late Medieval Florence*, Chicago-London, The University of Chicago Press.

HENDERSON, John, 2006. *The Renaissance Hospital. Healing the Body and Healing the Soul*, New Haven-London, Yale University Press.

HENDERSON, John, 2019. *Florence Under Siege: Surviving Plague in an Early Modern City*, New Haven-London, Yale University Press.

HERLIHY, David; KLAPISCH-ZUBER, Christiane, 1985. *Tuscans and Their Families: A Study of the Florentine Catasto of 1427*, New Haven-London, Yale University Press.

NARDI, Jacopo, 1842. *Istorie della città di Firenze*, ed. Lorenzo Arbib, Florence.

PASSERINI, Luigi, 1853. *Storia degli stabilmenti di beneficenza e d'istruzione elementare gratuita della città di Firenze*, Florence, Le Monnier.

STEVENS-CRAWSHAW, Jane, 2012. *Plague Hospitals: Public Health for the City in Early Modern Venice*, Farnham, Ashgate.

TOGNOTTI, Eugenia, 2018. *L'altra faccia di Venere. La sifilide dalla prima età moderna all'avvento dell'Aids (XV-XX sec.)*, Rome, FrancoAngeli.

WRAY, Shona, 2004. "Boccaccio and the doctors: medicine and compassion in the face of plague", *Journal of Medieval History*, 30: 301-322.

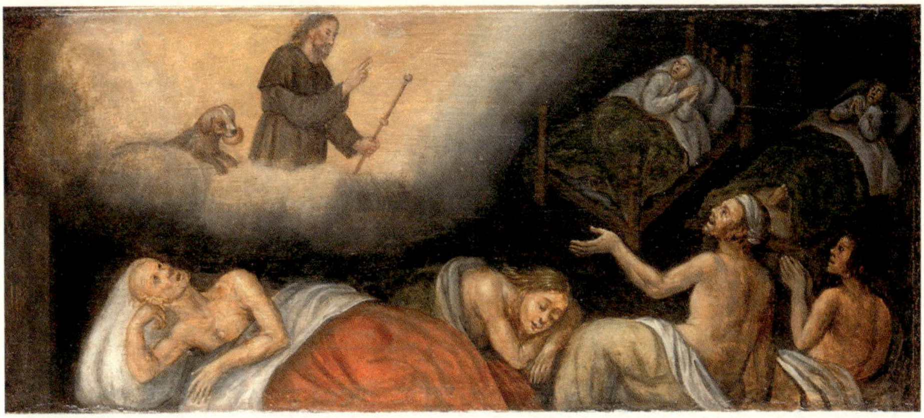

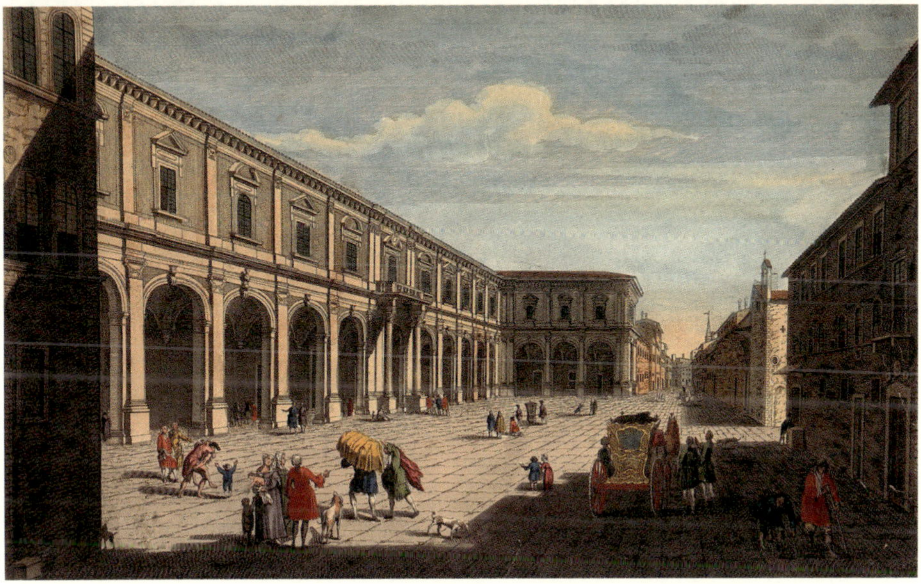

Fig. 1. "San Rocco visits plague victims in a *Lazaretto*", c.1580-c.1620 (London, Wellcome Collection: Public Domain Mark).
Fig. 2. Giuseppe Zocchi: "Ospedale di Santa Maria Nuova", Florence (coloured line engraving by N. Parr), c. 1794 (London: Wellcome Collection, Public Domain Mark).

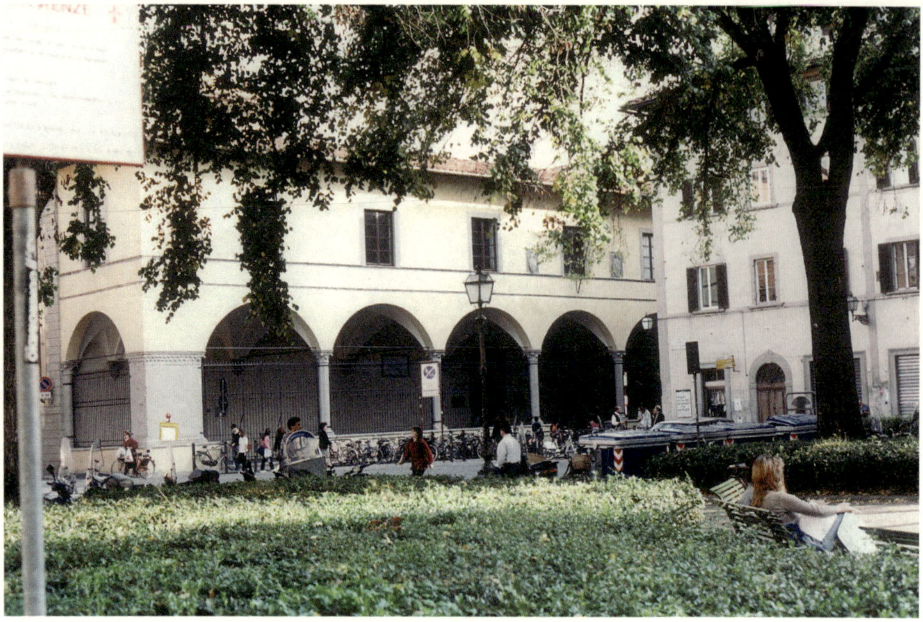

Fig. 3. The Hospital of San Matteo, Piazza San Marco, Florence. Photograph by author.

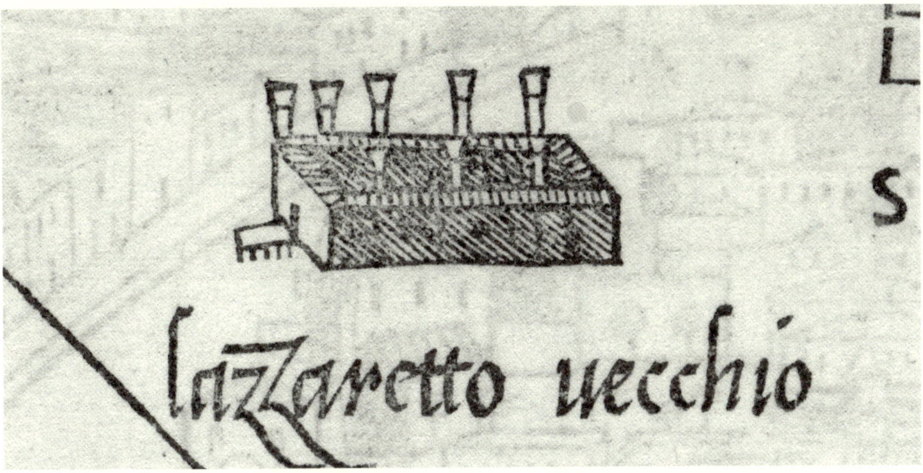


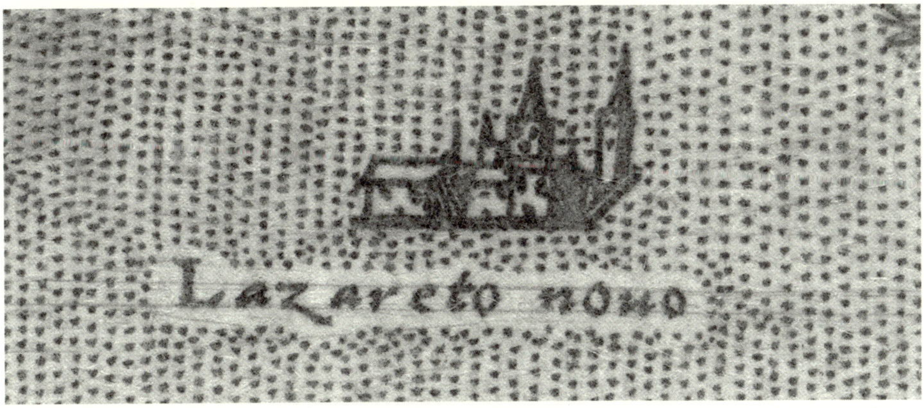


Fig. 4. "The *Lazaretto Vecchio*", Venice. Detail from *L'isole piv famose del mondo descritte e intagliate da Girolamo Porro* by Thomaso Porcacchi, 1590 (London: Wellcome Collection, Public Domain Mark).
Fig. 5. "The *Lazaretto Nuovo*", Venice. Detail from *L'isole piv famose del mondo descritte e intagliate da Girolamo Porro* by Thomaso Porcacchi, 1590 (London: Wellcome Collection, Public Domain Mark).

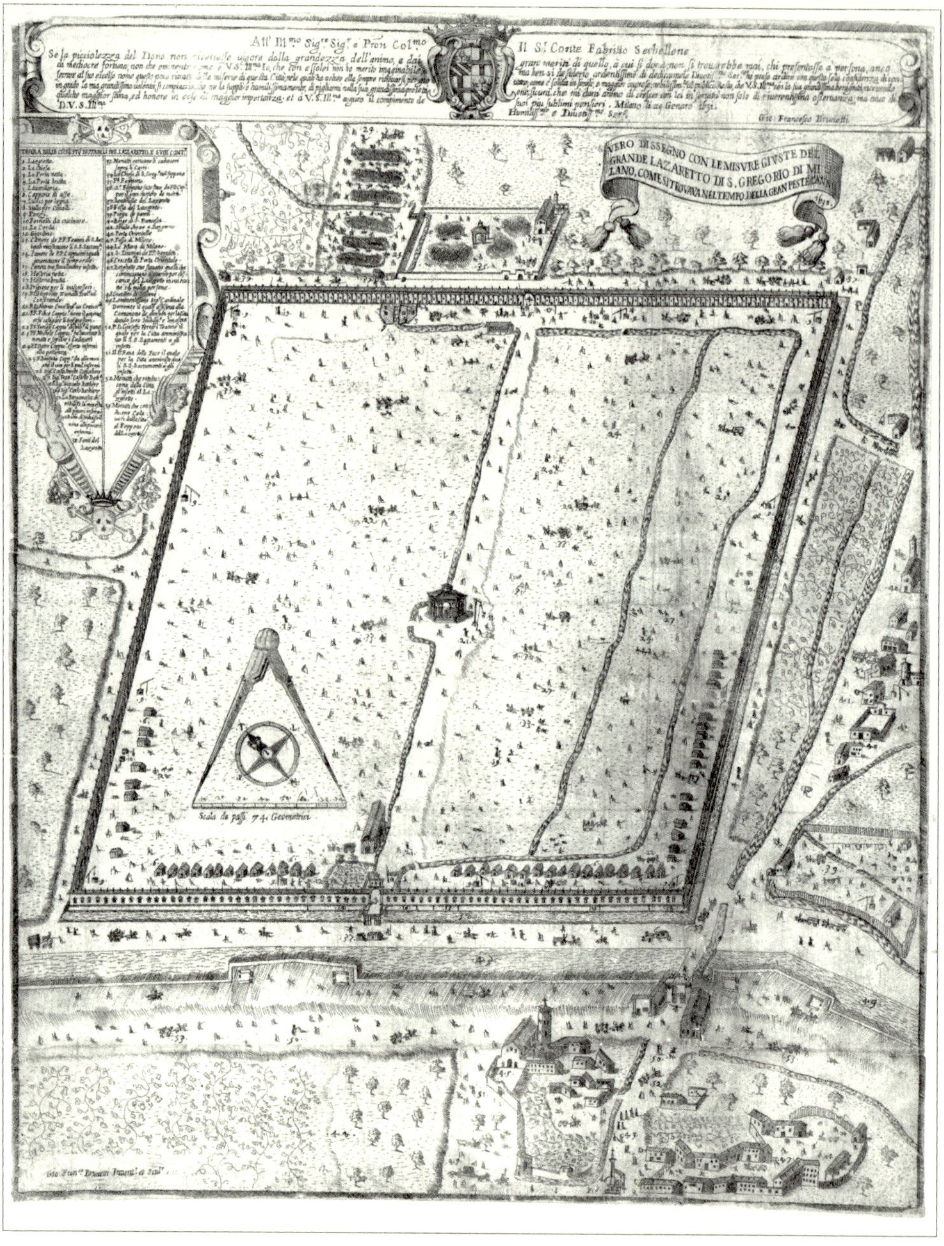

Fig. 6. Giovanni Francesco Brunetti, *Vero dissegno con le misure giuste del grande lazaretto di S. Gregorio di Milano come si trovava nel tempo della gran peste l'anno 1630*, 1631 (Wikimedia Commons).

Finito di stampare
nel mese di novembre 2023
da The Factory s.r.l.
Roma